D1278405

CLINICAL PHARMACOLOGY AND THERAPEUTICS OF HYPERTENSION

PUBLISHED VOLUMES IN THE SERIES

SERIES EDITORS: W. H. BIRKENHÄGER AND J. L. REID

Volume 25

CLINICAL PHARMACOLOGY AND THERAPEUTICS OF HYPERTENSION

Editor

Gordon T. McInnes
Professor of Clinical Pharmacology and Honorary Consultant Physician
Section of Clinical Pharmacology and Stroke Medicine
Division of Cardiovascular and Medical Sciences
Gardiner Institute
Western Infirmary
Glasgow, UK

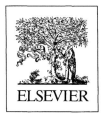

ELSEVIER

EDINBURGH LONDON NEW YORK OXFORD
PHILADELPHIA ST LOUIS SYDNEY TORONTO 2008

ELSEVIER B.V.

Radarweg 29, 1043 NX, Amsterdam, The Netherlands

First published 2008

ISBN: 978 0 444 51757 9 (Vol 25)

ISBN: 978 0 444 90341 9 (Series)

British Library Cataloguing in Publication Data
A catalogue record for this book is available from the British Library

Library of Congress Cataloging in Publication Data
A catalog record for this book is available from the Library of Congress

Notice

Knowledge and best practice in this field are constantly changing. As new research and experience broaden our knowledge, changes in practice, treatment and drug therapy may become necessary or appropriate. Readers are advised to check the most current information provided (i) on procedures featured or (ii) by the manufacturer of each product to be administered, to verify the recommended dose or formula, the method and duration of administration, and contraindications. It is the responsibility of the practitioner, relying on their own experience and knowledge of the patient, to make diagnoses, to determine dosages and the best treatment for each individual patient, and to take all appropriate safety precautions. To the fullest extent of the law, neither the Publisher nor the Editor assumes any liability for any injury and/or damage to persons or property arising out or related to any use of the material contained in this book.

The Publisher

Transferred to digital print 2009

Printed and bound in Great Britain by CPI Antony Rowe, Chippenham and Eastbourne

Contributors

I. Aursnes
Professor of Medicine,
Department of Pharmacology,
Oslo, Norway

H.R. Black
Clinical Professor of Internal Medicine,
New York University School of
Medicine, New York,
New York, USA

C.J. Calderwood
Consultant in Obstetrics and
Gynaecology, Women's and
Children's Services, Lothian NHS
Trust St John's Hospital, Livingston
and Royal Infirmary of Edinburgh,
Edinburgh, UK

S.G. Carruthers
Dean, The Faculty of Medicine and
Health Sciences
University of the United Arab
Emirates, Al Ain, United Arab
Emirates

M. de Gasparo
MG Consulting Company,
Rossemaison, Switzerland

P.W. du Leeuw
Professor of Medicine and Hypertension,
Department of Medicine,
University Hospital Maastricht and
Cardiovascular Research Institute,
Maastricht, The Netherlands

R. Dell'Oro
Assistant of Medicine, Clinical
Medica, Dipartimento di Clinica
Medicina, Prevenzione e
Biotecnologie Sanitarie, Università
Milano-Bicocca, Monza (Milan), Italy

H.L. Elliott
Senior Lecturer, Department of
Medicine and Therapeutics, Gardiner
Institute, Western Infirmary,
Glasgow, UK

W.J. Elliott
Department of Preventative
Medicine, RUSH Medical College of
RUSH University, RUSH University
Medical Center, Chicago, USA

F. Feihl
Professor of Medicine, Division of
Clinical Pathophysiology, University
Hospital, Lausanne, Switzerland

G. Grassi
Professor of Medicine, Clinical
Medica, Dipartimento di Clinica
Medicina, Prevenzione e
Biotecnologie Sanitarie, Università
Milano-Bicocca, Monza (Milan), Italy

D.S. Hanes
Associate Professor of Medicine,
Division of Nephrology, University
of Maryland Hospital, Baltimore,
Maryland, USA

D. Johnston
Department of Therapeutics,
Queen's University, Belfast,
Northern Ireland, UK

C. Jones-Burton
Assistant Professor of Medicine,
Division of Nephrology, University
of Maryland Hospital, Baltimore,
Maryland, USA

S.E. Kjeldsen
Professor of Cardiology and
Cardiovascular Medicine, Department
of Cardiology, University of Oslo,
Oslo, Norway

A.A. Kroon
Associate Professor of Internal
Medicine, Department of Internal
Medicine, University Hospital
Maastricht and Cardiovascular
Research Institute, Maastricht,
The Netherlands

L. Liaudet
Professor of Medicine, Division of
Clinical Pathophysiology, University
Hospital, Lausanne, Switzerland

P. Lund-Johansen
Professor of Medicine, Department of
Heart Disease, Haukeland University
Hospital, Bergen, Norway

T.M. MacDonald
Department of Medicine and
Therapeutics, Division of Clinical
Pharmacology, Ninewells Hospital,
University of Dundee, Dundee, UK

G.T. McInnes
Section of Clinical Pharmacology and
Stroke Medicine, Division of
Cardiovascular and Medical
Sciences, Gardiner Institute, Western
Infirmary, Glasgow, UK

G. Mancia
Professor of Medicine, Clinical
Medica, Dipartimento di Clinica
Medicina, Prevenzione e
Biotecnologie Sanitarie, Università
Milano-Bicocca, Monza (Milan),
Italy

P.A. Meredith
Department of Medicine and
Therapeutics, University of Glasgow,
Western Infirmary, Glasgow, UK

C. Nelson-Piercy
Consultant Obstetric Physician,
Guy's and St Thomas' Foundation
Trust, Queen Charlotte's and Chelsea
Hospital, London, UK

M.G. Nicholls
Department of Internal Medicine,
Faculty of Medicine and Health
Sciences, University of United Arab
Emirates, Al Ain, United Arab
Emirates

S. Oparil
Director, Vascular Biology and
Hypertension Program, School of
Medicine, University of Alabama at
Birmingham, Birmingham, Alabama,
USA

I. Os
Professor of Nephrology,
Department of Nephrology,
Ullevaal Hospital, University of Oslo,
Oslo, Norway

H.K. Parthasarathy
Specialty Registrar, Department of
Cardiology, Norfolk and Norwich
University Hospital, Norwich, UK

G. Petroianu
Department of Pharmacology and
Therapeutics, Faculty of Medicine
and Health Sciences, University of
the United Arab Emirates, Al Ain,
United Arab Emirates

M. Pratt-Ubanama
Vascular Biology and Hypertension
Program, University of Alabama at
Birmingham, Birmingham, Alabama,
USA

B.N.C. Prichard
Emeritus Professor of Clinical
Pharmacology, Centre for
Clinical Pharmacology,
University College London,
London, UK

J.L. Reid
Division of Cardiovascular and
Medical Sciences, Gardiner Institute,
Western Infirmary, Glasgow,
UK

S. Ross
Clinical Lecturer, Department of
Medicine and Therapeutics,
University of Aberdeen,
Aberdeen , UK

L.M. Ruilope
Hypertension Unit, Hospital 12 de
Octobre, Madrid, Spain

D.A. Sica
Division of Clinical Pharmacology
and Hypertension, Medical College
of Virginia, Richmond,
Virginia, USA

A.-E. Stenehjem
Consultant Nephrologist, Department
of Nephrology, Ullevaal University
Hospital, Oslo, Norway

F. Quarti-Trevano
Assistant of Medicine Clinical Medica,
Dipartimento di Clinica Medicina,
Prevenzione e Biotecnologie Sanitarie,
Università Milano-Bicocca, Monza
(Milan), Italy

P.A. van Zwieten
Clinical Pharmacologist, Emeritus
Professor of Pharmacology,
Department of Cardiovascular
Surgery, Academic Medical Centre,
University of Amsterdam,
Amsterdam, The Netherlands

B. Waeber
Professor of Medicine, Division of
Clinical Pathophysiology, University
Hospital, Lausanne, Switzerland

J. Webster
Consultant Physician, Clinical
Pharmacology Unit, Aberdeen Royal
Infirmary, Aberdeen, UK

M.R. Weir
Professor of Medicine, Division of
Nephrology, University of Maryland
Hospital, Baltimore, Maryland, USA

Foreword

This volume of the Handbook of Hypertension is the 25th in a series of authoritative books published since 1983 on aspects of hypertension, its causes and consequences. This volume on the Clinical Pharmacology and Therapeutics of Hypertension provides an update on the drug treatment of high blood pressure. Over the last 50 years the development of innovative pharmacological agents which modify mechanisms regulating blood pressure have been introduced, evaluated and shown to not only control blood pressure but reduce or even reverse the increased risk of heart disease, stroke and renal failure associated with raised blood pressure.

We have included three previous volumes in the series on the basic and clinical aspects of drugs used to treat hypertension. These include volume 3 on the Pharmacology of Hypertension edited by Peter Van Sweeten and volume 4 on the Clinical Pharmacology of Antihypertensive Drugs edited by Austin Doyle. Austin Doyle updated and revised the volume on Clinical Pharmacology (volume 11) in 1988 in recognition of the dramatic developments in antihypertensive therapy that had occurred in that decade.

Although in recent years the pace and intensity of new drug discovery and introduction of novel classes of treatment has perhaps slowed, there is accumulating evidence of the benefits of long term therapy and an increasing evidence base for guidance on therapeutic decision making in blood pressure treatment. Gordon McInnes has brought together a very distinguished group of international clinical scientists to provide an update on the Clinical Pharmacology and Therapeutics of Hypertension for the 21st century.

This volume includes authoritative up to date reviews on all the classes of antihypertensive drugs used today together with contemporary reviews on the evidence base for hypertension treatment from published clinical trials and meta analyses. Therapeutic strategies for long term drug use as well as specific aspects of the management of some special groups of hypertensive patients are also included.

In spite of the enormous successes in hypertension therapy there remain a number of opportunities and challenges. Although we have achieved major benefits in preventing complications of hypertension by drug treatment, a failure even now to understand many aspects of the basic mechanisms controlling blood pressure leave possible exciting opportunities for new therapeutic developments based on innovative basic research. In addition the challenges of obesity, diabetes and metabolic syndrome which increase cardiovascular risk need to be addressed.

WILLEM H BIRKENHÄGER, Rotterdam
JOHN L REID, Glasgow

Preface

A revised volume devoted to the clinical pharmacology and therapeutics of antihypertensive drugs is long overdue. In the two decades since the publication of Volume 11, new classes of antihypertensive agents have been introduced, notably angiotensin receptor blockers in the mid 1990s and in the first decade of the new millennium direct renin inhibitors. Furthermore, calcium channel blockers, ACE inhibitors, angiotensin receptor blockers and other antihypertensive drug classes are now widely utilized in the management of hypertension.

The last decade has seen the publication of several large-scale outcome trials that have defined the place of newer drugs in hypertension treatment regimens. In addition, clinical studies have provided insights into the appropriate use of antihypertensive drugs based on sound clinical pharmacological principles. We now have a much clearer idea of how to use blood pressure lowering strategies to attenuate the atheromatous consequences of hypertension.

Thus, a volume which reviews comprehensively the present understanding of the clinical pharmacology and therapeutics of currently available antihypertensive agents, following a standard format, is timely. This is doubly relevant since we now appear to be entering an era when fewer new molecules are entering development. As well as reflecting on what is known about existing drugs, it is appropriate to contemplate the promise of new approaches. These are likely to depend on utilizing established agents more efficiently and fully realizing their potential through a greater understanding of molecular biology and pharmacogenomics. These considerations provide a real hope of a bright new future for the clinical pharmacology and therapeutics of antihypertensive therapy.

GORDON T. MCINNES

Contents

General considerations

1 | Classification of antihypertensive drugs and pharmacological considerations: historical perspective and future prospects

John L. Reid and Gordon T. McInnes

INTRODUCTION

There were no effective, clinically useful drugs for control of blood pressure (BP) until the 1950s. BP had been measured for over 100 years and the link between high BP and adverse clinical outcomes was recognized. The first association was with chronic kidney disease (Bright's disease), but insurance and other actuarial data collected in the early years of the 20th century provided evidence of an incremental risk of stroke, renal failure and heart disease with increasing BP.[1] By the 1940s there was a recognition of the adverse effects of raised BP, but there was no means of lowering BP in an acceptable manner. Thus the cause–effect relationship between BP and risk of stroke or heart disease could not be confirmed with certainty.

The scope of hypertension treatment has evolved over the intervening 50 years, from the short-term care of a few hospitalized patients with severely elevated BP and extensive target organ damage (small volume – high unit cost) to a major long-term community health problem involving a substantial proportion of the population (high volume – low unit cost). At one time, it appeared that the mechanisms involved in the pathogenesis of hypertension could be identified by a limited array of circumspect and straightforward tests. This is now clearly not so. It is apparent that there are many aetiological factors and each only contributes to a small and variable extent to human hypertension.

At the same time, it has become clear that effective and widespread use of antihypertensive drugs can improve stroke outlook,[2] although this has not yielded the full expected fall in the incidence of atherosclerotic disease in hypertensive individuals.[3] The shortfall has provided a major stimulus for research into the relationship between hypertension and atheroma. The fruits of such an approach might be anticipated to be a driving force in the continuing search for new therapeutic agents.

MECHANISM OF HYPERTENSION AND ANTIHYPERTENSIVE DRUGS

BP is the composite of several physiological variables. The principal components are cardiac output and peripheral vascular resistance.[4] However, therapeutics decisions are based upon the level of BP rather than measurement of cardiac output and peripheral resistance.

Extensive basic research in physiology and pharmacology in the first half of the 20th century identified the sympathetic nervous system (SNS) as a factor maintaining BP, at least in the short term. Further studies identified the link between sodium uptake and BP, with identification of the key role of the renin–angiotensin–aldosterone system (RAAS). These discoveries provided putative mechanisms for hypertension and targets for interventions to lower BP (and became the sources for candidates for antihypertensive drugs). The weakness of this approach was (and remains) that, in the absence of a full understanding of the mechanisms that underpin the development and maintenance of hypertension in man, modification of the SNS and RAAS may fall short of complete control and/or reversal of the underlying process.

An early objective was selectivity, initially identifying drugs that would block the SNS without having the disabling effect of a parasympathetic blockade. Guanethidine, bethanidine and debrisoquine were products of this endeavour.[5] All were potent antihypertensive drugs without significant parasympathetic activity, although orthostatic hypertension persisted.

Serendipity remained an important source of new drug development. α-methyldopa was synthesized originally to inhibit dopa-decarboxylase, and was widely believed to block the peripheral synthesis of norepinephrine;[6,7] only later were the central actions understood. Insights into the pharmacological actions of methyldopa and the centrally acting drug, clonidine, led to major advances in the identification of the mechanism involved in the central control of BP.

It is striking that nearly 60 years after the first effective drug candidates were introduced, antihypertensive drug therapy is still based largely on:

(1) prevention of vasoconstriction (or vasodilatation) directly or via blockade of the SNS or angiotensin mediated vasoconstriction
(2) increased excretion of sodium by the kidney or via interference in the RAAS.[4]

Successful modern long-term management of hypertension is based on regimens using both these approaches with multiple drugs or drugs with more than one action.

CLASSIFICATION OF ANTIHYPERTENSIVE DRUGS

From the available drugs, there are agents that alter the responses of all known control systems, often at more than one point (Table 1.1). The best reason for preferring one drug class over another would be specific reversal of an aetiological factor, e.g. spironolactone in a patient with primary hyperaldosteronism; however, such individuals are a tiny minority of those considered for treatment. In most instances, the aetiology of hypertension is unknown and the

Table 1.1 Classes of antihypertensive drugs 1950–2000

(1)	Ganglion blockers
(2)	Sympathetic peripheral neurone blockers
(3)	Reserpine
(4)	Diuretics
	a. Thiazide and related compounds
	b. Loop diuretics
	c. Aldosterone antagonists and other potassium sparers
(5)	Centrally acting drugs, e.g. methyldopa and clonidine
(6)	Adrenoceptor antagonists
	a. α-blockers
	b. β-blockers
(7)	Vasodilators, e.g. hydralazine and minoxidil
(8)	Calcium channel blockers
	a. Dihydropyridines
	b. Non-dihydropyridines
(9)	Renin–angiotensin system blockers
	a. ACE inhibitors
	b. Angiotensin receptor blockers
	c. Renin inhibitors
(10)	Others
	a. Serotonin antagonists, e.g. ketanserin
	b. Endothelin antagonists
	c. Endopeptidase inhibitors

choice of drug is made empirically, the chosen drug producing a relatively high degree of inhibition of one of the control mechanisms. This almost always has the consequence that other control mechanisms are activated to oppose the BP reduction, e.g. the rise in plasma renin and angiotensin that accompanies treatment with a thiazide diuretic. Thus, the fall in BP is usually bought at the price of appreciable physiological imbalance.

Centrally acting agents

The brain is the main site of action of several different antihypertensive drugs, e.g. methyldopa, reserpine and the $α_2$-agonists, clonidine and guanfacine.[7] β-blockers also have a central action, but this is unlikely to be important since lipophilic and hydrophilic compounds that penetrate the brain slowly are equally efficacious as antihypertensive agents.[8]

Drugs that lower BP by a central action are associated with troublesome dose-related side effects, e.g. sedation with clonidine and methyldopa, and depression with reserpine. As a consequence, use of these drugs has declined in favour of agents with less annoying side effects. More recently, centrally acting drugs that interact with a specific imidazoline binding site (rilmenidine and moxonodine) are claimed to lower BP with fewer side effects.[7]

Drugs that alter cardiac output

In the early stages of hypertension, cardiac output[4] is often raised while peripheral resistance is unchanged. In such (mainly younger) individuals, it would appear logical to use drugs with a main mode of action to reduce cardiac output. β-blockers are the major class of antihypertensive drugs with this mode of action.

The antihypertensive effect of β-blockers is not confined to individuals with raised cardiac output and normal peripheral resistance.[6] Most people have BP reduction following β-blockade. The effect appears to be less in blacks and in older people than in other patient groups; this may be related to lower plasma renin levels in such individuals.

Several vasodilators (hydralazine, minoxidil, calcium channel blockers) can raise cardiac output secondary to baroreflex cardiac activation.[9–11] Preload and afterload are reduced, but these haemodynamic changes can have detrimental effects, since angina may be worsened.

Drugs that affect peripheral vascular resistance

Direct vasodilators have variable patterns of response depending on the vessel type targeted.[5] Hydralazine is predominantly an arteriolar vasodilator (decreased afterload) while sodium nitroprusside mainly dilates veins (decreased preload). Selective α-blockers dilate both arterioles and veins, perhaps explaining the lesser tendency to reflex tachycardia and renin release compared with hydralazine.[12] However, α-blockers are associated with postural hypertension, which may be lessened by agents with pharmacokinetics that favour more gradual onset and longer duration of action. Sympathetic inhibitors (e.g. clonidine, methyldopa or guanethidine) also reduce peripheral vascular resistance.[7] Sexual dysfunction and postural side effects can be associated with some of these agents. β-blockers cause an acute increase in peripheral vascular resistance, predominately via baroreflex activation, but, in the long term, peripheral resistance tends to fall to the pre-treatment value.[8]

ACE inhibitors and angiotensin receptor blockers reduce peripheral vascular resistance by attenuation of circulating angiotensin II concentrations or blockade of angiotensin II receptors respectively.[13,14] The advantages of these drugs include the absence of reflex tachycardia and of circulatory adjustments on standing or during exercise. Thus, orthostatic hypotension is not a problem.

Calcium channel blockers act directly on vascular smooth muscle calcium channels to promote vasodilatation.[15] This in turn results in reflex cardiac activation to an extent that depends on the direct cardiac effects of these drugs. Dihydropyridines (amlodipine and nifedipine) are relatively selective for the peripheral circulation and, therefore, reflex tachycardia is prominent. In contrast, non-dihydropyridines (diltiazem and verapamil) also have marked cardioinhibitory effects and reflex tachycardia is blocked. Indeed, these calcium channel blockers are associated with modest bradycardia and have a role in patients with tachyarrhythmias. In the peripheral circulation, calcium channel blockers have a predominant effect on pre-capillary vessels. The lack of an action of calcium channel blockers on post-capillary vessels explains the tendency to peripheral oedema with these drugs. This side effect is more marked with the dihydropyridines.

Diuretics also reduce peripheral vascular resistance.[16] The acute effect of diuretics is to reduce extracellular volume and this is responsible for the early antihypertensive response. In the long term, extracellular fluid volume returns to the pre-treatment value and peripheral resistance fall. A change in the ionic composition of vascular smooth muscle has been suggested. Drugs with widely different chemical structures and sites of action, including spironolactone and amiloride, reduce BP.[17] Salt depletion caused by diuretics increases plasma renin and this tends to offset or limit the antihypertensive action. Although the exact mechanism is unclear, thiazide and loop diuretics cause dose-related sexual dysfunction and metabolic side effects including new onset diabetes.

Drugs that modify the renin–angiotensin system

Early proof of principle came from animal studies with intravenous angiotensin antagonists and renin inhibitors.[13,14] These findings have been amply confirmed with newer orally active agents. ACE inhibitors reduce circulating angiotensin II and aldosterone with increasing angiotensin I and renin.[14] Angiotensin receptor blockers antagonize the action of angiotensin II by selective action at the AT_1 receptor.[13] As a consequence, aldosterone is reduced to a variable extent. Inhibition of the negative feedback loop that controls renin release leads to increased renin and angiotensin II levels. ACE inhibitors and angiotensin receptor blockers have excellent tolerability, although ACE inhibitors are associated commonly with cough and rarely with angio-oedema, which can be life threatening. Both classes show enhanced antihypertensive efficacy when combined with diuretics or calcium channel blockers.

Specific renin inhibitors have been difficult to develop.[18] The recently introduced direct renin inhibitors have similar effects on the renin–angiotensin–aldosterone axis with the exception that renin is also reduced. As with ACE inhibitors, circulating angiotensin II levels are decreased, but the breakthrough renin-driven escape of angiotensin II concentrations, returning levels to pretreatment levels, with long-term ACE inhibition is avoided. There is some evidence that plasma renin is an independent cardiovascular risk factor.[19] However, whether direct renin inhibitors will demonstrate clinically important advantages remains untested. β-blockers also reduce circulating renin (and angiotensin II), but the extent to which this contributes to antihypertensive efficacy is controversial.[8]

Vasodilators and diuretics elevate plasma renin levels by different mechanisms (sympathetic activation of the baroreflex and volume depletion, respectively).[10,16] Elevation of renin levels limits the antihypertensive action of drugs from both classes.

Drugs that affect plasma volume

Diuretics reduce plasma volume, although the long-term effect is small (about 5%).[8] It is unknown to what extent this contributes to the antihypertensive action. Several drugs (guanethidine, methyldopa and minoxidil) cause fluid retention by a mechanism that is not clearly established.[5] Fluid retention can be controlled by concomitant use of diuretics. The peripheral oedema associated with calcium channel blockers does not reflect plasma volume expansion.[15] Diuretics are relatively ineffective in controlling this symptom.

PERSISTING PROBLEMS WITH ANTIHYPERTENSIVE DRUGS AND DRUG DEVELOPMENT

These can be summarized thus:

(1) There is a continued failure to fully understand the pathophysiological mechanisms of hypertension, the links to vascular disease and the precise interactions of individual drug classes.

(2) In the early years, use of monotherapy in heroically high doses with attempts to control BP in all (or most) individuals with a simple one drug regimen resulted in failure (in the majority) and the common occurrence of symptomatic side effects, with limited acceptability/compliance.

The evolution of clinical pharmacology over more than half a century is reflected in the development of antihypertensive drugs. The era began with the synthesis and characterization of the polymethylene bistrimethylaminion compounds, rapidly followed by the description of the potent ganglion-blocking properties of the pento- and hexamethylene members of the series. Early clinical evaluation of these compounds was discouraging. Major problems included incomplete oral absorption leading to erratic and variable effects. Furthermore, blockade of the sympathetic ganglia caused marked orthostatic hypotension, while interference of transmission at parasympathetic ganglia induced major symptomatic side effects, such as inhibition of salivation, interference with visual accommodation, constipation, urine retention and impotence.

The practical use of these compounds was achieved after realization that only incomplete ganglion blockade was required for antihypertensive efficacy. The necessary precise dose regimen required parenteral administration. With this approach, side effects due to sympathetic and parasympathetic blockade were reduced in severity.[5] Another clinical pharmacological principle employed was the enhancement of the desired sympathetic blockade by the use of low-sodium diet, and later by its combined use with reserpine or hydralazine. These manoeuvres allowed the desired degree of sympathetic blockade to be achieved at doses sufficiently low to have much less effect on the parasympathetic ganglia, thus minimizing side effects.

Although the treatment regimen was complex and side effects were still major limitations, the therapeutic effects were very impressive. Malignant hypertension could be arrested, fundal changes resolved, heart failure reversed and the incidence of cerebral haemorrhage reduced. These achievements led to acceptance of the importance of the level of BP as a cause of the vascular complications of hypertension and emphasized the value of BP reduction as a major goal of treatment.

Therapeutic approaches

The aim of antihypertensive therapy is to reduce the risk of hypertensive cardiovascular disease while keeping the adverse effects of treatment to a minimum.[8] The balance of benefit versus risk depends on the severity of hypertension. Unwanted effects of treatment that are entirely acceptable for the treatment of accelerated hypertension may be quite unacceptable in someone with grade I hypertension. The risks of hypertension comprise not only those associated with cardiovascular morbidity and mortality, but also the burden of symptomatic side effects and the awareness of ill-health associated with long-term drug therapy.

The choice of treatment regimen is greatly influenced by the need to minimize unwanted effects in symptomless individuals. The facilitating effect of non-pharmacological approaches should not be ignored. Alone, these are unlikely to be sufficient in most subjects, but careful attention to lifestyle factors can reduce the dose and number of antihypertensive drugs required to achieve control.[20]

RECENT DEVELOPMENTS

It can be argued that advances in drug treatment of hypertension over the last 50–60 years have been the consequence of a series of 'lucky breaks':

(1) There was no sound basis for the antihypertensive action of β-blockers. This was identified as a result of clinical observation.[8]
(2) Diuretics were used in the management of hypertension before it was realized that low doses of thiazides are as effective as high doses in BP reduction, but with low doses metabolic effects are less marked.[16] Furthermore, high-ceiling loop diuretics are no better than low-dose thiazides and carry the risk of more symptomatic problems.
(3) The development of stepped care therapy with logical low doses of two or more drugs and the emergence of rational fixed low-dose combinations was slow.[21]

The value of β-blockers in the treatment of hypertension illustrates some of the major distinctions between pharmacology and clinical pharmacology and therapeutics.[8] From the pharmacological knowledge at the time when these drugs became available, it could not be predicted that β-blockers would reduce BP, and even now the precise mechanism of action remains unknown.

The development of β-blockers was accompanied by renewed interest in drugs that dilate vascular smooth muscle, since the combination of these two drug classes prevents the reflex tachycardia, which limited the widespread use of vasodilators alone.[21] Additionally, the use of β-blockers stimulated studies of pharmacodynamic–pharmacokinetic relationships, accompanied by the development of sophisticated methods for the estimation of drug concentrations in biological fluids.[8]

Likewise, the ACE inhibitors have proved to be much more generally effective drugs than could have been predicted from pharmacology.[14] ACE inhibitors reduce BP in individuals who do not have high plasma renin activity, a finding that suggests that the RAAS may contribute to the pathogenesis of hypertension in a manner considerably more important, yet more subtle than seemed to be the case. These findings reinforce the likely clinical benefits of angiotensin receptor blockers and direct renin inhibitors.

The pharmacological effects of drugs that block calcium entry into cardiac and vascular smooth muscle resulted in much speculation.[8] Expected benefits beyond those attributable to BP reduction have failed to emerge, but calcium channel blockers have been demonstrated to be highly effective antihypertensive agents. Although these drugs are classified as one group, there are major differences between agents in the spectrum of activity. As further knowledge about the calcium channel blockers accumulated, clues about the controlling mechanisms of smooth muscle contractility emerged.

A further major advance was the introduction of thiazide diuretics.[16] Oral diuretic therapy confirmed the earlier experience of the value of salt depletion as an adjunct to antihypertensive drugs. While at least one functioning kidney is a prerequisite for action, whether the major antihypertensive effect of diuretics is mediated via sodium and volume depletion or more subtle actions on vascular smooth muscle is not yet fully resolved.

The focus on the natriuretic effect of diuretics as the mechanism for the antihypertensive action led to the use of thiazides at doses that would be considered industrial by present standards.[16] While such doses are effective in lowering BP, the incidence of side effects, mainly metabolic, is high. After many years, it was recognized that the dose–response for metabolic complications is steep while that for BP is shallow. Diuretic-induced natriuresis stimulates the RAAS and this offsets the antihypertensive effect. The recognition that low-dose diuretic therapy retains the bulk of the antihypertensive effect, but largely eliminates metabolic complications has been a major advance in the therapeutics of hypertension.

Factors affecting the pharmacodynamic response

The extent of antihypertensive response produced by a particular drug is determined partly by the activity or tone in the target physiological BP control mechanism. In particular, plasma renin concentration may be an important determinant of response.[4] High plasma renin activity tends to be a feature of younger hypertensive individuals, while low renin status characterizes long-standing hypertension and hypertension in black people. High renin subjects respond well to ACE inhibitors, angiotensin receptor blockers and low doses of β-blockers. In contrast, those with low renin hypertension respond particularly well to calcium channel blockers or diuretics.

On the basis of these considerations, it has been proposed that hypertensive individuals can be divided for therapeutic purposes into two groups: those in whom plasma volume expansion is the predominant mechanism and those in whom peripheral vasoconstriction is predominant.[4] These groups approximate to those with low renin hypertension and those with high renin hypertension, respectively. Accordingly, the former group would respond best to calcium channel blocker or diuretic therapy and the latter group would respond best to ACE inhibitor/angiotensin receptor blocker or β-blocker. This mechanism-specific approach is conceptually extremely attractive, but there remains some doubt about the general applicability of renin profiling as a method of selecting antihypertensive drug therapy.

Even when it is not possible to reverse a specific aetiological factor, it may be feasible to reduce cardiac output if it is the main reason for hypertension or peripheral resistance if it is the more important component.[4] In younger individuals (aged <55 years), the haemodynamic pattern is characterized by elevated peripheral resistance and normal or low cardiac output (activated RAAS), while older individuals tend to have raised cardiac output with little consistent change in peripheral vascular resistance (low plasma renin). Younger patients tend to respond better to drugs that block the RAAS (β-blockers and ACE inhibitors or angiotensin receptor blockers), while older patients have preferential response to diuretics and calcium channel blockers.

Therapeutic application

Over the years, many therapeutic regimens for the management of hypertension have been advocated. Initially, clinical pharmacologists expressed a strong preference for monotherapy rather than drug combinations. Problems with this purist approach are that the dose–antihypertensive response is usually shallow; the dose required is often high and, even then, insufficient to achieve control, while side effects often have a steep dose–response relationship. Gradually, a consensus was formed that it is better to combine two or more drugs with different pharmacological actions, such that antihypertensive effects are additive, but side effects, which are specific to the mode of action, are less than additive. Furthermore, the majority of hypertensive individuals require at least two drugs to achieve the currently recommended rigorous BP targets.[20]

Traditionally, the first step in this combined approach was a thiazide diuretic, the second a β-blocker and the third a vasodilator.[8] The unwanted effects of diuretics (hypokalaemia, hyperuricaemia and hyperglycaemia), β-blockers (fatigue and cold limbs) and vasodilators (headache, flushing and palpitation) are all dose-related. Therefore, limitation of the dose of each drug will minimize these problems. Furthermore, β-blockers tend to reduce the hypokalaemia caused by diuretics and the reflex tachycardia induced by vasodilators. Low-dose diuretic-based stepped care is still recommended in US guidelines.[3]

Three-drug, stepped-care regimens have been remarkably effective in controlling BP in the majority of hypertensive individuals, with an acceptable burden of side effects. However, the advent of ACE inhibitors, angiotensin receptor blockers, calcium channel blockers and selective α-blockers challenged this approach. As well as replacing older vasodilators as third-line agents, a case can be made for using these drugs as initial therapy. ACE inhibitors and angiotensin receptor blockers cause very few symptomatic side effects or biochemical disturbances and are advocated as monotherapy.[13,14] Calcium channel blockers[15] and α-blockers[12] can also be used as first-line agents, although symptoms are more common at high doses, particularly in the case of α-blockers. Again with these agents, addition of other drugs, usually diuretics or β-blockers, is often needed for adequate BP control. These considerations underpin current European guidelines, which offer a free choice of first-line therapy between diuretics, β-blockers, ACE inhibitors, angiotensin receptor blockers, calcium channel blockers or α-blockers.[22]

A problem with the stepped-care approach is that it takes no account of inter-individual variability in the response to individual drugs. Thus, the eventual antihypertensive regimen may include one or more drugs which has little activity in that individual. Much effort has been expended in identifying factors that may predict individual responses to drugs and to allow better selection of agents. Younger people tend to have activated RAAS and, therefore, respond well to drugs that block that system. In contrast, older individuals and blacks tend to respond better to drugs that address the volume component of hypertension. These principles form the basis of the British Hypertension Society ABCD algorithm:[20] A (ACE inhibitor or angiotensin receptor blocker) or B (β-blocker) as first-line therapy in individuals aged <55 years and C (calcium channel blocker) or D (diuretic) in individuals aged >55 years or black people of any age. To achieve target BP, drugs are combined (A or B plus C or D) in a logical sequence. In its most recent iteration, the algorithm has been shortened to ACD.[23] The reason for this change is accumulating evidence that suggests that β-blockers are less effective than other drugs in protecting against cardiovascular events, particularly stroke,[24] and the realization that β-blockers increase the risk of progression to new onset diabetes.[25,26]

Choice between drugs

The principal factor that would enable choice of one drug over another would be if one agent had a particularly favourable effect on morbidity and mortality. Failing that, the factors in order of importance, might be: efficacy, side effects and cost.

The clinical trial evidence that underpins the management of hypertension has blossomed in the last 25 years. Numerous trials in many thousands of individuals have demonstrated benefits of antihypertensive drugs against placebo or control[2] and have compared different therapeutic approaches.[27–30] The latter studies have demonstrated few important differences, although some drug classes may have particular advantages in certain patient populations. The importance of rigorous BP control has been demonstrated repeatedly and consistently.[28–30] Thus, what you do appears to be much more important than the way that you do it. Since rigorous BP control usually involves combination therapy, the focus has shifted from the choice of first-line therapy to the selection of treatment regimen.

One conclusion that emerged early is that the reduction in cardiovascular events achieved by treating mild hypertension is modest;[31] if 850 mildly hypertensive individuals are given antihypertensive therapy for 1 year, only one stroke will be prevented. Certainly, at this rate, the benefit to be gained does not appear to be worthwhile in an individual who may have to tolerate appreciable side effects.

Since the benefits in terms of morbidity and mortality are small in mild hypertension, the secondary considerations of efficacy, side effect profile and cost become important. These issues are particularly relevant since mild hypertension is highly prevalent. For such high volume therapy to be attractive to health authorities, unit cost must be low. In most countries, cost containment has become decisive in planning and limiting the health budget.

Furthermore, the need to avoid side effects in an essentially asymptomatic population has led to a drive towards choosing antihypertensive agents on the less definable, but clearly important criterion of effect on 'quality of life'. Much work still needs to be done to refine methods of assessment, but newer drugs (such as ACE inhibitors) appear preferable in this respect to older drugs such as methyldopa or propranolol.[32] It is much more difficult to demonstrate differences in the effects on quality of life between contemporary drugs used at currently recommended doses.[33]

Findings from the clinical trials have encouraged consideration that different drugs may be indicated in different population subgroups.[30] These findings have also led to an appreciation that the benefits of therapy may not be large enough to warrant treatment in individuals with mild hypertension and a propensity to side effects. However, the priorities in the treatment of hypertension are still making the best choice of drug regimen, changing the constituent drugs or doses if side effects occur and retaining an active concern about the individual over many years of treatment. These undramatic aspects of clinical life have as much influence upon the outcome and quality of life for treated hypertensive individuals as does erudite knowledge of pathophysiology and pharmacology. Unfortunately, these aspects are often ignored.

FUTURE PROSPECTS

Predicting the future is generally a futile exercise. However, there are three areas where antihypertensive therapy is likely to evolve in the forthcoming decades:

(1) Combination therapy, including low-dose multi-drug combination therapy and combinations with other cardioprotective agents.
(2) Pharmacogenetics/pharmacogenomics to enhance prediction of response in populations and eventually individuals, with the goal of improved efficacy and safety.
(3) Novel molecules derived from greater understanding of mediators for hypertension and mechanisms providing new targets for the interface between hypertension and vascular disease.

Combination therapy

It is increasingly recognized that to achieve modern treatment targets, combination therapy with two or more antihypertensive agents is usually necessary.[34,35] As recently as 10 years ago, prescribers favoured monotherapy, with only 40% of treated hypertensive individuals receiving multiple drugs.[36] This pattern has changed dramatically, with only a minority now receiving a single antihypertensive drug.

There is much speculation about the appropriate constituents of combination therapy. It is generally recommended that drugs with complementary actions should be prescribed, i.e. a drug with primary action on peripheral resistance (e.g. ACE inhibitor) together with a drug with predominant action on plasma volume (e.g. diuretic). A meta-analysis of over 300 trials provides little support for this hypothesis.[37] This suggests that all commonly used antihypertensive drugs have strictly additive effects on BP. However, very few studies have been designed to adequately assess whether antihypertensive drugs have additive, more than additive (mistakenly referred to as synergistic) or less than additive effects when used in combination. Happily, few antihypertensive agents have detrimental effects when used in combination. The exceptions are β-blockers plus verapamil (or diltiazem) where there is a real risk of bradyarrhythmias and even sudden death, and possibly potassium sparing agents with other drugs which increase potassium levels. Recent findings suggest the latter combination is well tolerated, provided serum potassium is monitored.[4,20]

Since increasing doses of antihypertensive drugs usually only modestly increase antihypertensive effects, low doses of constituent drugs are advocated to reduce the incidence of side effects.[34,35] In combination therapy, low doses are appropriate, as with diuretics, where there is a steep dose–adverse-effect relationship. This consideration does not apply to ACE inhibitors and angiotensin receptor blockers where side effects are not dose-dependent. Furthermore, the antihypertensive efficacy of high doses of diuretics is limited by activation of the RAAS. Higher doses may be appropriate where the RAAS is blocked (e.g. in combination with an ACE inhibitor) and blockade of the RAAS attenuates some of the metabolic effects of diuretics.[4,20] Reduction in aldosterone levels with ACE inhibitors and angiotensin receptor blockers ameliorates diuretic-induced hypokalaemia and recent evidence indicates that these drugs lessen the risk of new onset diabetes in diuretic-treated patients.[25,38] Therefore, the most appropriate doses of the constituent drugs in combination therapy remain to be established.

Currently, there is controversy about when combination therapy should be introduced. The most recent US guidelines[3] recommend that low-dose combination therapy including a thiazide diuretic should be considered as initial therapy for hypertensive individuals with BP 20/10 mmHg above the on-treatment target BP, since monotherapy is unlikely to be adequate in such people. There is some support for this from studies such as ASCOT[39] and VALUE[40] where BP differences early during therapy could not be compensated by adding further drugs over several years of therapy. Among explanations for this phenomenon is the hypothesis that failure to control BP by initial therapy results in compensatory mechanisms, which make control more difficult to achieve in the long term. Testing this hypothesis is very difficult, but several protocols are in development.

Another unsettled issue is whether multiple drugs should be prescribed as free combination or fixed dose combinations in a single tablet.[41] Fixed-dose combinations might be expected to improve compliance and, therefore, enhance achieved BP control. In cash-strapped health systems cost will always be a problem. For widespread adoption, fixed-dose combinations must be similar in cost (or even cheaper) than the constituents taken as separate pills. Furthermore, fixed-dose combinations are often introduced by drug companies towards the end of the patent-life of a drug, leading to suspicion that these are marketing devices to extend the product life. Demonstration of a real advantage of a fixed-dose combination in terms of efficacy, side effects and compliance is a major challenge. The task may be most relevant for those with co-morbidities when multiple drugs are indicated.

Many hypertensive patients have co-morbidities such as hyperlipidaemia and are at high cardiovascular risk.[3] Theoretically, a combination of drugs that addresses not only BP, but also those other co-morbidities, would have a greater impact on cardiovascular outcomes. This 'polypill' approach suggests that while antihypertensive therapy alone would be expected to reduce cardiovascular risk by 25%, a pill comprising a low-dose thiazide, ACE inhibitor, statin and aspirin might reduce risk by over 60%.[42] Findings from trials such as ASCOT,[39,43] which examined antihypertensive therapy with or without a statin in people with relatively 'normal' serum cholesterol levels, support this hypothesis. Rigorous antihypertensive therapy plus atorvastatin, and aspirin in high-risk individuals, reduced cardiovascular risk by more than 50% compared with imputed placebo.

With the 'polypill' approach, the devil is in the detail. Which drugs and at what doses should be included in the fixed dose combination? Few would question the inclusion of low-dose thiazide and possibly an ACE inhibitor or angiotensin receptor blocker at appropriate 'high' dose. Other constituents are more controversial. Clinical trial evidence supports the use of a statin regardless of baseline serum cholesterol,[44] but many are concerned about possible side effects. Aspirin is effective and cheap, but not cheerful. Serious and even fatal haemorrhage is relatively common and safe use necessitates risk assessment; net benefit if 10-year cardiovascular risk is at least 20%, but net harm if risk is 10% or less.[20] Other suggested constituents such as folic acid have no evidence base.

Pharmacogenetics/pharmacogenomics

Much recent effort has been devoted to understanding the genetics of hypertension, in the hope of finding genotypes that predict the antihypertensive response in populations or individuals. The objective is targeting appropriate therapy to improve efficacy and safety. Thus, a particular drug would be used to treat individuals with a genotype that predicts a good antihypertensive effect and no side effects. Wasteful therapy that results in little BP lowering, but may increase the burden of side effects, would be avoided.

This approach may lead to unexpected complications. Since any drug would be restricted in its market on the basis of genotyping to a relatively small proportion of individuals, the economics of hypertension management would return to a low volume – high cost strategy. Furthermore, it is now clear that hypertension is associated with many more genotypes than anticipated and each predicts BP variability much less than expected.[45,46] Alleles are distributed unevenly and the impact is heterogeneous.

To establish the clinical utility of pharmacogenomics, prospective studies that satisfy certain criteria are required. The starting point is a well documented major candidate gene that is functionally relevant for all aspects of pharmacology and toxicology. Global and regional variation must be considered. Demographics are environmental factors that have to be included as co-variables. Rigorous assessment of drug exposure and compliance must be carried out. The study should have adequate power to take multiple gene effects into consideration. Even then a positive result requires prospective testing in a further population and cost–benefit analysis.

Pharmacogenetic analysis has scored some successes in picking the low hanging fruit of rare simple diseases. For common complex diseases, such as hypertension, studies have not advanced much beyond fishing expeditions. The promise of predictive tests to assist therapeutic choices is far down the line. The expectations of personalized medicines and individualized prescriptions are, so far, largely based on extrapolations from small retrospective studies reported by enthusiasts.

To date, the reality of pharmacogenetics is that promise is unfulfilled. The factors determining desired and unwanted drug effects are complex. Genes are important but so too are environment and behaviour. Therapeutic failure and adverse drug effects can usually be attributed to poor prescribing skills, drug interactions and lack of adherence with therapy.

Pharmacogenomics has provided more questions than answers. Early reports of positive associations between genotype and phenotype have not been replicated in larger studies. Studies have had low power, making false positive results likely. Since multiple genes are each responsible for small risks, allowance for multiple testing is needed but has seldom been considered.

The current status of pharmacogenomics has led to a proliferation of pseudoscience with direct-to-consumer marketing. Genetic testing is now available on the internet. The consequences can be unnecessary anxiety or false reassurance.

Several ethical dilemmas have arisen. There is potential for loss of individual freedom and ownership of genetic material requires safeguards. Disclosure of genetic information for health insurance purposes is particularly sensitive. The risks of increased premiums or refusal to insure are obvious concerns. However, the result may place the individual on a slippery slope; as precision of outcome becomes more assured, the principle of mutuality, which underpins health insurance, is invalidated. Those involved in pharmacogenetics must take responsibility for wider education and for ethical issues.

These concerns should not be taken to deny that some progress has been made. Recent successes include the identification of the genotype that appears to be associated with failure to respond to ACE inhibitors.[47] However, much work needs to be done. It can be predicted that widespread use of pharmacogenomics will not be possible for many decades.

Novel molecules

Novel mediators of BP continue to appear (and to disappear). Ten years ago, there was much interest in atrial natriuretic peptides and endothelin. Drugs which modify these mediators have been developed but proved to be less effective and/or less well tolerated than predicted. No doubt, further targets will be identified but, at present, few novel molecules are close to the clinic.

Potential mechanisms that provide targets for the interface between hypertension and vascular disease may be more promising. There is clustering between high BP, dyslipidaemia, blood sugar (diabetes) and obesity. Individuals with all four markers of cardiovascular risk (sometimes known as the metabolic syndrome) are exquisitely sensitive to blood-pressure reduction in prevention of cardiovascular risk.[3] This observation suggests that hitherto unidentified mechanisms are important in mediating the association between BP and cardiovascular disease. Preliminary evidence supports a role for drugs that block the RAAS, but more specific molecules targeting candidate mechanisms are in development.

CONCLUSIONS

The development of understanding of the clinical pharmacology of drugs that reduce BP has been a major factor in improved insights into the pathogenic process not only of hypertension, but also of cardiovascular disease. At the same time, the development of new drugs that are safer and induce fewer side effects than earlier agents has allowed the treatment of hypertension to move from the management of severely ill patients to the use of these drugs, together with other cardioprotective agents, as major components in the widespread prevention of cardiovascular disease. Advances in drug therapy will continue thanks to the ingenuity of molecular biologists working in collaboration with the pharmaceutical industry.

References

1. May O. Hyperpiesia IV: mortality in relation to hyperpiesia. *BMJ* 1925;ii:116–117.
2. Collins R, MacMahon S. Blood pressure, antihypertensive drug treatment and the risks of stroke and of coronary heart disease. *Br Med Bull* 1994;50:272–298.
3. Chobanian AV, Bakris GE, Black HR, et al. The National High Blood Pressure Education Program Coordinating Committee. The seventh report of the Joint National Committee on Prevention, Detection, and Treatment of High Blood Pressure. The JNC 7 Report. *JAMA* 2003;289:2560–2572.
4. Brown MJ, Cruickshank JK, Dominiczak AF, et al. Better blood pressure control: how to combine drugs. *J Hum Hypertens* 2003;17:81–86.

5. McInnes G. Potent vasodilators. In: Birkenhäger WH, Reid JL, eds. *Handbook of hypertension. Clinical pharmacology and therapeutics of antihypertensive drugs, Vol 24*. Amsterdam: Elsevier; 2007.

6. Reid JL, Elliott HL. Methyldopa in Handbook of Hypertension. In: Birkenhäger WH, Reid JL, eds. *Handbook of hypertension. Clinical pharmacology of antihypertensive drugs, Vol 11*. Amsterdam: Elsevier; 1988:103–124.

7. Pritchard BNC, Van Zweiten PA. Methyldopa and imidazoline agonists. In: Birkenhäger WH, Reid JL, eds. *Handbook of hypertension. Clinical pharmacology and therapeutics of antihypertensive drugs, Vol 24*. Amsterdam: Elsevier; 2007.

8. Struthers AD, Dollery CT. Antihypertensive drugs: pharmacokinetics, pharmacodynamics, metabolism, side-effects, drug interactions. In: Birkenhäger WH, Reid JL, eds. *Handbook of hypertension. Clinical pharmacology of antihypertensive drugs, Vol 11*. Amsterdam: Elsevier; 1998:1–40.

9. Koch-Weser J. Hydralazine. *N Engl J Med* 1976;295:320–323.

10. Koch-Weser J. Vasodilator drugs in the treatment of hypertension. *Arch Intern Med* 1974;133:1017–1027.

11. Swales JD, Bing RF, Heagerty AM, et al. Treatment of refractory hypertension*Lancet* 1982;1:894–896.

12. Meredith P. Alpha-blocking drugs in Handbook of Hypertension. (Ser eds: Birkenhäger WH, Reid JL) *Clinical Pharmacology and Therapeutics of Antihypertensive Drugs* Vol 24 (Vol ed: McInnes GT) Amsterdam; Elsevier; 2007.

13. de Gaspero M, McInnes G. Angiotensin receptor blockers in Handbook of Hypertension. (Ser eds: Birkenhäger WH, Reid JL) *Clinical Pharmacology and Therapeutics of Antihypertensive Drugs* Vol 24 (Vol ed: McInnes GT) Amsterdam; Elsevier; 2007.

14. Nicholls M, Petrioianu G, Carruthers JG. Angiotensin converting enzyme inhibitors in Handbook of Hypertension. (Ser eds: Birkenhäger WH, Reid JL) *Clinical Pharmacology and Therapeutics of Antihypertensive Drugs* Vol 24 (Vol ed: McInnes GT) Amsterdam; Elsevier; 2007.

15. Elliott HL. Calcium channel blockers in Handbook of Hypertension. (Ser eds: Birkenhäger WH, Reid JL) *Clinical Pharmacology and Therapeutics of Antihypertensive Drugs* Vol 24 (Vol ed: McInnes GT) Amsterdam; Elsevier; 2007.

16. Pratt-Ubanama M, Oparil S. Thiazides and loop diuretics in Handbook of Hypertension. (Ser eds: Birkenhäger WH, Reid JL) *Clinical Pharmacology and Therapeutics of Antihypertensive Drugs* Vol 24 (Vol ed: McInnes GT) Amsterdam; Elsevier; 2007.

17. Krishnan PH, MacDonald T. Aldosterone antagonists in Handbook of Hypertension. (Ser eds: Birkenhäger WH, Reid JL) *Clinical Pharmacology and Therapeutics of Antihypertensive Drugs* Vol 24 (Vol ed: McInnes GT) Amsterdam; Elsevier; 2007.

18. Staessen JA, Li Y, Richart T. Oral renin inhibitors. *Lancet* 2006;368:1449–1456.

19. Alderman MH, Madhavan SH, Ooi WL, et al. Association of the renin-sodium profile with the risk of myocardial infarction in patients with hypertension. *N Engl J Med* 1991;324:1098–1104.

20. Williams B, Poulter NR, Brown M, et al. Guidelines for management of hypertension: report of the fourth working party of the British Hypertension Society, 2004 - BHS IV. *J Human Hypertens* 2004;18:139–185.

21. Zacest R, Gilmore E, Koch-Weser J. Treatment of essential hypertension with combined vasodilation and beta adrenergic blockade. *N Engl J Med* 1972;286:617–622.

22. Guidelines Committee. European Society of Hypertension - European Society of Cardiology guidelines for the management of arterial hypertension. *J Hypertens* 2003;21:1011–1053.

23. National Institute for Health and Clinical Excellence. Clinical Guidelines Hypertension: management of hypertension in adults in primary care: 2006. Available at *http://www.nice.org. uk/CG034*.

24. Lindholm LH, Carlberg B, Samuelsson O. Should β blockers remain first choice in the treatment of primary hypertension? A meta-analysis. *Lancet* 2005;366:1545–1553.

25. Elliott WJ, Meyer PM. Incident diabetes in clinical trials of antihypertensive drugs: a network meta-analysis. *Lancet* 2007;369:201–207.

26. Mason JM, Dickinson HO, Nicolson DJ, et al. The diabetogenic potential of thiazide-type diuretics and beta-blocker combinations in patients with hypertension*J Hypertens* 2005;23:1777–1781.

27. Blood Pressure Lowering Treatment Trialists' Collaboration. Effects of ACE inhibitors, calcium antagonists, and other blood-pressure-lowering drugs: results of prospectively designed overviews of randomised trials. *Lancet* 2000;355:1955–1964.

28. Blood Pressure Lowering Treatment Trialist Collaboration. Effects of different blood-pressure-lowering regimens on major cardiovascular events: results of prospectively-designed overviews of randomised trials. *Lancet* 2003;362:1527–1535.

29. Staessen JA, Wang JG, Thijs L. Cardiovascular protection and blood pressure reduction: a meta-analysis. *Lancet* 2001;358:1305–1315.

30. Verdecchia P, Reboldi G, Angeli A, et al. Angiotensin-converting enzyme inhibitors and calcium channel blockers for coronary heart disease and stroke prevention. *Hypertension* 2005;46:386–392.

31. Medical Research Council Working Party MRC trial of treatment of mild hypertension: principal results. *Br Med J* 1985;291:97–104.

32. Croog SH, Levine S, Testa MA, et al. The effects of antihypertensive therapy on quality of life. *N Engl J Med* 1986;314:1657–1664.

33. Herrick AL, Waller PC, Berkin KE, et al. Comparison of enalapril and atenolol in mild to moderate hypertension. *Am J Med* 1989;86:421–426.

34. Mahmud A, Feely J. Low-dose quadruple antihypertensive combination: more efficacious than individual agents - a preliminary report. *Hypertension* 2007;49:272–275.

35. Reid JL. Fall and rise of polypharmacy? *Hypertension* 2007;49:266–267.

36. Primatesta P, Brookes M, Poulter NR. Improved hypertensive management and control: results from the health survey of England 1998. *Hypertension* 2001;38:827–832.

37. Law MR, Wald NJ, Morris JK, Jordan RE. Value of low dose combination treatment with blood pressure lowering drugs: analysis of 354 randomised trials. *BMJ* 2003;326:1427–1435.

38. Scheen AJ, Prevention of type 2 diabetes mellitus through inhibition of the renin-angiotensin system. *Drugs* 2004;64:2537–2565.

39. Dahlof B, Sever PS, Poulter NR, et al; for the ASCOT investigators. Prevention of cardiovascular events with an antihypertensive regimen of amlodipine adding perindopril as required, in the Anglo-Scandinavian Cardiac Outcomes Trial - Blood Pressure Lowering Arm (ASCOT-BPLA): a multicentre randomised controlled trial. *Lancet* 2005;366:895–906.

40. Julius S, Kjeldsen SE, Weber M, et al; for the VALUE trial group. Outcomes in hypertensive patients at high cardiovascular risk treated with regimens based on valsartan or amlodipine the VALUE randomised trial. *Lancet* 2004;363:2022–2031.

41. Reid JL. The treatment of hypertension: a therapeutic philosophy for the 1990s. *J Cardiovasc Pharmacol* 1991;18(Suppl 2):S64–S67.

42. Wald NJ, Law MR. A strategy to reduce cardiovascular disease by more than 80%. *BMJ* 2003;326:1419–1423.

43. Sever PS, Dahlöf B, Poulter NR, et al. Prevention of coronary and stroke events with atorvastatin in hypertensive patients who have average or lower-than-average cholesterol concentration in the Anglo Scandinavian Cardiac Outcomes Trial in Lipid Lowering Arm (ASCOT-LLA): a multicentre randomised controlled trial. *Lancet* 2003;361:1149–1158.

44. Cholesterol Treatment Trialists' Collaboration. Efficacy and safety of cholesterol-lowering treatment: prospective meta-analysis to date from 90,056 participants in 14 randomised trials of statins. *Lancet* 2005;366:1267–1278.

45. Caulfield M, Munroe P, Pembroke J, et al. Genome-wide mapping of human loci for essential hypertension. *Lancet* 2003;361:2118–2123.

46. Harrap SB. Where are all the blood-pressure genes? *Lancet* 2003;361:2149–2151.

47. Padmanabhan S, Wallace C, Munroe PB, et al. Chromosome 2p shows significant linkage to antihypertensive response in the British Genetics of Hypertension Study. *Hypertension* 2006;47(part 2):603–608.

2 | Interaction of antihypertensive drugs with mechanisms of blood pressure regulation

Peter W. de Leeuw and Abraham A. Kroon

INTRODUCTION

High blood pressure (BP) contributes substantially to cardiovascular complications such as cerebrovascular accidents and myocardial infarction. Peripheral vascular disease, heart failure and renal insufficiency have also been identified as major sequelae of the hypertensive process. Fortunately, many studies have shown that adequate antihypertensive treatment will reduce the number of cardiovascular complications, with risk reductions of about 40% for cerebrovascular events and approximately 20% for cardiac endpoints. However, epidemiologic investigations such as the Framingham Study have also shown that an elevated BP tends to cluster with other (metabolic) risk factors, such as diabetes and hyperlipidaemia, which markedly enhance the risk carried by the increased pressure itself. It is essential, therefore, that the practising physician takes care of hypertension and other risk factors at the same time.

Because antihypertensive treatment, once instituted, must be maintained for many years, the decision to treat or not should not be taken lightly. According to current guidelines and recommendations this requires the assessment of overall risk, which means that one tries to estimate the chance that a patient will sustain a major cardiovascular event within a certain time frame. If overall risk is low, it is justifiable to withhold treatment for a while and to keep the patient under surveillance. However, when risk exceeds a certain (arbitrary) level the patient should be treated with antihypertensive drugs. Currently, the most important of these are diuretics, β-blockers, calcium antagonists, angiotensin converting enzyme inhibitors and angiotensin II type 1 receptor blockers, because of their favourable effect on long-term prognosis.[1] It is not an easy task to choose among the various categories. In coming to a sound decision, the physician may take several courses, approaching the problem from a drug-related or a patient-related perspective. In this chapter we will focus on the mechanisms of BP regulation with which antihypertensive drugs can interfere.

MECHANISMS OF BLOOD PRESSURE CONTROL AS TARGETS FOR TREATMENT

Figure 2.1 provides a simplified scheme of the most important systems that are involved in blood-pressure control. Theoretically, all these systems are potential targets for therapeutic intervention. Haemodynamically, hypertension can be considered as an increase in systolic and diastolic BP or mean arterial pressure (MAP), the latter representing a 'static' component of the circulation. Alternatively, an increase in pulse pressure ('dynamic' component) can be taken as the most important haemodynamic abnormality in hypertension.[2] From a circulatory point of view, MAP is determined by cardiac output (CO) and systemic vascular resistance (SVR), while pulse pressure (PP) is largely dependent upon ventricular ejection and the stiffness of the arterial tree. Theoretically, all these components are amenable to pharmacological modulation.

In the normal individual, BP is kept within certain limits by an extensive array of stabilizing mechanisms, with the sympathetic nervous system and the kidney as the most important regulators. Short-term changes in BP can be effectively buffered by the baroreflex and the sympathetic nervous system, but in the long term it is the kidney that will determine at what level BP will be maintained.[3] This Guytonian concept of circulatory control thus predicts that no intervention will be able to produce a sustained drop in BP unless the renal volume–pressure relationship (pressure-natriuresis or renal function curve) is reset.

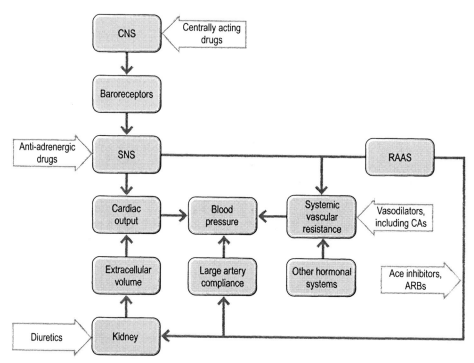

Fig. 2.1 Simplified scheme of the mechanisms involved in the control of the circulation and the site of action of various classes of drugs. CNS = central nervous system; SNS = sympathetic nervous system; RAAS = renin–angiotensin–aldosterone system.

Table 2.1 Main (primary) effect of various classes of antihypertensive agents

Class of drug	Effect
Centrally acting drugs	Reduced sympathetic outflow
Anti-adrenergic drugs	
- ganglion blockers	Inhibition of neurotransmission
- neuron blockers	Depletion of neurotransmitters
- α-adrenoceptor blockers	Antagonism of α-adrenoceptors
- β-adrenoceptor blockers	Antagonism of β-adrenoceptors
ACE inhibitors	Reduced formation of Ang II
ARBs	Antagonism of type 1 receptors for Ang II
Vasodilators	Potassium channel opening; activation of guanylate cyclase (but not always known)
Calcium antagonists	Reduced intracellular calcium concentration
Diuretics	Increased urinary sodium output

ACE=angiotensin converting enzyme; Ang=angiotensin; ARB=angiotensin II type 1 receptor blocker

Basically, both the regulation of fluid volume balance and that of vascular resistance can be attacked. In practice, however, most antihypertensive drugs act on multiple systems so that it is not always evident which mechanisms are actually responsible for a certain fall in BP. Moreover, any direct drug effect may be compensated for by counterregulatory (and not necessarily renal) systems, which can even totally offset an initial decline in pressure. In the long term, therefore, the efficacy of each antihypertensive agent is determined not only by its primary pharmacological effect, but also by the efficiency of such compensatory mechanisms.

Based on current pathophysiological concepts, drugs have been designed that can lower cardiac output or vascular resistance, increase urinary sodium output or modulate vessel wall properties. In general, the primary pharmacological action of available drugs is straightforward (Table 2.1), but the compensatory mechanisms that are elicited are not always obvious. Consequently, for most antihypertensive drugs the *long-term* actions have not been defined so clearly. However, since the kidney responds to a fall in pressure by retaining more sodium, no antihypertensive drug can work effectively if sodium excretion is not facilitated, either directly or via modulation of neurohumoral systems with a bearing on renal sodium handling.

While the aim of treatment has always been to lower systolic, diastolic and mean arterial pressure, we are now increasingly aware that not only the 'static' components of pressure, but also pulse pressure should be reduced.[2] An ideal antihypertensive drug, therefore, not only lowers MAP but also PP. In the following, the mechanisms by which various classes of antihypertensive drugs interfere with BP regulatory systems will be discussed in more detail.

INTERFERENCE WITH SYSTEMIC HAEMODYNAMICS

Since mean arterial pressure is the product of cardiac output and systemic vascular resistance, it follows that drugs that are to lower pressure must do so by affecting either CO or SVR or both. The ways by which such haemodynamic changes are accomplished may vary considerably however, and can involve direct effects on the heart (e.g. β-blockers) or the vessels (e.g. so-called direct vasodilators) or indirect actions. As both the sympathetic nervous system and the renin–angiotensin system play a key role in regulating haemodynamics, it is not surprising that many antihypertensives act via one of these systems. Alternatively, drugs may interfere directly with the vascular contraction process, for example by inhibiting the inflow of calcium ions or by blocking the excitation–contraction coupling. In recent years there has been increasing interest in agents that, besides lowering vascular resistance, enhance the dynamic properties of the vasculature (compliance, distensibility).

Cardiac output as the primary target

Although CO may be elevated in a subgroup of especially young patients,[4] the common finding in hypertension is a normal or slightly reduced CO.[5] At first sight, therefore, there seems to be no point in reducing cardiac output any further. Yet, drugs that lower CO, such as β-blocking agents, have become a mainstay in the treatment of hypertension with a definite benefit on prognosis.[1] Thus, a fall in CO is not a priori harmful.

Acute administration of β-blocking drugs is associated with an immediate fall in heart rate and CO, but BP does not change appreciably because SVR rises at the same time. However, with prolonged treatment this haemodynamic picture changes with SVR gradually falling to its initial level or even below. At that time, BP also drops.[6] Man in 't Veld has summarized the acute and chronic haemodynamic effects of a variety of β-blocking agents in over 900 patients.[7] This analysis yielded a fairly consistent pattern: cardiac output initially falls, but less so when the drug possesses more partial agonistic activity. In the long term, peripheral resistance is invariably reduced. Prospective data seem to confirm this sequence of events.[6] Up to now, however, the causes of the secondary drop in resistance remain elusive. Table 2.2[8] lists several potential mechanisms, but none of these has been unequivocally proven to be the cause of the vasodilatory effect. One of the prevailing theories is that β-blockers inhibit the facilitation of noradrenaline release from nerve terminals by presynaptic β-adrenoceptors. As a consequence, α-mediated vasoconstriction would be reduced. As attractive as this theory may appear, a fundamental problem is that the presynaptic β-adrenoceptor is a β_2 receptor, while the most effective β-blockers have a high degree of β_1 selectivity. Alternatively, suppression of renin (via the β_1 adrenoceptor) may be of importance, as conditions in which

Table 2.2 Potential mechanisms by which β-blockers may lower systemic vascular resistance

Inhibition of β-1 mediated renin release
Inhibition of central autonomic nervous system
Resetting of the baroreflex
Increase in natriuretic peptides
Effect on prejunctional β-receptors: reduction in noradrenaline release
Reduction in venous tone
Reduction in plasma volume
Attenuation of the pressor effect of catecholamines
Increase in vasodilator prostaglandins

(Adapted from: ref. (8).)

renin is low have often been associated with lesser response to β-blockers. Although this supposition has not been universally reproduced and, although the hypotensive effect of β-blockers does not correlate well with changes in renin, it is interesting that black people in whom renin is almost invariably suppressed consistently exhibit a reduced responsiveness to β-blockade.[9] There must also be a role, albeit a modest one, for prostaglandins, as non-steroidal anti-inflammatory drugs that inhibit prostaglandin synthesis are able to attenuate the blood-pressure-lowering effect of β-blockers by a few mmHg.[10]

In the past, several attempts have been made to define subgroups of patients in whom β-blockers would be particularly useful, i.e. those with an elevated cardiac output and/or high renin levels. While a few studies do, indeed, support these claims, the number of exceptions is too great, presumably indicating that we still do not know precisely how β-blockers lower pressure. Unfortunately, there are at present no distinct pathophysiological features that are able to predict precisely the degree of responsiveness to β-blockade. The recent claim that some β-blocking agents have effects on the prognosis of hypertensive patients that are less favourable than others,[11] seems premature and needs confirmation. If this is found to be true, then this casts doubt on a uniform mechanism for all β-blockers.

While beta-adrenergic blockers primarily lessen heart rate and myocardial contractility, they generally do not or only marginally lower stroke volume. The latter may be diminished, however, by drugs which reduce venous return. As well as nitrates and nitrate-like substances, diuretics, α-blockers, ACE inhibitors and centrally acting antihypertensives may induce venodilation and diminish cardiac preload. Whether this is a favourable mechanism depends on many factors, including the haemodynamic status of the patient. Thus, under certain conditions a fall in stroke volume may help to lower pressure. However, it is also possible that CO falls too much and that orthostatic intolerance ensues. Therefore, drugs with high selectivity for the venous system without other beneficial effects have no significant role in the treatment of hypertension.

Peripheral vasculature as the primary target

As, eventually, all forms of hypertension are related to an increase in SVR, it seems only logical to treat the disorder by lowering arteriolar tone. In fact, as a general rule, no drug will lower pressure unless it is able to elicit, directly or as a secondary phenomenon, a fall in vascular resistance. Vasodilation can be achieved in various ways. First of all, drugs may reduce the overall activity of pressor systems (sympathetic nervous system, renin–angiotensin–aldosterone system (RAAS)). Secondly, drugs could interfere with specific receptors in the vascular wall that mediate the effects of these systems. Thirdly, drugs may modulate voltage- or receptor responsive channels in the cell membrane that play a role in the initiation of the contraction of the vascular smooth muscle cell. Lastly, the contraction process in itself can be the target for interference.

Although it is a matter of semantics, drugs which lower SVR by modulating 'extravascular' mechanisms are not normally classified as vasodilators, even though their hypotensive potential may depend entirely upon the relaxation of precapillary arterioles (cf. the secondary fall in systemic vascular resistance during long-term β-blockade). These agents will be discussed elsewhere under the appropriate headings (see below). The term (direct) vasodilator has been reserved for drugs that activate intracellular guanylate cyclase. This convention will also be followed here. Sometimes, calcium antagonists are also classified as vasodilators, but this is less appropriate in view of their different mode of action.

Vasodilators may act on the arterial as well as the venous side of the circulation. Probably, there are no drugs with an exclusive effect on either the arteries or the veins; there is always a mixture of arteriolar and venular effects. It is the relative balance of pre- and postcapillary resistance reduction that determines whether BP, heart rate and/or cardiac output will fall, remain unchanged or increase. Nitrates, for instance, predominantly dilate the venous system, thereby reducing atrial pressure, stroke volume and cardiac output, but at higher doses nitrates may also cause some dilation of resistance vessels and a drop in systemic BP.[12,13] Usually, the greatest changes are seen in systolic pressure with no or very little alteration in diastolic pressure. The latter suggests that nitrates act more on the large conduit arteries (improving compliance) than on arteriolar vessels. This alleged property makes nitrates an interesting tool for the treatment of patients with (isolated) systolic hypertension.[14]

The mechanism by which nitrates dilate blood vessels involves the generation of nitric oxide (NO) from the drug molecules, although the precise steps in this pathway are not well understood. NO is thought to stimulate cytosolic guanylate cyclase, which, in turn, increases the intracellular concentration of cyclic guanosine monophosphate (cGMP). The latter inhibits the inositol pathway and reduces intracellular calcium. As a result, the vascular smooth muscle cell relaxes. Because the formation of NO is independent of the endothelium, nitrates still work when the vascular endothelium is damaged.

A similar mechanism holds for sodium nitroprusside that has a more balanced effect on arteriolar and venular tone. Due to venous dilatation, stroke volume falls. In comparison with nitrates, nitroprusside lowers BP and afterload more and slightly stimulates CO. Because the drug can only be administered intravenously, it is mainly used when BP needs to be lowered rapidly as in conditions where rapid unloading of the heart is essential.

Other direct vasodilators acting via different mechanisms are hydralazine, minoxidil and diazoxide. These agents primarily dilate arterioles while exerting little, if any, effect on the venous side of the circulation. Recent data suggest that such drugs increase the intracellular concentration of cGMP, by acting as potassium channel openers. ATP-dependent potassium channels in the sarcolemmal membrane are believed to be involved in the maintenance of basal vessel wall tone in several vascular beds.[15] Opening of these channels causes efflux of potassium and membrane hyperpolarization. Subsequently, calcium influx is reduced and the vascular smooth muscle cell relaxes.

Clinically, the use of direct vasodilators as monotherapy is greatly limited by hyperadrenergic symptoms and marked fluid retention. These 'side effects' are related to enhanced sympathetic activity and fluid retention secondary to activation of the RAAS. The rise in cardiac output that is observed during treatment with a direct vasodilator together with the expansion of the extracellular volume, may then completely offset the initial fall in BP. Nicorandil has potassium channel opening and nitrate-like properties. It lowers both preload and afterload with little effect on heart rate or cardiac output.[16]

INTERFERENCE WITH PRESSOR MECHANISMS

Despite a wealth of mechanisms that are involved in the regulation of cardiac output and vascular tone, presently only the sympathetic nervous system and the RAAS are of major clinical importance. In this part of our review, therefore, we will restrict ourselves to a discussion of those drugs that interfere with these systems. This is not to negate the role of, for example, prostaglandins, brady-kinin or other humoral factors, but to date these systems have not been the primary target of the currently available antihypertensive drugs.

Sympathetic nervous system as the primary target

Pharmacologically, the sympathetic nervous system (SNS) can be 'attacked' at several levels: centrally, at the level of preganglionic or postganglionic neurons, and at the receptor level. Ganglion-blocking drugs interrupt the transmission of sympathetic activity at the site where pre- and postganglionic nerve fibres communicate. Although these agents are extremely potent as antihypertensives, use should now be considered as obsolete (unless in very severe cases) because of intolerable side effects. Since both sympathetic and parasympathetic ganglia are blocked, a wide array of physiological functions is disturbed, leading to such problems as orthostatic hypotension, constipation, impaired micturition and loss of accommodation. Orthostatic hypotension and various other adverse effects may also be seen with adrenergic neuron-blockers and reserpine, which cause long-lasting depletion of noradrenaline stores in postganglionic sympathetic nerve endings. The limited use of these agents in the current treatment of hypertension does not justify an extensive discussion of these drugs in this chapter. Presently, only the centrally acting agents and the adrenoceptor blockers remain relevant for clinical practice.

Centrally acting antiadrenergic drugs

Centrally acting drugs inhibit sympathetic outflow via stimulation of α_2-adrenoceptors or type-1 imidazoline (I_1) receptors. These receptors are located in the nucleus tractus solitarii and the rostral ventrolateral medulla respectively. Methyldopa is the classic example of an α_2-agonist, while moxonidine and rilmenidine primarily stimulate I_1-receptors and have much weaker affinity for α_2-adrenoceptors. Clonidine has a mixed action and stimulates both types of receptors. Although it is difficult to obtain direct evidence for a central sympatholytic effect of these compounds in humans, a compelling observation was made by Reid and coworkers in tetraplegic patients with physiologically complete chronic cervical spinal cord transsection.[17] In such patients, a single oral dose of clonidine, 300 µg, which is effective in control subjects, did not lower BP, although heart rate still fell and 'peripheral' side effects still occurred. These data are at least consistent with a central mechanism of action and suggest that the hypotensive effect of clonidine in humans is dependent on intact descending bulbospinal pathways. In patients with an intact sympathetic system clonidine also lowers resting plasma noradrenaline concentrations, as would be expected if the drug reduces sympathetic activity. In fact, the fall in BP correlates well with the decline in plasma noradrenaline levels.[18] In addition, the noradrenaline response to a cold pressor stimulus is reduced.[19] Besides a central action clonidine has also been shown to interact with a variety of other receptors, including α_1-adrenoceptors and histaminergic receptors as well as with opioidergic mechanisms.[20] Based on a number of animal experiments and the observation of clinical behaviour equivalent to that of clonidine,[18] the central action of methyldopa is also beyond dispute. For moxonidine and rilmenidine, the evidence mainly rests on experimental data, although moxonidine has also been shown to reduce plasma noradrenaline levels.[21,22] In humans, cumbersome side effects, such as sedation and dry mouth, are less frequently seen with these drugs than with clonidine, presumably because these are related to the stimulation of α_2-receptors and not the I_1-receptors.

The haemodynamic profile of centrally acting antihypertensives is favourable: SVR falls with little change or sometimes a minute fall in heart rate and/or CO. The bradycardic effect may be enhanced by simultaneous activation of the parasympathetic system. Importantly, levels of renin and aldosterone are also reduced. Methyldopa has sometimes been found to lower venous tone, but it is uncertain whether this plays a role in humans. With all agents, reversal of left ventricular hypertrophy has been observed during long-term treatment.

One other phenomenon has been consistently associated with the use of clonidine, namely an immediate pressor effect when the drug is administered intravenously. This is usually explained by a direct effect of the agent on peripheral, postsynaptic α_2-adrenoceptors, leading to vasoconstriction.[23] At higher doses of the drug this pressor effect even surpasses the BP lowering effect. If the central and peripheral effects are both operative, either simultaneously or sequentially, clonidine must produce a complex haemodynamic pattern. This is evident, for instance, in the study by Mitchell and associates, who reported on the immediate haemodynamic responses following intravenous administration of a single dose of clonidine of about 300 mg in 28 normal volunteers.[24] Using impedance cardiography to measure cardiac output, they observed a profound fall in this variable that could be accounted for mostly by a substantial reduction in stroke volume. Total peripheral vascular resistance showed a biphasic pattern with an immediate, short-lasting decline that was followed by a gradual increase. The initial reduction in vascular resistance was explained by a vasodilatory action on the vascular wall (possibly involving nitric oxide) while the secondary rise in resistance was thought to be the result of baroreceptor-mediated reflex vasoconstriction. As attractive as these explanations may seem, there are other possibilities that need to be considered. Indeed, in the dosage used, clonidine must have been able to stimulate *presynaptic* α_2-adrenoceptors, the result of which is inhibition of noradrenaline release from nerve terminals. This mechanism, together with an immediate central effect, could account for the early fall in vascular resistance. Additionally, it is difficult to see why primary vasodilation would not be associated with baroreceptor-mediated increases in heart rate and cardiac output. It is very likely, therefore, that clonidine exerted an immediate sympatholytic effect leading to a decline in both cardiac output and vascular resistance. More complicated pharmacological experiments employing various agonists and antagonists or such manoeuvres as orthostatic stress would be needed to elucidate whether the effect is primarily central or peripheral. Other explanations for the secondary rise in vascular resistance are also possible. Earlier observations suggested that clonidine could 'sensitize' the arterial baroreceptors, meaning that at a given level of BP afferent firing would be increased.[25] This would lead to greater inhibition of sympathetic outflow. However, this sensitization occurs at relatively high dosages of the drug. Probably more important is the observation that clonidine facilitates reflex baroreceptor slowing. Indeed, clonidine-induced cardiac slowing is reduced following baroreceptor denervation.[26] What, then, could explain the vasoconstriction? The most attractive hypothesis is probably the rise in vascular resistance secondary to stimulation of *postsynaptic* α_2-adrenoceptors. This would then further stimulate the baroreceptor-mediated fall in cardiac output. Thus, most of the findings of Mitchell et al.[24] could be explained entirely by an effect of clonidine on pre- and postsynaptic α_2-adrenoceptors. Nevertheless, it is noteworthy that such observations have not been made with the other centrally acting sympatholytics. This suggests that there are some more subtle differences between the various representatives of this class.

Peripherally acting antiadrenergic drugs

In the periphery, only blockers of postsynaptic α- and β-adrenoceptors are relevant for the treatment of hypertension. As β-blockers have already been discussed (see above), we will confine ourselves here to α-adrenoceptor blocking agents. Unfortunately, only a few drugs in this category are available. Moreover, popularity has declined significantly, not only because of side effects, but also because of an alleged (and not totally well founded) adverse effect on cardiovascular prognosis.[27,28] In routine clinical practice, non-selective α-adrenoceptor blocking drugs (e.g. phentolamine) have no place. Prazosin and doxazosin, on the other hand, are selective blockers of the α_1-adrenoceptor and these agents are discussed here in greater detail. The mode of action seems straightforward: competitive inhibition of noradrenaline at the postsynaptic receptor. Drugs may differ, however, in relative potency for a variety of other receptors. These agents do not block the presynaptic α-adrenoceptor (of the α_2-type) and, therefore, leave the presynaptic modulation of neurotransmitter release (inhibition by α_2-adrenoceptor stimulation) from nerve terminals intact. Since α_1-adrenoceptors are present in both resistance and capacitance vessels, the antagonists produce arterial as well as venous dilation. As a result, BP falls by virtue of a drop in SVR without major changes in CO. Venous dilation may contribute to the frequently observed orthostatic hypotension. As expected, volume depletion aggravates the postural response. Tachycardia may occur but is usually mild. Although not very frequent, a troublesome side effect may be sodium retention, which occurs despite the lack of significant activation of renin and aldosterone. There may be some increase in extracellular volume due to enhanced renal sodium reabsorption, but this observation is disputed. If true, however, this may contribute to the allegedly higher incidence of congestive heart failure that has been observed in clinical trials.[27,28]

A few drugs combine α_1-adrenoceptor blocking activity with other effects, such as blockade of β-adrenoceptors (labetalol), central $5HT_{1A}$-serotonergic receptors (urapidil) or $5HT_2$-serotonergic receptors (ketanserin).

Renin–angiotensin–aldosterone system as the primary target

The RAAS can be inhibited at several levels. Firstly, the secretion of renin can be inhibited via blockade of β_1-adrenoceptors. Since β-blockers have already been discussed (see above), these drugs will not be dealt with here. Secondly, the action of renin can be inhibited directly, thus producing a fall in the levels of angiotensin I (Ang I) and angiotensin II (Ang II). In the past attempts to design effective renin inhibitors have not been successful. Newer renin inhibitors have potential.[29,30] The third level to inhibit the RAAS is by blocking angiotensin converting enzyme (ACE), which converts Ang I into Ang II. Finally, the action of Ang II can be antagonized at the level of its receptor by means of an angiotensin II type 1 receptor blocker (ARB). Specific blockers of aldosterone also exist, but these agents leave the effects of Ang II on the circulation untouched. Only ACE inhibitors and ARBs are now clinically available to antagonize the RAAS in hypertensive patients.

Superficially, the mode of action for ACE inhibitors is clear: diminished activity of the enzyme will eliminate plasma Ang II and thereby reduce peripheral vasoconstriction. Indeed, acute administration of an ACE-inhibitor is associated with a fall in BP that correlates with the decrement in plasma Ang II.[31] However, during continued treatment plasma Ang II and aldosterone tend to rise again, sometimes to values that are not different from pre-treatment values, even though BP remains reduced. Such observations make plasma Ang II a less likely candidate to explain the hypotensive effect of ACE inhibitors. Accumulation of bradykinin (less degradation by ACE) and continued suppression of tissue ACE are among the most popular explanations for the long-term efficacy of these drugs. An alternative possibility is enhanced formation of the vasodilatory peptide Ang(1–7). Regardless of the immediate interruption of the RAAS by ACE inhibitors, Ang II has a number of indirect effects and via these pathways an additional effect on BP can be achieved. For instance, the drop in aldosterone may increase natriuresis or at least prevent reactive sodium retention. In addition, the stimulating effect of Ang II on the sympathetic nervous system will disappear during ACE inhibition. The latter may be responsible for the lack of a baroreceptor-mediated rise in sympathetic activity during ACE inhibition. Suppression of endothelin secretion[32] and improvement in endothelial function[33] may also contribute to a sustained reduction in pressure. ACE inhibitors have also been shown to improve arterial compliance, notably in the aorta.[34]

Haemodynamically, ACE inhibitors produce a fall in SVR without significant changes in heart rate or CO. Cardiac filling pressures also tend to decline,[31] possibly as a result of ACE-inhibitor-mediated venodilation.[35] These drugs, therefore, reduce preload and afterload, and thus exert a favourable effect on the circulation, without orthostatic hypotension. ACE inhibitors have important effects on regional vascular beds. For instance, in the coronary circulation these drugs improve flow reserve and in the cerebral vasculature shift the lower limit of autoregulation towards lower BP levels so that cerebral blood flow is maintained even under conditions of a low perfusion pressure.[36–38] Finally, in the kidney ACE inhibitors lower postglomerular resistance and intraglomerular pressure and by that mechanism may reduce proteinuria. Renal blood flow is usually maintained or increases to a variable extent.

Nowadays, ACE inhibitors have to compete with ARBs in the treatment of hypertension. These receptor blockers interact with aminoacids in the transmembrane domains of AT1 receptors and occupy space among the seven helices, thereby preventing the binding of Ang II.[39] The antagonist-receptor complex is not internalized and hence does not influence the receptor population on the cell surface. Differences between various ARBs observed in the laboratory (e.g. surmountable versus insurmountable antagonism) seem to be irrelevant in the clinical context. Overall, the effects of ARBs are similar to those of ACE inhibitors. The most conspicuous difference, however, lies in their effect on Ang II levels. While these tend to be reduced during ACE inhibition, they increase in response to ARB treatment. As ARBs only block the AT1 receptor, the AT2 receptor remains accessible to Ang II. Possibly (although this has not been proven unequivocally), the AT2 receptor mediates several of the advantageous effects of ARBs (such as vascular remodelling).

The haemodynamic effects of ARBs closely resemble those of ACE inhibitors: BP and vascular resistance fall while cardiac output remains largely unchanged.[40] Also, the renal effects of these classes of drug are similar. It is uncertain whether it is useful to combine an ACE inhibitor and an ARB. The rationale for such an approach is that during ACE inhibitor treatment alone, Ang II can still be formed via non-ACE pathways while during ARB treatment alone elevated levels of Ang II may overcome receptor blockade. Although a few attempts have been made to evaluate the combination, most studies have not utilized full doses of the drugs. Therefore, the claim made by some that the combination produces additive effects[41–43] needs further substantiation. Clinically, it remains uncertain whether the combination confers more benefit than either drug alone.

ACE inhibitors and ARBs have a favourable effect on the microcirculation. That this effect may be responsible for or contribute to an improvement in insulin sensitivity. As β-blockers and diuretics often have opposite effects on the microcirculation, insulin sensitivity usually deteriorates during treatment with those drugs. The different microcirculatory actions of the various agents may well account for the different incidences of new-onset diabetes mellitus observed in large-scale trials. The number of patients with new diabetes is consistently lower when treatment is based on an ACE inhibitor or an ARB.[44–46]

Calcium influx as the primary target

Calcium antagonists (CA) are drugs that inhibit the influx of calcium into vascular smooth muscle cells by blocking plasma membrane calcium channels. Although some calcium antagonists may block T-type or N-type channels, these are less relevant for clinical practice. The CAs that are used for the treatment of hypertension have the slow L-type voltage-gated channels as target. These channels are present in vascular smooth muscle cells, in the myocardium and in atrioventricular nodal tissue. Three types of CAs have found their way to the clinic: the phenylalkylamine verapamil, the benzothiazepine diltiazem and the large group of dihydropyridines. The common effect of these drugs is a decrease in the cytosolic calcium concentration, which leads to relaxation of the smooth muscle cell. In addition, CAs mitigate the response to vasoconstrictor hormones such as endothelin, Ang II and noradrenaline. In chronic therapy, CAs may also exert positive effects on the structure of the vascular wall. An example of this effect has been demonstrated by Schiffrin and Deng who investigated the effects of the CA nifedipine GITS and the β-blocker atenolol on the structure and function of resistance arteries in normotensive and hypertensive people.[47] Vessel specimens were obtained from gluteal sub-cutaneous biopsies. Their data show that hypertensive patients with well-controlled BP after treatment for more than 1 year with nifedipine GITS exhibit normal structure and function of gluteal subcutaneous small arteries, whereas similar patients with BP equally well controlled by the β-blocker atenolol have thicker small arteries with abnormal endothelium-dependent relaxation and altered contractility. Whether this finding also applies to other vascular beds, could not be determined from this study.

The various CAs show clear-cut differences in haemodynamics. Verapamil, for instance, has a greater affinity for cardiac than for vascular tissue and pairs vasodilation with a degree of negative inotropy/chronotropy. Heart rate usually slows modestly, while myocardial contractility and atrioventricular conduction are more markedly depressed by this drug. Diltiazem has about equal affinity for cardiac and vascular calcium channels, but has haemodynamic actions that resemble those of verapamil. Dihydropyridines, in contrast, have far greater affinity for vascular tissue and primarily induce vasodilation. Some increases in heart rate and cardiac output may ensue, secondary to baroreceptor-mediated sympathetic activation, but these are usually transient. A side effect frequently seen during treatment with a dihydropyridine is the development of oedema, which seems to be the result of altered haemodynamic forces in the microcirculation. Since these drugs mainly dilate precapillary vessels, a relatively greater portion of systemic pressure is transmitted into the capillary system. As a consequence, and even in the face of a reduced systemic pressure, intracapillary pressure rises leading to extravasation of fluid. The same increase in transcapillary pressure, when it occurs in the kidney, may be responsible for a (transient) rise in albumin excretion. The corollary of these changes is that the addition of a drug that dilates the postcapillary vessels (e.g. an ACE inhibitor) should reduce the incidence of oedema. Indeed, this was observed in a large, double-blind trial on the combination of a CA and an ACE inhibitor.[48] The development of oedema does not seem to result from enhanced sodium retention; rather, CAs stimulate natriuresis, at least in the early stage of therapy. The reason why CAs do so has not been fully elucidated, but may involve relative suppression of aldosterone. CAs are usually somewhat less effective in terms of BP lowering when the patient is on a low salt diet or simultaneously uses a diuretic. An explanation for this phenomenon may be that the natriuretic effect will be less pronounced when the patient adheres to a low rather than to a high salt intake.

Finally, dihydropyridine calcium antagonists may activate the sympathetic nervous system, although this effect is variable and drug-dependent. With long-acting agents that produce a gradual and sustained fall in BP, sympathetic activation hardly occurs.[49]

INTERFERENCE WITH RENAL FUNCTION

As stated earlier, the tendency of the kidney to retain sodium upon a fall in BP must be counteracted if the change in BP is to persist. Obviously, many of the compounds described above must act on the kidney, although the mechanism is far from clear. Based on the principles of Guyton, the renal function curve (pressure-natriuresis curve) must have shifted leftwards. However, this does not necessarily have to be the case when drugs are administered that force the kidney to excrete more sodium, as when diuretics are given.

Like β-blockers, diuretics have been in the forefront of hypertension treatment for many years. The increasing knowledge about their potential to improve overall prognosis has, unfortunately, not been matched by concurrent insight into mode of action. It is known that the different classes of diuretics interfere with sodium reabsorption in the renal tubules. Loop diuretics, such as furosemide, inhibit the Na-K-2Cl cotransporter in the ascending limb of the loop of Henle, while thiazides block the basolateral sodium-chloride cotransporter in the distal convoluted tubule. Amiloride and triamterene directly inhibit sodium channels while aldosterone antagonists have a similar effect via antagonism of the nuclear aldosterone receptor. Drugs that act in the proximal tubule, such as the carbonic anhydrase inhibitors, are not generally used in hypertension because of low efficacy.

Diuretic treatment is associated with a biphasic response. Initially, renal sodium output increases leading to a fall in plasma and extracellular volume. This phase is characterized by renal vasoconstriction, a modest decline in glomerular filtration rate (GFR) and slight elevation of filtration fraction.[50] Various counterregulatory mechanisms are then activated, among which is the RAAS. These mechanisms are needed to limit the loss of body sodium. The adaptation to diuretic treatment and the re-establishment of a steady state between intake and output occur swiftly and may precede any fall in BP. After several weeks of treatment, cardiac output is reduced with the greatest effect occurring after approximately 3 months.[51] Although it is tempting to attribute the hypotensive effect of diuretics to this decline in cardiac output, observations during prolonged treatment as well as comparisons between responders and non-responders argue against this notion. Indeed, with continued administration of a thiazide diuretic, plasma volume is partially restored while cardiac output rises again.[51–53] Nevertheless, extracellular volume remains low.[53] In this phase of treatment, the fall in BP is due mainly to a reduction in systemic vascular resistance. The picture is even more compelling when responders and non-responders are compared. For instance, Van Brummelen and coworkers contrasted the haemodynamic findings in responders (greater than 10% fall in mean arterial pressure) with those in non-responders (less than 10% fall) and observed strikingly different patterns.[51,54] In responders the initial fall in cardiac output was followed by a return to pretreatment levels, whereas in non-responders it was permanently reduced. Consequently, total peripheral resistance was lowered only in responders. Non-responders also tended to show a greater degree of plasma volume depletion and greater stimulation of renin and aldosterone. The latter may have contributed to the elevated peripheral resistance. These data show that changes in cardiac output are unlikely to be of decisive importance in the ultimate reduction of BP in responders to thiazide therapy. Thus, the secondary fall in SVR seems to be the prime mechanism whereby diuretics lower the pressure. Why this vasorelaxant effect occur has not been fully elucidated. In experiments with aortic and pulmonary artery rings from male Wistar rats, Abrahams and associates found various diuretic preparations to possess vasorelaxing properties that were endothelium independent.[55] This effect was expressed only when plasma had been added to the bath. This suggests that diuretic compounds need a cofactor from plasma in order to obtain vasodilatory potential. On the other hand, there is evidence to show that diuretics are able to activate potassium channels in vascular smooth muscle cells leading to hyperpolarization and a reduction in intracellular calcium.[56,57]

With continued treatment both renal blood flow and glomerular filtration rate rise substantially, while renal vascular resistance and filtration fraction fall. This sequence of events was observed in patients who were treated with a rather high dose of hydrochlorothiazide (50 mg twice daily) and who had only mild reductions in sodium intake. In contrast Scaglione and coworkers treated 13 essential hypertensive patients who were maintained on a normal sodium diet (150 mmol/day for 8 weeks with hydrochlorothiazide (25 mg once a day)). Using somewhat less reliable methods to measure renal plasma flow and glomerular filtration rate they showed a significant fall in renal vascular resistance without changes in flow, filtration rate and filtration fraction at the end of the study period.[58] Despite differences in methodology between studies, the various data by and large point in the same direction: long-term treatment with a thiazide drug induces a favourable renal haemodynamic response whereby renal function is maintained.

CONCLUSION

Today, many antihypertensive agents are at the disposal of the practising physician. Not infrequently, though, the prescribing doctor is more interested in the clinical efficacy (i.e. the final drop in pressure) than in the mechanisms whereby drugs are exerting these effects. Still, detailed knowledge of these mechanisms is essential to understand why a drug works or not. This knowledge will help to find either suitable alternatives or appropriate combinations of drugs in patients who do not respond to the initial therapy.

References

1. Neal B, MacMahon S, Chapman N. Effects of ACE inhibitors, calcium antagonists, and other blood-pressure-lowering drugs: results of prospectively designed overviews of randomised trials. Blood Pressure Lowering Treatment Trialists' Collaboration. *Lancet* 2000;356: 1955–1964.
2. Safar ME. Mechanical factors predicting cardiovascular risk and drug treatment of hypertension. *J Hypertens* 2002;20:349–352.
3. Guyton AC, Hall JE, Coleman TG, et al. The dominant role of the kidneys in long-term arterial pressure regulation in normal and hypertensive states. In: Laragh JH, Brenner BM, eds. *Hypertension. Pathophysiology, Diagnosis, and Management*. New York: Raven Press; 1995. pp. 1311–1326.
4. Julius S, Krause L, Schork NJ, et al. Hyperkinetic borderline hypertension in Tecumseh, Michigan. *J Hypertens* 1991;9:77–84.
5. Birkenhäger WH, De Leeuw PW, Schalekamp MADH. *Control mechanisms in essential hypertension*. Amsterdam: Elsevier Biomedical Press; 1982.
6. van den Meiracker AH, Man in 't Veld AJ, van Eck HJ, et al. Hemodynamic and hormonal adaptations to beta-adrenoceptor blockade. A 24-hour study of acebutolol, atenolol, pindolol, and propranolol in hypertensive patients. *Circulation* 1988;78:957–968.
7. Man in 't Veld AJ, Van den Meiracker AH, Schalekamp MADH. Do β-blockers really increase peripheral vascular resistance? Review of the literature and new observations under basal conditions. *Am J Hypertens* 1988;1:91–96.
8. Frishman WH. *Clinical Pharmacology of the Beta-Adrenoceptor Blocking Drugs*. Norwalk. CT: Appleton-Century-Crofts; 1984.

9. Saunders E, Weir MR, Kong BW, et al. A comparison of the efficacy and safety of a beta-blocker, a calcium channel blocker, and a converting enzyme inhibitor in hypertensive blacks. *Arch Intern Med* 1990;150:1707–1713.

10. De Leeuw PW. Nonsteroidal anti-inflammatory drugs and hypertension. The risks in perspective. *Drugs* 1996;51:179–187.

11. Carlberg B, Samuelsson O, Lindholm LH. Atenolol in hypertension: is it a wise choice? *Lancet* 2004;364:1684–1689.

12. Kawakami H, Sumimoto T, Hamada M, et al. Acute effect of glyceryl trinitrate on systolic blood pressure and other hemodynamic variables. *Angiology* 1995;46:151–156.

13. Pannier BM, Kando T, Safarian AA, et al. Altered hemodynamic response to isosorbide dinitrate in essential hypertension. *J Clin Pharmacol* 1990;30:127–132.

14. Safar ME, London GM. Therapeutic studies and arterial stiffness in hypertension: recommendations of the European Society of Hypertension. The Clinical Committee of Arterial Structure and Function. Working Group on Vascular Structure and Function of the European Society of Hypertension. *J Hypertens* 2000;18:1527–1535.

15. Pollesello P, Mebazaa A. ATP-dependent potassium channels as a key target for the treatment of myocardial and vascular dysfunction. *Curr Opin Crit Care* 2004;10:436–441.

16. Purcell H, Patel D, Mulcahy D, et al. In: Messerli FH, *Cardiovascular Drug Therapy*, Philadelphia: WB Saunders Company; 1996. pp. 1638–1645.

17. Reid JL, Wing LM, Mathias CJ, et al. The central hypotensive effect of clonidine. Studies in tetraplegic subjects. *Clin Pharmacol Ther* 1977;21:375–381.

18. Struthers AD, Brown MJ, Adams EF, Dollery CT. The plasma noradrenaline and growth hormone response to alpha-methyldopa and clonidine in hypertensive subjects. *Br J Clin Pharmacol* 1985;19:311–317.

19. Koshiji M, Ito H, Minatoguchi S, et al. A comparison of guanfacine, bunazosin, atenolol and nadolol on blood pressure and plasma noradrenaline responses to cold pressor testing. *Clin Exp Pharmacol Physiol* 1992;19:481–488.

20. Jarrott B. Clonidine and related compounds. In: Doyle AE, *Clinical Pharmacology of Antihypertensive Drugs*. Amsterdam: Elsevier Science Publishers BV; 1988. pp. 125–186.

21. Mitrovic V, Patyna W, Huting J, Schlepper M. Hemodynamic and neurohumoral effects of moxonidine in patients with essential hypertension. *Cardiovasc Drugs Ther* 1991;5:967–972.

22. Kirch W, Hutt HJ, Planitz V. Pharmacodynamic action and pharmacokinetics of moxonidine after single oral administration in hypertension patients. *J Clin Pharmacol* 1990;30:1088–1095.

23. Prichard BN. Principles and practice of α-antiadrenergic therapy. In: Messerli FH, *Cardiovascular Drug Therapy*. Philadelphia: WB Saunders Company; 1996. pp. 601–616.

24. Mitchell A, Buhrmann S, Opazo Saez A, et al. Clonidine lowers blood pressure by reducing vascular resistance and cardiac output in young healthy males. *Cardiovasc Drugs Ther* 2005; 19(1):49–55.

25. Aars H. Effects of clonidine on aortic diameter and aortic baroreceptor activity. *Eur J Pharmacol* 1972;20:52–59.

26. Shaw J, Hunyor SN, Korner PI. The peripheral circulatory effects of clonidine and their role in the production of arterial hypotension. *Eur J Pharmacol* 1971;14:101–111.

27. Sica DA. Doxazosin and congestive heart failure. *Congest Heart Fail* 2002;8:178–184.

28. The ALLHAT Officers and Coordinators for the ALLHAT Collaborative Research Group. Major cardiovascular events in hypertensive patients randomized to doxazosin vs chlorthalidone: the antihypertensive and lipid-lowering treatment to prevent heart attack trial (ALLHAT). *JAMA* 2000;283:1967–1975.

29. Azizi M, Menard J, Bissery A, et al. Pharmacologic demonstration of the synergistic effects of a combination of the renin inhibitor aliskiren and the AT1 receptor antagonist valsartan on the angiotensin II-renin feedback interruption. *J Am Soc Nephrol* 2004;15:3126–3133.

30. Gradman AH, Schmieder RE, Lins RL, et al. Aliskiren, a novel orally effective renin inhibitor, provides dose-dependent antihypertensive efficacy and placebo-like tolerability in hypertensive patients. *Circulation* 2005;111:1012–1018.

31. Brunner HR, Waeber B, Nussberger J. Angiotensin-converting enzyme inhibitors. In: Messerli FG, *Cardiovascular Drug Therapy*. Philadelphia: WB Saunders Company; 1996. pp. 690–711.

32. Brunner F, Kukovetz WR. Postischemic antiarrhythmic effects of angiotensin-converting enzyme inhibitors. Role of suppression of endogenous endothelin secretion. *Circulation* 1996;94:1752–1761.

33. Mancini GB, Henry GC, Macaya C, et al. Angiotensin-converting enzyme inhibition with quinapril improves endothelial vasomotor dysfunction in patients with coronary artery disease. The TREND (Trial on Reversing ENdothelial Dysfunction) Study. *Circulation* 1996;94:258–265.

34. Topouchian J, Brisac AM, Pannier B, et al. Assessment of the acute arterial effects of converting enzyme inhibition in essential hypertension: a double-blind, comparative and crossover study. *J Hum Hypertens* 1998;12:181–187.

35. Zarnke KB, Feldman RD. Direct angiotensin converting enzyme inhibitor-mediated venodilation. *Clin Pharmacol Ther* 1996;59:559–568.

36. Dyker AG, Grosset DG, Lees K. Perindopril reduces blood pressure but not cerebral blood flow in patients with recent cerebral ischemic stroke. *Stroke* 1997;28:580–583.

37. Lartaud I, Makki T, Bray-des-Boscs L, et al. Effect of chronic ANG I-converting enzyme inhibition on aging processes. IV. Cerebral blood flow regulation. *Am J Physiol* 1994;267: R687–694.

38. Motz W, Strauer BE. Improvement of coronary flow reserve after long-term therapy with enalapril. *Hypertension* 1996;27:1031–1038.

39. Goodfriend TL, Elliott ME, Catt KJ. Angiotensin receptors and their antagonists. *N Engl J Med* 1996;334:1649–1654.

40. Bauer JH, Reams GP. The angiotensin II type 1 receptor antagonists. A new class of antihypertensive drugs. *Arch Intern Med* 1995;155:1361–1368.

41. Azizi M, Guyene TT, Chatellier G, et al. Additive effects of losartan and enalapril on blood pressure and plasma active renin. *Hypertension* 1997;29:634–640.

42. Mogensen CE, Neldam S, Tikkanen I, et al. Randomised controlled trial of dual blockade of renin-angiotensin system in patients with hypertension, microalbuminuria, and non-insulin dependent diabetes: the candesartan and lisinopril microalbuminuria (CALM) study. *BMJ* 2000;321:1440–1444.

43. Stergiou GS, Skeva II, Baibas NM, et al. Additive hypotensive effect of angiotensin-converting enzyme inhibition and angiotensin-receptor antagonism in essential hypertension. *J Cardiovasc Pharmacol* 2000;35:937–941.

44. Dahlof B, Devereux RB, Kjeldsen SE, et al. Cardiovascular morbidity and mortality in the Losartan Intervention For Endpoint reduction in hypertension study (LIFE): a randomised trial against atenolol. *Lancet* 2002;359:995–1003.

45. Julius S, Kjeldsen SE, Weber M, et al. Outcomes in hypertensive patients at high cardiovascular risk treated with regimens based on valsartan or amlodipine: the VALUE randomised trial. *Lancet* 2004;363:2022–2031.

46. The ALLHAT Officers and Coordinators for the ALLHAT Collaborative Research Group. Major outcomes in high-risk hypertensive patients randomized to angiotensin-converting enzyme inhibitor or calcium channel blocker vs diuretic: The Antihypertensive and Lipid-Lowering Treatment to Prevent Heart Attack Trial (ALLHAT). *JAMA* 2002;288:2981–2997.

47. Schiffrin EL, Deng LY. Structure and function of resistance arteries of hypertensive patients treated with a beta-blocker or a calcium channel antagonist. *J Hypertens* 1996;14:1247–1255.

48. Messerli FH, Oparil S, Feng Z. Comparison of efficacy and side effects of combination therapy of angiotensin-converting enzyme inhibitor (benazepril) with calcium antagonist (either nifedipine or amlodipine) versus high-dose calcium antagonist monotherapy for systemic hypertension. *Am J Cardiol* 2000;86:1182–1187.

49. Ruzicka M, Leenen FH. Relevance of 24 h blood pressure profile and sympathetic activity for outcome on short- versus long-acting 1,4-dihydropyridines. *Am J Hypertens* 1996;9:86–94.

50. Van Brummelen P, Woerlee M, Schalekamp MA. Long-term versus short-term effects of hydrochlorothiazide on renal haemodynamics in essential hypertension. *Clin Sci (Lond)* 1979;56:463–469.

51. Van Brummelen P, Man in 't Veld AJ, Schalekamp MA. Haemodynamics during long-term thiazide treatment in essential hypertension: differences between responders and non-responders. *Clin Sci (Lond)* 1979;57 Suppl 5:359s–362s.

52. Conway J, Lauwers P. Hemodynamic and hypotensive effects of long-term therapy with chlorothiazide. *Circulation* 1960;21:21–27.

53. Van Brummelen P, Schalekamp MA. Body fluid volumes and the response of renin and aldosterone to short- and long-term thiazide therapy of essential hypertension. *Acta Med Scand* 1980;207:259–264.

54. Van Brummelen P, Man in 't Veld AJ, Schalekamp MA. Hemodynamic changes during long-term thiazide treatment of essential hypertension in responders and nonresponders. *Clin Pharmacol Ther* 1980;27:328–336.

55. Abrahams Z, Tan LL, Pang MY, et al. Demonstration of an in vitro direct vascular relaxant effect of diuretics in the presence of plasma. *J Hypertens* 1996;14:381–388.

56. Calder JA, Schachter M, Sever PS. Direct vascular actions of hydrochlorothiazide and indapamide in isolated small vessels. *Eur J Pharmacol* 1992;220:19–26.

57. Pickkers P, Hughes AD, Russel FG, et al. Thiazide-induced vasodilation in humans is mediated by potassium channel activation. *Hypertension* 1998;32:1071–1076.

58. Scaglione R, Indovina A, Parrinello G, et al. Antihypertensive efficacy and effects of nitrendipine on cardiac and renal hemodynamics in mild to moderate hypertensive patients: randomized controlled trial versus hydrochlorothiazide. *Cardiovasc Drugs Ther* 1992;6:141–146.

Antihypertensive drugs: pharmacokinetics, pharmacodynamics, metabolism, side effects and drug interactions

Domenic A. Sica

INTRODUCTION

There is no clear consensus on which is the best drug class with which to begin the treatment of hypertension. This may, however, be a moot point since one-drug therapy often fails to bring blood pressure (BP) to goal, thus calling for the addition of a second antihypertensive medication. An inability of selected two-drug regimens to bring BP to goal qualifies a hypertensive patient as being difficult-to-manage. Several next steps can be taken with such patients including: a preliminary assessment for secondary forms of hypertension, evaluation for medication non-compliance, as well as a determination of how the pharmacokinetics/pharmacodynamics of the agents in use might have some play in an inadequate BP-lowering response. This chapter addresses those pharmacological issues that most commonly influence the response to drug therapy in the patient with hypertension.

PHARMACODYNAMICS AND PHARMACOKINETICS

Pharmacokinetic properties of a drug are those related to its absorption, distribution and elimination. For most drugs and the majority of patients, pharmacokinetic considerations are of inconsequential importance in that they are already reflected in the approved dose ranges and dosing intervals. Pharmacokinetic differences are most readily apparent in the use of certain drugs in subpopulations with impaired systemic clearance. For example, a drug that is water soluble and principally eliminated by glomerular filtration often requires dosage adjustment in patients with renal impairment in order to avoid its systemic accumulation. From a practical point of view, however, it is the pharmacodynamic properties of a drug (i.e. characteristics that describe its biological effects) that are of greatest import in the majority of patients.

DOSING INTERVALS AND PEAK:TROUGH EFFECTS

Antihypertensive drugs are pharmacokinetically evaluated after a single dose to determine an 'area-under-the-curve' or AUC. This computation is then linked to the time course and duration of the drug response. Because this particular indicator is so burdensome to obtain, a pharmacodynamic measure of peak and trough BP effects is usually substituted for AUC determinations. Trough BP readings, values that are best derived from ambulatory BP monitoring studies, are particularly useful in defining whether BP control has been effectively maintained throughout a dosing interval. An antihypertensive drug is viewed as approvable for once-daily use if its peak effect is substantially different from placebo and its trough effect (usually BP lowering at 24 hours after the last dose) is at least 50% of its peak effect.[1]

DOSE–RESPONSE RELATIONSHIPS

A fundamental concept in therapeutics is that of the log-linear dose–response curve, which is vital to an accurate understanding of the effects of a given drug (Fig. 3.1). In the case of an adrenergic receptor antagonist, for example, receptor occupancy can vary from 0% to 100%. The effect of the antagonist is correlated with the logarithm of its concentration and, by extension, the logarithm of the dose. In the case of a true log-linear relationship, a 10-fold increase in dose would be needed to double the effect (point A to B in Fig. 3.1); doubling the dose would then be expected to increase the effect by the logarithm of 2 (about 0.3, i.e. from point A to C). If the relationship were ln-linear, a fourfold dose increase would be needed to double the effect. In either case, it can be readily seen that small titration steps (increasing the existing dose by less than 100%) would be expected to have relatively little effect on a patient's BP.[2]

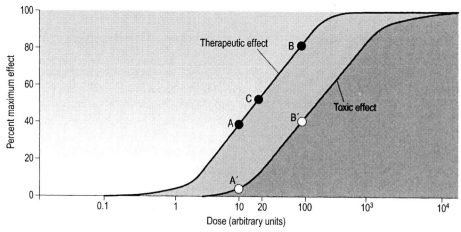

Fig. 3.1 Prototypical dose–response and dose–toxic effect curve. A 10-fold increase in dose is needed to double the effect (point A to B); doubling the dose would then be expected to increase the effect by the logarithm of 2 (about 0.3, i.e. from point A to C). The latter (moving from point A to C) results in minimal additional BP lowering but significant additional concentration-dependent side effects.

A corollary to the dose–response principle is that a drug exhibits a log-dose response for its toxic effects that is typically parallel and to the right of its therapeutic effect curve. Thus, at any given clinical dose of an approved agent, the therapeutic effect is expected to be greater than the toxic effect (equivalent to moving from point B to B[1]). Decreasing the medication dose tends to decrease both therapeutic and toxic effects, but may result in a relatively greater decrease in toxicity (point A to A[1]). The difference between the therapeutic and toxic curves is sometimes termed the 'therapeutic window' of a drug.[2]

FACTORS AFFECTING DOSE–RESPONSE RELATIONSHIPS

Pharmacodynamic differences between drugs

Dose–response relationships can be pictured in a number of ways. In the case of the angiotensin-receptor blockers (ARBs), or angiotensin converting enzyme (ACE) inhibitors the contour of the curve ranges from shallow to flat as the dose increases beyond the initial effect dose.[3] Thiazide diuretics typically display a moderate response at low doses, which quickly flattens thereafter. Dihydropyridine calcium channel blockers (CCBs), such as the immediate-release form of nifedipine, have an unusually steep response curve. A rough guide to the effectiveness of dose titration (or 'steepness' of the dose–response relationship) for antihypertensive drug classes is: sympatholytics > CCBs > diuretics > β-blockers = ACE inhibitors = ARBs.[2,3]

Pharmacodynamic differences in endpoint responsiveness

In the same individual different clinical endpoints may have dissimilar dose–response relationships for a given drug; for example, the ARB and ACE inhibitor dose required to maximally reduce proteinuria is higher than that which yields maximal BP reduction.[4] In other instances, dose-ranging studies are not undertaken and the lone dose employed in a randomized, controlled clinical trial is accepted by default as the optimal effect dose (or not) when, in fact, it merely represents the drug dose having been studied. Such would be the case for the ACE inhibitors ramipril (10 mg/day and a positive study) and trandolapril (4 mg/day and a negative study) in the Heart Outcomes Prevention Evaluation (HOPE) and Prevention of Events with ACE inhibition (PEACE) studies, respectively.[5,6]

Drug–drug interactions

In virtually all cases, addition of a diuretic to a preexisting drug regimen enhances the antihypertensive response, typically reflected by (1) a leftward shift of the curve (less drug required to effect the same reduction in BP), (2) a greater peak (sometimes called plateau) response, or (3) a steepening of the response slope at its midpoint.[7] In contrast, addition of a non-steroidal anti-inflammatory drug (NSAID) to a given regimen may oppose the effect(s) of various BP-lowering medications. Pulse-rate lowering compounds typically can be expected to improve the dose–response to an antihypertensive medication administration of which engenders a tachycardic response.[8] A similar sequence of events unfolds with compounds that diminish sympathetic nervous system (SNS) and renin–angiotensin–aldosterone system (RAAS) activity if these axes have been activated by preceding therapies.[7]

Drug–host interactions

A number of 'host' factors are known to influence the dose–response to a particular antihypertensive medication. Some are 'immutable' and thereby predictable (e.g. genetic predispositions), while some fluctuate with changes in the host's environment. Until recent years, the former consideration – pharmacogenetics of antihypertensive medications – has dealt chiefly with pharmacokinetic variations: cytochrome P_{450} polymorphisms were responsible for a varying hydroxylation status for several β-blockers;[8–10] variations in N-acetyltransferase led to a slow-acetylation status and a much greater risk of a lupus-like syndrome with hydralazine;[11] and polymorphisms of catechol O-methyltransferase caused low-methylators to be overly responsive to the antihypertensive effects of low doses of α-methyldopa.[12]

Recent studies have focused on specific *pharmacodynamic* drug–gene interactions in attempting to provide more predictability to drug response in the individual patient. As genotypic information has become more readily available, mechanisms operative in the pathogenesis of hypertension (sodium [Na^+] sensitivity, SNS stimulation, RAAS activation) can be utilized to generate candidate genes from these pathways (e.g. endothelial Na^+ channel, β-adrenergic receptor, angiotensinogen), which may then be studied for common polymorphisms. Diuretics, ACE inhibitors, ARBs and β-blockers are the drug classes most carefully studied by these methods.[13]

As an example, significant patient-to-patient variation exists in the response to ACE inhibitors.[14,15] This has prompted examination of RAAS polymorphisms in the hope of identifying genetic markers that might better forecast the response to ACE inhibition; however, the most extensively studied common polymorphisms of the RAAS (ACE insertion/deletion [I/D], angiotensinogen [AGT Met235Thr], angiotensin receptor [AT1R, A1166C]) have failed to reliably predict the BP response to ACE inhibition.[13]

Thus, although variability in the BP response to therapy is well established, pharmacogenomic data have yet to yield any consist culprit polymorphisms. The failure thus far to identify genetic targets for a 'magic bullet' antihypertensive drug or drug class is not entirely surprising, given the multiple systems involved in BP regulation. Although many studies show that BP response to a given class of antihypertensive medications varies by polymorphic genotypes, so far none has been identified that without fail predict BP response.[13,16]

Population subgroups and drug responses

Black hypertensives are generally less responsive to low doses of ACE inhibitors or ARBs presumably, in part, because they have a low renin/volume expanded state;[14,15] however, if doses are increased, the level of response seen more closely approximates that seen in white hypertensives.[17] Similar response characteristics are observed in black hypertensives with the use of β-blockers and possibly peripheral α-blockers.[18,19] Such response characteristics to these drug classes are shared (to a certain extent) with other low renin subgroups, such as elderly individuals and/or diabetics.

Dietary changes

Sodium balance is the most obvious factor affecting the response to antihypertensive medications on a day-to-day basis in that an excess dietary Na^+ intake blunts the effect of most antihypertensive drugs (except perhaps CCBs).[20,21] Conversely, dietary Na^+ restriction (or concomitant diuretic therapy) enhances the effect of other antihypertensive drugs.[7] Potassium has the opposite effect on BP in that an increased intake of this cation typically reduces BP.[22] An increase in K^+ intake per se may not enhance the effect of antihypertensive medications except in the instance of diuretic-related hypokalaemia with K^+ supplementation (average increase in serum K^+ of 0.56 mmol/L) in hypokalaemic (serum K^+– values <3.5 mmol/L) diuretic-treated patients being followed by a 5.5 mmHg average fall in mean arterial pressure.[23]

Pseudotolerance

Another consideration in the pharmacodynamic dose–response relationship for an antihypertensive medication is the extent to which BP counterregulatory mechanisms are activated in the course of BP lowering. Acute and chronic BP reduction can activate an interlinked series of mechanisms intended to return BP to pre-therapy levels. Reflex increases in cardiac output and Na^+ retention can result from baroreflex-mediated activation of the SNS and/or the RAAS. These responses are most likely when certain vasodilating compounds – such as hydralazine, minoxidil, dihydropyridine CCBs are used. High-dose diuretics by virtue of volume contraction activate both the SNS and the RAAS. Alternatively, drug classes such as β-blockers, peripheral α-blockers, and central α-agonists can trigger significant Na^+ retention as the primary basis for pseudotolerance.[2,7]

Clinically, it can be difficult to gauge the extent to which counterregulatory systems are activated. A relatively reliable sign is an unexplained loss of previously established BP control. A clinically relevant increase in pulse rate (>10%) should prompt consideration of either lowering the dose of the provoking agent or adding a β-blocker. Sodium retention, as a means by which BP control is lost, is easy to recognize if peripheral oedema develops. Sodium retention can still have occurred, however, without peripheral oedema being present. If volume expansion is suspected a diuretic can be started empirically or if a diuretic is already being used its dose can be increased sufficient to effect a weight loss in the order of 1–2% of body weight.

Other physiologic adaptations

Some differences in responsiveness between acute and chronic dosing may occur as a result of metabolic changes such as hypokalaemia or possibly by way of changes in receptor populations. True tachyphylaxis, in which enzyme induction steps up drug metabolism, is, however, generally not observed with antihypertensive drugs.

Duration of therapy

Very few long-term studies are available, but it appears that the full effects of some drugs may not be apparent until months after therapy is begun. It has been speculated that favourable remodelling of the heart and blood vessels, a process that takes much longer than acute haemodynamic effects, can occur with certain agents, such as ACE inhibitors and ARBs. Thus, a dose–response relationship for an individual compound must generally be evaluated as a function of time.[24]

Overdosing errors

Several antihypertensive medications were originally introduced at doses higher than those currently recommended, including: thiazide diuretics, β-blockers, α-methyldopa, hydralazine, and captopril. The use of these very high doses derived from studies in which doses had been increased at regular intervals until the desired antihypertensive effect was achieved or until unacceptable adverse effects developed.[25] The administration of inappropriately large doses of these medications resulted in an impressive array of adverse effects either not seen with conventional medication doses (e.g. proteinuria with captopril)[26] or due to the higher blood levels caused by a medication (sedation and depression with α-methyldopa and a lupus-like syndrome with hydralazine). With thiazide-type diuretics, the currently advocated lower doses – which appear equally effective and safer than higher doses – were only determined by trial and error long after these agents had been approved for use.[27]

Underdosing errors

Lack of data on maximal therapeutic doses

Complete dose–response curves are rarely generated for antihypertensive drugs in their initial developmental phase. There is a prevailing reluctance on the part of drug developers to push the dose of an investigational drug to its toxic limits for fear that the side effects that emerge would contaminate its tolerability perception. This developmental sticking point is most obvious in the case of ARBs, where there has been unwillingness to explore more carefully the response to higher doses, despite a drug toxic effect profile little different from that of placebo.

Inadequate titration with a failure to recognize dose–response effects

Characteristic dose–response relationships for many antihypertensive drugs are often obscured during drug development because of the scientific inadequacy of typical endpoint-limited dose-titration trials. Such trials fail to recognize the bias inherent in a heterogeneous response to a test agent and the consequences of not testing all patients at each available dose. In an endpoint-limited dose-titration trial, a prespecified endpoint (e.g. failure to achieve a nominal BP reduction >10 mmHg or to reach a final BP <140/90 mmHg) is used as the criterion for each titration. As such, responder status (to the starting and lowest dose) can be arbitrarily classified into poor or hyporesponders, normal responders, and hyper-responder categories, with all hyper-responders excluded from any additional dose escalation by having met the predetermined criteria for response.

If a second titration step occurs, the individuals ultimately receiving this higher dose are the ones who are inherently most resistant. The result of this systematic selection bias is that the dose–response curve becomes artificially flat (i.e. a limited maximal effect or plateau). Such bias is further exaggerated by the degree of heterogeneity of population responses (e.g. age- and race-dependent responses to ACE inhibitors and ARBs, which are incorrectly believed to have 'essentially flat' dose–response curves). Many of the pooled dosing studies on currently available ACE inhibitors and ARBs in reality demonstrate an 'enigmatic' reduction in BP effect at the highest tested dose – further evidence of the impact of dose-selection bias.

DIET AND PHARMACOKINETICS AND PHARMACODYNAMICS

Meal-related effects and antihypertensive medication action

The majority of clinically relevant food–drug interactions are caused by food-induced changes in the drug's bioavailability. Since the bioavailability and clinical effect of most drugs are closely correlated, bioavailability is an important pharmacokinetic parameter. The most important interactions that decrease treatment effect arise if bioavailability is significantly reduced in the fed state; however, with a few exceptions this is unusual for antihypertensive medications. In addition, if food is to reduce the bioavailability of an antihypertensive medication it will do so at the lowend of the dose range when insufficient drug would then have been absorbed to arrive at the medication effect threshold.

The bioavailability of antihypertensive medications typically does not change with alterations in gastric acid secretion and/or food-induced increases in drug solubility. Antihypertensive medications are also not ordinarily chelated by food constituents; an exception is quinapril, which reduces the absorption of tetracycline by $\approx 35\%$, possibly related to the high magnesium (Mg^{++}) content of quinapril tablets. Food–drug interactions slowing the rate of drug absorption (without changing the extent of absorption) can sometimes be used to minimize concentration-dependent adverse effects.

Food can reduce the bioavailability of hydralazine by 50–60%, which is sufficient to reduce its vasodepressor effect.[28] Fluctuations in hydralazine effect are best prevented by ingesting the drug at consistent times in relationship to meals. The bioavailability of furosemide is reduced inconsistently (as much as 50%) when taken with food, making the food–drug interaction for furosemide for the most part of minimal clinical importance;[29] however, the occasional reduction in response to furosemide when ingested with food may explain why some individuals with resistance to furosemide respond better to bumetanide – a compound without a food–drug interaction.

Food intake also decreases the bioavailability of captopril by about 50%. This interaction generally is of limited haemodynamic relevance unless insufficient drug is available for the desired effect.[30] Finally, concomitant intake of nisoldipine coat-core tablets with high-fat, high-calorie foods results in as much as a 300% increase in the maximum plasma concentrations of nisoldipine; however, total absorption may decrease since presystemic gut-wall metabolism (greatest in the proximal portions of the small intestine) may come into play. The food-effect can be avoided by administration of the coat-core tablet up to 30 minutes before the intake of food.[31]

Nutrients and their effects on blood pressure

Whereas drug–drug interactions are commonly recognized occurrences in the hypertensive population, drug–nutrient interactions are more poorly appreciated. The fresh grapefruit juice – CCB interaction is one that has been known since 1989.[32] The basis for this interaction has been diligently explored and appears to relate to both flavanoid and non-flavanoid components of grapefruit juice interfering with enterocyte CYP3A4 activity. In the process, pre-systemic clearance of susceptible drugs decreases and bioavailability increases.

Although several CCBs are liable to this interaction, it appears that it occurs most prominently with felodipine.[32,33] In that regard, one glass of grapefruit juice more than doubles the bioavailability of standard and extended-release felodipine, but with significant interindividual variability. Amlodipine and nifedipine and non-dihydropyridine CCBs have better inherent bioavailability and hence are less affected by grapefruit juice with only a 20–30% increase in blood levels.

Patients receiving an established CCB dose, in whom an unexpected BP response and/or vasodilator side effect is noted, should be questioned with regard to their intake of grapefruit juice.[33] Alternatively, the question can also be raised as to whether there is a therapeutic role for grapefruit juice in the hypertensive patient receiving a CCB. Unfortunately, no guiding principle exists for which grapefruit juice brand (and thereby the amount ingested) is best matched to the particular CCB being used by a patient.

CONSIDERATIONS IN SYSTEMIC DRUG ELIMINATION

Cytochrome P_{450} system

Two major pathways exist for cytochrome P_{450}-mediated drug interactions: enzyme induction and inhibition. Induction refers to increased synthesis or decreased degradation of cytochrome P_{450} isozymes, events that step up conversion to inactive metabolites, decrease plasma levels of the substrate and thereby reduce the pharmacodynamic effect. Examples of inducing substances include rifampin and phenobarbital. The converse applies to substances that are inhibitors of cytochrome P_{450}-metabolized compounds.[34–36]

A number of cytochrome P_{450}-related interactions can occur with antihypertensives, which with the exception of suppression of CYP3A4 activity by drugs such as verapamil and diltiazem, are typically of little consequence (Table 3.1).[34,35] The cytochrome P_{450} interaction with verapamil and diltiazem can be put to clinical use. For example, ciclosporin is an expensive drug and the coadministration of diltiazem or verapamil with ciclosporin slows its metabolism, which necessitates lowering its dose to prevent toxic blood levels from developing. This dose manipulation translates into considerable cost savings.[37]

Although several compounds are capable of stimulating/suppressing the P_{450} isozymes responsible for metabolism of the ARB losartan, none appears not to change the plasma levels of losartan in a meaningful manner.[38]

Table 3.1 Antihypertensive medications and the cytochrome P_{450} system

Drug class	Cytochrome P_{450} interaction potential	Interactions
ACE inhibitors	No significant interactions; most ACE inhibitors are prodrugs that undergo hepatic and/or enterocyte metabolism	Prodrug conversion to active diacid ACE inhibitors is minimally impacted by hepatic disease as occurs in heart failure
Diuretics	Hydrochlorothiazide and chemically related diuretics are not metabolized. Furosemide and spironolactone are metabolized to glucuronide and sulphated metabolites, respectively. Eplerenone is metabolized by CYP3A4	No significant effect on the cytochrome P_{450} system. Coadministration of verapamil with eplerenone results in an $\approx$ twofold ↑ in the area-under-the curve for eplerenone
Angiotensin-receptor blockers	Losartan and irbesartan are primarily metabolized by CYP2C9. Losartan undergoes metabolism to an active metabolite E-3174 via CYP2C9, which creates the potential for interaction with inhibitors or stimulators of this P_{450} isozyme	Co-administration of losartan with enzyme inducers such as rifampin and phenobarbital reduces losartan and E-3174 levels whereas enzyme inhibitors such as fluconazole decrease the levels of E-3174. These changes are inconsequential and seem not to affect the BP lowering effect of losartan
β-adrenergic blocking agents	The pharmacokinetics of a number of β-adrenergic blocking agents are strongly affected by cytochrome P_{450} inducers and inhibitors as relates to CYP2D6	Rifampin increases propranolol clearance two- to threefold; quinidine and diphenhydramine increase blood levels of β-blockers such as timolol or metoprolol
Calcium channel blockers (CCBs)	These drugs serve as substrates for and inhibitors of CYP3A4. Verapamil and diltiazem are known inhibitors of CYP3A4. Symptomatic hypotension can occur when CYP3A4 inhibitors are given with dihydropyridine CCBs	The concomitant use of azole anti-fungals with dihydropyridine CCBs should be with caution; most CCBs inhibit the metabolism of ciclosporin; diltiazem inhibits the metabolism of triazolam and methylprednisolone

The ability to metabolize a drug through a specific cytochrome P_{450} pathway is also modulated by genetic polymorphisms, with some individuals being poor (slow) and others extensive (rapid) metabolizers.[39] Although these polymorphisms have major effects on the pharmacokinetic profiles of commonly used antihypertensive drugs, such as metoprolol, and lesser used drugs, such as hydralazine, α-methyldopa and minoxidil, polymorphisms have not been shown to influence variation in the antihypertensive effect of these drugs at conventional doses; however, slow metabolizers of β-blockers can have exaggerated β-blocker effects at low doses.[39,40]

RENAL CLEARANCE

Serum creatinine (S_{creat}) remains the most common means of appraising renal function; however, assigning a specific glomerular filtration rate (GFR) to any

Table 3.2 Pharmacokinetics of antihypertensives in renal disease

Drug class	Comments
Peripheral α-blockers	Pharmacokinetics of prazosin, terazosin, and doxazosin are not altered in chronic kidney disease (CKD)
Central α-agonists	Guanfacine is mainly cleared hepatically and does not accumulate in CKD. Clonidine undergoes modest renal clearance. Its plasma half-life is prolonged in CKD. No specific recommendations for dosage adjustment of clonidine in CKD
β-blockers	Water-soluble drugs such as atenolol, betaxolol, bisoprolol and sotalol undergo modest renal clearance, with the other β-blockers undergoing exclusive hepatic clearance. Empiric dose reduction of water-soluble β-blockers
Calcium-channel blockers	Hepatically cleared without meaningful accumulation in CKD
ACE inhibitors	Exclusively renally-cleared with the exception of fosinopril and trandolapril. Dose adjustment for renally-cleared ACE inhibitors in product information but seldom implemented
Angiotensin-receptor blockers	Class members are all cleared hepatically (at least 50%) with clearance sufficient to avoid meaningful accumulation in CKD

one S_{creat} value requires careful consideration, since S_{creat} values are influenced by both the GFR and muscle mass. Because of the latter, a S_{creat} value may fall within an established range for population values and it does not follow automatically that renal function is normal; thus, S_{creat} values should not be the basis for determining when and to what degree renally cleared drugs (antihypertensive medications amongst others) should have their dose reduced. Any of the several urine-free formulae currently in use to estimate GFR can better guide the adjustment of drug dosing in chronic kidney disease (CKD).

Medication dose adjustment in CKD may involve one (or both) of two approaches. To maintain a therapeutic drug level and, at the same time, avoid drug accumulation and possible concentration-dependent toxicity in a patient with CKD, the maintenance dose of a medication is reduced and/or the time interval between doses is extended. In practice, dose adjustment should match the degree of which renal function is reduced; however, in the case of antihypertensive medications this is seldom necessary (Table 3.2). Antihypertensive medications are typically dosed until the desired effect is achieved and dosage reduction is only considered when goal BP has been reached and/or drug concentration-dependent side effects appear.[41]

DELIVERY SYSTEM CONSIDERATIONS IN HYPERTENSION

Since the early 1980s, there have been increasing numbers of pharmaceutical products using novel drug delivery systems. Although many extended-release formulations have been criticized as being no more than patent-life extenders, these do have the potential for increasing the duration of drug action; thus allowing an otherwise short half-life compound to avoid a compliance disadvantage in the treatment of hypertension (Table 3.3).[42] More recently, delivery systems that are both delayed and sustained-release have been developed for

Table 3.3 Delivery system considerations in the treatment of hypertension

Advantage of extended release preparations
Increased efficacy
Improved medication adherence and/or compliance
Decreased administration frequency
Nocturnal dosing with the possibility of targeting early morning blood pressure
Targeted blood concentrations with avoidance of high peak plasma concentrations
Reduced peak concentration adverse effects
Decreased dispensing costs

Disadvantages of extended release preparations
Delayed attainment of pharmacological effect on initiating therapy
Dosing inflexibility
Possibility of dose dumping with tablet cutting or crushing
Altered absorption with derangements in gastrointestinal motility
Sustained adverse effects
Adverse reactions due to the delivery system
Increased cost compared to immediate-release preparations, which are more often generic

night-time administration. Drugs such as verapamil, diltiazem, and propranolol are available in such formulations.[43,44] These particular formulations are chronotherapeutically directed in that they match the highest blood concentrations of a medication to morning BP surges.[43,44] To date, however, such therapies have not been shown to have an outcomes benefit beyond that observed with conventional delivery systems.[45]

Clonidine is the only antihypertensive medication that can be given via the transdermal route. Average clonidine concentrations are higher with application of the skin devices to the chest or upper arm than when applied to the thigh; this is the basis for recommending patch application to the upper arm or torso.[46] Pharmacokinetic studies with transdermal clonidine show plasma levels to increase gradually, reach steady-state by the third day, and remain relatively constant throughout the remainder of the time that the system is worn. This delay in the onset of action should be kept in mind when transdermal clonidine replaces other antihypertensive therapy, particularly in patients with more severe forms of hypertension. The slow onset of action with transdermal clonidine makes this product inappropriate for the acute management of hypertensive urgencies. Transdermal clonidine can be of particular utility in patients who cannot receive orally administered medications. Unlike oral clonidine, transdermal clonidine is infrequently associated with rebound hypertension. This probably relates to an 'autotapering' feature attributable to residual drug found in the skin where the removed patch was previously affixed.[47]

SIDE EFFECTS AND DRUG INTERACTIONS

Adverse reactions and drug–drug interactions are common occurrences with many drug classes and, in particular, with antihypertensive medications. These consequences take many forms including electrolyte changes, alterations in level of renal function, non-specific or idiosyncratic side effects, and side effects that specifically relate to drug levels. There is considerable interplay between several antihypertensive compounds and the CYP_{450} system, and an understanding of this system is needed to avoid what can sometimes be life-threatening drug–drug interactions with antihypertensive medications. In many instances the reported side effect or drug–drug interaction reflects a class effect, but side effects are sometimes drug and not class specific.

DIURETICS

Much of the negative biochemical and metabolic experience with diuretics was related to the very high doses, e.g. hydrochlorothiazide (100–200 mg/day) that had previously been in common use. The frequency of metabolically negative side effects, such as hypokalaemia, hypomagnesaemia, glucose intolerance, and/or hypercholesterolaemia, is much less with low-dose diuretic therapy (Table 3.4). Hyponatraemia is an uncommon but serious complication of diuretic therapy.[48] Thiazide diuretics are more apt than loop diuretics to cause

Table 3.4 Diuretic-related side effects

Compound	Comments
Thiazides and thiazide-like diuretics	
Chlorthalidone	More prolonged effect than hydrochlorothiazide; greater likelihood of hypomagnesaemia, hypokalaemia
Hydrochlorothiazide	Short-acting diuretic; impotence is not uncommon (class effect); decreases urine calcium excretion and is used in nephrolithiasis and adjunctively in osteoporosis management (class effect); decreases lithium clearance in lithium-treated patients with an increased risk of lithium toxicity; diuretic-related hyponatraemia more common (class effect) than with loop diuretics
Indapamide	Suggestion but little evidence that this may cause less hypokalaemia than other thiazide diuretics
Metolazone	Effective at GFR <40 mL/minute unlike thiazide diuretics and can be used together with a loop diuretic in diuretic resistant states. Combination therapy can be accompanied by significant volume losses and hypokalaemia/hypomagnesaemia
Loop diuretics	
Bumetanide	Short acting loop diuretic; associated with significant hypercalciuria (class-effect for loop diuretics)
Furosemide	Shorter duration of action – multiple daily dosing to avoid rebound sodium retention (same for bumetanide)
Torsemide	Long duration of action; independent vasodepressor effect
Ethacrynic acid	Only non-sulphonamide diuretic; ototoxicity
Potassium-sparing	
Amiloride	Hyperkalaemia; decreases urine calcium excretion above and beyond that with hydrochlorothiazide; magnesium-sparing (class effect) and useful in the hypomagnesaemia associated with cis-platinum or amphotericin; reduces polyuria associated with lithium
Spironolactone	Dose-dependent gynaecomastia; hyperkalaemia; increases digoxin levels by interference with assay.
Triamterene	Hyperkalaemia, triamterene stones can occur; increased risk of nephrotoxicity when administered together with non-steroidal anti-inflammatory drugs (NSAIDs); interferes with the tubular secretion of creatinine (like creatinine it is an organic cation) and thereby reduces the reliability of serum creatinine as a marker of renal function

hyponatraemia.[27] Mild metabolic alkalosis is a common feature of thiazide diuretic therapy, particularly at high doses. Severe metabolic alkalosis is much less frequent and typically occurs more often with loop diuretic therapy.

Photosensitivity dermatitis occurs rarely secondary to thiazide or furosemide therapy.[49] Hydrochlorothiazide causes photosensitivity more commonly than the other thiazide-type diuretics.[50] Cross-sensitivity with sulphonamide drugs may occur with all diuretics, with the exception of ethacrynic acid; however, the frequency with which cross-sensitivity occurs is much less common than was first thought and appears to be due to a predisposition to allergic reactions rather than to specific cross-reactivity with sulphonamide-based drugs; thus, patients with a sulphonamide allergy that was not 'extreme' (such as Stevens-Johnson syndrome or a necrotizing vasculitis) in its original presentation can be given a thiazide or a loop diuretic with caution.[51]

Loop diuretics can potentiate aminoglycoside nephrotoxicity.[52] By causing hypokalaemia, diuretics increase the risk of digitalis toxicity.[53] Plasma lithium (Li^+) concentrations can increase with thiazide therapy due to a volume-dependent increase in Li^+ absorption.[54] NSAIDs can both antagonize the effects of diuretics and predispose diuretic-treated patients to a form of functional renal insufficiency. The combination of indometacin and triamterene may be particularly dangerous in that a slowly reversible form of acute renal failure can develop.[55]

DIRECT VASODILATORS

Hydralazine and minoxidil cause dose-dependent tachycardia and/or salt-and-water retention. The former can provoke cardiac ischaemia and the latter can cause symptomatic volume overload. Minoxidil use is frequently accompanied by an increase in left ventricular mass, a process that can be prevented by co-administration of an ACE inhibitor. Pericardial effusions have also been reported in as many as 3% of patients treated with minoxidil.[56] In many cases a minoxidil-related pericardial effusion is simply an extension of the generalized volume overload that can accompany therapy; however, in some instances it is idiopathic (and volume-independent) and recurs with minoxidil rechallenge.[57]

Hypertrichosis is common with minoxidil and can be cosmetically disfiguring, particularly in women.[58] Hair growth begins within 3 to 6 weeks of starting therapy, occurring over the temples and eyebrows initially, spreading to areas between the eyebrows and hairline or sideburn regions, to finally involve the trunk, extremities and scalp. Hypertrichosis disappears within a few weeks of discontinuing minoxidil, though in some cases there is less hair than before the drug was started.[59] Generalized hair growth in areas that are not 'bald' can also occur with any of the topical minoxidil solutions, which are currently available in both 2 and 5% solutions. For this to occur it generally requires application of the topical solution in amounts exceeding current recommendations.[60]

In slow acetylators, women, and HLA-DR 4 phenotypes, there appears to be a correlation with the lupus-like syndrome and high doses of hydralazine (greater than 200 to 400 mg/day), although patients receiving smaller doses have also developed the lupus-like syndrome. Generally, the syndrome occurs early in therapy, but can occur after many years of treatment.[61] In severe cases of hydralazine-induced lupus, the syndrome may be accompanied by pulmonary oedema or pneumonia, pericardial tamponade and renal failure. Hydralazine increases the oral bioavailability of metoprolol, propranolol and oxprenolol (high clearance and lipophilic β-blockers) by means of a reduction in first-pass metabolism. This occurs more frequently in a fasting state and appears not to occur with sustained-release β-blockers.[62]

PERIPHERAL α-ANTAGONISTS

Side effects of peripheral α1-adrenergic blockers are dose-dependent and commonly include dizziness, lethargy, and fatigue.[63] Postural hypotension is another common finding with drugs in this class, occurring in up to 10% of treated patients.[64] Postural hypotension with peripheral α1-adrenergic blockers is more common when administered with β-blockers (due to suppression of compensatory heart rate responses) or phosphodiesterase-5 inhibitors such as sildenafil (mechanism unknown).[65,66]

In women, urinary incontinence may be triggered by α1-adrenergic antagonists, a side effect reversible upon withdrawal of the offending drug.[67] Finally, there appears to be a greater incidence of heart failure with doxazosin-based therapy (without concomitant diuretic treatment) in older hypertensives.[68] Aetiological considerations in this process include plasma volume expansion, sympathetic nervous system activation, inadequate BP control and suboptimal regression of left ventricular mass.[69]

CENTRAL α-AGONISTS

Clonidine is the most commonly used drug in this class. This drug supplanted α-methyldopa, in part, because clonidine avoids an array of troublesome side effects. Other side effects with α-methyldopa include: autoimmune haemolytic anaemia, drug fever, and/or liver dysfunction.[70,71]

Dose titration of clonidine beyond 0.4 mg per day is often followed by bothersome side effects, such as lethargy and dry mouth, although these side effects can occur at lower doses. Such side effects are less frequent with transdermal clonidine, but this mode of delivery is limited by the occurrence of skin irritation.[72] A number of studies indicate bradycardia is a potential adverse effect with clonidine, particularly when given in the setting of CKD.[73]

Rebound hypertension occurs with oral clonidine if the drug is terminated suddenly, particularly in patients with excessive adrenergic tone, who require high medication doses, or who are receiving clonidine together with a β-blocker and inadvertently continue β-blocker therapy while discontinuing clonidine.[74] Clonidine overdose will produce paradoxical hypertension due to peripheral α2-adrenergic receptor stimulation, which supersedes the BP lowering effect of central α2-adrenergic receptor stimulation.[75]

ANGIOTENSIN-RECEPTOR BLOCKERS

Side effects are uncommon with ARBs and do not relate to dose; accordingly, higher doses of ARBs are now used routinely (Table 3.5).[3,4] The relative

Table 3.5 Angiotensin receptor blocker-related side effects

First-dose hypotension – particularly if volume contracted
Small changes in serum creatinine (e.g. a 20% increase) can occur as a normal physiological response in renal failure patients. Therapy need not be stopped
Anaemia secondary to decrease in erythropoietin levels
Angio-oedema (rare)
Contraindicated in pregnancy secondary to fetopathy potential
Interaction between telmisartan and digoxin with increases in digoxin levels – monitoring of digoxin level advised with start or increase in the dose of digoxin
Decreased renal lithium clearance with potential for toxicity
Use with caution in patients with bilateral renal artery stenosis or unilateral stenosis with a solitary functional kidney. Increase in serum potassium but less than that seen with ACE inhibitors (class effect)

absence of side effects with this drug class is further borne out by the observation that certain side effects, such as headache, are even less common in ARB than in placebo-treated patients.[76] Cough does not occur with ARBs and angio-oedema is a rare occurrence. If ARB therapy is considered in a patient with prior ACE-inhibitor-related angio-oedema there should be some justification for use, such as the presence of heart failure or proteinuric nephropathic states.[77]

The occurrence of functional renal insufficiency with an ARB does not preclude a patient from future therapy with an ARB unless high-grade bilateral renal artery stenosis is present. Hyperkalaemia appears to be less likely with ARBs than with ACE inhibitors.[78]

ARBs are contraindicated in the 2nd and 3rd trimester of pregnancy because a fetopathy can occur. The fetal effects of ARBs during the 1st trimester are controversial. Any observed effects may represent the after effects of fetal hypoperfusion and not a teratogenic effect per se.[79]

To date, few clinically relevant drug–drug interactions have been described with ARBs.[80] Of note, there is a 49% increase in digoxin peak plasma concentration and a 20% increase in trough digoxin concentration when co-administered with telmisartan. The mechanism is unknown and is not thought to be related to the CYP_{450} system.[81] There is evidence that ARBs may substantially increase steady-state plasma Li^{++} levels, and sometimes result in Li^{++} toxicity. This drug–drug interaction likely relates to an increase in proximal tubular Li^{++} reabsorption prompted by ARB-related changes in renal haemodynamics.[82]

ACE INHIBITORS

Non-specific side effects of ACE inhibitors are infrequent, with the exception of leukopenia, skin rash and dysgeusia, which are more common with captopril. Hypotension is not a specific side effect of ACE inhibitors; rather, it represents a physiological extension of the drug's expected effect and is more common when dehydration is present. Hyperkalaemia is an uncommon finding with ACE inhibitors unless a specific predisposition to hyperkalaemia exists, such as diabetes, heart failure with renal insufficiency (receiving K^+-sparing diuretics or K^+ supplements).[83,84]

A dry, irritating, non-productive cough is common with ACE inhibitors. The incidence of cough is quite variable (range 0–44%), but averages 15% in the largest and best-conducted studies. Cough is a class phenomenon with ACE inhibitors and has been attributed to an increase in bradykinin and/or other vasoactive peptides, such as substance P. No therapy to suppress or eliminate ACE inhibitor-associated cough has been successful.[85] Angioneurotic oedema is a potentially life-threatening complication of ACE inhibitors, and is about three times more common in blacks.[86] The incidence is greatest within the first 2–4 weeks of starting ACE inhibitor therapy, but its onset can sometimes be delayed many months. When patients with a history of ACE inhibitor-related angio-oedema are given an ARB, angio-oedema can reappear, but it is generally milder and rarely life threatening.[77] Angio-oedema of the intestine, which is more common in women, can also occur with ACE inhibitor therapy.[87]

Shortly after their release, ACE inhibitors were associated with a syndrome of 'functional renal insufficiency' in patients with critical renal artery stenosis and a solitary functioning kidney. ACE inhibitors can have similar adverse renal effects when predisposing conditions, such as dehydration, NSAID use, heart failure and/or microvascular renal disease exist.[83] A complication analogous to that of 'functional renal insufficiency' is exposure to ACE inhibitors during the second or third trimester of pregnancy. This has resulted in a 'Black Box Warning' for all ACE inhibitors and all ARBs. With such exposure BP and renal perfusion drop in tandem, with resultant in utero acute renal failure. Oligohydramnios develops thereafter, along with specific abnormalities thought to be secondary to reduced amniotic fluid volume (limb deformities, cranial ossification defects, lung hypoplasia and tubular dysgenesis) (Table 3.6).[79]

ACE inhibitors have also been associated with anaemia. These drugs suppress the production of erythropoietin in a dose-dependent manner, which presents a particular problem when ACE inhibitors are administered in the presence of heart failure and/or CKD.[88] ACE inhibitor-related anaemia is, in part, related to N-acetyl-seryl-aspartyl-lysyl-proline accumulation in plasma. This substance is mainly degraded by ACE and is a potent natural inhibitor of haematopoietic stem cell proliferation. Finally, the combination of captopril

Table 3.6 ACE inhibitor-related side effects

First-dose hypotension – particularly if volume contracted

Neutropenia, skin rash, and dysgeusia occur more frequently with captopril than with other ACE inhibitors; increased risk of developing hypoglycaemia with captopril

Suppresses red blood cell production, a property may that be useful in post-transplant erythrocytosis

Hyperkalaemia – suggested to be less with renally/hepatically cleared ACE inhibitors

Aspirin may interfere with the haemodynamic effect of ACE inhibitors in severe coronary heart failure (CHF) as well as to reduce their antihypertensive effect

ACE inhibitors may cause fetal or neonatal injury or death when used during pregnancy. Hypotension, neonatal skull hypoplasia, anuria, and renal failure have occurred in fetuses and neonates

Angio-oedema is a potentially life-threatening event. Rechallenge should never occur with any ACE inhibitor

Decreased renal lithium clearance with potential for toxicity

Quinapril reduces the absorption of tetracycline by ≈35% possibly due to the high magnesium tablet content

Small changes in serum creatinine (e.g. a 20% increase) can occur as a normal physiological response in renal failure patients (class effect). Therapy need not be stopped

Diarrhoea, which can be related to angio-oedema of the gut

and allopurinol is associated with a higher risk of hypersensitivity reactions, such as Stevens–Johnson syndrome.[89] Quinapril reduces the absorption of tetracycline by $\approx 35\%$, which may be due to the high Mg^{++} content in its tablets.

β-BLOCKERS

Adverse effects with β-blockers fall into two categories: those from known pharmacological consequences of β-blockade and other reactions independent of β-blockade.

The first type includes asthma, heart failure, limited recognition of hypoglycaemia, bradycardia and heart block, and Raynaud's phenomena. Side effects of the second category are more uncommon. β-blockers vary considerably in pharmacological features and efficacy. Side effect profiles that specifically link to β-blockade will vary depending on the particular compound and the drug delivery system being used (Table 3.7). For example, compounds with intrinsic sympathomimetic activity (ISA) do not decrease the risk of a second myocardial infarction as well as β-blockers without this characteristic.[90] In addition; $β_1$-cardioselective agents may have some side effect advantages for $β_2$-mediated side effects, but only at low-end doses. These include a risk of paradoxical pressor effects during major stresses less than that with non-selective β-blockade and a lesser change in bronchial tone in patients with reactive airway disease and/or chronic airways obstruction.[91] As much as 2/3 of an ophthalmically administered β-blocker may enter the nasolacrimal duct only to be swallowed and absorbed, with ensuing systemic β-blockade representing an unrecognized source of β-blockade.[40]

β-blocker use can also be associated with a number of non-specific side effects including: depression, fatigue and sexual dysfunction. The frequency with which these side effects occur is not nearly as great as conventionally believed.[92] Dreams, hallucinations, and insomnia are suggested to be more common with lipid-soluble β-blockers, such as propranolol and metoprolol, but this has not been a verifiable finding in clinical trials.[93] Non-selective β-blockers can raise triglycerides and reduce high-density lipoprotein cholesterol, effects not seen with β-blockers with partial agonist activity and combined α–β-blockers such as carvedilol.[94]

Table 3.7 β-blocker-related side effects

Lupus-like reactions reported with acebutolol – close monitoring is indicated during therapy (this is not a class-effect for β-blockers)
Diminished effectiveness of adrenaline (epinephrine) in the setting of anaphylaxis
Rebound hypertension or withdrawal symptomatology upon abrupt discontinuation. Abrupt withdrawal of clonidine while receiving a β-blocker may exaggerate the rebound hypertension due to unopposed α-stimulation
Diphenhydramine inhibits the metabolism of metoprolol in extensive metabolizers, thereby prolonging the negative chronotropic and inotropic effects of the drug
Increases serum potassium by blocking $β_2$-mediated intracellular flux of potassium – most prominent when chronic kidney disease (CKD) limits potassium excretion
Cimetidine may increase the blood levels of propranolol by as much as twofold (due to decreased metabolism); hydralazine increases the bioavailability of short-acting forms of propranolol
Attenuated antihypertensive effect with non-steroidal anti-inflammatory drugs (NSAIDs)

A number of drug–drug interactions of a pharmacokinetic and pharmacodynamic nature can occur with β-blockers.[95] Flecainide plasma levels may increase by as much as 30% when propranolol is co-administered.[96] Cimetidine has been reported to increase propranolol, metoprolol, and labetalol levels two-fold, but not atenolol, nadolol or pindolol levels.[97] The clinical significance of the interaction is unknown since most studies report no change in heart rate or BP when cimetidine is concurrently given with a β-blocker. Concomitant administration of metoprolol and diphenhydramine leads to prolonged negative chronotropic and inotropic effects of metoprolol in extensive, but not poor metabolizers.[98] Finally, β-blockers given together with non-dihydropyridine CCBs can have added negative inotropic and chronotropic effects.

CALCIUM CHANNEL BLOCKERS

The side effect profiles of all drugs in this class are similar and in many instances are dose-dependent. Side effects associated with CCBs are typically vasodilatory in nature and include headaches, flushing and dependent oedema. The latter relates to CCBs being more potent arteriolar than venodilators and is both dose-dependent and more common in women. The peripheral oedema with CCBs does not occur as a consequence of salt-and-water retention; thus, it is poorly responsive to diuretic therapy. The co-administration of venodilators, such as ACE inhibitors, ARBs or nitrates, generally reduces or eliminates CCB-induced peripheral oedema.[99] CCBs as a class can also be associated with gastro-oesophageal reflux and gingival hyperplasia.[100] Most side effects of CCBs are class-specific, with the exception of constipation and atrioventricular block, which occur more commonly with verapamil; atrioventricular block is also seen with diltiazem.

An additional consideration with CCBs relates to the issue of drug interactions. Concomitant administration of CCBs (nifedipine, diltiazem, nicardipine, verapamil) and digitalis glycosides (digoxin) can result in up to a 50% increase in serum digoxin concentrations.[101] In addition, verapamil and diltiazem inhibit the CYP3A4 isozyme and thereby slow the metabolism of drugs such as ciclosporin, nifedipine, simvastatin, quinidine and theophylline. These drug–drug interactions present as an exaggeration of the pharmacological effect of the index drug (e.g. theophylline toxicity or additive BP reduction when verapamil or diltiazem is given together with nifedipine) or with concentration-related side effects (e.g. the increased risk of rhabdomyolysis when diltiazem is co-administered with simvastatin).[102] Such drug–drug interactions may prove beneficial (e.g. the reduced dose of ciclosporin required when it is given together with verapamil or diltiazem).[103]

CONCLUSION

The treatment of hypertension remains as much an art as it is a science. The blueprint for success in any antihypertensive regimen requires that there be an ongoing careful assessment of the pharmacokinetic and pharmacodynamic interplay of the various medications. A number of 'host' factors influence the dose-response to an antihypertensive medication and these should be assessed carefully when the BP-lowering response to an antihypertensive regimen is either inadequate or excessive. Thereafter, the unique interplay between many medications has to be considered, particularly when the observed response falls outside predetermined therapeutic boundaries and/or when intolerable side effects occur.

References

1. Zannad F, Radauceanu A, Parati G. Trough-to-peak ratio, smoothness index and morning-to-evening ratio: why, which and when? *J Hypertens* 2003;21:851–854.
2. Izzo J, Sica DA. Antihypertensive drugs: Pharmacologic Principles and Dosing Effects. In: Izzo J, Black H, eds. *Hypertension primer, 3rd edn.* Dallas, TX: American Heart Association; 2003:405–408.
3. Sica DA. Pharmacotherapy Review. Angiotensin-receptor blockers. *J Clin Hypertens* 2005;7:681–684.
4. Schmieder RE, Klingbeil AU, Fleischmann EH, et al. Additional antiproteinuric effect of ultrahigh dose candesartan: a double-blind, randomized, prospective study. *J Am Soc Nephrol* 2005;16:3038–3045.
5. Yusuf S, Sleight P, Pogue J, et al. Effects of an angiotensin-converting enzyme inhibitor, ramipril, on cardiovascular events in high-risk patients. The Heart Outcomes Prevention Evaluation Study Investigators. *N Engl J Med* 2000;342:145–153.
6. The PEACE Trial Investigators. Angiotensin-converting-enzyme inhibition in stable coronary artery disease. *N Engl J Med* 2004;351:2058–2068.
7. Sica DA. Rationale for fixed-dose combinations in the treatment of hypertension: the cycle repeats. *Drugs* 2002;62:243–262.
8. Gonzalez FJ, Skoda RC, Kimura S, et al. Characterization of the common genetic defect in humans deficient in debrisoquine metabolism. *Nature* 1988;331:442–446.
9. Shah RR, Oates NS, Idle JR, Smith RL. Beta blockers and drug oxidation status. *Lancet* 1982;1:1019–1020.
10. Zanger UM, Raimundo S, Eichelbaum M. Cytochrome P450 2D6 overview and update on pharmacology, genetics, biochemistry. *Naunyn Schmiedebergs Arch Pharmacol* 2004;369:23–37.
11. Uetrecht JP, Woosley RL. Acetylator phenotype and lupus erythematosus. *Clin Pharmacokinet* 1981;6:118–134.
12. Campbell NR, Dunnette JH, Mwaluko G, et al. Platelet phenol sulfotransferase and erythrocyte catechol-O-methyltransferase activities: correlation with methyldopa metabolism. *Clin Pharmacol Ther* 1984;35:55–63.
13. Mellen PB, Herrington DM. Pharmacogenomics of blood pressure response to antihypertensive treatment. *J Hypertens* 2005;23:1311–1325.
14. Mokwe E, Ohmit SE, Nasser SA, et al. Determinants of blood pressure response to quinapril in black and white hypertensive patients: the Quinapril Titration Interval Management Evaluation Trial. *Hypertension* 2004;43:1202–1207.
15. Sehgal AR. Overlap between whites and blacks in response to antihypertensive drugs. *Hypertension* 2004;43:566–572.
16. Schelleman H, Stricker BH, De Boer A, et al. Drug-gene interactions between genetic polymorphisms and antihypertensive therapy. *Drugs* 2004;64:1801–1816.
17. Weir MR, Gray JM, Paster R, Saunders E. Differing mechanisms of action of angiotensin-converting enzyme inhibition in black and white hypertensive patients. The Trandolapril Multicenter Study Group. *Hypertension* 1995;26:124–130.
18. Prisant LM, Mensah GA. Use of beta-adrenergic receptor blockers in blacks. *J Clin Pharmacol* 1996;36:867–873.
19. Saunders E. The safety and efficacy of terazosin in the treatment of essential hypertension in blacks. *Am Heart J* 1991;122:936–942.
20. Chrysant SG, Weder AB, McCarron DA, et al. Effects of isradipine or enalapril on blood pressure in salt-sensitive hypertensives during low and high dietary salt intake. MIST II Trial Investigators. *Am J Hypertens* 2000;13:1180–1188.
21. Weir MR, Chrysant SG, McCarron DA, et al. Influence of race and dietary salt on the antihypertensive efficacy of an angiotensin-converting enzyme inhibitor or a calcium channel antagonist in salt-sensitive hypertensives. *Hypertension* 1998;31:1088–1096.
22. Whelton PK, He J, Cutler JA, et al. Effects of oral potassium on blood pressure. Meta-analysis of randomized controlled clinical trials. *JAMA* 1997;277:1624–1632.
23. Kaplan NM, Carnegie A, Raskin P, et al. Potassium supplementation in hypertensive patients with diuretic-induced hypokalemia. *N Engl J Med* 1985;312:746–749.

24. Schiffrin EL, Touyz RM. From bedside to bench to bedside: role of renin-angiotensin-aldosterone system in remodeling of resistance arteries in hypertension. *Am J Physiol Heart Circ Physiol* 2004;287:H435–446.

25. Case DB, Atlas SA, Mouradian JA, et al. Proteinuria during long-term captopril therapy. *JAMA* 1980;244:346–349.

26. Johnston GD. Dose-response relationships with antihypertensive drugs. *Pharmacol Ther* 1992;55:53–93.

27. Sica DA. Diuretic related side-effects: development and treatment. *J Clin Hypertens* 2004;6:532–540.

28. Shepherd AM, Irvine NA, Ludden TM. Effect of food on blood hydralazine levels and response in hypertension. *Clin Pharmacol Ther* 1984;36:14–18.

29. Beermann B, Midskov C. Reduced bioavailability and effect of furosemide given with food. *Eur J Clin Pharmacol* 1986;29:725–727.

30. Salvetti A, Pedrinelli R, Magagna A, et al. Influence of food on acute and chronic effects of captopril in essential hypertensive patients. *J Cardiovasc Pharmacol* 1985;7:S25–S29.

31. Heinig R. Clinical pharmacokinetics of nisoldipine coat-core. *Clin Pharmacokinet* 1998;35:191–208.

32. Bailey DG, Spence JD, Munoz C, Arnold JM. Interaction of citrus juices with felodipine and nifedipine. *Lancet* 1991;337:268–269.

33. Sica DA. Interaction of grapefruit juice and calcium channel blockers. *Am J Hypertens* 2006;19:768–773.

34. Flockhart DA, Tanus-Santos JE. Implications of cytochrome P450 interactions when prescribing medication for hypertension. *Arch Intern Med* 2002;162:405–412.

35. Dresser GK, Spence JD, Bailey DG. Pharmacokinetic-pharmacodynamic consequences and clinical relevance of cytochrome P450 3A4 inhibition. *Clin Pharmacokinet* 2000;38:41–57.

36. Michalets EL. Update: clinically significant cytochrome P-450 drug interactions. *Pharmacotherapy* 1998;18:84–112.

37. Campana C, Regazzi MB, Buggia I, Molinaro M. Clinically significant drug interactions with cyclosporine: an update. *Clin Pharmacokinet* 1996;30:141–179.

38. Sica DA, Gehr TW, Ghosh S. Clinical pharmacokinetics of losartan. *Clin Pharmacokinet* 2005;44:797–814.

39. Schwartz GL, Turner ST. Pharmacogenetics of antihypertensive drug responses. *Am J Pharmacogenomics* 2004;4:151–160.

40. Sica DA. Ophthalmically administered beta blockers and their cardiopulmonary effects. *J Clin Hypertens (Greenwich)* 2001;3:175–178.

41. Sica DA. Hypertension, renal disease, and drug considerations. *J Clin Hypertens (Greenwich)* 2004;6(Suppl 2):24–30.

42. Prisant LM, Elliott WJ. Drug delivery systems for treatment of systemic hypertension. *Clin Pharmacokinet* 2003;42:931–940.

43. Hermida RC, Smolensky MH. Chronotherapy of hypertension. *Curr Opin Nephrol Hypertens* 2004;13:501–505.

44. Sica DA, Weber M, Neutel J. The antihypertensive efficacy and safety of a chronotherapeutic formulation of propranolol in patients with hypertension. *J Clin Hypertens* 2004;6:231–241.

45. Black HR, Elliott WJ, Grandits G, et al. Principal results of the Controlled Onset Verapamil Investigation of Cardiovascular End Points (CONVINCE) trial. *JAMA* 2003;289:2073–2082.

46. Langley MS, Heel RC. Transdermal clonidine. A preliminary review of its pharmacodynamic properties and therapeutic efficacy. *Drugs* 1988;35:123–142.

47. Metz S, Klein C, Morton N. Rebound hypertension after discontinuation of transdermal clonidine therapy. *Am J Med* 1987;82:17–19.

48. Chow KM, Szeto CC, Wong TY, et al. Risk factors for thiazide-induced hyponatraemia. *Q J Med* 2003;96:911–917.

49. Addo HA, Ferguson J, Frain Bell W. Thiazide-induced photosensitivity: A study of 33 subjects. *Br J Dermatol* 1987;116:749–760.

50. Diffey BL, Langtry J. Phototoxic potential of thiazide diuretics in normal subjects. *Arch Dermatol* 1989;125:1355–1358.

51. Strom BL, Schinnar R, Apter AJ, et al. Absence of cross-reactivity between sulfonamide antibiotics and sulfonamide nonantibiotics. *N Engl J Med* 2003;349:1628–1635.

52. Lawson DH, Macadam RF, Singh MH, et al. Effect of furosemide on antibiotic-induced renal damage in rats. *J Infect Dis* 1972;126:593–600.

53. Shapiro S, Slone D, Lewis GP, et al. The epidemiology of digoxin toxicity. A study in three Boston hospitals. *J Chronic Dis* 1969;22:361–371.

54. Petersen V, Hvidt S, Thomsen K, et al. Effect of prolonged thiazide treatment on renal lithium clearance. *Br Med J* 1974;3:143–145.

55. Favre L, Glasson P, Vallotton MB. Reversible acute renal failure from combined triamterene and indomethacin: a study in healthy subjects. *Ann Intern Med* 1982;96:317–320.

56. Martin WB, Spodick DH, Gins GR. Pericardial disorders occurring during open-label study of 1,869 severely hypertensive patients treated with minoxidil. *J Cardiovasc Pharmacol* 1980;2: S217–S227.

57. Reichgott MJ. Minoxidil and pericardial effusion: an idiosyncratic reaction. *Clin Pharmacol Ther* 1981;30:64–70.

58. Burton JL, Marshall A. Hypertrichosis due to minoxidil. *Br J Dermatol* 1979;101:593–595.

59. Kidwai BJ, George M. Hair loss with minoxidil withdrawal. *Lancet* 1992;340:609–610.

60. Gonzalez M, Landa N, Gardeazabal J, et al. Generalized hypertrichosis after treatment with topical minoxidil. *Clin Exp Dermatol* 1994;19:157–158.

61. Russell GI, Bing RF, Jones JA, et al. Hydralazine sensitivity: clinical features, autoantibody changes and HLA-DR phenotype. *Q J Med* 1987;65:845–852.

62. Lindeberg S, Holm B, Lundborg P, et al. The effect of hydralazine on steady-state plasma concentrations of metoprolol in pregnant hypertensive women. *Eur J Clin Pharmacol* 1988;35:131–135.

63. Carruthers SG. Adverse effects of alpha 1- adrenergic blocking drugs. *Drug Saf* 1994;11:12–20.

64. Young RA, Brogden RN. Doxazosin: a review of its pharmacodynamic and pharmacokinetic properties, and therapeutic efficacy in mild to moderate hypertension. *Drugs* 1988;35:525–541.

65. Pomara G, Morelli G, Pomara S, et al. Cardiovascular parameter changes in patients with erectile dysfunction using pde-5 inhibitors: a study with sildenafil and vardenafil. *J Androl* 2004;25:625–629.

66. Elliott HL, McLean K, Sumner DJ, et al. Immediate cardiovascular responses to oral prazosin: effects of concurrent beta-blockers. *Clin Pharmacol Ther* 1981;29:303–309.

67. Marshall HJ, Beevers DG. α-adrenoceptor blocking drugs and female urinary incontinence: prevalence and reversibility. *Br J Clin Pharmacol* 1996;42:507–509.

68. Davis BR, Cutler JA, Furberg CD, et al. Relationship of antihypertensive treatment regimens and change in blood pressure to risk for heart failure in hypertensive patients randomly assigned to doxazosin or chlorthalidone: further analyses from the Antihypertensive and Lipid-Lowering Treatment to Prevent Heart Attack Trial. *Ann Intern Med* 2002;137:313–320.

69. Sica DA. Doxazosin and congestive heart failure. *Congest Heart Fail* 2002;8:178–184.

70. Furhoff A-K. Adverse reactions with methyldopa – a decade's reports. *Acta Med Scand* 1978;203:425–428.

71. Lawson DH, Gloss D, Jick H. Adverse reactions to methyldopa with particular reference to hypotension. *Am Heart J* 1978;96:572–579.

72. Sica DA, Grubbs R. Transdermal clonidine: therapeutic considerations. *J Clin Hypertens* 2005;7:558–562.

73. Byrd BF III, Collins HW, Primm RK. Risk factors for severe bradycardia during oral clonidine therapy for hypertension. *Arch Intern Med* 1988;148:729–733.

74. Mehta JL, Lopez LM. Rebound hypertension following abrupt cessation of clonidine and metoprolol. Treatment with labetalol. *Arch Intern Med* 1987;147:389–390.

75. Marruecos L, Roglan A, Frati ME, Artigas A. Clonidine overdose. *Crit Care Med* 1983;11:959–960.

76. Hansson L, Smith DH, Reeves R, Lapuerta P. Headache in mild-to-moderate hypertension and its reduction by irbesartan therapy. *Arch Intern Med* 2000;160:1654–1658.

77. Sica DA, Black HR. ACE inhibitor-related angioedema: can angiotensin-receptor blockers be safely used? *J Clin Hypertens (Greenwich)* 2002;4:375–380.

78. Bakris GL, Siomos M, Richardson D, et al. ACE inhibition or angiotensin receptor blockade: impact on potassium in renal failure. VAL-K Study Group. *Kidney Int* 2000;58:2084–2092.

79. Quan A. Fetopathy associated with exposure to angiotensin converting enzyme inhibitors. *Early Hum Dev* 2006;82:23–28.

80. Unger T, Kaschina E. Drug interactions with angiotensin receptor blockers: a comparison with other antihypertensives. *Drug Saf* 2003;26:707–720.

81. Stangier J, Su C, Hendriks M, et al. The effect of telmisartan on the steady-state pharmacokinetics of digoxin in healthy male volunteers. *J Clin Pharmacol* 2000;40:1373–1379.

82. Leung M, Remick R. Potential drug interaction between lithium and valsartan. *J Clin Pharmacol* 2000;20:392–393.

83. Schoolwerth AC, Sica DA, Ballermann BJ, Wilcox CS. Renal considerations in angiotensin converting enzyme inhibitor therapy: a statement for healthcare professionals from the Council on the Kidney in Cardiovascular Disease and the Council for High Blood Pressure Research of the American Heart Association. *Circulation* 2001;104:1985–1991.

84. Palmer B. Managing hyperkalemia caused by inhibitors of the renin-angiotensin-aldosterone system. *N Engl J Med* 2004;351:585–592.

85. Sica DA, Brath L. Angiotensin-converting enzyme inhibition-emerging pulmonary issues relating to cough. *Congest Heart Fail* 2006;12:223–226.

86. Kostis JB, Packer M, Black HR, et al. Omapatrilat and enalapril in patients with hypertension: The Omapatrilat Cardiovascular Treatment vs. Enalapril (OCTAVE) trial. *Am J Hypertension* 2003;17:103–111.

87. Orr KK, Myers JR. Intermittent visceral edema induced by long-term enalapril administration. *Ann Pharmacother* 2004;38:825–827.

88. Ishani A, Weinhandl E, Zhao Z, et al. Angiotensin-converting enzyme inhibitor as a risk factor for the development of anemia, and the impact of incident anemia on mortality in patients with left ventricular dysfunction. *J Am Coll Cardiol* 2005;45:391–399.

89. Pennell DJ, Nunan TO, O'Doherty MJ. Fatal Stevens-Johnson syndrome in a patient on captopril and allopurinol (letter). *Lancet* 1984;1:463.

90. Freemantle N, Cleland J, Young P, et al. Beta blockade after myocardial infarction: systematic review and meta-regression analysis. *BMJ* 1999;318:1730–1737.

91. Salpeter SR, Ormiston TM, Salpeter EE. Cardioselective ß-blockers in patients with reactive airway disease: a meta-analysis. *Ann Intern Med* 2002;137:715–725.

92. Ko DT, Hebert PR, Coffey CS, et al. Beta-blocker therapy and symptoms of depression, fatigue, and sexual dysfunction. *J Am Med Assoc* 2002;288:351–357.

93. McAinsh J, Cruickshank JM. Beta-blockers and central nervous system side effects. *Pharmacol Ther* 1990;46:163–197.

94. Bakris GL, Fonseca V, Katholi RE, et al. Metabolic effects of carvedilol vs metoprolol in patients with type 2 diabetes mellitus and hypertension: a randomized controlled trial. *J Am Med Assoc* 2004;292:2227–2236.

95. Opie LH. Adverse cardiovascular drug interactions. *Curr Probl Cardiol* 2000;25:621–676.

96. Holtzman JL, Kvam DC, Berry DA, et al. The pharmacodynamic and pharmacokinetic interaction of flecainide acetate with propranolol: effects on cardiac function and drug clearance. *Eur J Clin Pharmacol* 1987;33:97–99.

97. Mutschler E, Spahn H, Kirch W. The interaction between H2-receptor antagonists and beta-adrenoceptor blockers. *Br J Clin Pharmacol* 1984;17(suppl 1):51S–57S.

98. Hamelin B, Bouayad A, Methot J, et al. Significant interaction between nonprescription antihistamine and the CYP2D6 substrate metoprolol in healthy men with high or low CYP2D6 activity. *Clin Pharmacol Ther* 2000;67:466–477.

99. Sica DA. Calcium channel blocker-related peripheral edema: can it be resolved? *J Clin Hypertens (Greenwich)* 2003;5:291–294.

100. Ellis JS, Seymour RA, Steele JG, et al. Prevalence of gingival overgrowth induced by calcium channel blockers: a community-based study. *J Periodontol* 1999;70:63–67.

101. Andrejak M, Hary L, Andrejak MT, et al. Diltiazem increases steady state digoxin serum levels in patients with cardiac disease. *J Clin Pharmacol* 1987;27:967–970.

102. Yeo KR, Yeo WW, Wallis EJ, et al. Enhanced cholesterol reduction by simvastatin in diltiazem-treated patients. *Br J Clin Pharmacol* 1999;48:610–615.

103. Smith CL, Hampton EM, Pederson JA, et al. Clinical and medicoeconomic impact of the cyclosporine-diltiazem interaction in renal transplant recipients. *Pharmacotherapy* 1994;14:471–481.

4 | Antihypertensive drugs: haemodynamic effects

Per Lund-Johansen

INTRODUCTION

During the last decade the interest in haemodynamics in untreated hypertension – as well as in the haemodynamic effects of antihypertensive drugs – seems to have been less than in the 1970s and 1980s.[1] However, the results of ALLHAT should remind us that the haemodynamic effects of the different classes of antihypertensive drugs differ widely and that incorrect use may lead to dangerous outcomes, particularly when shifting abruptly from one class to another (i.e. from diuretic directly to α-receptor blocker).[2] The use of rapid-release formulations may induce myocardial infarction in special categories of patients, while slow release formulations are less hazardous owing to different effects on haemodynamics.[3,4]

HAEMODYNAMICS IN UNTREATED HYPERTENSION

Extensive reviews of haemodynamics in essential hypertension have been published.[5–9] Very briefly, essential or primary hypertension may be due to several pathophysiologic mechanisms: (1) increased sympathetic activity, (2) abnormalities in sodium handling and (3) disturbances in calcium transport, leading to increased intracellular calcium concentration and augmented contraction of smooth muscles in the walls of resistance vessels.[5,6] Whether this mechanism is important in most patients with essential hypertension is unclear.[5] However, it is well documented by accurate invasive studies that in nearly all patients who need drug therapy for essential hypertension, total peripheral resistance (TPR) is elevated and arteriolar resistance is increased in most tissues.[7–9] Cardiac output (CO), the other main determinant of blood pressure (BP), is usually unchanged or slightly reduced at rest. During exercise, however, cardiac output is usually suppressed because of insufficient increase in stroke volume.[7]

In elderly hypertensives, and particularly in those with systolic hypertension, reduced arterial compliance contributes to the increased systolic pressure. The haemodynamic disturbances in symptom-free patients with essential hypertension in their 60s compared to those in their 20s are widely different, even if they have the same mean arterial pressure (MAP) at rest (Fig. 4.1).

Prospective invasive 20-year follow-up studies in subjects with untreated essential hypertension have shown that the cardiac output drops and the TPR increases over the years more than would be expected from normal ageing (Fig. 4.2). It is likely that these changes reflect a gradual restructuring of the

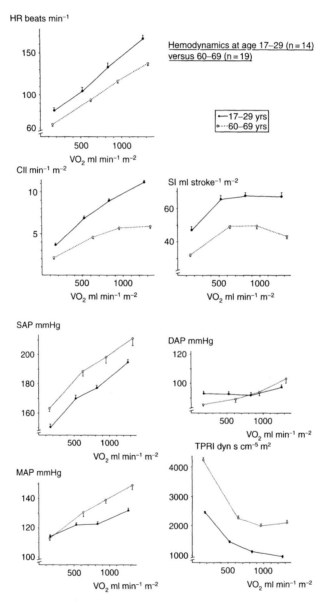

Fig. 4.1 Contrasting haemodynamics in young and elderly hypertensives with identical intraarterial mean arterial pressure (MAP) during rest, sitting. HR = heart rate; CI = cardiac index; SI = stroke index; SAP = systolic arterial pressure; DAP = diastolic arterial pressure; VO_2 = oxygen consumption; TPRI = total peripheral resistance index. Note the very much higher TPRI and lower SI and CI in the oldest group. *(Modified from ref. (7)).*

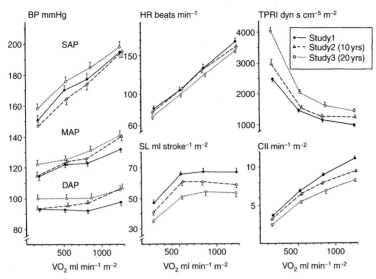

Fig. 4.2 Changes in central haemodynamics in untreated hypertension over 20 years during rest and exercise. Invasive methods. Age at first study 17–29 years. Note the marked increase in TPRI and fall in SI – in spite of only moderate changes in blood pressure. *(Modified from ref. (7)).*

high pressure compartment in hypertension – according to Folkow's concept.[8] It is important to know to what extent these changes are reversible by drug treatment.

HAEMODYNAMIC EFFECTS OF ANTIHYPERTENSIVE DRUGS

Antihypertensive agents reduce BP by decreasing either TPR or cardiac output or both. Sometimes acutely and chronically induced haemodynamic changes differ. The antihypertensive agents fall into four main categories:

(1) Diuretics
(2) Drugs acting on the nervous system
(3) Vasodilators (including calcium antagonists)
(4) Angiotensin converting enzyme (ACE) inhibitors and angiotensin II receptor blockers (ARB).

Initially antihypertensive agents lower BP through very different mechanisms: e.g. reduction in cardiac output via increased diuresis and fall in plasma volume by diuretics; reduction in cardiac output and TPR via changes in nervous tone to the heart or resistance vessels by α- and β-blockers; reduction in TPR via direct effect on the arteriolar wall by hydralazine or via decreased angiotensin II effect by ACE inhibitors on ARB or via interference with Ca^{2+} transport in the smooth muscle cell in the arteriolar wall.

These initial effects may be counteracted by immediate compensatory reflex mechanisms, such as increase in heart rate and cardiac output. During long-term use the pressure reduction may itself induce secondary changes in cardiac output and TPR, which are most likely due to reversal of structural changes in the heart and in the resistance vessels.[10] The haemodynamic profile is greatly influenced by whether studies are made when the patient is actually receiving the drug and the plasma concentration is within the therapeutic range, or whether they are made days (or weeks) after the last dose. However, it seems that vasodilation and not just BP reduction is important for improvement of the structure in the resistance vessels.[11]

DIURETICS

A breakthrough in drug treatment of hypertension was made with the discovery of the thiazide diuretics in 1957. The diuretics used today in the therapy of hypertension are (1) thiazides and similar compounds, (2) short-acting, highly potent diuretics and (3) potassium-sparing diuretics.

Thiazide diuretics

It is generally agreed that all thiazides lower BP through the same mechanisms, although doses and duration of effects vary.[12,13] The thiazide diuretics block the reabsorption of Na^+ and Cl^- in the distal convoluted tubules of the kidneys; K^+ excretion is also increased. After an oral dose the diuretic effect is apparent after 2–4 hours with maximum effect after 6–8 hours. Total duration of action is about 12–24 hours (for polythiazide 24–48 hours). The dose–response curve for the thiazides is relatively flat.[12] However, less than 25 mg hydrochlorothiazide daily as monotherapy induces only minor BP reduction compared with placebo.[14]

Acute haemodynamic effects

When chlorothiazide 500–1000 mg was injected intravenously in patients with essential hypertension a rapid drop in cardiac output occurred due to reduction in stroke volume without any change in heart rate. TPR increased and BP remained unchanged or was only slightly reduced.[15,16] After some hours there was a decrease in plasma volume.[17,18] A direct reduction in myocardial contractility has also been proposed.[19] However, when the thiazides are given orally for several days important readjustment reactions take place. The TPR gradually decreases and BP falls. Cardiac output remains reduced because of persistent decrease in the stroke volume and heart rate is unchanged.[20] The plasma volume is reduced by about 10–15%.[20–23] A reduced pressor response to catecholamines has been demonstrated in this phase.[24]

Chronic haemodynamic effects

During prolonged thiazide therapy adjustment reactions continue.[25] In 1970 we showed that hydrochlorothiazide 50 mg twice daily for 1 year reduced TPR (Fig. 4.3). Heart rate, stroke volume and cardiac output remained at the pre-treatment level during rest and muscular exercise, and partial correction of the abnormal haemodynamics was achieved.[26] A study with polythiazide gave similar results. Plasma volume remained 7% or 240 mL lower than before treatment, similar to the observations by Wilson and Freis in 1959.[27] Sudden

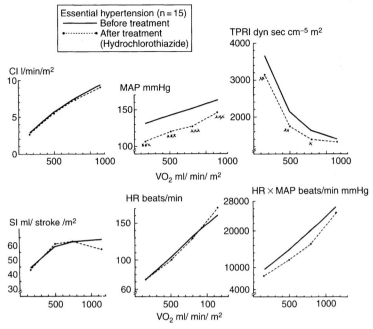

Fig. 4.3 Haemodynamic changes induced by 1-year treatment with hydrochlorthiazide. Note the marked decrease in TPRI during rest as well as during exercise and maintained CI. xxx = $p < 0.001$, xx = $p < 0.01$, x = $p < 0.05$. *(Redrawn from ref. (26)).*

withdrawal of a thiazide causes an increase in plasma volume – sometimes in the order of 300–400 mL – and a rise in BP.[28,29]

As a consequence of the reduction in plasma volume, plasma renin and angiotensin levels are increased. In some patients this might lead to vasoconstriction and/or fluid retention via an increase in aldosterone secretion.[29–31]

Although the thiazides have been cornerstones in the treatment of hypertension for about 50 years, it is still not agreed how these drugs reduce TPR during long-term use. Since plasma volume is reduced, it is possible that this will decrease the effect of various pressor stimuli and enhance the effect of depressor stimuli. A direct effect on the vessel wall such as that of the thiazide-like vasodilatator, diazoxide, seems unlikely because of its slow onset. A gradual reversal of the hypertrophy in the arteriolar wall as a consequence of a long-term reduction in pressure could be possible. Changes in the ionic composition of the arteriolar wall have also been suggested.[30,31] Normalization of renal haemodynamics has been demonstrated.[31]

Chlorthalidone

Chlorthalidone differs from most thiazides in having a longer effect (24–48 hours). The dose range is 25–50 mg every day or 50–100 mg every second day.

In a long-term study of patients with essential hypertension, treated with chlorthalidone 100 mg every second day, the reduction in BP was associated with a persistent decrease in cardiac output and stroke volume, no change in heart rate and, contrary to experience with thiazides, no change in TPR.[26] The cause of this difference between thiazides and chlorthalidone during long-term use is unknown.

Short-acting, highly potent loop diuretics

The short-acting, highly potent diuretics (furosemide, etacrynic acid and bumetanide) also lower BP.[32–34] The haemodynamic effects are thought to be the same as for the thiazide diuretics. These drugs are very useful in acute situations such as hypertensive crisis, hypertension with pulmonary oedema, and also in hypertension associated with renal failure.[34]

Spironolactone

Spironolactone inhibits the action of aldosterone in distal tubules and collecting ducts of the kidneys, induces increased excretion of NaCl and water, and reduction in potassium excretion. The drug is used in patients with primary aldosteronism, permanently or prior to surgical therapy[35,36] and, in recent years, for heart failure. Although overproduction of aldosterone is uncommon in patients with essential hypertension, spironolactone 25–50 mg once or twice daily also lowers BP in most hypertensives, mainly due to reduction in TPR.[36]

DRUGS ACTING ON THE CENTRAL NERVOUS SYSTEM AND THE SYMPATHETIC AND PARASYMPATHETIC GANGLIA (α-METHYLDOPA, CLONIDINE, RESERPINE, GANGLIONIC BLOCKERS)

Drugs interfering with the nervous control of the heart and blood vessels were used quite extensively in therapy of hypertension for about 35 years. Modes of action vary, some drugs acting centrally in the hypothalamus or vasomotor centres, others in the sympathetic and parasympathetic ganglia. Some agents have several modes of action. As far as we know, these drugs do not correct any abnormalities in the nervous system in hypertensive patients, but rather disturb the metabolism or storage of noradrenaline (norepinephrine) or interfere with receptors normally stimulated by noradrenaline (norepinephrine).[37–41] Since these drugs often induce side effects like tiredness and dry mouth, such agents are now seldom used and have been replaced with newer drugs with fewer side effects. Therefore, these agents are not discussed further in this chapter, and the readers are referred to the 1988 edition of *Handbook of Hypertension*,[42] where the haemodynamic effects of the older drugs are described.

β-ADRENOCEPTOR BLOCKING AGENTS (β-BLOCKERS)

The main effect of the β-blockers on the heart is a reduction in heart rate and contractility, reducing cardiac output.[1,43] Since the cardiac output is not increased in the majority of patients with established essential hypertension, the introduction of β-blockers in treatment of hypertension by Prichard and Gillam in 1964[44] was referred to as a 'paradox'. Apart from being simple to use, the β-blockers have been shown to control BP at rest and during muscular exercise.[45–48]

Non-cardioselective β-blockers without intrinsic sympathomimetic activity (ISA) [Partial agonist activity (PAA)]

Injection of propranolol 10–15 mg intravenously causes an immediate decrease in heart rate, a small reduction in stroke volume and consequently a fall in cardiac output. The TPR increases, but BP is unchanged.[49–51] A similar response occurs with timolol.[52]

During long-term treatment, important readjustments take place. The TPR gradually falls with unchanged heart rate and cardiac output, and as a consequence BP is reduced.[47,53,54] It should be emphasized that TPR is usually not reduced below the pre-treatment level.[47–63]

During muscular exercise BP is reduced (compared with pre-treatment level) and the haemodynamic mechanisms are mainly the same as those at rest. TPR remains at the pre-treatment level or is slightly increased. The reduction in both heart rate and BP causes a dramatic fall in the workload on the heart. The BP × heart rate product is often reduced by 40% at rest and during exercise (Fig. 4.4).[47–54] Oxygen consumption is not changed and the chronic reduction in cardiac output is associated with an increase in arteriovenous oxygen difference[45,47] owing to increased tissue oxygen uptake. Studies of the regional circulation have shown that the blood flow is reduced in the kidneys at rest and during exercise.[60]

Other β-blockers

The non-cardioselective β-blockers with ISA (PAA) such as alprenolol[48,65] and the cardioselective blockers such as atenolol[64,65] and metoprolol[66] seem to reduce BP largely by the same mechanisms as those of propranolol or timolol.[1] A 5-year follow-up study in patients treated with atenolol showed that the haemodynamic changes after 5 years resembled those seen after 1 year.[67] No further fall in TPR or increase in stroke volume was found (Fig. 4.5). β-blockers with ISA (PAA) such as pindolol cause less depression of heart rate at rest as well as during exercise,[47,62] but in contrast with propranolol, timolol and metoprolol, these agents do not protect against re-infarction and death in post-myocardial-infarction patients, and are seldom used today.

Apart from in young subjects with mild essential hypertension, the β-blockers do not change central haemodynamics towards normal, particularly not during exercise; nor do these agents normalize the structure in the arterioles.[11] The chronic depression of cardiac output is usually well tolerated, although a reduction in the blood flow to the liver, skeletal muscles[68] and the kidneys has been demonstrated.[60] Most patients on chronic treatment are able to perform ordinary physical exercise without problems even if muscular fatigue is common at the beginning of the treatment.[69] However, during long-lasting severe physical exercise the endurance is reduced.[70,71] For this reason β-blockers should be avoided in subjects who are physically very active. An unexpected development in the use of β-blockers was the observation that these drugs improve symptoms and prognoses in patients with congestive heart failure (CHF), when added in a very small dose to diuretics and ACE inhibitor (ACEI), with cautious upward titration if well tolerated. This is explained by a reduced sympathetic drive to the failing heart.

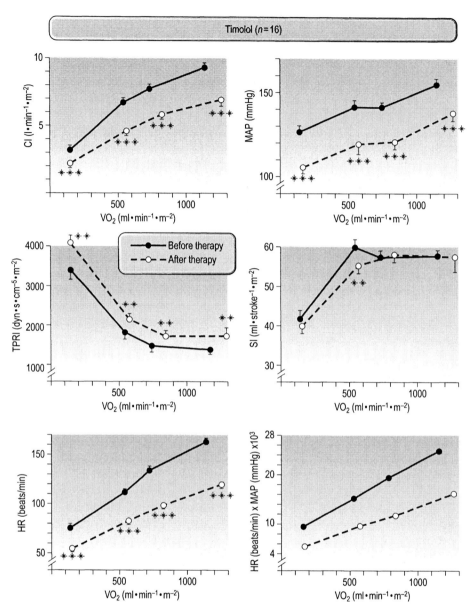

Fig. 4.4 Haemodynamic changes induced by 1-year treatment with timolol. Note dramatic decrease in heart rate, cardiac index, heart rate × mean arterial pressure product and increase in total peripheral resistance index. Bars = Standard error or mean (SEM); ** = $p < 0.01$; *** = $p < 0.001$. For further explanation see Figure 4.1. *(Redrawn from ref. (58))*.

α-ADRENOCEPTOR BLOCKING AGENTS (α-BLOCKERS)

Phentolamine, phenoxybenzamine

Since resistance vessels are mainly controlled by α-adrenergic receptors, α-blockade would seem to be a logical approach to treatment in most forms of hypertension. However, although BP will be reduced by compounds such as phentolamine and phenoxybenzamine, long-term treatment is usually not

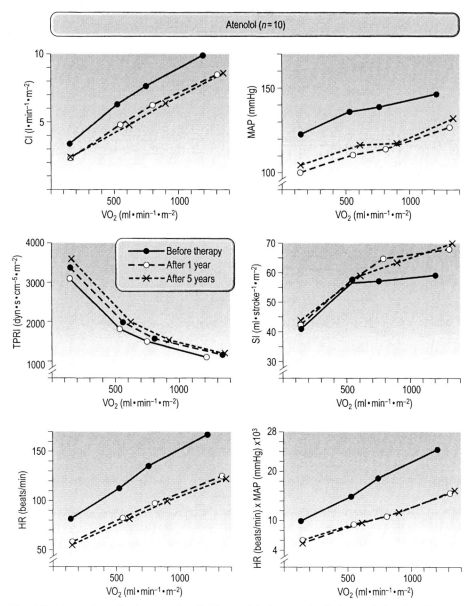

Fig. 4.5 Haemodynamic changes at rest sitting and during exercise before and after 1 and 5 years of treatment with atenolol. For explanation see Figure 4.1. *(Redrawn from ref. (67)).*

successful due to reflex increase in heart rate and cardiac output.[72] This led to the development of the postsynaptic α-adrenergic receptor blockers.

Prazosin, trimazosin, doxazosin

These drugs block selectively the postsynaptic α-adrenergic receptors, and prevent the reflex rise in heart rate which occurs with presynaptic α-blockers (and with vasodilators).[73,74] This unique haemodynamic effect underpinned the use of the first drug, prazosin, as an agent in the treatment of hypertension. Haemodynamic studies have shown that the acute and chronic effects were largely the

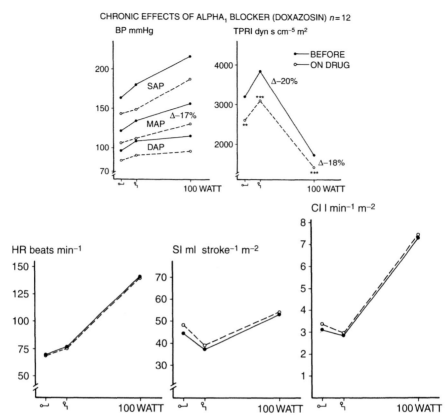

Fig. 4.6 Haemodynamic changes induced by 1-year treatment with doxazosin during rest supine and sitting, and during 100 watt exercise. Note that the reduction in BP is entirely due to fall in total peripheral resistance index – with no depression in heart pump function. *(Redrawn from ref. (79)).*

same. The fall in BP was associated with a marked decrease in TPR, no change or only a slight increase in cardiac output and no significant change in heart rate.[75] Thus, prazosin seemed to correct the central haemodynamic disturbances in hypertension and renal blood flow was preserved.[76] More recent β-blockers, trimazosin[77,78] and doxazosin,[79] have similar modes of action. Figure 4.6 shows the effects of doxazosin.[79] Prazosin had to be administered three times daily and has been replaced by doxazosin GITS, which may be given only once daily.[80] Like pure vasodilators, doxazosin causes increase in plasma volume and extracellular fluid volumes.[79] In patients with latent heart failure on diuretic treatment a sudden switch from diuretic to doxazosin could induce marked fluid retention and cause manifest heart failure. It is likely that these effects explain the observation of increased 'heart failure' in the doxazosin arm compared with the diuretic arm in ALLHAT.[2]

β-BLOCKERS WITH VASODILATOR EFFECTS

Labetalol

Labetalol blocks both α- and β-receptors.[81] After intravenous doses of 50–100 mg or oral doses of about 200–800 mg, BP is reduced by about 20% – at rest as well as during exercise. In acute studies the BP decreases rapidly and is associated with a marked decrease in TPR and a moderate decrease in heart

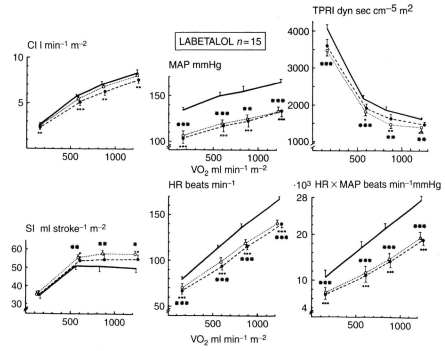

Fig. 4.7 Haemodynamic changes induced by labetalol after 1 year (***, small stars) and after 6 years (***, big stars). The beta blocking effect (reduction in HR) is maintained, but since total peripheral resistance index has fallen and stroke index increased, cardiac index after 6 years is no longer reduced. *(Redrawn from ref. (86))*.

rate and cardiac output.[82–84] Long-term studies have shown a substantial reduction in BP associated with significant decrease in TPR and a modest reduction in heart rate and cardiac output.[85] After 6 years of treatment, cardiac output was no longer reduced and TPR had fallen almost to normal levels at rest as well as during exercise (Fig. 4.7).[86] Thus, labetalol has a rather pronounced antihypertensive effect associated with an acute and chronic reduction in TPR and only a modest reduction in heart rate and cardiac output. Glomerular filtration rate is preserved.[87] To avoid hypotension, the starting dose should be low (12.5 or 25 mg daily).

Carvedilol

This compound was initially claimed to be an antihypertensive agent with marked vasodilator action and a moderate β-blocking effect. In acute studies the drug clearly differs from the non-selective β-blockers like propranolol. During the first hours after an oral dose of 50 mg the BP fell – mainly due to fall in the total perfusion: total peripheral resistance index (TPRI), but thereafter the fall in heart rate and cardiac index dominated.[88,89]

During chronic treatment the drug clearly had a marked β-blocking effect (Fig. 4.8).[90] Like the conventional β-blockers carvedilol has become a useful drug in congestive heart failure in patients with or without previous hypertension – on top of diuretic and ACE inhibitors therapy.[91]

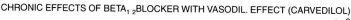

CHRONIC EFFECTS OF BETA$_{1,2}$BLOCKER WITH VASODIL. EFFECT (CARVEDILOL)

$n=9$

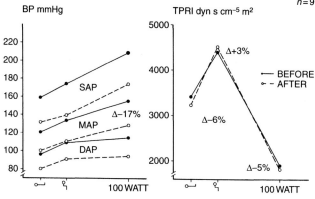

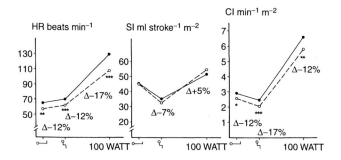

Fig. 4.8 Haemodynamic changes induced by 1-year treatment with carvedilol. Note the marked reduction in heart rate due to the β-blocking effect and a modest reduction in total peripheral resistance index (N.S.). *(Redrawn from ref. (90)).*

VASODILATORS

The term 'vasodilators' refers to drugs acting directly on the smooth muscles of the arterioles. Vasodilators may act also on capacitance vessels. In the latter case a reduction in venous return and in cardiac output could contribute to the fall in BP.[92] Unfortunately, the drop in BP with vasodilators is often counteracted by a reflex increase in heart rate and cardiac output. This can be abolished by co-administration of a β-blocker.[93,94]

Hydralazine

Hydralazine has a direct effect on the myogenic tone of the resistance vessels. Since the sympathetic innervation of the resistance and capacitance vessels is not affected, there is no orthostatic hypotension. After injection of hydralazine there is an immediate fall in BP due to a marked decrease in TPR. A marked fall in vascular resistance in the forearm is also seen. Heart rate increases, as does cardiac output. This counteracts the fall in BP.[95,96] Hydralazine should not be used alone, but with a β-blocker or similar drug. Since there is an increase in the blood flow to the kidneys, the drug was used in patients with hypertension and decreased renal function,[96] but in recent years ACE inhibitors or Angiotensin receptor blockers (ARBs) have reduced this role.

Diazoxide, minoxidil

These drugs are occasionally used acutely in very severe hypertension. Injection of diazoxide 300–600 mg reduces BP in most patients with severe hypertension associated with a fall in TPR and a simultaneous rise in cardiac output and heart rate.[97,98] Since a fall in BP may occur too quickly, it should be used with great caution. Haemodynamic studies of minoxidil have demonstrated a similar reaction pattern.[99] Hypertrichosis and fluid retention is often a problem with this drug, which is seldom used today.

CALCIUM ANTAGONISTS

This class of drugs has been claimed to interfere specifically with abnormal calcium transport, possibly present in patients with essential hypertension.[100–104] The calcium antagonists inhibit calcium influx in muscle cells, in the heart and in resistance vessels. The latter effect causes vasodilatation. In addition, some calcium antagonists depress pacemaker activity and prolong impulse transmission in the heart, while others (the dihydropyridine derivatives) do not show this effect in vivo. Calcium antagonists have been used in treatment of angina pectoris for several decades and more recently in treatment of hypertension. Many calcium antagonists have been found to be effective in lowering BP. Most data are available for verapamil, diltiazem and nifedipine.[105] Some calcium antagonists decrease the rate of artificial arteriosclerosis in certain animal models.[106]

Non-dihydropyridines

Verapamil

Verapamil 80–160 mg three times daily reduces BP by about 15/15 mmHg.[107,108] At rest in the supine position, the effect on heart rate is modest, but during 24 hours of ambulatory monitoring a reduction in heart rate is seen for most of the day.[109]

After oral intake of 160 mg the BP falls in the next 3 hours due to a decrease in TPR, without any significant changes in heart rate or cardiac output.[110] In patients with mild-to-moderate essential hypertension, verapamil 240 mg per day for 1 year reduced the BP at rest and during exercise by about 13/12 mmHg.[111] At rest, TPR was decreased and cardiac output did not show any significant change. Heart rate was moderately decreased at rest and during exercise, but this was compensated by an increase in stroke volume.

In hypertensive patients with abnormal left ventricular performance, improvement after verapamil has been demonstrated by echocardiography.[112] A reduction in renal vascular resistance with unchanged renal blood flow has also been demonstrated.[113] Due to its effect on the sinus and atrioventricular node, it should usually not be combined with a β-blocker (risk of severe bradycardia).

Diltiazem

The acute and chronic haemodynamic effects of diltiazem at rest and during exercise resemble those induced by verapamil.[114,115] The acute effects of diltiazem on central and peripheral haemodynamics were a fall in TPR and dilatation of large arteries.[116] Cardiac output and heart rate increased initially, but returned to pretreatment values while TPR remained reduced. Other studies have shown similar results.[117,118] In a 1-year invasive study in patients with moderately severe hypertension we found that diltiazem normalized central haemodynamics and increased exercise performance (Fig. 4.9).[119]

Dihydropyridine derivatives (nifedipine, nisoldipine, nitrendipine, felodipine, lacidipine, lercanidipine, nimodipine, amlodipine, isradipine)

These compounds differ from verapamil and diltiazem in immediate effect on heart rate. Initial reflex tachycardia is seen with all these compounds, although to a lesser degree with the slow release formulations. In vivo, dihydropyridines do not affect the sinus or atrioventricular node.[120]

Nifedipine

Nifedipine was first used in a capsule preparation (10–20 mg) with resultant immediate reduction in vascular resistance and marked reflex tachycardia and increase in cardiac output.[121,122] Significant reduction in forearm resistance has been demonstrated.[123,124] BP falls within a few minutes, with a maximal effect usually after 30–60 minutes. Due to this rapid effect, associated with a marked reduction in vascular resistance and no depression in heart pump function, the drug was used in treatment of hypertensive crisis.[125,126]

After nifedipine became available as tablets and in sustained-release preparations reflex tachycardia was less prominent, and during long-term treatment it disappears. In a long-term study in 15 subjects with mild-to-moderate essential hypertension, systolic, diastolic and mean arterial pressure fell by about 17% at rest, a little less during exercise.[127] In all circumstances the fall in BP was associated with a statistically significant reduction in TPR. There were no significant changes in oxygen consumption, heart rate, cardiac output or stroke index (Fig. 4.10).

Other dihydropyridine derivatives

During the last two decades several dihydropyridine calcium antagonists have been developed and found effective in trials on hypertensive patients. Such compounds include nisoldipine,[128] amlodipine,[129] nitrendipine,[130] felodipine,[131,132] lacidipine,[133] and lercanidipine.[134] These drugs all reduce TPRI, without depression of heart pump function.

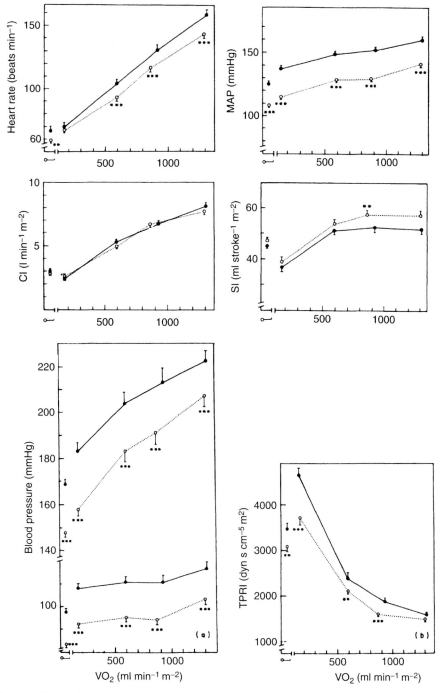

Fig. 4.9 Haemodynamic changes induced by 1-year treatment with diltiazem. Note that heart rate is decreased – particularly during exercise – but due to an increase in stroke index, cardiac index is maintained. Total peripheral resistance index is significantly reduced. *(Redrawn from ref. (119)).*

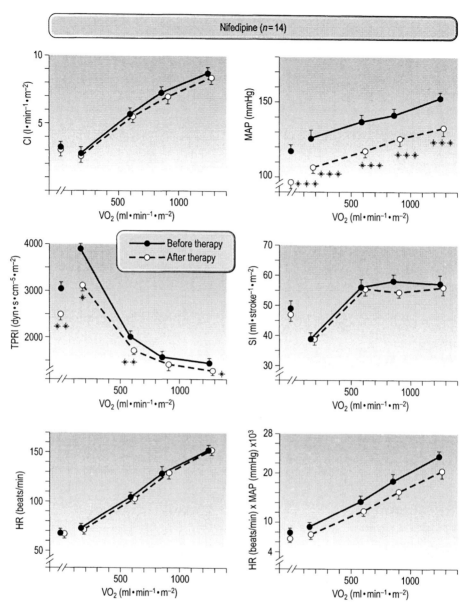

Fig. 4.10 Haemodynamic changes induced by 1-year treatment with nifedipine. The values to the left of each diagram are mean values at rest supine, the others are at rest sitting and at 50, 100 and 150 W exercise loads. Note particularly that the heart rate values after 1 year are identical to the pretreatment values. *(Redrawn from ref. (127)).*

Calcium antagonists and oedema

A common side effect of all calcium antagonists, but mainly the dihydropyridine derivatives, is ankle or leg oedema – seen in at least 25% of patients. This is due to the effect of these drugs on the regional circulation in the lower extremities. More recent compounds, like lacidipine and lercanidipine, seem to induce less oedema than seen with earlier drugs.[132,133]

ANGIOTENSIN CONVERTING ENZYME (ACE) INHIBITORS

The renin–angiotensin system plays an important role in BP control. In patients with essential hypertension a wide range of plasma renin activity (PRA) is found. Interference with the renin–angiotensin system by decreasing the formation of angiotensin II with ACE inhibitors or by blocking the angiotensin II receptor reduces BP in several forms of hypertension even if pretreatment values for PRA and angiotensin II are not increased.[135] Several ACE inhibitors have been developed, including captopril, lisinopril, enalapril, ramipril and trandolapril.

Captopril

Captopril reduces BP in renal hypertension and in a large proportion of patients with essential hypertension. The dose range is 25–150 mg three times daily. In about half of patients the addition of diuretic is necessary to obtain adequate BP control.[136–138] When captopril 25–50 mg is given orally to patients with essential hypertension, the BP falls after 1–2 hours by 15–25 mmHg. This is due to a decrease in TPR with no change in cardiac output or heart rate.[139–143] Thus reflex tachycardia is not typical (in contrast to the dihydropyridines) and during ergometer bicycling a reduction in exercise BP is seen, owing to TPR reduction without any changes in cardiac output.

In patients with essential and renovascular hypertension captopril 10–1000 mg daily for days or weeks reduced BP in most patients and cardiac output determined by echocardiography was not changed. TPR fell by an average of 19%.[143]

Omvik and Lund-Johansen[144] studied central haemodynamics following captopril at rest and during exercise in patients with severe therapy-resistant hypertension. In addition, plasma volume, blood volume and extracellular fluid volume were measured. Most patients were also given a diuretic. After 6–8 months BP was reduced by 35/17 mmHg at rest supine and by 25/17 mmHg during 50 Watt exercise. TPR was significantly reduced at rest, but not during exercise.

Enalapril

Enalapril was the second ACE inhibitor to become available commercially. In patients with essential or renovascular hypertension, an oral dose of 10–20 mg reduces BP within 2–3 hours due to reduction in TPR, without changes in heart rate or cardiac output.[145–149]

In a long-term study of 19 patients with moderately severe essential hypertension, enalapril 10–50 mg (mean 33 mg) daily (+25–50 mg hydrochlorothiazide in seven patients) reduced BP at rest by 19% and was associated with a 14% fall in TPR, with no significant reduction in cardiac output. During exercise the same pattern was seen (Fig. 4.11).[150]

Thus, in contrast to calcium antagonists of the dihydropyridine type, the fall in BP on enalapril is usually more gradual, and reflex tachycardia, flushing and palpitation are not commonly observed.[148,149] Biopsy studies in hypertensive patients have shown that the fall in TPR is due to regression of arteriolar wall hypertrophy.[11] ACE inhibitors are also effective in reversing left

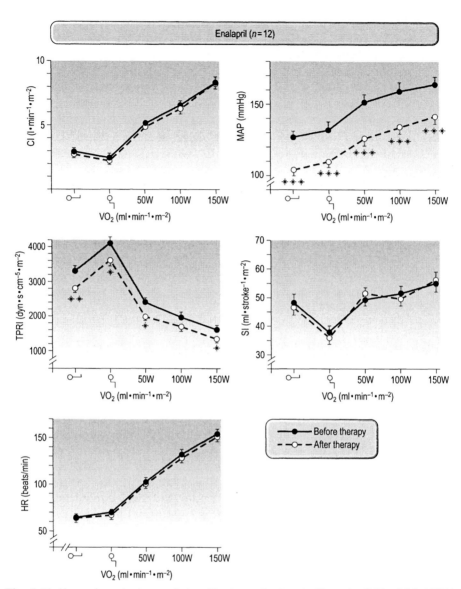

Fig. 4.11 Haemodynamic changes induced by 1-year treatment with enalapril. The fall in MAP is due to reduction in total peripheral resistance index with maintained heart pump function. *(Redrawn from ref. (150)).*

ventricular hypertrophy and, like captopril and enalapril, other more recent ACE drugs have been found very useful in the treatment of congestive heart failure, owing to an effect on preload as well as on afterload.[151–153]

Angiotensin II receptor blockers (ARB)

During the last decade several ARB drugs have been developed (losartan, candesartan, eprosartan, valsartan, irbesartan and others). This class of drugs is very effective and has fewer side effects than seen with ACE inhibitors

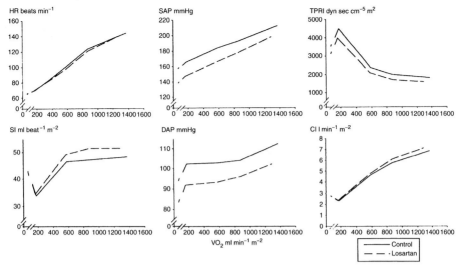

Fig. 4.12 Haemodynamic changes induced by 1-year treatment with losartan. Note the similarity to the effect of the ACE inhibitors enalapril. *(Redrawn from ref. (158).)*

(particularly free of the dry cough which is quite common on ACE inhibitors).[153,154] Many have recently been studied in large scale clinical long-term trials (i.e. LIFE,[155] VALUE,[156] SCOPE[157]) and have been associated with few side effects.

In an invasive haemodynamic study of losartan in patients with moderately severe hypertension, losartan reduced BP by about 10% owing to a reduction in TPR.[158] A slight improvement in heart pump function at rest and during exercise was observed (Fig. 4.12).

Losartan has also proved to be very useful in patients with left ventricular hypertrophy (LVH), reducing LVH more effectively than after atenolol.[159] Improvement of cerebral blood flow has also been demonstrated.[160]

GUIDELINES FOR PRACTICAL TREATMENT BASED ON HAEMODYNAMIC EFFECTS

Although many factors need to be considered when choosing the drug to start with in the treatment of essential hypertension, haemodynamic factors should not be neglected. The haemodynamic mechanisms responsible for increased BP may differ widely. Thus, even though they both have a BP of 170/110 mmHg, a man in his 20s may have different haemodynamic problems from those of someone in his 60s. In the young subject a relatively high heart rate and cardiac output, and an almost normal TPR is typical, whilst in the elderly man the cardiac output may be just half that of the young man and the resistance twice as high. During exercise, however, both subjects have decreased cardiac output. Antihypertensive agents inducing widely different haemodynamic changes are often used without considering the prevailing haemodynamics. Many elderly hypertensive patients have other additional diseases, so that the appropriate selection of antihypertensive drugs is very important, whereas in relatively young subjects such problems are less frequent and tolerance to various haemodynamic alterations is greater. From a strictly haemodynamic point of view, the logical treatment in the majority of patients would be to reduce TPR without any decrease in cardiac output or plasma volume, using α-receptors, calcium antagonists, ACE inhibitors, ARB, or combined α- and β-blockade. The β-blockers on the other hand induce reduction in heart pump function at rest and particularly during relatively short-term exercise. Work performance is not reduced, although in subjects performing heavy exercise for several hours, endurance time is reduced.[69–71] Thus, in physically very active subjects β-blockers should probably be avoided. These drugs should also be avoided in patients who develop side effects from reduced blood flow, such as cold hands and feet, and antihypertensive agents that do not reduce peripheral blood flow should be used. These latter agents include diuretics, doxazosin, calcium antagonists, ACE inhibitors and ARBs. Apart from these general rules, it is important to consider particular patient groups:[161]

Hypertension and angina pectoris

Patients in this category (particularly if resting heart rate is increased) will generally benefit greatly from a β-blocker. The fall in heart rate and BP often reduces the work load on the heart by 40%, and angina is relieved, sometimes completely. When patients in this category develop side effects or do not tolerate β-blockers, a calcium antagonist would seem to be a good alternative.[162]

Hypertension and heart failure

Treatment for this group of patients has been radically changed and improved during the last decade. ACE inhibitors or ARB, usually with a diuretic added, is standard treatment. On top of that, a small dose of a β-blocker should be added – with cautious increase of the dose. When looking back to the previous warning not to use β-blockers in congestive heart failure, this has been a most unexpected discovery.[161]

Isolated systolic hypertension (ISH)

As the hypertensive population lives longer, and systolic arterial pressure (SAP) increases and diastolic arterial pressure (DAP) falls with ageing, treatment of ISH has become a great challenge. Improvement of the compliance of the aorta should lead to falls in SAP and pulse pressure. Calcium antagonists, ARBs and chlorthalidone have been useful in several large clinical studies.[163,164]

Hypertension and renal failure

This category of patients should not have the renal blood flow decreased further. Most β-blockers and thiazide diuretics are unsuitable, whereas ACE inhibitors or ARBs have been shown to maintain renal blood flow – if a diuretic is necessary, furosemide should be used.

Hypertension and cardioprotection

In patients less than 50 years old with mild and moderate essential hypertension living in Western societies, the most important complications are early myocardial infarctions or sudden death. It is now well established that in patients who have survived a myocardial infarction, long-term treatment with β-blockers is indicated whether the patient is hypertensive or not.[165,166,167,168] It is possible that a lipophilic β-blocker (propranolol, timolol or metoprolol) should be preferred.[169,170]

CONCLUSION

Meta-analysis of large-scale studies comparing the effects of the different classes of antihypertensive agents on mortality and cardiovascular disease have shown no or only small differences between the different groups.[171,172] Selection of an appropriate drug or drug combination in patients with hypertension will obviously depend on many factors other than just the haemodynamic effects. Nevertheless, it should always be remembered that treatment of hypertension is not just a question of reducing BP. The haemodynamic aspects should always be recognized in patients who develop side effects related to the haemodynamic effects of a certain drug. Selection of a compound from another class of antihypertensive agents may sometimes solve the problem, but since most patients will need more than one class of drug, appropriate selection of the combined therapy is important.

References

1. Man in 't Veld AJ, Meiracker AH. Effects of antihypertensive drugs on cardiovascular haemodynamics. In: Laragh JH, Brenner BM, eds. *Hypertension pathophysiology. Diagnosis and management.* New York: Raven Press; 1995:2753–2763.
2. ALLHAT Officers and Coordinators for the ALLHAT Collaborative Research Group. Major cardiovascular events in hypertensive patients randomized to doxazosin vs chlorthalidone: the antihypertensive and lipid-lowering treatment to prevent heart attack trial (ALLHAT). *JAMA* 2000;283:1967–1975.
3. Psaty BM, Heckbert SR, Koepsell TD, et al. The risk of myocardial infarction associated with antihypertensive drug therapies. *JAMA* 1995;274:620–625.
4. Furberg CD, Psaty BM, Meyer JV. Nifedipine: dose-related increase in mortality in patients with coronary heart diseases. *Circulation* 1995;92:1326–1331.
5. Folkow B. Physiological aspects of primary hypertension. *Physiol Rev* 1982;62:347–504.
6. Conway J. Haemodynamic aspects of essential hypertension in humans. *Physiol Rev* 1984;64:617–660.
7. Lund-Johansen P. Haemodynamics of essential hypertension. In: Swales DJ, ed. *Textbook of hypertension.* London: Blackwell Scientific Publications; 1994:61–76.
8. Folkow B. Considering "the mind" as a primary cause. In: Birkenhäger WH, Robertson JIS, Zanchetti A, eds. *Handbook of hypertension. Hypertension in the twentieth century.* Edinburgh: Elsevier; 2004:59–80.
9. Lund-Johansen P. Haemodynamic concepts of hypertension: cardiac output versus peripheral vascular resistance. In: Birkenhäger WH, Robertson JIS, Zanchetti A, eds. *Handbook of hypertension. Hypertension in the twentieth century.* Edinburgh: Elsevier; 2004:151–171.
10. Jennings GL, Esler M, Korner PI. Effect of prolonged treatment on haemodynamics of essential hypertension before and after autonomic block. *Lancet* 1980;2:166.
11. Christensen KL, Mulvany MJ. Vasodilatation, not hypotension, improves resistance vessels design during treatment of essential hypertension: a literary survey. *J Hypertens* 2001;19:1001–1006.
12. Kaplan NM. Diuretics in the therapy of hypertension. In: Hunt JC, ed. *Hypertension update: mechanisms, epidemiology, evaluation, management.* Bloomfield: Health learning systems; 1980:209.
13. Mudge GH. Diuretics and other agents employed in the mobilization of edema fluid. In: Goodman LS, Gilman A, eds. *The pharmacological basis of therapeutics* New York: MacMillan Publishing; 1976:817.
14. Jounela AJ, Lilja M, Lumme J, et al. Relation between low dose of hydrochlorothiazide, antihypertensive effect and adverse effects. *Blood Pressure* 1994;3:231–235.

15. Crosley AP, Cullen RC, White D, et al. Studies of the mechanism of action of chlorothiazide in cardiac and renal disorders. *J Lab Clin Med* 1960;55:182.

16. Villareal H, Exaire JE, Revollo A, et al. Effects of chlorothiazide on systemic haemodynamics in essential hypertension. *Circulation* 1962;36:405.

17. Dustan H, Cumming CR, Cocoran AC. A mechanism of chlorothiazide-enchanced effectiveness of antihypertensive ganglioplegic drugs. *Circulation* 1959;19:300.

18. Frohlich ED, Schnaper HW, Wilson IM, et al. Hemodynamic alterations in hypertensive patients due to chlorothiazide. *N Engl J Med* 1960;262:1261.

19. Greene ED, Boltax AJ, Scherr ES. Acute effects of intravenous chlorothiazide upon cardiovascular hemodynamics. *Am Heart J* 1961;62:659.

20. Van Brummelen P, Man in 't Veld AJ, Schalekamp MADH. Hemodynamic changes during long-term thiazide treatment of essential hypertension in responders and nonresponders. *Clin Pharmacol Ther* 1980;27:328.

21. Hansen J. Hydrochlorothiazide in the treatment of hypertension. *Acta Med Scand* 1968;183:317.

22. Leth A. Changes in plasma and extracellular fluid volumes in patients with essential hypertension during long-term treatment with hydrochlorothiazide. *Circulation* 1970; 42:479.

23. Varnauskas E, Cramaer G, Malmcrona R, et al. Effect of chlorothiazide on blood pressure and blood flow at rest and on exercise in patients with arterial hypertension. *Clin Sci* 1961;20:406.

24. Eckstein JW, Wendling MG, Abboud FM. Effect of prolonged-treatment with chlorothiazide on cardiovascular responses to norepinephrine. *J Lab Clin Med* 1964;64:853.

25. Conway J, Lauwers P. Hemodynamic and hypotensive effects of long-term therapy with chlorothiazide. *Circulation* 1960;21:21.

26. Lund-Johansen P. Hemodynamic changes in long-term diuretic therapy of essential hypertension. *Acta Med Scand* 1970;187:509.

27. Wilson IM, Freis ED. Relationship between plasma and extracellular fluid volume depletion and the antihypertensive effect of chlorothiazide. *Circulation* 1959;20:1028.

28. Dustan HP, Tarazi RC, Bravo EL. False tolerance to antihypertensive drugs. In: Sambhi MP, ed. *Systemic effects of antihypertensive agents*. New York: Symposia Specialists; 1976:51.

29. Tarazi RC. Diuretic drugs: mechanisms of antihypertensive action. In: Onesti G, Kim KE, Moyer JH, eds. *Hypertension: mechanisms and management*. New York: Grune and Stratton; 1973:251.

30. Freis ED. Hemodynamic changes during acute and chronic administration of thiazide diuretics. In: Sambhi MP, ed. *Systemic effects of antihypertensive agents*. Symposia specialists: New York; 1976:41.

31. Van Brummelen P, Woerlee M, Schalekamp MADH. Long-term versus short-term effects of hydrochlorothiazide on renal haemodynamics in essential hypertension. *Clin Sci* 1979;56:463.

32. Atkins LL. Long-term use of furosemide alone in hypertension. In: Onesti G, Kim KE, Moyer JH, eds. *Hypertension: mechanisms and management*. New York: Grune and Stratton; 1973:273.

33. Hesse B, Nielsen I, Lund-Jacobsen H. The early effects of intravenous frusemide on central haemodynamics, venous tone and plasma rennin activity. *Clin Sci Mol Med* 1975;49:551.

34. Ramsey LE, Silas JH, Freestone S. Diuretic treatment of resistant hypertension. *Br Med J* 1980;281:1101.

35. Ganguly A, Luetscher JA. Spironolactone therapy in primary aldosteronism diagnostic and therapeutic implications. In: Sambhi MP, ed. *Systemic effects of antihypertensive agents*. New York: Symposia Specialists; 1976:383.

36. Weinberger MH, Grim E. Effects of spironolactone and hydrochlorothiazide on blood pressure and plasma renin activity in hypertension. In: Sambhi MP, ed. *Systemic effects of antihypertensive agents*. New York: Symposia Specialists; 1976:481.

37. Van Zwieten PA. The central action of antihypertensive drugs mediated via central receptors. *J Pharm Pharmacol* 1973;25:89.

38. Nickerson M, Collier B. Drugs inhibiting adrenergic nerves and structures innervated by them. In: Goodman LS, Gilman A, eds. *The pharmacological basis of therapeutics*. New York: MacMillan Publishing; 1976:533.

39. Henning M. New trends in pharmacology. *Acta Med Scand* 1977;606(Suppl 87).

40. Lund-Johansen P. Haemodynamic effects of antihypertensive agents. In: Freis ED, ed. *The treatment of hypertension*. Lancaster: MTP Press; 1978:61.

41. Scriabine A. Methyldopa. In: Scriabine A, ed. *Pharmacology of antihypertensive drugs*. New York: Raven Press; 1980:43.

42. Lund-Johansen P. Hemodynamic effects of antihypertensive agents. In: Birkenhäger WH, Robertson JIS, eds. *Handbook of hypertension. Clinical pharmacology of antihypertensive drugs*. Amsterdam: Elsevier; 1988:41.

43. Prichard BNC, Cruickshank JM, Graham BR. Beta-adrenergic blocking drugs in the treatment of hypertension. *Blood Pressure* 2001;10:366–386.

44. Prichard BNC, Gillam PMS. The use of propranolol in the treatment of hypertension. *Br Med J* 1964;2:725.

45. Lund-Johansen P. The effect of beta-blocker therapy on chronic hemodynamics. *Prim Cardiol* 1980;6(Suppl 1):20.

46. Franz IW. Differential antihypertensive effect of acebutolol and hydrochlorothiazide/amiloride hydrochloride combination on elevated exercise blood pressures in hypertensive patients. *Am J Cardiol* 1980;46:301.

47. Lund-Johansen P. Central haemodynamic effects of beta-blockers in hypertension. A comparison between atenolol, metoprolol, timolol, penbutolol, alprenolol, pindolol, and bunitrolol. *Eur Heart J* 1983; (Suppl D):1.

48. Johnsson G, Guzman M, Bergman H, et al. The haemodynamic effects of alprenolol and propranolol at rest and during exercise in hypertensive patients. *Pharmacol Clin* 1969;2:34.

49. Hansson L. Beta-adrenergic blockade in essential hypertension. *Acta Med Scand* 1973; (Suppl 7): 550.

50. Tarazi RC, Dustan HP. Beta adrenergic blockade in hypertension. *Am J Cardiol* 1972;29:633.

51. Ulrych M, Frohlich ED, Dustan HP, et al. Immediate hemodynamic effects of beta-adrenergic blockade with propranolol in normotensive and hypertensive men. *Circulation* 1968;37:411.

52. Franciosa JA, Freis ED, Conway J. Antihypertensive and hemodynamic properties of the new beta adrenergic blocking agent timolol. *Circulation* 1973;48:118.

53. Frohlich ED, Tarazi RC, Dustan HP, et al. The paradox of beta-adrenergic blockade in hypertension. *Circulation* 1968;37:417.

54. Simon G, Kiowski W, Julius S. Effect of systemic autonomic inhibition on the hemodynamic response to antihypertensive therapy with timolol. *Int J Clin Pharmacol Biofarm* 1979;17:507.

55. Ferlinz J, Easthope JL, Hughes D, et al. Right ventricular performance in essential hypertension after beta-blockade. *Br Heart J* 1981;46:23.

56. Lydtin H, Kusus T, Daniel W, et al. Propranolol therapy in essential hypertension. *Am Heart J* 1972;83:589.

57. Dunn FG, De Carvalho JGR, Frohlich ED. Hemodynamic, reflexive, and metabolic alterations induced by acute and chronic timolol therapy in hypertensive man. *Circulation* 1978;37:140.

58. Lund-Johansen P. Hemodynamic long-term effects of timolol at rest and during exercise in essential hypertension. *Acta Med Scand* 1976;199:263.

59. Aronow WS, Ferlinz J, Del Vicario M, et al. Effect of timolol versus propranolol on hypertension and hemodynamics. *Circulation* 1976;54:47.

60. Pedersen EB. Abnormal renal haemodynamics during exercising young patients with mild essential hypertension without treatment and during long-term propranolol therapy. *Scand J Clin Lab Invest* 1978;38:567.

61. Lund-Johansen P. Hemodynamic changes at rest and during exercise in long-term beta-blocker therapy of essential hypertension. *Acta Med Scand* 1974;195:117.

62. Atterhög JH, Dunèr H, Pernow B. Haemodynamic effects of pindolol in hypertensive patients. *Acta Med Scand* 1977;606(Suppl 55).

63. Reybrouck T, Amery A, Billiet L. Hemodynamic response to graded exercise after chronic beta-adrenergic blockade. *J Appl Physiol* 1977;42:133.

64. Lund-Johansen P. Hemodynamic long-term effects of a new beta-blocker atenolol (ICI 66082). *Br J Clin Pharmacol* 1976;3:445.

65. Ibrahim MM, Madkour MA, Mossallan R. Effect of atenolol on left ventricular function in hypertensive patients. *Clin Sci* 1980;59:473.

66. Lund-Johansen P, Ohm O-J. Hemodynamic long-term effects of metoprolol at rest and during exercise in essential hypertension. *Br J Clin Pharmacol* 1977;4:147.

67. Lund-Johansen P. Hemodynamic consequences of long-term beta-blocker therapy: a 5-year follow-up study of atenolol. *J Cardiovasc* 1979;1:487.

68. Trap-Jensen J, Clausen JP, Noer I, et al. The effects of beta-adrenoceptor blockers on cardiac output, liver blood flow and skeletal muscle blood flow in hypertensive patients. *Acta Physiol Scand* 1976;440(Suppl):30.

69. Kaiser P Physical performance and muscle metabolism during beta-adrenergic blockade in man. *Acta Physiol Scand* 1984; (Suppl 536):1.

70. Lundborg P, Åström H, Bengtsson C, et al. Effect of beta-adrenoceptor blockade on exercise performance and metabolism. *Clin Sci* 1981;61:299.

71. Lund-Johansen P. Exercise and antihypertensive therapy. *Am Heart J* 1987; (Suppl 59):98A.

72. Taylor SH, Sutherland GR, MacKenzie GJ, et al. The circulatory effects of intravenous phentolamine in man. *Circulation* 1965;31:741.

73. Constantine JW. Analysis of the hypotensive action of prazosin. In: Cotton DWK, ed. *Prazosin - evaluation of a new antihypertensive agent.* Amsterdam: Excerpta Medica; 1974:16.

74. Davey MJ. Relevant features of the pharmacology of prazosin. *J Cardiovasc Pharmacol* 1980;2 (suppl 3):287.

75. Lund-Johansen P. Haemodynamic changes at rest and during exercise in long-term prazosin therapy of essential hypertension. In: Cotton DWK, ed. *Prazosin -Evaluation of a new antihypertensive agent.* Amsterdam: Excerpta Medica; 1974:43.

76. De Leeuw PW, Wester A, Strienstra R, et al. Hemodynamic and endocrinological studies with prazosin in essential hypertension. In: Lund-Johansen P, Mason DT, eds. *Recent advances in hypertension and congestive heart failure - prazosin.* Amsterdam: Excerpta Medica; 1978:11.

77. Chrysant SG, Miller RF, Brown JL, et al. Long-term hemodynamic and metabolic effects of trimazosin in essential hypertension. *Clin Pharmacol Ther* 1981;30:600.

78. Pool PE, Seagren SC, Salel AF. Clinical hemodynamic profile of trimazosin in hypertension. *Am Heart J* 1983;106:1237.

79. Lund-Johansen P, Omvik P, Haugland H. Acute and chronic haemodynamic effects of doxazosin in hypertension at rest and during exercise. *Br J Clin Pharmacol* 1986;21:45.

80. Lund-Johansen P, Kirby RS. Effect of doxazosin GITS on blood pressure in hypertensive and normotensive patients: a review of hypertensive and BPH studies. *Blood Press* 2003; (Suppl 1): 5–13.

81. Louis WJ, McNeil JJ, Drummer OH. Labetalol and other vasodilator/β-blocking drugs. In: Birkenhäger WH, Robertson JIS, eds. *Handbook of hypertension. Clinical pharmacology of antihypertensive drugs.* Amsterdam: Elsevier; 1988:244–273.

82. Rønne-Rasmussen JO, Andersen GS, Bowal Jensen N, et al. Acute effect of intravenous labetalol in the treatment of systemic arterial hypertension. *Br J Clin Pharmacol* 1976;3 (suppl):805.

83. Omvik P, Lund-Johansen P. Acute hemodynamic effects of labetalol in severe hypertension. *J Cardiovasc Pharmacol* 1982;4:915.

84. Fagard F, Amery A, Reybrouck T, et al. Response of the systemic and pulmonary circulation to alpha- and beta-receptor blockade (labetalol) at rest and during exercise in hypertensive patients. *Circulation* 1979;60:1214.

85. Lund-Johansen P, Bakke OM. Haemodynamic effects and plasma concentrations of labetalol during long-term treatment of essential hypertension. *Br J Clin Pharmacol* 1979;7:169.

86. Lund-Johansen P. Pharmacology of combined a-ß-blockade II. Hemodynamic effects of labetalol. *Drugs* 1984;28(suppl 2):35.

87. Rasmussen S, Nielsen PE. Blood pressure, body fluid volumes and glomerular filtration rate during treatment with labetalol in essential hypertension. *Br J Clin Pharmacol* 1981;12:349.

88. Omvik P, Lund-Johansen P. Acute haemodynamic effects of carvedilol in essential hypertension at rest and during exercise. *Eur Heart J* 1991;12:736–740.

89. Eggertsen R, Andren L, Sivertsson R, et al. Acute haemodynamic effects of carvedilol (BM 14190), a new combined beta-adrenoceptor blocker and precapillary vasodilating agent, in hypertensive patients. *Eur J Clin Pharmacol* 1984;27:19.

90. Lund-Johansen P, Omvik P. Chronic haemodynamic effects of carvedilol in essential hypertension at rest and during exercise. *Eur Heart J* 1992;13:281–286.

91. Dargie HJ, Colucci WS, Ford I, et al. Effect of carvedilol on outcome after myocardial infarction in patients with left-ventricular dysfunction: The CAPRICORN randomised trial. *Lancet* 2001;357:1385–1390.

92. Gross F. Drugs. Drugs acting on arteriolar smooth muscle (vasodilator drugs). In: Gross F, ed. *Antihypertensive agents.* Berlin: Springer Verlag; 1977:397.

93. Hansson L, Oleander R, Aberg H, et al. Treatment of hypertension with propranolol and hydralazine. *Acta Med Scand* 1971;190:531.

94. Sannerstedt R, Stenberg J, Johnsson G, et al. Hemodynamic interference of alprenolol with dihydralazine in normal and hypertensive man. *Am J Cardiol* 1971;28:316.

95. Zachest R, Reece P. Hydralazine. In: Birkenhäger WH, Robertson JIS, eds. *Handbook of hypertension.* Amsterdam: Elsevier; 1988:341–381.

96. Koch-Weser J. Drug therapy: hydralazine. *N Engl J Med* 1976;295:320.

97. Mroczek WJ, Leibel BA, Davidov M, et al. The importance of the rapid administration of diazoxide in accelerated hypertension. *N Eng J Med* 1971;285:603.

98. Bhatia SK, Frohlich ED. Hemodynamic comparison of agents useful in hypertensive emergencies. *Am Heart J* 1973;85:367.

99. Bryan RK, Hoobler SW, Rosenzweig J, et al. Effect of minoxidil on blood pressure and hemodynamics in severe hypertension. *Am J Cardiol* 1977;39:796.

100. Dargie H, Rowland E, Krikler D. Role of calcium antagonists in cardiac therapy. *Br Heart J* 1981;46:8.

101. Aoki K, Kawaguchi Y, Sato K, et al. Clinical and pharmacological properties of calcium antagonists in essential hypertension in humans and spontaneously hypertensive rats. *J Cardiovasc Pharmacol* 1982;4:298.

102. Opie LH.*Calcium antagonists and cardiovascular disease.* New York: Raven Press; 1984:1–365.

103. Aoki K, Sato K, Kawaguchi Y. Increased cardiovascular responses to norepinephrine and calcium antagonists in essential hypertension compared with normotension in humans. *J Cardiovasc Pharmacol* 1985;7(suppl 6):S182.

104. Halperin AK, Cubeddu LX. The role of calcium channel blockers in the treatment of hypertension. *Am Heart J* 1986;111:363.

105. Lund-Johansen P. Hemodynamic effects of calcium antagonists in hypertension. In: Epstein M, ed. *Calcium antagonists in clinical medicine*. Philadelphia: Hanley & Belfus; 2002:317–337.

106. Fleckenstein A, Frey M, Fleckenstein-Grün G. Antihypertensive and arterial anticalcinotic effects of calcium antagonists. *Am J Cardiol* 1986;57:1D.

107. Doyle AE, Anavekar SN, Oliver LE. A clinical trial of verapamil in treatment of hypertension. In: Zanchetti A, Krikler DM, eds. *Calcium antagonism in cardiovascular therapy: experiences with verapamil*. Amsterdam: Excerpta Medica; 1981:252.

108. Leonetti G, Sala C, Bianchi C, et al. Antihypertensive and renal effects of orally administered verapamil. *Eur J Clin Pharmacol* 1980;18:175.

109. Gould BA, Mann S, Kieso H, et al. The 24-hour ambulatory blood pressure profile with verapamil. *Circulation* 1982;65:22.

110. Muiesan G, Agabiti-Rosei E, Alicandri C, et al. Influence of verapamil on catacholamines, renin and aldosterone in essential hypertensive patients. In: Zanchetti A, Krikler DM, eds. *Calcium antagonism in cardiovascular therapy: experiences with verapamil*. Amsterdam: Excerpta Medica; 1981:238.

111. Lund-Johansen P. Hemodynamic long-term effects of verapamil in essential hypertension at rest and during exercise. *Acta Med Scand* 1984;681:109.

112. Hanrath P, Kremer P. Effect of verapamil on abnormal left ventricular diastolic performance in patients with secondary left ventricular hypertrophy due to systemic hypertension. In: Zanchetti A, Krikler DM, eds. *Calcium antagonism in cardiovascular therapy: experiences with verapamil*. Amsterdam: Excerpta Medica; 1981:222.

113. De Leeuw PW, Smout AJ PM, Willemse PJ, et al. Effects of verapamil in hypertensive patients. In: Zanchetti A, Krikler DM, eds. *Calcium antagonism in cardiovascular therapy: experiences with verapamil*. Amsterdam: Excerpta Medica; 1981:233.

114. Chaffman M, Brogden RN. Diltiazem: A review of its pharmacological properties and therapeutic efficacy. *Drugs* 1985;29:387.

115. Aoki K, Sato K, Kondo S, et al. Hypotensive effects of diltiazem to normals and essential hypertension. *Eur J Clin Pharmacol* 1983;25:475.

116. Safar ME, Simon ACH, Levenson JA, et al. Haemodynamic effects of diltiazem in hypertension. *Circ Res* 1983;52(suppl 1):169.

117. Klein W, Brandt D, Vrecko K, et al. Role of calcium antagonists in treatment of essential hypertension. *Circ Res* 1983;52(suppl 1):174.

118. Pool PE, Seagren SC, Salel AF, et al. Effects of diltiazem on serum lipids, exercise performance and blood pressure: randomized, double-blind, placebo-controlled evaluation for systemic hypertension. *Am J Cardiol* 1985;56:86H.

119. Lund-Johansen P, Omvik P. Effect of long-term diltiazem treatment on central haemodynamics and exercise endurance in essential hypertension. *Eur Heart J* 1990;11:543–551.

120. Yamakado T, Oonishi N, Nakao T, et al. Effects of nifedipine and diltiazem on hemodynamic responses at rest and during exercise in hypertensive patients. *Jpn Circ J* 1985;49:415.

121. Olivan MT, Bartorelli C, Polese A, et al. Treatment of hypertension with nifedipine, a calcium antagonist agent. *Circulation* 1979;59:1056.

122. Soto ME, Thibonnier M, Sire O. Antihypertensive and hormonal effects of single oral doses of captopril and nifedipine in essential hypertension. *Eur J Clin Pharmacol* 1981;20:157.

123. Lederballe Pedersen O, Christensen NJ, Rämsch KD. Comparison of acute effects of nifedipine in normotensive and hypertensive man. *J Cardiovasc Pharmacol* 1980;2:357.

124. Bühler FR, Bolli P, Erne P, et al. Position of calcium antagonists in antihypertensive therapy. *J Cardiovasc Pharmacol* 1985;7(suppl 4):S21.

125. Kuwajima I, Ueda K, Kamata C, et al. A study on the effects of nifedipine in hypertensive crises and severe hypertension. *Jpn Heart J* 1978;19:455.

126. Houston MC. Treatment of hypertensive urgencies and emergencies with nifedipine. *Am Heart J* 1986;3:963.

127. Lund-Johansen P, Omvik P. Haemodynamic effects of nifedipine in essential hypertension at rest and during exercise. *J Hypertens* 1983;1:159.

128. Lund-Johansen P, Omvik P, Haugland H. Acute and chronic hemodynamic effects of nisoldipine in essential hypertension at rest and during exercise. *Acta Med Scand* 1986; 714(suppl):183.

129. Lund-Johansen P, Omvik P, White W, et al. Long-term haemodynamic effects of amlodipine at rest and during exercise in essential hypertension. *J Hypertens* 1990;8:1129–1136.

130. Franz I-W, Wiewel D. Antihypertensive effects on blood pressure at rest and during exercise of calcium antagonists, beta-receptor blockers, and their combination in hypertensive patients. *J Cardiovasc Pharmacol* 1984;6:1037.

131. Clement DL, De Pue NY. Effect of felodipine and metoprolol on muscle and skin arteries in hypertensive patients. *Drugs* 1985;29(suppl 2):137.

132. Lorimer AR, McAlpine HM, Rae AP, et al. Effects of felodipine on rest and exercise heart rate and blood pressure in hypertensive patients. *Drugs* 1985;29(suppl 2):154.

133. Andrèsdòttir MB, van Hamersvelt HW, van Helden MJ, et al. Ankle edema formation during treatment with the calcium channel blockers lacidipine and amlodipine: A single-centre study. *J Cardiovasc Pharmacol* 2000;35(suppl 1):525–530.

134. Lund-Johansen P, Stranden E, Helberg S, et al. Quantification of leg oedema in postmenopausal hypertensive patients treated with lercanidipine or amlodipine. *J Hypertens* 2003;21:1003–1010.

135. Laragh JH. Position paper: the renin-angiotensin-aldosterone system for blood pressure regulation and for subdividing patients to reveal and analyse different forms of hypertension. In: Laragh JH, Bühler FR, Seldin DW, eds. *Frontiers in hypertension research*. New York: Springer Verlag; 1981:183.

136. Heel RC, Brogden RN, Speight TM, et al. Captopril: a preliminary review of its pharmacological properties and therapeutic efficacy. *Drugs* 1980;20:409.

137. Streeten DHP, Anderson Jr. GH. Angiotensin-receptor blocking drugs. In: Birkenhäger WH, Robertson JIS, eds. *Handbook of hypertension. Clinical pharmacology of antihypertensive drugs*. Amsterdam: Elsevier; 1988:274–300.

138. Johnston CI. Angiotensin converting enzyme inhibitors. In: Birkenhäger WH, Robertson JIS, eds. *Handbook of hypertension. Clinical pharmacology of antihypertensive drugs*. Amsterdam: Elsevier; 1988:301–326.

139. Liebau G, Riegger AJG, Steilner H. Hemodynamic effects of captopril in patients with congestive heart failure and hypertension. In: Brunner HR, Gross F, eds. *Recent advances in hypertension therapy: captopril*. Amsterdam: Excerpta Medica; 1980:76.

140. Tarazi RC, Bravo EL, Fouad FM, et al. Hemodynamic and volume changes associated with captopril. *Hypertension* 1980;2:576.

141. Fagard R, Bulpitt C, Lijnen P, et al. Response of the systemic and pulmonary circulation to converting-enzyme inhibition (captopril) at rest and during exercise in hypertensive patients. *Circulation* 1982;65:33.

142. Sullivan JM, Ginsburg BA, Ratts TE, et al. Hemodynamic and antihypertensive effects of captopril, an orally active angiotensin converting enzyme inhibitor. *Hypertens* 1979;1:397.

143. De Bruyn JHB, Man in 't Veld AJ, Wenting GJ, et al. Haemodynamic profile of captopril treatment in various forms of hypertension. *Eur J Clin Pharmacol* 1981;20:163.

144. Omvik P, Lund-Johansen P. Combined captopril and hydrochlorothiazide therapy in severe hypertension: long-term hemodynamic changes at rest and during exercise. *J Hypertens* 1984;2:73–80.

145. Todd PA, Heel RC. Enalapril. A review of its pharmacodynamic and pharmacokinetic properties, and therapeutic use in hypertension and congestive heart failure. *Drugs* 1986;31:198.

146. Dunn FG, Oigman W, Ventura HO, et al. Enalapril improves systemic and renal haemodynamics and allows regression of left ventricular mass in essential hypertension. *Am J Cardiol* 1983;53:105.

147. Fouad FM, Tarazi RC, Bravo EL. Cardiac and haemodynamic effects of enalapril. *J Hypertens* 1983;1(suppl 1):135.

148. McFate Smith W, Kulaga SF, Moncloa F, et al. Overall tolerance and safety of enalapril. *J Hypertens* 1984;2(suppl 2):113.

149. Gavras H, Waeber B, Gravras I, et al. Antihypertensive effect of the new oral angiotensin converting enzyme inhibitor 'MK-421'. *Lancet* 1981;2:543.

150. Lund-Johansen P, Omvik P. Long-term hemodynamic effects of enalapril at rest and during exercise in essential hypertension. *Scand J Urol Nephrol* 1984; (Suppl 79):87.

151. Agabiti-Rosei E, Muiesan ML. Hypertension and the heart: from left ventricular hypertrophy to ischemia to congestive heart failure. In: Birkenhäger WH, Robertson JIS, Zanchetti A, eds. *Handbook of hypertension. Hypertension in the twentieth century*. Amsterdam: Elsevier; 2004:339–366.

152. Remme WJ, Svedberg K. Guidelines for the diagnosis and treatment of chronic heart failure. *Eur Heart J* 2001;22:1527–1560.

153. Burnier M, Brunner Hr. Comparative antihypertensive effects of angiotensin II receptor antagonists. *J Am Soc Nephrol* 1999;10(suppl 12):S278–S282.

154. Sebastian JL, MaKinney WP, Kaufmann J, et al. Angiotensin-converting enzyme inhibitors and cough. *Chest* 1991;99:36–39.

155. Dahlöf B, Devereux RB, Kjeldsen SE, et al. Cardiovascular morbidity and mortality in the losartan intervention for endpoint reduction in hypertension study (LIFE); a randomised trial against atenolol. *Lancet* 2002;359:995–1003.
156. Julius S, Kjeldsen SE, Weber M, et al. Outcomes in hypertensive patients at high cardiovascular risk treated with regimens based on valsartan or amlodipine: the VALUE randomised trial. *Lancet* 2004;363:2022–2031.
157. Lithell H, Hansson L, Skoog I, et al. The study on cognition and prognosis in the elderly (SCOPE): principal results of a randomized double-blind intervention trial. *J Hypertens* 2003;21:875–886.
158. Omvik P, Gerdts E, Myking OI, et al. Long-term central haemodynamic effects at rest and during exercise of losartan in essential hypertension. *Am Heart J* 2000;140:624–630.
159. Devereux RB, Dahlöf B, Gerdts E, et al. Regression of hypertensive left ventricular hypertrophy by losartan compared with atenolol: the losartan intervention for endpoint reduction in hypertension (LIFE) trial. *Circulation* 2004;110(11):1456–1462.
160. Moriwaki H, Uno H, Nagakane Y, et al. Losartan, an angiotensin II (AT(1)) receptor antagonist, preserves cerebral blood flow in hypertensive patients with history of stroke. *J Hum Hypertens* 2000;18(10):683–699.
161. Kaplan NM. Tailoring antihypertensive therapy to the individual patient. In: Birkenhäger WH, Robertson JIS, Zanchetti A, eds. *Handbook of hypertension. Hypertension in the twentieth century*. Amsterdam: Elsevier; 2004:541–554.
162. Lund-Johansen P. Blood pressure and heart rate responses during physical stress in hypertension: modifications by drug treatment. *Eur Heart J* 1999;1(suppl B):10–17.
163. Staessen J, Fagard I, Thijs I, et al. Randomised double-blind comparison of placebo and active treatment for older patients with isolated systolic hypertension in Europe. *Lancet* 1997;350:757–764.
164. Kostis JB, Davis BR, Cutler J, et al. Prevention of heart failure by antihypertensive drug treatment in older persons with isolated systolic hypertension. *JAMA* 1997;273:212–216.
165. Medical Research Council Working Party. MRC trial of treatment of mild hypertension principal results. *Br Med J* 1985;291:97.
166. IPPPSH Collaborative Group. Cardiovascular and risk factors in a randomized trial of treatment based on the beta-blocker oxprenolol: the International Prospective Primary Prevention Study in Hypertension. *J Hypertens* 1985;3:379.
167. The Norwegian Multicenter Study Group. Timolol-induced reduction in mortality and reinfarction in patients surviving acute myocardial infarction. *N Engl J Med* 1981;304:801.
168. Hampton JR. Beta-blockers in the prevention of myocardial infarction. *Practitioner* 1984;228:55.
169. Aronow WS. Might losartan reduce sudden cardiac death in diabetic patients with hypertension? *Lancet* 2003;362:591–592.
170. Carlberg B, Samuelsson O, Lindholm LH. Atenolol in hypertension: is it a wise choice? *Lancet* 2004;364:1684–1689.
171. Turnbull F. Blood Pressure Lowering Treatment Trialists' Collaboration. Effects of different blood-pressure-lowering regimens on major cardiovascular events: results of prespectively-designed overviews of randomised trials. *Lancet* 2003;362:1527–1535.
172. Cushman WC. Are there benefits to specific antihypertensive drug therapy? *Am J Hypertens* 2003;16(suppl 11):31–35.

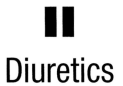

Diuretics

5 | Thiazide and loop diuretics

Monique Pratt-Ubanama and Suzanne Oparil

INTRODUCTION

Diuretics have been used to treat essential hypertension for more than 30 years and are the most widely prescribed class of antihypertensive agents.[1] Diuretics are classified according to their primary site of action within the renal tubule, starting from the proximal portion and moving to the collecting duct.[2] The major classes of diuretics are: (1) carbonic anhydrase inhibitors, which act on the proximal convoluted tubule (PCT) and have limited antihypertensive effect, (2) loop diuretics, which act on the thick ascending limb (TAL) of Henle's loop, (3) thiazide and thiazide-like compounds, which act on the distal convoluted tubule (DCT) and (4) potassium-sparing agents, which act on the collecting duct (CD) (Fig. 5.1). Thiazide and thiazide-like diuretics are the most commonly used diuretic agents in the treatment of hypertension and are recommended as first-line therapy or as a component of multi-drug therapy for most patients.[3] Loop diuretics have potent natriuretic/diuretic effects, but limited antihypertensive efficacy when compared with the thiazides. These agents are usually reserved for patients with chronic kidney disease, heart failure or hypertensive emergencies, in whom thiazide diuretics are rarely effective.[4] This chapter will focus on the thiazide and thiazide-like diuretics and the loop diuretics because the potassium-sparing agents are covered elsewhere and the carbonic anhydrase inhibitors are rarely used in the treatment of hypertension. Clinical data on the antihypertensive efficacy and the adverse effects of diuretics, as well as outcome data on the use of diuretics in hypertension, will be emphasized.

RENAL REGULATION OF SODIUM CHLORIDE BALANCE: THE SUBSTRATE OF DIURETIC ACTION

The nephron is the basic urine-forming unit of the kidney, consisting of a filtering apparatus, the glomerulus, connected to a long tubular portion.[5] An ultra-filtrate of plasma (tubular fluid) is delivered sequentially to the PCT, Henle's

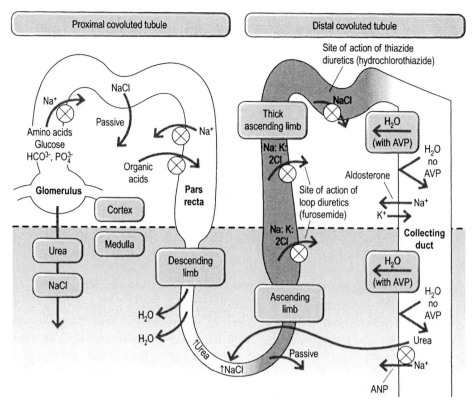

Fig. 5.1 Transport functions of the various anatomic segments of the mammalian nephron. Sites of action of thiazide and loop diuretics and AVP are shown. *(Reproduced with permission of McGraw-Hill Companies, Inc. from ref. (6).)*

loop, the DCT, the connecting tubule and the CD (Fig. 5.1).[2,6] Each segment of the renal tubule reabsorbs a fraction of the delivered sodium chloride (NaCl). Approximately 50–55% of filtered Na^+ is reabsorbed in the PCT. Most of the filtered bicarbonate (HCO_3^-), amino acids, glucose and phosphate (PO_4^{3-}) are also reabsorbed in the PCT.[6] The pars recta of the PCT is capable of active transport of NaCl independent of organic solute transport. As the tubular fluid enters the thin descending limb of Henle's loop, approximately 35–40% of filtered NaCl is reabsorbed.[5] This segment is highly permeable to H_2O and impermeable to NaCl because of its inability to actively transport NaCl from the tubular lumen into the interstitium. Water is, therefore, passively reabsorbed as the tubular fluid approaches the bend of Henle's loop. The resultant hypertonic tubular fluid with a greater NaCl concentration than the surrounding interstitium enters the thin ascending limb of Henle's loop. This segment is largely impermeable to H_2O and urea, but highly permeable to NaCl and permits passive outward diffusion of NaCl from the tubular lumen into the surrounding interstitium.[6]

As the tubular fluid enters the TAL of Henle's loop, NaCl is actively transported across this H_2O-impermeable segment via the $Na^+{:}K^+{:}2Cl^-$ cotransporter (NKCC2). Thus, the tubular fluid becomes dilute and the medullary interstitium hypertonic. The tubular fluid that enters the DCT is hypoosmotic irrespective of the final osmolality of the urine. At the DCT, active transport of NaCl from the tubular lumen to the surrounding interstitium occurs via a $Na^+:Cl^-$ (NCC) cotransporter. The tubular fluid then enters the collecting duct (CD), the primary site where arginine vasopressin (AVP), also known as antidiuretic hormone (ADH), exerts its primary effect. If ADH is absent, the CD is H_2O-impermeable and the hypotonic tubular fluid becomes dilute urine. However, in the presence of ADH, H_2O is reabsorbed from the tubular lumen into the surrounding interstitium and then into the blood, resulting in hypertonic urine.

The renal tubular epithelium, like other epithelial cells, has an apical surface and a basolateral surface held together by tight junctions (Fig. 5.2). In general, solutes can be reabsorbed or secreted across renal tubular cells via the transcellular pathway or between cells by moving across the tight junctions and intercellular spaces by way of the paracellular pathway.[7] Na^+ moves through both routes, although most is transported via the transcellular pathway.

For reabsorption to occur, NaCl must cross the apical and basolateral surfaces of the renal tubular epithelium and enter the peritubular interstitium. This transcellular absorption requires transporters or channels in the apical and basolateral membranes because charged ions cannot pass freely through the lipid membrane bilayer.[5] The basolateral transport pathway is the same for each of the renal tubular segments, namely the $Na^+:K^+:ATPase$, which actively transports 3 Na^+ out of the cell into the peritubular interstitium, and 2 K^+ ions into the cell (Figs 5.2 & 5.3). In contrast, the transport of ions from tubular fluid into cells across the apical surface is mediated by distinct pathways in different tubular segments. At the apical membrane of the DCT cell, Na^+ enters via a $Na^+:Cl^-$ cotransporter (NCC) (Fig. 5.2). It is this entry mechanism on the apical side of the DCT cell that is affected by thiazide and thiazide-like

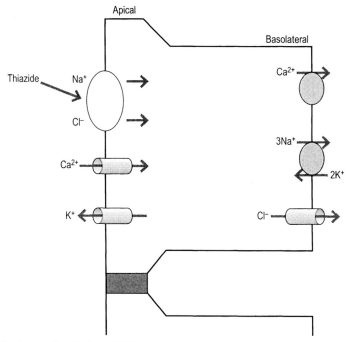

Fig. 5.2 Distal convoluted tubule (DCT) cell showing sites of action of thiazide and thiazide-like drugs. *(Modified with permission of Blackwell Publishing from ref. (10).)*

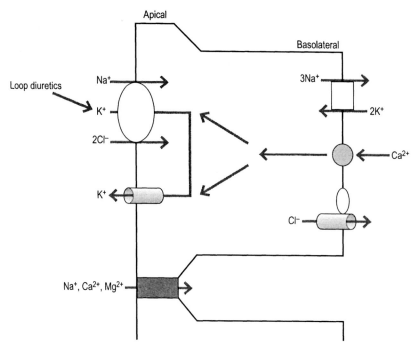

Fig. 5.3 Thick ascending limb (TAL) cell showing sites of action of loop diuretics. *(Modified with permission of Blackwell Publishing from ref. (10).)*

diuretics. In contrast, the major pathway for Na^+ reabsorption in the apical membrane of the TAL of Henle's loop is the NKCC2 (Fig. 5.3). It is at this site where loop diuretics act.

THIAZIDES AND THIAZIDE-LIKE DIURETICS

The thiazide diuretics are inhibitors of the NCC. These drugs are sulphonamides and many are analogues of 1,2,4-benzothiadiazine-1,1-dioxide.[5] Drugs that are pharmacologically similar to thiazide diuretics, but are not thiazides, are called thiazide-like diuretics. Thiazide and thiazide-like diuretics are regarded by many as the cornerstone of antihypertensive therapy, based on their efficacy in reducing both blood pressure (BP) (an intermediate endpoint) and cardiovascular morbidity and mortality, the real endpoints on which antihypertensive drugs are judged. The pathophysiologic basis of this approach is that control of NaCl balance, which is largely dependent on regulation of NaCl excretion by the kidney, is an important regulator of BP.[8] Further, many forms of hypertension, including those for which single gene mutations are responsible, are associated with abnormalities in Na^+ and Cl^- transport along the renal tubule.[9]

MECHANISMS OF ACTION

Diuresis/natriuresis

Thiazide and thiazide-like diuretics act primarily at the level of the DCT to block the NCC, thereby increasing Na^+ and Cl^- excretion (Fig. 5.2). In the

DCT, as in other nephron segments, the Na^+:K^+:ATPase on the basolateral membrane of the tubular cells provides the electrochemical gradient that allows Na^+ to be transported from the lumen to the interstitial space.[10] The free energy in the electrochemical gradient for Na^+ is harnessed by the NCC in the apical membrane, which moves Cl^- into the epithelial cell against its electro-chemical gradient.[5] Cl^- then passively exits the basolateral membrane via a Cl^- channel. Thiazide and thiazide-like diuretics inhibit the NCC, apparently by competing for the Cl^- binding site.[11]

The NCC from urinary bladder of the winter flounder, dogfish shark rectal gland, rat and human has been cloned.[10,12,13] In mammals, the NCC is expressed mainly in the kidney and localized to the apical membrane of the DCT epithelial cells.[14–17] Expression of the NCC is induced by aldosterone.[18–20] Gain of function mutations of the NCC cause Gitelman syndrome, an autosomal recessive disorder characterized by a form of hypokalaemic alkalosis result-ing from a defect in the distal renal tubule thiazide-sensitive NCC.[21] The NCC has also been implicated in the pathophysiology of a salt-dependent hypertension syndrome known as pseudohyperaldosteronism type II (PHAII) or Gordon's syndrome.[2] This syndrome is an autosomal dominant disorder owing to mutations in the gene encoding a particular serine/threonine kinase named WNK4, resulting in arterial hypertension accompanied by hyperkalaemic metabolic acidosis.[22]

Ca^{2+} reabsorption

Thiazide diuretics acting on the distal nephron increase Ca^{2+} reabsorption and thus reduce Ca^{2+} excretion.[23] In the DCT, NaCl and Ca^{2+} reabsorption are related reciprocally.[2] Blocking or reducing the activity of the NCC with a thia-zide increases Ca^{2+} reabsorption, while increased expression or activity of the NCC reduces Ca^{2+} reabsorption.[23] The precise mechanism by which diuretics affect the reabsorption of Ca^{2+} remains unclear, but most evidence suggests that thiazide action and Ca^{2+} reabsorption may be linked functionally through an indirect mechanism. Thiazides reduce NaCl entry at the apical membrane, thus reducing intracellular Na^+ concentration. As a consequence, DCT cells become hyperpolarized, increasing the electrochemical driving force for Ca^{2+} entry at the apical membrane through Ca^{2+} channels.[2,24,25] This effect of thia-zides on Ca^{2+} reabsorption is thus secondary to natriuretic action and constitu-tes the basis for their usefulness in preventing the formation of calcium-containing renal stones. This action may also explain the protective effect of thiazides in osteoporosis.[26,27]

Blood pressure reduction

The BP reducing effects of thiazides and related compounds can be separated into three phases: (1) an acute phase, in which a volume/diuretic-related effect occurs within 1–2 weeks of treatment, (2) a subacute phase at approximately 6–8 weeks of therapy, during which volume returns to slightly less than pre-treatment levels and resistance factors also contribute and (3) a chronic phase several months after instituting therapy in which the BP lowering effect appears to be vascular (reduced peripheral vascular resistance) (Fig. 5.4).[28]

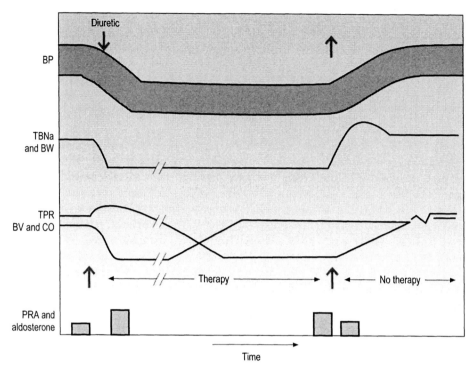

Fig. 5.4 Haemodynamic and hormonal effects of diuretic therapy. At the initiation of treatment (the acute phase), diuretic-induced blood pressure (BP) reduction is associated with a reduction in total body sodium (TBNa), reflected by loss of body weight (BW), reductions in blood volume (BV) and cardiac output (CO), and an increase in total peripheral resistance (TPR). The diuretic-mediated salt depletion is accompanied by a compensatory activation of the renin–angiotensin–aldosterone system (PRA-plasma renin activity). During chronic therapy, the antihypertensive effect persists together with the negative sodium balance, but both BV and CO return to near pretreatment values. With time, however, a reduction in TPR occurs. *(Modified with permission from Waeber B, Brunner H. In: Braunwald E, Hollenberg NK, eds.* Atlas of heart disease: hypertension. *Current Medicine LLC 2002.)*

A landmark study of the mechanism of antihypertensive action of thiazide diuretics was carried out in patients with essential hypertension who received hydrochlorothiazide (50 mg orally twice daily) and were subjected to measurements of haemodynamic parameters, i.e. cardiac output, plasma and extracellular fluid volume (ECF), as well as an assessment of total peripheral resistance (TPR) on four occasions: before treatment and 48 hours after beginning treatment to determine acute effects, and at 6 and 8 weeks post-treatment to assess subacute effects.[29] The acute phase (first 24–48 hours) of treatment with hydrochlorothiazide was characterized by a net Na[+] loss and a reduction in total ECF of 12%, which amounts to a 1–2L decrease in ECF volume, with a related fall in cardiac output.[29,30] Plasma volume was reduced similarly, indicating that acute volume loss arises proportionally from both plasma and interstitial compartments.[31] The decrease in plasma volume both reduced venous return and diminished cardiac output, providing the basis for the initial BP fall.[29] Diuretic-mediated reductions in plasma volume and NaCl depletion stimulate compensatory activation of both the sympathetic nervous and renin–angiotensin–aldosterone systems (RAAS). The degree to which these systems are activated modulates the magnitude of BP decrease with either thiazide diuretic monotherapy or with thiazides administered in combination with agents that interrupt the RAAS.[32]

The subacute phase of thiazide diuretic treatment is a transitional period during which both volume and resistance factors contribute to the continued reduction in BP.[29,33] The study above demonstrated that after 6–8 weeks of treatment with hydrochlorothiazide, cardiac output returned to near pretreatment values; TPR was only slightly reduced, and ECF was reduced by only 20% and 24% respectively when compared to pretreatment levels.[29]

The chronic phase of diuretic treatment is characterized by arteriolar vasodilation, which reduces TPR, and thus sustains the reduction in BP.[30,33] In a study of hypertensive subjects, haemodynamic parameters were assessed at 4, 12, 24 and 36 weeks of treatment with hydrochlorothiazide 50 mg orally twice daily. Maximal reductions in mean arterial pressure were seen after 12 weeks of treatment. In the first 4 weeks, the fall in BP in those who eventually responded to treatment (i.e. >10% fall in mean arterial pressure) was not significantly different from that in non-responders (i.e. <10% fall in BP). Only responders showed a further decrease thereafter, and the difference from non-responders became significant.[30] Further, only responders had a significant fall in TPR after 12 weeks; TPR remained elevated in the non-responders. The chronic reduction in TPR with a resultant reduction in BP has made thiazides and related compounds the mainstay of antihypertensive therapy.[34]

Several mechanisms, supported by experimental evidence from both animals and humans, have been suggested to explain the reduction in TPR with thiazide diuretic use.[29,34,35] Adjustments in Na^+/Ca^{2+} balance in vascular smooth muscle cells with the acute volume contraction are seen during the first several days of diuretic therapy in humans. It is unclear how this phenomenon translates into a reduction in TPR, but effects on BP can be seen for several weeks even after thiazide diuretics are withdrawn.[36,37]

In vitro studies in isolated animal and human resistance arteries have demonstrated a direct vasodilator effect of thiazide diuretics.[38–41] The vasodilator effect is mediated by opening vascular Ca^{2+}-activated K^+ channels (K_{Ca}), thereby hyperpolarizing and reducing intracellular Ca^{2+} concentrations in vascular smooth muscle cells. The vascular action of thiazides is inhibited by K_{Ca} blockers such as tetraethylammonium (TEA), charybdotoxin, a 37-amino acid peptide present in the venom of the scorpion *Leiurus quinquestriatus hebraeus*, and iberiotoxin, a peptide from the venom of the scorpion *Buthus tamulus* that shares 70% homology with charybdotoxin and is an even more highly selective inhibitor of K_{Ca}. In contrast, blockers of other vascular K^+ channels do not inhibit the vasodilator effects of the thiazides.[39,40,42,43] These findings support the selectivity of the large-conductance Ca^{2+}-activated K^+ channel (K_{Ca}) in accounting for thiazide-induced vasodilation.

A more recent study tested whether hydrochlorothiazide has a direct vasodilator effect in intact normotensive and hypertensive humans and whether the observed vascular effect of the thiazide is related to K_{Ca} channel activation and/or inhibition of the NCC.[35] Forearm vasodilator responses to infusions of increasing doses of hydrochlorothiazide (8, 25 and 75 mcg $min^{-1} \cdot dL^{-1}$) or placebo into the brachial artery of normotensive and hypertensive subjects were measured and recorded as forearm blood flow (FBF). FBF with increasing doses of hydrochlorothiazide was also measured in patients with Gitelman syndrome, who lack the thiazide-sensitive NCC, to determine if hydrochlorothiazide exerts a direct vasodilator effect independent of its documented action on the NCC. Further, in normotensive subjects FBF was recorded after local administration of tetraethylammonium (TEA) to determine the role of K_{Ca} channel activation in hydrochlorothiazide-induced vasodilation. Hydrochlorothiazide infusion elicited a dose-dependent vasodilator response that was similar in normotensive and hypertensive persons and in those with Gitelman syndrome (Fig. 5.5). The finding of a vasodilator response in the Gitelman patients indicates that hydrochlorothiazide exerts a direct vasodilator action that is independent of its effect on the NCC. Further, the vasodilator effect of hydrochlorothiazide in normotensive volunteers was inhibited by TEA, demonstrating its K_{Ca} dependence (Fig. 5.6).

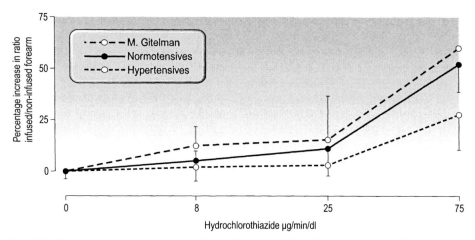

Fig. 5.5 Percentage change in forearm blood flow ratio (infused/non-infused arm) during graded intrabrachial infusions of hydrochlorothiazide compared with placebo infusion as measured by venous occlusion plethysmography (mean±SEM). Direct vasoactivity of hydrochlorothiazide in normotensives (n=6), hypertensives (n=6), and patients with Gitelman syndrome (n=2). *(Adapted with permission of Lippincott, Williams & Wilkins from ref. (35).)*

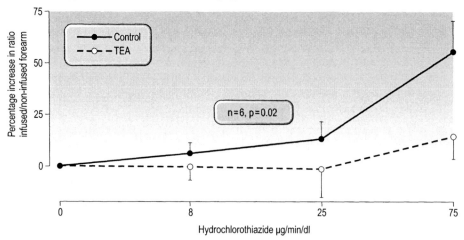

Fig. 5.6 Direct vasoactivity of hydrochlorothiazide in normotensive subjects in the absence and in the presence of the potassium channel blocker TEA. p value refers to the statistical difference as analyzed by ANOVA with repeated measures over the complete dose–response curve. Direct vasoactivity of hydrochlorthiazide: p=0.013; inhibition by TEA: p=0.02. *(Adapted with permission of Lippincott, Williams & Wilkins from ref. (35).)*

This study demonstrated that hydrochlorothiazide exerts a direct acute vasodilator effect in the human forearm at supratherapeutic plasma levels and that this action is mediated by activation of K_{Ca} channels, not by inhibition of a putative vascular NCC. The key unanswered question is whether the direct vasodilator effect of K_{Ca} channel activation contributes to the BP lowering seen with chronic hydrochlorothiazide administration to hypertensive patients.

Several limitations of the study described above, acknowledged by the authors, call into question the importance of K_{Ca} channel activation at the peripheral vascular level in mediating the chronic antihypertensive effect of hydrochlorothiazide: (1) vasodilation occurred only at plasma levels of hydrochlorothiazide higher than those achieved during chronic oral treatment, (2) the increase in FBF reached steady state within 1–2 minutes of hydrochlorothiazide administration, whereas the antihypertensive effect of thiazide diuretics is slow in onset, (3) vasodilation occurred in both normotensive and hypertensive subjects and even tended to be less in the latter group, (4) there was no correlation between pretreatment BP or forearm vascular resistance and the vasodilator effect of hydrochlorothiazide. The authors pointed out the possibilities that accumulation of hydrochlorothiazide in vascular smooth muscle cells over time, as documented in previous studies, as well as prevention of fluid and Na^+ retention, normal counterregulatory effects of vasodilation, by its diuretic action could amplify the vasodilator potency of chronically administered hydrochlorothiazide. Further studies of the effects of selective inhibitors of K_{Ca} channels in hypertensive patients treated chronically with hydrochlorothiazide are needed to assess the role of direct arterial dilation via K_{Ca} channel activation in the chronic antihypertensive effects of this drug.

Indapamide, a lipophilic thiazide-like agent that lowers BP at doses that have minimal diuretic effects,[44] had no vasodilator effect when infused directly into the brachial artery of either normotensive or hypertensive subjects. This negative finding is consistent with results of ex vivo studies in isolated arteries of human origin.[38] Experiments in animal tissues have shown that indapamide has calcium channel antagonist effects, inhibiting slow inward Ca^{2+} current in vascular smooth muscle[45] and resulting in reduced Ca^{2+} uptake and relaxation in arteries preconstricted with norepinephrine or a depolarizing K^+ solution.[46] Thus, hydrochlorothiazide and indapamide have different mechanisms of vasodilator action and different species specificities.

PHARMACOKINETICS

Thiazide diuretics and related compounds are generally well absorbed from the gastrointestinal tract, but there is substantial variability in oral bioavailability between individual drugs in this class (Table 5.1). For example, indapamide has 93% bioavailability when taken orally, while hydrochlorothiazide, chlorthalidone and metolazone are 65–70% absorbed, and chlorothiazide has a wide range of dose-dependent oral bioavailability.[5] Once absorbed, thiazide diuretics are bound to plasma proteins, but the binding varies considerably between individual agents. The extent of protein binding determines the contribution that filtration makes to tubular delivery of a specific thiazide diuretic.[5] Thiazide and thiazide-like diuretics are also secreted in the PCT by the organic acid secretory pathway because these sulphonamide compounds are organic acids.

VOL 25 CLINICAL PHARMACOLOGY AND THERAPEUTICS OF HYPERTENSION

Table 5.1 Inhibitors of Na⁺Cl⁻ (NCC) cotransporter. Thiazide and thiazide-like diuretics commonly used and referred to in JNC7 hypertension treatment guidelines are shown

Drug	Structure	Relative potency	Oral availability	t$_{1/2}$ (Hours)	Route of elimination
Chlorothiazide (DIURIL)	R$_2$ = H, R$_3$ = H, R$_6$ = Cl (Unsumurated between C3 and N4)	0.1	9–56% (dose-dependent)	~1.5	R
Hydrochlorothiazide (HYDRODIURIL)	R$_2$ = H, R$_3$ = H, R$_6$ = Cl	1	~70%	~2.5	R
Polythiazide (RENESE)	R$_2$ = CH$_3$, R$_3$ = CH$_2$SCH$_2$CF$_3$, R$_6$ = Cl	25	~100%	~25	~25% R, ~75% U
Chlorthalidone (HYGROTON)		1	~65%	~47%	~65% R, ~10% B, ~25% U
Indapamide (LOZOL)		20	~93%	~14	M
Metolazone (MYKROX, ZAROXOLYN)		10	~65%	ID	~80% R. ~10% B, ~10% M

Abbreviations: R, renal excretion of intact drug: M, rectabolism: B, excretion of intact drug into bile: U, unknown pathway of elimination: ID, insufficient data.

Chlorothiazide and hydrochlorothiazide are entirely excreted intact in the urine, while 65% of chlorthalidone and 80% of metolazone are excreted in the urine intact. Indapamide is completely metabolized before delivery to the nephron.

ADVERSE EFFECTS ASSOCIATED WITH THIAZIDE AND THIAZIDE-LIKE DIURETICS

Thiazide and thiazide-like diuretics are associated with a variety of adverse effects (Table 5.2), generally related to volume depletion, electrolyte disturbances or metabolic effects.[47] Sensitivity reactions are less common and are usually attributed to the sulphonamide moieties in these drugs. We will discuss here the clinically most important adverse effects of thiazides, i.e. hypokalaemia, insulin resistance/diabetes, dyslipidaemia and sexual dysfunction.

Hypokalaemia

Potassium is secreted into the urine in the DCT and CD. As Na^+ is reabsorbed, a lumen-negative gradient is established that favours secretion of K^+ (Fig. 5.2). Thiazide and thiazide-like diuretics increase Na^+ delivery to these regions and are thus kaliuretic.[48] Diuretic-induced hypokalaemia and volume reduction result in secondary hyperaldosteronism, which enhances the loss of K^+ at the DCT and CD. Levels of dietary NaCl also play a role in K^+ loss, because as NaCl intake increases, distal delivery of Na^+ remains high indefinitely and K^+ secretion is favoured.[48] Chloride depletion also promotes urinary loss of K^+ with thiazide diuretic use.[49,50]

Hypokalaemia is more common with the thiazides than with the loop diuretics and is a particular problem with long-acting agents such as chlorthalidone. Diuretic-induced hypokalaemia has been implicated in the adverse metabolic effects of these drugs, i.e. increased insulin resistance and new onset diabetes (to be discussed below), as well as increased coronary events (sudden cardiac death), and limiting the outcome benefits of diuretic therapy.

Table 5.2 Adverse effects related to the use of thiazide and thiazide-like diuretics

Volume depletion	**Sexual dysfunction**
Fatigue	Impotence
Dizziness	Decreased libido
Electrolyte disturbances	**Sensitivity reactions**
Hypokalaemia	Skin rashes
Hyponatraemia	Photosensitivity
Hypomagnesaemia	Vasculitis
Hypocalciuria	Bone marrow aplasia
Hypericaemia	
Metabolic alkalosis	
Metabolic	
Insulin resistance/diabetes	
Dyslipidaemia	

(Modified from ref. (47).)

Multiple lines of evidence have shown that high-dose diuretic therapy, while helpful in preventing stroke and heart failure, is less effective in preventing coronary heart disease (CHD) and even increases the risk of some coronary events, e.g. sudden cardiac death. For example, in the Multiple Risk Factor Intervention Trial (MRFIT), 12 866 men at high risk for CHD were randomly assigned to either a special intervention programme (SI) that included stepped-care treatment for hypertension that began with either hydrochlorothiazide or chlorthalidone, or to their usual sources of health care in the community (UC).[51] After 7 years of follow-up, CHD mortality was not different in the two treatment groups overall. However, for hypertensive men who had baseline ECG abnormalities, CHD mortality was higher in the SI group. The authors suggested that this reflected an unfavourable response to antihypertensive therapy with diuretics, but cautioned that the data came from a post hoc subgroup analysis and emphasized the need for further study.

Further support for the concept that high-dose diuretic therapy may have an adverse effect on cardiovascular disease outcomes was provided by a population-based case-control study that examined the association between thiazide treatment for hypertension and the occurrence of primary cardiac arrest.[52] The study included 114 cases of primary cardiac arrest (sudden cardiac death) that occurred between 1977 and 1990 in persons that were being treated for hypertension. The risk of sudden cardiac death among patients receiving combined thiazide and K^+-sparing diuretic (hydrochlorothiazide and triamterene or spironolactone) therapy was lower than that among persons treated with a thiazide (hydrochlorothiazide or chlorthalidone) alone. Combined therapy with low-dose thiazide (25 mg hydrochlorothiazide daily) and a K^+-sparing agent (triamterene or amiloride) was associated with a reduced risk of cardiac arrest among patients treated with single or multiple antihypertensive drugs. Moderate-dose thiazide therapy (50 mg daily of either chlorthalidone or hydrochlorothiazide) was associated with a moderate increase in risk, while high-dose therapy (100 mg daily) was associated with a large increase in risk when compared to low-dose therapy.

This observation suggests that the dose-related hypokalaemic effect of thiazides is a plausible explanation for the increased risk of sudden cardiac death in diuretic-treated hypertensive patients and that K^+-sparing agents, when administered with a thiazide diuretic, may have a beneficial role in reducing the risk of sudden cardiac death in hypertensive patients. Although these findings do not come from a prospective randomized trial, attempts should probably be made to prevent or minimize the fall in serum K^+ in patients treated with thiazides or thiazide-like diuretics by using smaller doses and/or administering a K^+-sparing diuretic or supplemental K^+.

The Systolic Hypertension in the Elderly Program (SHEP) trial analyzed data from 4126 elderly patients with isolated systolic hypertension (systolic BP (SBP) 160–219 mmHg and diastolic BP (DBP) <90 mmHg) to determine whether hypokalaemia with long-term diuretic administration is associated with a reduced benefit in terms of cardiovascular events.[53] Participants were randomized to active treatment with chlorthalidone 12.5 mg or 25 mg, or placebo and followed for 5 years. After 1 year of active treatment, K^+ levels decreased significantly in the active treatment group, i.e. 7.2% of those randomized to active treatment had hypokalaemia (serum K^+ <3.5 mmol/L) compared with 1% of participants randomized to placebo. Compared with

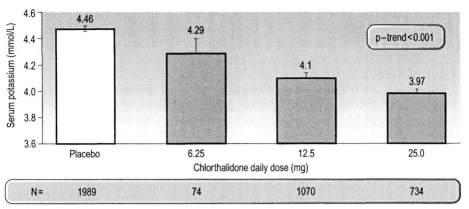

Fig. 5.7 Serum potassium at 1 year of the Systolic Hypertension in the Elderly Program (SHEP) trial, according to chlorthalidone dose. The numbers at the bottom of the figure indicate the number of participants in each group. *(Adapted with permission of Lippincott, Williams & Wilkins from ref. (53).)*

placebo, chlorthalidone at doses of 6.25, 12.5 or 25 mg per day resulted in significantly lower serum K^+ levels, and the chlorthalidone dose was inversely associated with serum K^+ levels at the first annual visit (Fig. 5.7). During the last 4 years of the study, after adjustments for known cardiovascular risk factors and study drug dose, participants randomized to chlorthalidone who became hypokalaemic had a two- to threefold increase in risk of CHD and stroke events compared to those in the active treatment group who remained normokalaemic. This clinical trial provides clear evidence that persistent diuretic-induced hypokalaemia has adverse effects on cardiovascular disease outcomes, although the conclusions again depended on sub-group retrospective analysis.

Insulin resistance/diabetes

Thiazide and thiazide-like diuretics are associated with small increases in serum glucose levels (3–4 mg/dL or 0.17–0.22 mmol/L) and accordingly with an increase in new onset diabetes in hypertensive patients.[54–59] It has been claimed that thiazide-induced glucose intolerance/hyperglycaemia/diabetes is attributable to K^+ depletion and can be prevented or reversed with maintenance of K^+ balance. Weight control, increased physical activity and caution when using β-blockers in combination therapy may be helpful in preventing dysglycaemia.[60,61] Small short-term mechanistic studies of the effects diuretic use has in healthy human subjects have generally shown reversible impairment in glucose tolerance that was related to reduced or delayed insulin release and not insulin resistance. In contrast, a larger randomized controlled trial comparing hydrochlorothiazide 25–50 mg to captopril 50–100 mg showed a 15% reduction in insulin sensitivity by glucose clamp with hydrochlorothiazide and 19% increase with captopril compared to baseline placebo levels; fasting blood glucose and insulin levels were increased in the hydrochlorothiazide group.[62]

Long-term studies of hypertensive patients treated with diuretics have shown inconsistent results: older studies in which higher dose diuretics were administered showed increases in fasting glucose levels and impaired glucose tolerance in association with reductions in serum K^+; later studies with lower diuretic doses ± K^+ replacement showed small effects on glucose metabolism and K^+. The large population-based Atherosclerosis Risk in Communities Study (ARIC) suggested that risk of diabetes was increased with antihypertensive treatment with β-blockers but not diuretics.[63] This finding may be related to a temporal trend toward lower dose diuretics in antihypertensive therapy.

Results of large randomized controlled trials of antihypertensive treatment have usually, but not always, shown a higher incidence of new diabetes in participants randomized to diuretics and β-blockers than in those randomized to other drug classes. Diabetes incidence was 6.9% with diuretics and β-blockers versus 6.1% with captopril ($p=0.04$) in the Captopril Prevention Project (CAPPP); 7.7% with diuretics versus 5.6% with nifedipine ($p=0.0001$) in the Intervention as a Goal in Hypertension Treatment study (INSIGHT); and 8% with atenolol versus 6% with losartan ($p=0.001$) in the Losartan Intervention for End-point Reduction (LIFE) study.[64–66] At the end of the Antihypertensive and Lipid-Lowering Treatment to Prevent Heart Attack Trial (ALLHAT), the incidence of new diabetes was 11.6% in the chlorthalidone group, 9.8% in the amlodipine group ($p=0.04$), and 8.1% in the lisinopril group ($p<0.001$).[67] In contrast, the incidence of new diabetes in the Swedish Trial in Old Patients with Hypertension-2 (STOP-2) study was 11.4% in the diuretics and/or β-blockers group, 10.7% in the ACE inhibitors group, and 10.5% in the calcium-channel blockers group ($p=0.77$).[56] Also, in the Nordic Diltiazem (NORDIL) study, incidence of new diabetes did not differ between the groups randomized to diuretics and β-blockers compared with the diltiazem group.[68] These somewhat discrepant findings underscore the need for randomized controlled trials specifically designed to test the effects of various thiazide-based regimens on glucose tolerance.

The overriding clinical question in considering thiazide-induced dysglycaemia is whether thiazide-induced diabetes carries the same ominous prognosis as naturally occurring diabetes.[54,55,57,69,70] This topic is being vigorously debated in the current literature. An early review of trials in which diuretics were used as antihypertensive treatment concluded that, while diuretics were associated with development of impaired glucose tolerance, the metabolic abnormality did not increase the risk of CHD.[71] A later observational study carried out in 686 hypertensive men found that thiazide ± β-blocker-related development of diabetes did not increase risk of CHD events over a 15-year treatment period, while diabetes at baseline was associated with CHD.[72] However, the confidence interval of the risk associated with drug-related diabetes was so wide that a clinically important effect on risk of myocardial infarction (MI) could not be excluded. In addition, results were not reported separately by drug class, and few participants remained on thiazide monotherapy throughout the follow-up period. Results of the ALLHAT trial confirmed the dissociation between diuretic-induced diabetes and CHD outcomes: the increased incidence of diabetes in the chlorthalidone group was not related to an increase in CHD events during the 5-year follow-up period of the trial.[67] Therefore, the ALLHAT investigators did not caution against diuretic use on this basis.[69]

Observational studies with long periods of follow-up that have assessed the relationship between diuretic therapy for hypertension and cardiovascular disease outcomes have drawn inconsistent conclusions, in part because of deficiencies in the data. The longitudinal population-based Uppsala study designed to identify risk factors for cardiovascular disease in men demonstrated a positive relationship between increase in blood glucose over time and MI, but only in those receiving antihypertensive treatment.[55] The cohort included 1860 men who were examined initially at age 50, re-examined at age 60 and followed for a mean of 17.4 years; 316 of these received antihypertensive treatment (21% thiazide diuretics, 30% thiazide-β-blocker combinations and 46% β-blockers). The incidence of MI was significantly greater in men treated for hypertension than in those without such treatment (23% vs. 13.5%, $p<0.0001$), and those who sustained an MI after age 60 showed a significantly larger increase in blood glucose between age 50 and 60 than those who were infarct-free. Increase in blood glucose was an independent risk factor for MI only in men receiving antihypertensive treatment at age 60. There was a significant interaction between baseline proinsulin concentration (a marker of insulin resistance) and antihypertensive treatment on increase in blood glucose between age 50 and 60. Both increase in blood glucose and in baseline proinsulin concentration were risk factors for MI in men receiving antihypertensive treatment with thiazide diuretics, β-blockers, or both, suggesting that both an insulin-resistant state and the metabolic effects of diuretics and β-blockers increase the risk of MI in middle-aged white men. Further study is needed to determine whether these findings can be generalized to other populations.

The Progetto Ipertensione Umbria Monitoraggio Ambulatoriale (PIUMA) study, an observational registry of morbidity and mortality in initially untreated persons with essential hypertension, assessed the prognostic value of incident type 2 diabetes in a cohort of 795 patients over a median of 6 years (range 1–16 years) of follow-up.[73] At follow-up, 5.8% (43 subjects) of initially non-diabetic participants had incident diabetes. Participants who developed incident diabetes were treated with antihypertensive drugs more often than those who remained diabetes free, and a logistic regression analysis showed that exposure to diuretics at follow-up and high baseline glucose concentration were the sole independent predictors of incident diabetes. The relative risk of cardiovascular disease events was increased in participants with incident diabetes, as well as those with diabetes at baseline compared with non-diabetic subjects (Fig. 5.8). While incident diabetes was an independent predictor of cardiovascular disease risk, diuretic use, albeit predictive of incident diabetes, was not an independent predictor of cardiovascular disease outcomes. Limitations of the study include the small proportion of participants (11%) treated with a diuretic/β-blocker alone and failure to report results for specific regimens separately. Nevertheless, the authors' recommendation of careful monitoring of hypertensive patients with high normal plasma glucose levels and those treated with diuretics to prevent new diabetes seems warranted.

Long-term (mean 14.3 years) follow-up data from the SHEP trial have called into question the clinical significance of incident diabetes in diuretic-treated hypertension.[74] Cardiovascular mortality rate was significantly lower in SHEP participants randomized to chlorthalidone (19%) compared with placebo (22%), and diabetes that developed in those on diuretic therapy was not associated with increased cardiovascular or total mortality. In contrast, incident diabetes in participants randomized to placebo was associated with increased cardiovascular outcomes and mortality rate, as was diabetes at baseline. Thus chlorthalidone-based treatment in SHEP improved long-term outcomes in both

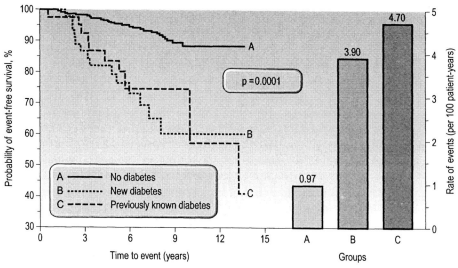

Fig. 5.8 Cardiovascular events in treated hypertensive subjects without diabetes (group A), new-onset diabetes (group B), and previously known diabetes (group C). *(Adapted with permission of Lippincott, Williams & Wilkins from ref. (73).)*

diabetic and non-diabetic persons, and those with incident diabetes associated with diuretic treatment had a better prognosis than those with pre-existing diabetes.

Limitations of this observational extension study include its retrospective design and the absence of any data on BP, treatment, non-fatal endpoints, and glycaemic status of participants after conclusion of the double-blind phase of SHEP. Further, if the author's assertion that more patients in the active treatment (chlorthalidone) group likely remained on active therapy than initiated therapy in the placebo group were true, persistent reductions in BP and target organ damage could account for the mortality benefits seen in the chlorthalidone group, overriding any deleterious effect of incident diabetes. The authors speculated that diuretic-induced hyperglycaemia was associated with lower cardiovascular risk than incident diabetes in the placebo group because of the modest degree of metabolic disturbance (small increases in fasting glucose, small alterations in cholesterol) in the former group and because of differences in underlying mechanisms: decreased glucose-stimulated insulin release due to hypokalaemia and insulin resistance related to increased sympathetic activity in the diuretic group[75–77] vs. physical inactivity, weight gain, ageing and genetic predisposition in the placebo group.[78] The latter are independent risk factors for accelerated atherosclerosis and cardiovascular disease events.

The clinical significance of diuretic-induced diabetes remains controversial. More long-term morbidity and mortality data with clearer documentation of ongoing treatment regimens are needed to resolve the controversy. Well-controlled studies of strategies to prevent and reverse the disorder, including maintaining K^+ balance, combining diuretics with other classes of antihypertensive drugs, and weight control and increased physical activity are also needed in order to optimize the benefits of diuretic therapy in high-risk hypertensives.

Dyslipidaemia

It has long been recognized that thiazide diuretics have unfavourable effects on serum lipids, at least in the short term. A meta-analysis of 475 studies of short-term effects of antihypertensive agents on lipids, 214 of which included thiazide-like diuretics, showed a significant increase in total and low-density lipoprotein cholesterol, but no change in high-density lipoprotein cholesterol in diuretic-treated patients.[79] The diuretic effects were dose-dependent. In contrast, the effects of thiazide diuretics on lipids in long-term studies were attenuated and did not seem to persist beyond 1 year.[80] Thus, the effects of thiazides on serum lipids appear to be small and of little clinical significance,[81] particularly in the era of potent and well-tolerated lipid lowering agents.

Sexual dysfunction

Antihypertensive medications have a long history of association with sexual dysfunction and this adverse effect has been a primary reason for premature withdrawal from hypertension trials. In the MRC trial of treatment of mild hypertension, which enrolled over 17 000 persons with mild-to-moderate hypertension, impotence was the principal reason for premature withdrawal from the study among men treated with the diuretic bendroflumethiazide.[82] In a long-term surveillance study of adverse effects of antihypertensive drugs carried out in 5000 participants, 8% of men discontinued therapy because of sexually related side effects, principally impotence and decreased libido; the rate of sexual problems was 21% in chlorthalidone-treated men.[83] These studies suggest that sexual dysfunction resulting from diuretic therapy is a potential reason for non-compliance.

Results of randomized placebo-controlled trials that included formal assessment of sexual dysfunction have also tended to support an association between diuretic therapy and sexual dysfunction. In a single-blind trial including 1000 men with mild-to-moderate hypertension who were given questionnaires about impotence at 12 weeks and 2 years after treatment with bendroflumethiazide, a β-blocker or placebo, complaints about impotence were 16% and 23% after 12 weeks and 2 years of bendroflumethiazide treatment, respectively, significantly greater than with placebo (9% and 10%, respectively) or β-blocker therapy (14% and 13%, respectively).[84] A randomized, placebo-controlled, double-blind study assessed sexual dysfunction using the Sexual Symptoms Distress Index in 176 hypertensive men between the ages of 35 and 70 years treated with a high-dose thiazide or thiazide-like diuretic alone (hydrochlorothiazide (HCTZ) or chlorthalidone 50 mg daily), or in combination with a K^+-sparing agent (HCTZ 50 mg-triamterene 100 mg daily), K^+ (HCTZ 50 mg-K^+ 40 mmol daily), magnesium oxide (HCTZ 50 mg-K^+ 40 mmol-magnesium oxide 20 mmol) or placebo.[85] Results from this study suggest that: (1) men taking diuretics had two to six times higher rates of sexual dysfunction compared with the placebo treatment and (2) the absolute rate of self-reported sexual dysfunction attributable to diuretic use was substantial: 50% reported new sexual dysfunction and 72% attributed this sexual dysfunction to the study medication.[85] Complaints about sexual dysfunction tended to occur early, within 2 months after initiating treatment.

The Treatment of Mild Hypertension Study (TOMHS), a double-blind, placebo-controlled, randomized trial, compared the effects of monotherapy with five antihypertensive medications of different classes with lifestyle modification (active placebo) on sexual dysfunction in over 900 participants with diastolic hypertension (557 men and 345 women).[86] Sexual function was ascertained by physician interviews at baseline and annually during the 4-year follow-up. At baseline, 12% of men and 2% of women reported sexual dysfunction (difficulty obtaining and/or maintaining an erection and having an orgasm, respectively). The incidence of erectile dysfunction (ED) in men at 24 and 48 months follow-up was 10% and 15% overall, and was related to type of antihypertensive therapy. Men randomized to chlorthalidone reported a significantly higher incidence of ED at 24 months compared to placebo (17% vs. 8%, $p=0.025$), but at 48 months this difference was attenuated (17% chlorthalidone, 12% placebo, $p=0.20$). Most of the men in the chlorthalidone group who developed ED experienced it in the first year, and a majority continued on the diuretic. The narrowing of the difference in ED incidence between the chlorthalidone and placebo groups was due to a greater incidence of new ED in the placebo group at 36 and 48 months of follow-up. In women, the incidence of sexual problems was low in all treatment groups, suggesting that sexual dysfunction is not a major concern in the treatment of hypertensive women. Results of TOMHS suggest that ED associated with diuretic use appears relatively early and is often tolerable. Occurrence after 2 years is unlikely.

The above large-scale studies depended primarily on the response to questionnaires or physician interviews for evaluating ED in hypertensive patients. Smaller mechanistic studies have used nocturnal penile tumescence tonometry to evaluate antihypertensive therapy-induced ED directly. In one study that included 12 patients, no significant difference for total mean tumescence, tumescence duration, or longest period of tumescence was found between patients after 4 weeks of treatment with hydrochlorothiazide, prazosin or placebo.[87] Thus, the relationship of diuretic therapy to ED remains unclear, especially since increasing age, physical and emotional stress may contribute to sexual dysfunction, particularly in the hypertensive patient.

The mechanism of the small but consistent increase in ED observed with use of thiazide and thiazide-like diuretics is unknown. Diuretics have no known central or autonomic nervous system effects that might impair erectile function.[86] ED has been linked to nitric oxide (NO) deficiency in patients with hypertension and other forms of cardiovascular disease.[88] NO is an essential mediator of penile erection, since it relaxes the corpus cavernosum. Diuretics, unlike ACE inhibitors and mineralocorticoid receptor antagonists, are not thought to play a major role in ameliorating endothelial dysfunction and enhancing NO availability in patients with vascular disease. Neither are these drugs thought to exacerbate endothelial dysfunction/NO availability. Thus the endothelium–NO mechanism does not account for the effect on ED.

INDIVIDUAL THIAZIDE AND THIAZIDE-LIKE DIURETICS

Hydrochlorothiazide and chlorthalidone

Hydrochlorothiazide and chlorthalidone are the agents that have been most commonly used in clinical trials and in clinical practice (Table 5.3). The drugs differ pharmacokinetically and pharmacodynamically.[89] Hydrochlorothiazide achieves a peak circulating concentration in approximately 2 hours and has a

Table 5.3 Commonly used oral thiazide and loop diuretics

	Oral antihypertensive drugs		
Class	*Drug (trade name)*	*Usual dose, range, mg/d*	*Daily frequency*
Thiazide diuretics	Chlorothiazide (Diuril)	125–500	1
	Chlorthalidone (generic)	12.5–25	1
	Hydrochlorothiazide (Microzide, HydoDIURIL)	12.5–50	1
	Polythiazide (Renese)	2–4	1
	Indapamide (Lozol)	1.25–2.5	1
	Metolazone (Mykrox)	0.5–1.0	1
	Metolazone (Zaroxolyn)	2.5–5	1
Loop diuretics	Bumetanide (Bumex)	0.5–2	2
	Furosemide (Lasix)	20–80	2
	Torasemide (Demadex)	2.5–10	1

(Modified from ref. (3) with permission.)

Table 5.4 Pharmacokinetic and pharmacodynamic comparisons of hydrochlorothiazide and chlorthalidone

Drug	**Onset (hours)**	**Peak (hours)**	**Half-life (hours)**	**Duration (hours)**
HCTZ	2	4–6	6–9 (single dose) 8–15 (long-term dose)	12 (single dose) 16–24 (long-term dose)
Chlorthalidone	2–3	2–6	40 (single dose) 45–60 (long-term dose)	24–48 (single dose) 48–72 (long-term dose)

half-life of 6–9 hours after a single oral dose, while chlorthalidone has a similar peak concentration time of about 2–6 hours but a much longer half-life (40 hours) after a single oral dose.[90–93] With long-term dosing hydrochlorothiazide and chlorthalidone have longer half-lives (8–15 hours and 45–60 hours, respectively) and longer durations of antihypertensive action (16–24 hours and 48–72 hours, respectively) (Table 5.4). The longer half-life of chlorthalidone has been attributed to its entry and concentration in erythrocytes, with slow release from this compartment.[94,95]

The usual starting daily dose of hydrochlorothiazide is 25 mg in younger patients with a maximum of 50 mg once daily, and 12.5 mg once daily in the elderly, to avoid side effects such as orthostatic hypotension and hypokalaemia.[3] Typical oral doses for chlorthalidone are 12.5 mg to 25 mg once daily (Table 5.3). As with hydrochlorothiazide, hypokalaemia associated with chlorthalidone is dose-related and lower doses of chlorthalidone, compared with the higher doses used in the past, offer a better efficacy-to-side effect ratio.[96–98]

Metolazone

Metolazone is a thiazide-like diuretic that differs from the typical thiazides in its chemical structure.[99] It is a heterocyclic variant of the benzothiadiazines, and because the thiazide ring system has been totally replaced by an alternate cyclic system, metolazone has distinctive characteristics. Metolazone retains its saliuretic potential in advanced renal failure, resembling the loop diuretics in this aspect. Direct inhibition of Na^+-dependent phosphate transport in the proximal tubule in vitro studies results in phosphaturia.[100,101] Metolazone also acts on the cortical diluting segment in a manner similar to the thiazides.[99,102,103]

Metolazone is well absorbed from the gastrointestinal tract with a 65% oral bioavailability.[5] Excretion is by secretion into the urine by the proximal tubular cells via the probenecid-sensitive organic acid pathway. Metolazone is excreted largely unchanged in the urine.[47,104,105]

Oral doses range from 2.5 to 5 mg daily.[3] Metolazone can be used in the treatment of hypertension either alone or in combination with other antihypertensive agents from a different class. However, use in hypertension is infrequent because of marked and rapid diuresis that may result in electrolyte imbalances, e.g. hyponatraemia, hypochloraemic alkalosis and hypokalaemia.[106] More common indications include treating oedematous states associated with congestive heart failure, renal and liver disease.

Indapamide

Indapamide is a thiazide-like diuretic that differs chemically from the thiazides in that it does not have a thiazide ring system and contains only one sulphonamide group.[106] This agent has 93% oral bioavailability.[5] Indapamide is approximately 70–80% bound to plasma protein and is preferentially and reversibly taken up by, and concentrated in, erythrocytes.[107] This drug is extensively metabolized, with only 5–7% recovered unchanged in the urine 48 hours after oral administration.[106,107] The usual daily dose for indapamide ranges from 1.25 mg to 2.5 mg.[3] Like metolazone, indapamide is indicated for the treatment of hypertension and oedematous states associated with congestive heart failure.

Indapamide has been implicated in a small number of case reports of severe hyponatraemia and hypokalaemia.[108] An Australian retrospective study reported that clinically significant hyponatraemia occurred more frequently with indapamide compared with the hydrochlorothiazide-amiloride combination or chlorothiazide, predominantly in elderly women.[109] The hyponatraemic effect of indapamide was dose-dependent, and approximately 85% of cases were related to use of the 2.5 mg dose. Hyponatraemia and hypokalaemia occurred in 21% and 22%, respectively, of all reported adverse drug reactions in which indapamide was the sole suspect drug.

Chlorothiazide

Chlorothiazide is the prototype thiazide diuretic, but is not commonly used today because of problems with bioavailability.[89] This diuretic is not metabolized and is eliminated rapidly by the kidney, with 10–15% of the drug excreted in the urine unchanged after oral dosing.[106] Usual oral doses for chlorothiazide range from 125 mg to 500 mg daily.[3] Indications include treatment of more severe forms of hypertension (either alone or to enhance the effectiveness of other antihypertensive agents) and adjunctive therapy in oedema associated with congestive heart failure, hepatic cirrhosis, renal failure, nephrotic syndrome and corticosteroid therapy.[106]

Polythiazide

Polythiazide is a benzothiadiazine derivative that shares indications with chlorothiazide: treating more severe forms of hypertension and oedematous states. There is complete oral bioavailability and the major route of elimination is in urine.[5] The usual oral daily dose for hypertension treatment is 2 mg to 4 mg.[3]

LOOP DIURETICS

The loop diuretics are used in clinical medicine mainly to remove excess NaCl and water in oedematous states such as heart failure, chronic kidney disease and liver disease. In addition, they are helpful in controlling BP in patients with chronic kidney disease in whom thiazides and thiazide-like agents are not effective.

Mechanisms of action

Diuresis/natriuresis

Loop diuretics are inhibitors of the type 2 $Na^+:K^+:2Cl^-$ cotransporter (NKCC2), the major pathway for Na^+ reabsorption in the apical membrane of the thick ascending limb (TAL) of the loop of Henle (Fig. 5.3). Na^+ enters the epithelial cells of the TAL by the participation of this cotransporter in the apical membrane, which allows Na^+, K^+, and $2Cl^-$ to enter simultaneously via Na^+ and $2Cl^-$ gradients. The loop diuretics act by competitively binding to one of the Cl^- binding sites on the apical aspect of the NKCC2, rapidly blocking transport. This cotransporter captures the energy in the Na^+ electrochemical gradient established by the basolateral $Na^+:K^+:ATPase$ pump and provides for 'uphill' transport of both K^+ and Cl^- into the cell.[5] K^+ recycles across the apical cell membrane, which is highly permeable to K^+, and thereby generates the positive potential in the tubule lumen. This positive potential difference repels cations (Na^+, Ca^{2+}, and Mg^{2+}) and, therefore, provides a driving force for the paracellular flux of these cations into the interstitium.[5] In addition, the basolateral membrane has a $Na^+:Cl^-$ cotransporter which permits the cotransport of Cl^- down the electrochemical gradient as well as the transport of Na^+ against an electrochemical gradient.

The NKCC from dogfish shark rectal gland, rabbit and humans has been cloned.[110,111] In mammals, the NKCC2 is of two varieties: (1) the 'absorptive' cotransporter (called ENCC2, NKCC2 or BSC1) expressed only in the kidney and localized to the apical membrane of the TAL and (2) the 'secretory' cotransporter (called ENCC3, NKCC1, or BSC2), which functions as a 'housekeeping' protein that is widely expressed and, in epithelial cells, is localized to the basolateral membrane.[112–116] Mutations in the genes coding for the absorptive NKCC2, the apical K^+ channel or the basolateral Cl^- channel give rise to Bartter's syndrome.[116] This autosomal recessive disorder is characterized by hypokalaemic metabolic alkalosis with salt wasting, arterial hypotension and nephrocalcinosis.[2]

Loop diuretics tend to increase renal blood flow without increasing filtration rate, especially after intravenous administration. When loop diuretics increase renal blood flow, blood flow is redistributed from the renal medulla to the cortex. As a result, acute diuresis increases intraluminal pressure and transiently reduces filtration rate.[117] This change in renal haemodynamics reduces fluid and electrolyte reabsorption in the proximal tubule and may augment the initial diuretic response to the loop diuretics.[118] However, this increase in renal blood flow is short-lived. Renal blood flow tends to decrease because of the reduction of extracellular fluid volume resulting from the drug-induced diuresis, allowing for increased reabsorption in the proximal tubule, a compensatory mechanism that limits delivery of solute to the TAL, thereby diminishing the diuresis.[118] This brings into question the minor proximal tubular action of loop diuretics. Some loop diuretics (like furosemide) can inhibit carbonic anhydrase, but the inhibitory action on the proximal tubule does not contribute to the diuresis, and effects have only been seen when massive doses of loop diuretic are given.[47]

Ca^{2+} reabsorption

Ca^{2+} is reabsorbed in parallel with Na^+ and Mg^{2+} at the apical membrane of the TAL (Fig. 5.3).[119] Loop diuretics, unlike the thiazides, enhance the excretion of Ca^{2+} and can, therefore, be used to treat hypercalcaemia. The calciuric action of loop diuretics is the basis for their use in symptomatic hypercalcaemia.[119] Volume depletion associated with hypercalcaemia should be corrected initially, as this alone may be sufficient to correct hypercalcaemia. If hypercalcaemia persists, loop diuretics can then be used. However, maintaining intravascular volume is imperative because of the vigorous diuresis that can result from these agents.[120]

Blood pressure reduction

Loop diuretics are occasionally used to treat hypertension, but are less effective than the thiazides in most hypertensive patients with well preserved renal function because of the ability of thiazides to produce a sustained reduction in TPR. There is weight loss during the first stage of therapy with loop diuretics because of resultant diuresis and loss of body fluids.[120] However, the diuretic and vasodilating effects are short-acting and can activate the sympathetic nervous system and cause an increase in afterload, a reduction in cardiac function and a rebound increase in BP.[121]

In essential hypertension, the short duration of action requires loop diuretics to be administered in multiple daily doses to control BP, and these drugs are, therefore, not favoured over the thiazides.[122] However, loop diuretics in combination therapy with other antihypertensive agents have been shown to be beneficial in controlling BP.[120] Most antihypertensive drugs have sodium-retaining properties associated with expansion of plasma and extracellular fluid volumes, and these volume changes may account for decreased responsiveness to antihypertensive therapy and the development of drug resistance.[123] Loop diuretics, especially at higher doses, block the sodium-retaining properties of other antihypertensive agents, thus allowing the latter to exert their full antihypertensive effect.[124] Loop diuretics, specifically furosemide or bumetanide, are often useful in treating hypertensive emergencies, both to lower BP by removing excess volume and to prevent the loss of potency of other antihypertensive agents that cause fluid retention.[125]

Pharmacokinetics

Loop diuretics are readily absorbed from the gastrointestinal tract, with an oral bioavailability of 60% for furosemide, and 80% for both bumetanide and torasemide (Table 5.5).[5] Like the thiazide diuretics, these drugs are highly bound to plasma proteins. Filtration of the loop diuretics is, therefore, limited. Loop diuretics are mainly secreted by the organic acid transport system in the proximal tubule, ultimately gaining access to their binding site on the NKCC2 in the luminal membrane of the TAL.[5] Furosemide and bumetanide are mainly excreted in the urine (65% and 62%, respectively). In contrast, torasemide is 80% metabolized.[5]

Adverse effects associated with loop diuretics

Loop diuretics share the adverse effects seen with thiazide and thiazide-like diuretics related to volume depletion, electrolyte disturbances or metabolic effects (Table 5. 2). Unlike the thiazides, loop diuretics can cause both auditory and vestibular toxicity, which can result in tinnitus and hearing loss.[34] This is usually associated with high doses, particularly in patients with renal insufficiency and in those receiving other ototoxic medications such as aminoglycoside antibiotics. Loop diuretic-induced ototoxicity is associated with loss of cochlear hair cells and alterations in electrolyte composition of the endolymph in the inner ear.[5,34] The risk of ototoxicity is greatest with ethacrynic acid, accounting for its low use compared with the other loop diuretics.[126,127] In contrast, ototoxicity is rare with the other loop diuretics, and large doses of furosemide, for example, can be administered without ototoxic effects.[128,129]

Allergic interstitial nephritis can occur with chronic use of loop diuretics.[34] Deterioration in renal function in a previously stable patient on chronic loop diuretic therapy may be an indication of this condition. If a loop diuretic is still required, an agent with a chemically different structure should be used.[34]

Individual loop diuretics

Furosemide

Furosemide is structurally similar to the thiazide class of diuretics in that it is also a sulphonamide derivative of anthranilic acid. This drug is strongly bound to plasma proteins and possesses low lipid solubility. Furosemide is poorly filtered and enters the tubular fluid mainly via secretion in the proximal tubule.[47] Probenecid can inhibit the secretion of furosemide at this site, thus reducing its diuretic effect. The diuretic effect of furosemide is short lived and is almost immediately reversed once the drug is discontinued.

Furosemide has a short half-life, which is responsible for its brief diuretic action. When administered intravenously, the response begins within a few minutes and lasts for 2–3 hours. If furosemide is given orally, diuresis occurs within about 30–90 minutes and continues for another 2–3 hours.[34] This brief duration of action requires furosemide to be administered multiple times in a day for adequate diuresis. Furosemide is available in 20, 40, and 80 mg tablets.[3] The initial dose in adults is 20 mg and can be repeated every 12 hours or as frequently as every 6 hours if there is no initial response.

Table 5.5 Inhibitors of Na$^+$-K$^+$-2Cl$^-$ cotransporter. Loop diuretics commonly used and referred to in JNC7 guidelines are shown

Drug	Structure	Relative potency	Oral availability	t$_{1/2}$ (Hours)	Route of elimination
Furosemide		1	~60%	~1.5	~65% R. ~35% M
Bumetanide		40	~80%	~0.8	~62% R. ~38% M
Torsemide		3	~80%	~3.5	~20% R, ~80% M

Abbreviations: R, renal excretion of intact drug; M, metabolism; ID, insufficient data.

Furosemide is useful for treating oedema of cardiac, renal or hepatic origin.[118] Oral administration is the preferred route, except in circumstances such as acute pulmonary oedema, where a rapid reduction in extracellular fluid is needed. In this case, intravenous administration is more effective. Loop diuretics are also useful in hypertensive crisis and in the setting of acute congestive heart failure, where severe elevations in systemic vascular resistance may precipitate left ventricular failure.[130] Sodium nitroprusside, administered in conjunction with oxygen, morphine and a loop diuretic is the treatment of choice.

Torasemide

Torasemide is an anilinopyridine sulphonylurea derivative that is pharmacologically similar to furosemide (Table 5.5).[131] Torasemide is as effective as furosemide in terms of its diuretic and saliuretic activity, with both drugs having a rapid onset of action when given intravenously. However, torasemide produces prolonged water and electrolyte excretion and is more likely to cause electrolyte disturbances, perhaps accounting for its limited clinical use.[132] Torasemide is indicated in the treatment of oedematous states, and at doses of less than 5 mg/day does not alter serum uric acid, K^+ or glucose levels.[131,133] Ototoxicity with torasemide is rare, even at high oral doses.[134]

Bumetanide

The sulphamoyl benzoic acid structure present in furosemide was altered in order to develop bumetanide.[99] The diuretic profile resembles that of furosemide, but it is 40 to 60 times more potent on a weight basis, i.e. 1 mg of torasemide is equivalent to 40 mg of furosemide orally.[47,135–137]

ROLE OF DIURETICS IN ANTIHYPERTENSIVE THERAPY

Thiazide and thiazide-like diuretics were the earliest class of antihypertensive drugs to be tested in outcome trials. Beginning with the V.A. Cooperative trial, conducted more than 35 years ago, antihypertensive regimens that included a thiazide-type diuretic have been tested for their ability to prevent cardiovascular disease (CVD) morbidity and mortality. The V.A. trial, which compared a fixed combination of hydrochlorothiazide, reserpine and hydralazine with placebo,[138] and the Hypertension Detection and Follow-up Program (HDFP), which compared stepped care with chlorthalidone, reserpine, methyldopa and hydralazine to usual care in the community,[139] were pioneering trials that documented the benefit on clinical outcomes of lowering BP with a thiazide-type diuretic-based regimen. Many subsequent trials have confirmed that finding. The largest of these, ALLHAT, randomized over 42 000 high-risk hypertensives to treatment with chlorthalidone, a calcium channel blocker, ACE inhibitor or α-blocker to test the hypothesis that the newer drug classes are more effective than the diuretics in preventing fatal CHD or non-fatal MI.[67] Results showed that thiazide diuretics are unsurpassed by representatives of the other major classes of antihypertensive agents in preventing fatal and non-fatal coronary events and are superior to other classes in preventing some of the cardiovascular complications of hypertension, including congestive heart failure (CHF) and stroke.

A network meta-analysis of data from 42 large, long-term outcome trials that included over 190 000 patients compared low-dose diuretics with placebo and each of five first-line active antihypertensive therapies.[140] The primary treatment strategies used a stepped-care approach and included: (1) placebo, untreated or usual care, (2) low-dose diuretic therapy (starting with 12.5 mg to 25 mg per day of chlorthalidone or hydrochlorothiazide), (3) β-blockers, (4) angiotensin-converting enzyme (ACE) inhibitors, (5) angiotensin receptor blockers (ARBs), (6) calcium channel blockers (CCBs) and (7) α-blockers. For all outcomes, including CHD, CHF, stroke, CVD events, CVD mortality and total mortality, low-dose diuretic therapy was superior to placebo (Fig. 5.9).[140] None of the other first-line treatment strategies was significantly better than low-dose diuretic therapy for any outcome. Low-dose diuretics were associated with reduced risks of: (1) CVD events compared with CCBs, (2) stroke, CHF and CVD events compared with ACE inhibitors, (3) CVD events compared with β-blockers and (4) CHF and CVD events compared with α-blockers. These results demonstrate that low-dose diuretics are the most effective first-line treatment for preventing CVD morbidity and mortality.[140]

Using the results from the above network meta-analysis, the placebo-controlled trials were divided into those that used chlorthalidone ($n=2$) and those that used other low-dose diuretic therapies ($n=3$).[140,141] Direct and indirect comparisons of low-dose chlorthalidone and non-chlorthalidone treatment on health outcomes were evaluated (Table 5.6). In these five trials, there were 214 CHD events and 660 deaths among the 7146 participants randomized to chlorthalidone, and 370 CHD events and 871 deaths among the 7940 participants randomized to other low-dose diuretics. Thus, major health outcomes with low-dose chlorthalidone and other thiazide-like drugs appear to be similar.[141] Based on these evidence-based findings and cost considerations, US, Canadian and WHO/ISH guidelines recommend thiazide-type diuretics as first-line treatment for most hypertensive patients, either alone or in combination with other antihypertensive agents.[3,142,143] British guidelines[144] provide an algorithm for choosing drugs/drug combinations based on the patient's age, race and comorbid conditions, while ESH/ESC guidelines[145] defer drug choices to the health care provider's judgment, with diuretics being one of the five major drug classes mentioned as acceptable options.

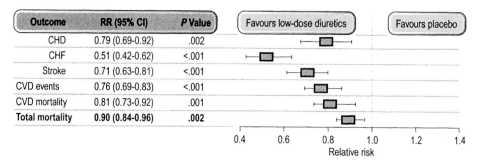

Outcome	RR (95% CI)	P Value
CHD	0.79 (0.69-0.92)	.002
CHF	0.51 (0.42-0.62)	<.001
Stroke	0.71 (0.63-0.81)	<.001
CVD events	0.76 (0.69-0.83)	<.001
CVD mortality	0.81 (0.73-0.92)	.001
Total mortality	0.90 (0.84-0.96)	.002

Fig. 5.9 Results from a network meta-analysis of first-line treatment strategy with low-dose diuretic therapy vs. placebo and health outcomes in randomized controlled clinical trials in hypertension. *(Modified with permission from ref. (140).)*

Table 5.6 Results from a meta-analysis of health outcomes of chlorthalidone vs. other thiazide diuretics

Outcome	RR (95% CI)		Indirect comparison SI (95% CI)*
	Chlorthalidone	Non-chlorthalidone	
Coronary disease	0.74 (0.58–0.95)	0.72 (0.54–0.95)	1.03 (0.71–1.48)
Stroke	0.64 (0.51–0.80)	0.71 (0.60–0.85)	0.90 (0.70–1.17)
Heart failure	0.53 (0.39–0.73)	NA	NA
Cardiovascular disease (CVD) events	0.70 (0.61–0.80)	0.76 (0.66–0.87)	0.92 (0.76–1.11)
CVD mortality	0.80 (0.61–1.04)	0.79 (0.65–0.94)	1.01 (0.74–1.39)
Total mortality	0.89 (0.75–1.06)	0.91 (0.79–1.03)	0.98 (0.79–1.21)

CI=confidence interval; NA=not available because of no data; RR=relative risk; SI=synergy index
*SI<1 suggests that chlorthalidone is superior to non-chlorthalidone diuretics for that outcome; SI>1 suggests that chlorthalidone is inferior to non-chlorthalidone diuretics for that outcome
(Adapted from ref. (141) with permission.)

Acknowledgements

National Heart, Lung, and Blood Institute Grant HL07457 (M.N.U.)

References

1. Health information update from IMS health 2001. Online. Available *http://www. imshealthcanada.com/htmen/3_1_5.htm.*
2. Knepper MA, Kleyman T, Gamba G. Diuretics: mechanism of action. In: Oparil S, Weber M, eds. *Hypertension: a companion to Brenner and Rector's the kidney, 2nd edn.* Philadelphia: Elsevier Sanders; 2005:638–652.
3. Chobanian AV, Bakris GL, Black HR, et al. The Seventh Report of the Joint National Committee on Prevention, Detection, Evaluation, and Treatment of High Blood Pressure. *JAMA* 2003;289:2560–2572.
4. Shah SU, Anjum S, Littler WA. Use of diuretics in cardiovascular disease: (2) hypertension. *Postgrad Med* 2003;80:271–276.
5. Jackson EK. Diuretics. In: Hardman JG, Limbird LE, Goodman Gilman A, eds. *Goodman & Gilman's The pharmacological basis of therapeutics.* New York: McGraw-Hill; 2001:757–787.
6. Brunner R, Brunner M. Adaptation to renal injury. In: Kasper D, Braunwald E, Fauci A, et al, eds. *Harrison's principles of internal medicine, 16th edn.* New York: McGraw Hill; 2002 Online. Available *http://www.harrisons.accessmedicine.com* 27 Aug 2002.
7. Guyton AC, Hall JE. Urine formation by the kidneys: II. Tubular processing of the glomerular filtrate. In: Guyton AC, Hall JE. *Textbook of medical physiology.* Philadelphia: Saunders; 1991:295–296.
8. Guyton AC. Blood pressure control – special role of the kidneys and body fluids. *Science* 1991;252:1813–1816.
9. Lifton RP, Gharavi AG, Geller DS. Molecular mechanisms of human hypertension. *Cell* 2001;104:545–556.
10. Gamba G. Molecular biology of distal nephron sodium transport mechanisms. *Kidney Int* 1999;56:1606–1622.
11. Beaumont K, Vaughn DA, Healy H. Thiazide diuretic receptors in the rat kidney: identification with ^{3}H metolazone. *Proc Natl Acad Sci U.S.A.* 1988;85:2311–2314.
12. Gamba G, Saltzberg SN, Lombardi M, et al. Primary structure and functional expression of cDNA encoding the thiazide-sensitive electroneutral sodium-chloride transporter. *Proc Natl Acad Sci U.S.A.* 1993;90:2749–2753.
13. Mastroianni N, De Fusco M, Zollo M, et al. Molecular cloning, expression pattern, and chromosomal localization of the human Na-Cl thiazide-sensitive cotransporter (SCL12A3). *Genomics* 1996;35:486–493.
14. Bachmann S, Velazquez H, Obermuller N, et al. Expression of a thiazide-sensitive Na-Cl cotransporter in rabbit distal convoluted tubule cells. *J Clin Invest* 1995;96:2510–2514.

15. Chang H, Tashiro K, Hirai M, et al. Identification of the cDNA encoding a thiazide-sensitive sodium-chloride cotransporter from the human and its mRNA expression in various tissues. *Biochem Biophys Res Commun* 1996;223:324–328.
16. Obermuller N, Kunchaparty S, Ellison DH, et al. Expression of the Na-K-2Cl cotransporter by the macula densa and thick ascending limb cells of rat and rabbit nephron. *J Clin Invest* 1996;98:635–640.
17. Plotkin MD, Kaplan MR, Verlander JW, et al. Localization of the thiazide-sensitive Na-Cl-cotransporter, rTSC1, in the rat kidney. *Kidney Int* 1996;50:174–183.
18. Bodtonjoglo M, Reeves WB, Reiley RF, et al. 11 β-hydroxysteroid dehydrogenase, mineralocorticoid receptor, and thiazide-sensitive Na-Cl cotransporter expression by distal tubules. *J Am Soc Nephr* 1998;9:1347–1358.
19. Kim GH, Masilamani S, Turner R, et al. The thiazide-sensitive Na-Cl cotransporter is an aldosterone-induced protein. *Proc Natl Acad Sci U.S.A.* 1998;14552–14557.
20. Velazquez H, Bartiss A, Bernstein P, et al. Adrenal steroids stimulate thiazide-sensitive NACl transport by rat renal distal tubules. *Am J Physiol* 1996;270:F211–F219.
21. Lemmink HH, van den Heuvel LP, van Dijk H, et al. Linkage of Gitelman syndrome to the thiazide-sensitive sodium-chloride cotransporter gene with identification of mutations in Dutch families. *Ped Nephrol* 1996;10:403–407.
22. Wilson FH, Disse-Nicodene S, Choate KA, et al. Human hypertension caused by mutations in WNK kinases. *Science.* 2001;293:1107–1112.
23. Costanzo LS. Localization of diuretic action in microperfused rat distal tubules: Ca and Na transport. *Am J Physiol (Renal Fluid and Electrolyte Physiology)* 1985;248:F527–F535.
24. Gesek FA, Friedman PA. Mechanism of calcium transport stimulated by chlorthiazide in mouse distal convoluted tubule cells. *J Clin Invest* 1992;90:429–438.
25. Stokes JB. Electroneutral NaCl transport in distal tubule. *Kidney Int* 1989;36:427–433.
26. Ray WA, Griffin MR, Downey W, et al. Long-term use of thiazide diuretics and risk of hip fracture. *Lancet* 1989;I:687–690.
27. Wanich R, Davis J, Ross P, et al. Effect of thiazide on rates of bone mineral loss: a longitudinal study. *Br Med J* 1990;310:1303–1305.
28. Roos JC, Boer P, Koomans HA, et al. Hemodynamic and hormonal changes during the acute and chronic diuretic treatment in essential hypertension. *Eur J Clin Pharmacol* 1981;19:107–112.
29. Shah S, Khatri I, Freis ED. Mechanism of antihypertensive effect of thiazide diuretics. *Am Heart J* 1978;95:611–618.
30. Van Brummelen P, Man in t'Veld AJ, Schalekamp MA. Hemodynamic changes during long-term thiazide treatment of essential hypertension in responders and nonresponders. *Clin Pharmacol Ther* 1980;279:328–336.
31. Tarazi RC, Dustan HP, Frohliich ED. Long-term thiazide treatment of essential hypertension in responders and non-responders. *Circulation* 1970;41:709–717.
32. Sica DA. Thiazide-type diuretics: Ongoing considerations on mechanism of action. *J Clin Hypertens* 2004;6:661–664.
33. Conway J, Lauers P. Hemodynamic and antihypertensive effects of long-term therapy with chlorthalidone. *Circulation* 1960;21:21–27.
34. Brater DC. Pharmacology of diuretics. *Am J Med Sci* 2000;319:38–50.
35. Pickkers P, Hughes AD, Franse GM, et al. Thiazide-Induced vasodilatation in humans is mediated by potassium channel activation. *Hypertension* 1998;32:1071–1076.
36. Levinson PD, Khari IM, Freis ED. Persistence of normal BP after withdrawal of drug treatment in mild hypertension. *Arch Intern Med* 1982;142:2265–2268.
37. Nelson MR, Reid CM, Krum H, et al. Short term predictors of maintenance of normotension after withdrawal of antihypertensive drugs in the second Australian National Blood Pressure Study (ANBP2). *Am J Hypertens* 2003;16:39–45.
38. Calder JA, Schachter M, Sever PS. Mechanisms of action of cicletanine in human guinea-pig resistance arteries. *J Cardiovasc Pharmacol* 1992;19:387–393.
39. Calder JA, Schachter M, Sever PS. Ion channel involvement in the acute vascular effects of thiazide diuretics and related compounds. *J Pharmacol Exp Ther* 1993;265:1175–1180.
40. Calder JA, Schachter M, Sever PS. Potassium channel opening properties of thiazide diuretics in isolated guinea-pig resistance arteries. *J Cardiovasc Pharmacol* 1994;24:158–164.
41. Pickkers P, Hughes AD. Relaxation and decrease in $[Ca^{2+}]_i$ by hydrochlorthiazide in guinea pig isolated mesenteric arteries. *J Cardiovasc Pharmacol* 1995;114:703–707.
42. Gimenez-Gallego GM, Navia MA, Reuben JP, et al. Purification, sequence and model structure of charybdotoxin a potent selective inhibitor of calcium activated potassium channels. *Proc Natl Acad Sci U.S.A.* 1988;85:3329–3333.
43. Longmore J, Newgreen DT, Weston AH. Effect of chromakalim, RF49256, diazoxide, glibenclamide and galanin in rat portal vein. *Eur J Pharmacol* 1990;190:75–84.

44. Campbell DB. The possible mode of action of indapamide: a review. *Curr Med Res Opin* 1983;8(Suppl 3):9–24.
45. Mironneau J. Indapamide-induced inhibition of calcium movement in smooth muscles. *Am J Med* 1988;84(Suppl 1B):10–14.
46. Del Rio M, Chulia T, Gonzalez P, et al. Effects of indapamide on contractile responses and $^{45}Ca^{2+}$ movements in various isolated blood vessels. *Eur J Pharmacol* 1993;250:133–139.
47. Morgan T. The use of diuretic drugs and aldosterone antagonists in hypertension. In: Birkenhäger WH, Reid JL, eds. *Handbook of hypertension, clinical pharmacology and hypertensive drugs,* Amsterdam: Elsevier; 1988:73–102.
48. Greenberg A. Diuretic complications. *Am J Med Sci* 2000;319:10–24.
49. Schwartz WB. Role of anions in metabolic alkalosis and potassium deficiency. *New Engl J Med* 1968;279:630–639.
50. Tannen RL. Diuretic-induced hypokalemia. *Kidney Int* 1985;28:988–1000.
51. Multiple Risk Factor Intervention Trial Research Group. Multiple risk factor intervention trial: risk factor changes and mortality results. *JAMA* 1982;248:1465–1477.
52. Siscovick DS, Raghunathan TE, Psaty BM, et al. Diuretic therapy for hypertension and the risk of primary cardiac arrest. *N Engl J Med* 1994;330:1852–1857.
53. Franse LV, Pahor M, Di Barig, et al. Hypokalemia associated with diuretic use and cardiovascular events in the Systolic Hypertension in the Elderly Program (SHEP). *Hypertension* 2000;35:1025–1030.
54. Gavras I, Gavras H. The debate goes on - What is your choice? *Am J Cardiol* 2005;95:53–54.
55. Dunder K, Lind L, Bjorn Z, et al. Increase in blood glucose concentration during antihypertensive treatment as a predictor of myocardial infarction: population based cohort study. *BMJ* 2003;326:1–5.
56. Hansson L, Lindholm LH, Ekborn T, et al. Randomized trial of old and new antihypertensive drugs in elderly patients: cardiovascular mortality and morbidity the Swedish Trial in Old Patients with Hypertension-2 study. *Lancet* 1999;354:1751–1756.
57. Padwal R, Laupacis A. Antihypertensive therapy and incidence of type 2 diabetes. *Diabetes Care* 2004;27:247–255.
58. SHEP Cooperative Research Group. Prevention of stroke by antihypertensive drug treatment in older persons with isolated systolic hypertension: Final results of the Systolic Hypertension in the Elderly Program (SHEP). *JAMA* 1991;265:3255–3264.
59. SHEP Cooperative Research Group. Influence of long-term, low-dose, diuretic-based, antihypertensive therapy on glucose, lipid, uric acid, and potassium levels in older men and women with isolated systolic hypertension: The Systolic Hypertension in the Elderly Program. *Arch Intern Med* 1998;13:741–751.
60. Knowles WC, Barrett-Connor E, Fowler SE, et al. Reduction in the incidence of type 2 diabetes with lifestyle intervention or metformin. *New Engl J Med* 2002;346:393–403.
61. Wilcox CS. Metabolic and adverse effects of diuretics. *Semin Nephrol* 1999;19:557–568.
62. Pollare T, Lithell H, Berbe C. A comparison of the effects of hydrochlorothiazide and captopril on glucose and lipid metabolism in patients with hypertension. *N Engl J Med* 1989;321: 868–873.
63. Gress TW, Nieto FJ, Shahar E, et al. Hypertension and antihypertensive therapy as risk factors for type 2 diabetes mellitus: atherosclerosis risk in communities study. *N Engl J Med* 2000;342:905–912.
64. Hansson L, Lindholm LH, Niskanen L, et al. Effect of angiotensin-converting-enzyme inhibition compared with conventional therapy on cardiovascular morbidity and mortality in hypertension: the Captopril Prevention Project (CAPPP) randomised trial. *Lancet* 1999;353: 611–616.
65. Brown MJ, Palmer CR, Castaigne A, et al. Morbidity and mortality in patients randomised to double-blind treatment with a long-acting calcium-channel blocker or diuretic in the International Nifedipine GITS study: Intervention as a Goal in Hypertension Treatment (INSIGHT). *Lancet* 2000;356:366–372.
66. Dahlof B, Devereux RB, Kjeldsen SE, et al. Cardiovascular morbidity and mortality in patients in the Losartan Intervention For Endpoint reduction in hypertension study (LIFE): a randomised trial against atenolol. *Lancet* 2002;359:1004–1010.
67. The ALLHAT Officers and Coordinators for the ALLHAT Collaborative Research Group. Major outcomes in high-risk hypertensive patients randomized to angiotensin-converting enzyme inhibitor or calcium channel blocker vs diuretic: The Antihypertensive and Lipid-Lowering Treatment to Prevent Heart Attack Trial (ALLHAT). *JAMA* 2002;288: 2981–2997.
68. Hansson L, Hedner T, Lund-Johansen P, et al. Randomised trial of effects of calcium antagonists compared with diuretics and beta-blockers on cardiovascular morbidity and mortality in hypertension: the Nordic Diltiazem (NORDIL) study. *Lancet* 2000;356:359–365.
69. Davis BR, Furberg CD, Wright JT, et al. ALLHAT: Setting the record straight. *Ann Intern Med* 2004;141:39–46.

70. Parmar M. Antihypertensive treatment, insulin resistance and risk of myocardial infarction.[Letter]. Bmj.com. 22 April 2003. Online. Available *http://bmj.com/cgi/letters/326/7391/681#31412.*

71. Ramsay LE, Yeo WW, Jackson PR, et al. Diabetes, impaired glucose tolerance and insulin resistance with diuretics. *Eur Heart J* 1992;13:68–71.

72. Samuelsson O, Pennert K, Andersson O, et al. Diabetes mellitus and raised serum triglyceride concentration in treated hypertension – are they of prognostic importance? Observational study. *BMJ* 1996;313:660–663.

73. Verdecchia P, Gianpaolo R, Fabio A, et al. Adverse prognostic significance of new diabetes in treated hypertensive subjects. *Hypertension* 2004;43:953–969.

74. Kostis JB, Wilson AC, Freudenberger RS, et al. Long-term effect of diuretic-based therapy on fatal outcomes in subjects with isolated systolic hypertension with and without diabetes. *Am J Cardiol* 2005;95:29–35.

75. Murphy MB, Lewis PJ, Kohner E, et al. Glucose intolerance in hypertensive patients treated with diuretics; a fourteen-year follow-up. *Lancet* 1982;2:1293–1295.

76. Plavinik FL, Rodrigues CI, Zanella MT, et al. Hypokalemia, glucose intolerance, and hyperinsulinemia during diuretic therapy. *Hypertension* 1992;19(Suppl):II26–II29.

77. Wilson PW, D'Agostino RB, Levy D, et al. Prediction of coronary heart disease using risk factor categories. *Circulation* 1988;97:1837–1847.

78. Swislocki AL, Hoffman BB, Reaven GM. Insulin resistance, glucose intolerance and hyperinsulinemia in patients with hypertension. *Am J Hypertens* 1989;2:419–423.

79. Kasiske BL, Ma JZ, Kalil RS, et al. Effects of antihypertensive therapy on serum lipids. *Ann Intern Med* 1995;122:133–141.

80. Grimm RHJ, Flack JM, Grandits GA, et al. Long-term effects on plasma lipids of diet and drugs to trest hypertension. Treatment of Mild Hypertension Study (TOHMS) Research Group. *JAMA* 1996;275:1549–1556.

81. Weir MR, Moser M. Diuretics and beta-blockers: is there a risk for dyslipidemia? *Am Heart J* 2000;139:174–183.

82. Medical Research Council Working Party. MRC trial of treatment of mild hypertension: principal results. *BMJ* 1985;291:97–104.

83. Curb JD, Borhani NO, Blaszkowski TP, et al. Long-term surveillance for adverse effects of antihypertensive drugs. *JAMA* 1985;253:3263–3268.

84. Report of Medical Research Council Working party on mild to moderate hypertension. Adverse reaction to bendrofluazide and propranolol for the treatment of mild hypertension. *Lancet* 1981;2:539–543.

85. Chang SW, Fine R, Siegel D, et al. The impact of diuretic therapy on reported sexual function and quality of life: TAIM study. *Ann Intern Med* 1991;114:613–620.

86. Grimm RH, Grandits GA, Prineas RJ, et al. Long-term effects on sexual function of five antihypertensive drugs and nutritional hygienic treatment in hypertensive men and women. Treatment of Mild Hypertension Study (TOMHS). *Hypertension* 1997;29:8–23.

87. Scharf MB, Maybleben DW. Comparative effects of prazosin and hydrochlorothiazide on sexual function in hypertensive men. *Am J Med* 1989;86(Suppl 1B):110–112.

88. Napoli C, Ignarro LJ. Nitric oxide-releasing drugs. *Annu Rev Pharmacol Toxicol* 2003;43: 97–123.

89. Carter BL, Ernst ME, Cohen JD. Hydrochlorothiazide versus chlorthalidone evidence supporting their interchangeablility. *Hypertension* 2004;43:4–9.

90. Giudicelli JF, Richer C, Mattei A. Pharmacokinetics and biological effects of captopril and hydrochlorothiazide after acute and chronic administration either alone or in combination in hypertensive patients. *Br J Clin Pharmacol* 1987;23(suppl 1):51S–63S.

91. Howes LG, Conway EL, Phillips PA, et al. Pharmacokinetic comparison of a combination tablet of enalapril and hydrochlorothiazide with enalapril and hydrochlorothiazide tablets administered together and separately. *Biopharm Drug Disposition* 1991;12:447–455.

92. McAinsh J, Bastain W, Young J, et al. Bioavailability in man of atenolol and chlorthalidone from a combination formula. *Biopharm Drug Disposition* 1981;2:147–156.

93. Riess W, Dubach UC, Burckhardt D, et al. Pharmacokinetic studies with chlorthalidone (Hygroton) in man. *Eur J Clin Pharmacol* 1977;12:375–382.

94. Colste P, Garle M, Rawlins MD, et al. Individual differences in chlorthalidone concentration in plasma and red cells of man after single and multiple doses. *European Journal of Clinical Pharmacology* 1976;9:319–325.

95. Tweedale MG, Olgilvie RI. Improved methods for estimating chlorthalidone in body fluids. *J Phar Sci* 1974;63:1065–1068.

96. Bengtsson C, Johnson G, Sannerstedt R, et al. Effects of different doses of chlorthalidone on blood pressure, serum potassium, and urate. *BMJ* 1975;1:197–199.

97. Grimm RH, Neaton JD, McDonald M, et al. Beneficial effects of systemic dosage reduction of the diuretic, chlorthalidone: a randomized study within a clinical trial. *Am Heart J* 1985;109: 858–864.

98. Morledge JH, Ettinger B, Aranda J, et al. Isolated systolic hypertension in the elderly: a placebo-controlled, dose-response evaluation of chlorthalidone. *J Am Geriatr Soc* 1986;34: 199–206.

99. Lant A. Diuretics: Clinical pharmacology and therapeutic use (part I). *Drugs* 1985;29:57–87.

100. Dargie HJ, Allison ME, Kennedy AC, et al. High dose metolazone in chronic renal failure. *BMJ* 1972;4:316–319.

101. Kempson SA, Kowalski JC, Puschett JB. Diuretic effect of metolazone on sodium-dependent transport across the renal brush-border membrane. *J Lab Clin Med* 1983;101:301–316.

102. Cangiaro JL. Effect of prolonged administration of metolazone in the treatment of essential hypertension. *Curr Ther Res* 1976;20:745.

103. Steinmuller SR, Puschett JB. Effects of metolazone on man:comparison with chlorothiazide. *Kidney Int* 1972;1:169.

104. Belair RA, Cohen AI, Yelnosky J. Renal excretion of metolazone, a new diuretic. *Br J Pharmacol* 1972;45:476–479.

105. Hinsvark ON, Zazulak W, Cohen AI. Liquid chromatography: its use in the biological characterization of metolazone-a new diuretic. *J Chromatography Sci* 1972;10:379–383.

106. Physicians Desk Reference, 59th Edition:1115–1116, 2222–2223;2038–2039.

107. Ackerman DM, Hook JB. Historical background, chemistry, and classification. In: Eknoyan G, Martinex-Maldonado M, eds. *The physiological basis of diuretic therapy in clinical medicine*, Orlando:Grune & Stratton; 1986:7–8.

108. Chan TY. Indapamide-induced severe hyponatremia and hypokalemia. *Ann Pharmacother* 1995;29:1124–1128.

109. Chapman MD, Hanrahan R, McEwen J, et al. Hyponatremia and hypokalemia due to indapamide. *Med J Aust* 2002;176:219–221.

110. Xu JC, Lytle TT, Payne JA, et al. Molecular cloning and functional expression of the bumetanide-sensitive Na-K-Cl cotransporter. *Proc Natl Acta Sci U.S.A.* 1994;91:2201–2205.

111. Payne JA, Forbush B. Alternatively spliced isoforms of the putative renal Na-K-Cl cotransporter are differentially distributed within the rabbit kidney. *Proc Natl Acad Sci U.S. A.* 1994;91:4544–4548.

112. Kaplan MR, Plotkin MD, Lee WS, et al. Apical localization of the Na-K-Cl cotransporter, RBSC1, on rat thick ascending limbs. *Kidney Int* 1996;49:40–47.

113. Lytle C, McManus, Haas M. A model of Na-K-2Cl cotransporter based on order ion binding and symmetry. *Am J Physiol* 1998;274:C299–C309.

114. Nielson S, Ecelbarger CA, Knepper MA. Ultrastructural localization of the Na-K-2Cl cotransporter in the thick ascending limb and macula densa of the rat kidney. *Am J Physiol* 1995;275:F885-F893.

115. Plata C, Mount DB, Rubia V, et al. Isoforms of the Na-K-2Cl cotransporter in murine TAL:II. Functional characterization and activation by cAmp. *Am J Physiol* 1999;276:F359-F366.

116. Simon DB, Lifton RP. Mutations in Na(K)Cl transporters in Gitelman's and Bartter's syndromes. *Curr Opin Cell Biol* 1998;10:450–454.

117. Mudge GH, Ciike WJ, Berndt WP. Electrolyte excretion and free-water production during onset of acute diuresis. *Am J Physiol* 1975;228:1304–1312.

118. Weiner IM. Diuretics and other agents employed in the mobilization of edema fluid. In: Hardman JG, Limbird LE, Goodman Gilman A, eds. *Goodman & Gilman's The pharmacological basis of therapeutics.* New York:McGraw-Hill; 2001:757–787.

119. Sutton RAL. Diuretics and calcium metabolism. *Am J Kidney Dis* 1985;5:4–9.

120. Mroczek WJ, Davidov M, Finnerty FA. Low dose furosemide therapy for hypertension. *Am J Cardiol* 1974;33:546–549.

121. Francis GS, Siel RM, Goldsmith SR, et al. Acute vasoconstrictor response to intravenous furosemide in patients with chronic congestive heart failure. *Ann Intern Med* 1985;103:1–6.

122. Kaplan N. *Clinical hypertension, 2nd edn.* Baltimore: Williams & Wilkins; 1978:117.

123. Mroczek WJ, Davidov M, Gavrilovich L, et al. Influence of the extracellular fluid volume on the antihypertensive drug response (abstract). *Clin Res* 1970;18:93.

124. Dustan HP, Tarazi RC, Bravo EL. Dependence of the arterial pressure on the intravascular volume in treated hypertensive patients. *N Engl J Med* 1972;286:861–866.

125. Kaplan N. *Clinical hypertension, 8th edn.* Philadelphia: Lippincott; 2002:353.

126. Cooperman LB, Rubin IL. Toxicity of ethacrynic acid and furosemide. *Am Heart J* 1973;85: 831–834.

127. Sheffield PA, Turner JS. Ototoxic drugs: a review of clinical aspects, histopathologic changes and mechanism of action. *South Med J* 1971;64:359–363.

128. Gerlag PGG, van Meijel JJM. High-dose furosemide in the treatment of refractory congestive heart failure. *Arch Intern Med* 1988;148:286–291.

129. Dormans TPJ, van Meyel JJM, Gerlag PGG, et al. Diuretic efficacy of high dose furosemide in severe heart failure: bolus injection versus continuous infusion. *J Am Coll Cardiol* 1996;28: 376–382.

130. Calhoun D. Hypertensive crisis. In: Oparil S, Weber M, eds. *Hypertension: A Companion to Brenner and Rector's.* The Kidney: WB Saunders; 2000:715–718.
131. Achhammer I, Metz P. Low dose loop diuretics in essential hypertension. Experience with torsemide. *Drugs* 1991;3:80–91.
132. Dunn CJ, Fitton A, Brogden RN. Torsemide: an update of its pharmacological properties and therapeautic efficacy. *Drugs* 1995;49:121–142.
133. Lehnert H, Schmitz H, Beyer J, et al. Control clinical trial investigating the influence of torsemide and furosemide on carbohydrate metabolism in patients with cardiac failure and concomitant type II diabetes. In: Puschett JB, Greenberg A, eds. *Diuretics IV: chemistry, pharmacology and clinical applications.* Philadelphia: Elsevier Science; 1993:271–274.
134. Clasen W, Khartabil T, Imm S, et al. Torsemide for diuretic treatment of advanced chronic renal failure. *Arzneimittel Forschung* 1988;38:209–211.
135. Asbury MJ, Gatenby PB, O'Sullivan S, et al. Bumetanide: Potent new 'loop' diuretic. *British Med J* 1972;1:211–213.
136. Branch RA, Read PR, Levine D, et al. Furosemide and bumetanide: A study of responses in normal English and German subjects. *Clin Pharm Ther* 1976;19:538–545.
137. Davies DL, Lant AF, Millard NR, et al. Renal action, therapeutic use, and pharmacokinetics of the diuretic bumetanide. *Clin Pharm Ther* 1974;15:141.
138. Veterans Administration Cooperative Study Group on Antihypertensive Agents. Effects of treatment on morbidity in hypertension: Results in patients with diastolic blood pressure averaging 115 through 129 mmHg. *JAMA* 1967;202:1028–1034.
139. Ramsay LE. The hypertension detection and follow-up program: 17 years on. *JAMA* 1997;277:167–170.
140. Psaty BM, Lumley T, Furberg CD, et al. Health outcomes associated with various antihypertensive therapies used as first-line agents. A network meta-analysis. *JAMA* 2003;289: 2534–2544.
141. Psaty BM. Meta-analysis of health outcomes of chlorthalidone-based vs nonchlorthalidone-based low-dose diuretic therapies (research letter). *JAMA* 2004;292:43–44.
142. Khan NA, McAlister FA, Campbell NR, et al. Canadian Hypertension Education Program. The 2004 Canadian recommendations for the management of hypertension: Part II-Therapy. *Can J Cardiol* 2004;20:41–54.
143. World Health Organization, International Society of Hypertension Writing Group. 2003 World Health Organization (WHO)/International Society of Hypertension (ISH) statement on management of hypertension. *J Hypertens* 2003;21:1983–1992.
144. Williams B, Poulter NR, Brown MJ, et al. British Hypertension Society Guidelines: Guidelines for management of hypertension: report of the fourth working party of the British Hypertension Society, 2004-BHS IV. *J Hum Hypertens* 2004;18:139–185.
145. Task Force for the Management of Arterial Hypertension of the European Society of Hypertension (ESH) and of the European Society of Cardiology (ESC). 2007 guidelines for the management of arterial hypertension. *J Hypertens* 2007;6:1105–1187.

6 | Aldosterone antagonists

Hari Krishnan Parthasarathy and Thomas M. MacDonald

INTRODUCTION

Aldosterone, first discovered by Simpson et al. in 1953, is a steroid hormone produced by the adrenal cortex. However, local synthesis in the heart, blood vessels and brain implies an alternative paracrine function. Aldosterone has been associated conventionally with fluid and electrolyte balance in the epithelial tissues, mainly the kidney and distal colon. The best known renal target sites for aldosterone are the cortical and outer medullary collecting tubules.[1–3] At the cortical collecting tubule, the principal role of mineralocorticoids is to enhance Na^+ reabsorption and K^+ secretion, while in the outer medullary collecting tubules, aldosterone stimulates H^+ secretion. There are three types of cells in these segments: principal cells, intercalated A cells and intercalated B cells. Principal cells reabsorb Na^+ through apical sodium channels and the basolateral Na^+:K^+:ATPase. H^+ is excreted by intercalated B cells, which have H^+-ATPase in the luminal membrane.[4] Aldosterone seems to have similar effects on Na^+ and K^+ transport in the colon.[5] The other epithelial targets for aldosterone are sweat glands, bile canalicula and the endolymphatic sac of the ear.[6,7] The role of aldosterone in these target organs is unclear.

In addition to its classical epithelial effects, aldosterone has a variety of non-epithelial effects, including induction of inflammatory processes, collagen formation, fibrosis and necrosis. Interest in these effects has recently resurfaced, having been noted as early as the 1940s by Selye.[8] Figure 6.1 shows the deleterious effects of aldosterone.

NON-EPITHELIAL DELETERIOUS EFFECTS OF ALDOSTERONE

In rat models of hypertension as well as in both primary and secondary hyperaldosteronism, aldosterone has been shown to induce accumulation of collagen and myocardial fibrosis.[10,11] Furthermore, in rats, aldosterone has been shown to induce severe coronary inflammatory lesions and subsequent myocardial

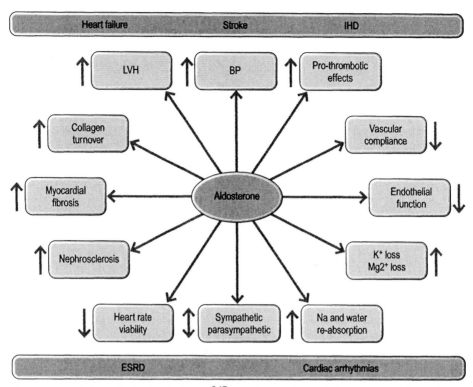

Fig. 6.1 Deleterious effects of aldosterone.[9,17] IHD=ischaemic heart disease; LVH=left ventricular hypertrophy; ESRD=end stage renal disease.

ischaemia and necrosis.[12] In human subjects with congestive cardiac failure, high baseline serum levels of markers of cardiac fibrosis, such as procollagen type III amino-terminal peptide (PIIINP), were significantly associated with poor outcome.[13] It has also been shown in various studies that left ventricular mass correlates with plasma aldosterone concentrations after adjustments for blood pressure (BP) in patients with hypertension and renal failure.[14,15] These effects of aldosterone can be blocked by both aldosterone receptor blockers and by reducing sodium chloride in the diet even when BP and other confounding factors are kept constant.

In the CONSENSUS trial involving subjects with congestive heart failure, a significant correlation was found between plasma aldosterone and mortality.[16] Angiotensin II and aldosterone reduction strategies with angiotensin converting inhibitors (ACE inhibitors) or angiotensin receptor blockers (ARBs) or their combination fail to completely block the renin–angiotensin–aldosterone system (RAAS) because of 'angiotensin II escape' or 'aldosterone escape'.[17] Findings from the recent Candesartan in Heart failure Assessment of Reduction in Mortality and morbidity study (CHARM-added limb) and Randomised Aldactone Evaluation Study (RALES) support these respective escape phenomena.[18,19]

Aldosterone induces endothelial dysfunction.[20,21] It also has been shown to contribute to the regulation of expression of plasminogen activator inhibitor (PAI-1), a regulator of fibrinolysis and extracellular matrix turnover.[22,23] Moreover there is recent evidence to show that increased aldosterone levels within the physiological range predispose to hypertension.[24]

There are currently three aldosterone antagonists licensed for use in clinical practice. These are spironolactone, potassium canrenoate and eplerenone.

Spironolactone

Spironolactone (proprietary name – Aldactone) is a non-specific mineralocorticoid receptor antagonist. The anti-mineralocorticoid activity of spironolactone was discovered in 1957 by Kagawa.[25]

Chemistry

Spironolactone (Fig. 6.2) (SC9420) is a synthetic steroid with chemical structure 17-hydroxy-7 α-mercapto-3-oxo-17 α-pregn-4-ene-21-carboxylic acid γ-lactone acetate; chemical formula $C_{24}H_{32}O_4S$ and molecular weight 416.57. The molecule is practically insoluble in water, but soluble in alcohol and readily soluble in benzene and chloroform.

Mechanism of action

Spironolactone acts as a competitive antagonist to aldosterone. The principal action is to compete for the intracellular mineralocorticoid receptors in the distal convoluted tubule and collecting ducts. The resultant spironolactone– receptor complex, unlike the aldosterone– receptor complex, is unable to attach to the DNA in the nucleus. This results in failure of induction of mediator proteins and subsequent inhibition of the primary sodium retaining effect of aldosterone. This consequently leads to inhibition of potassium and hydrogen ion secretion into the tubular lumen. Spironolactone and its metabolites may have similar effects on other target epithelial cells including sweat glands, colon, endolymphatic sac of the ear and biliary canalicula.[6,7]

Pharmacokinetics

Spironolactone is well absorbed from the gastrointestinal tract with bioavailability greater than 90%. Absorption is enhanced to nearly 100% by concomitant food intake.[26] In a pharmacokinetic study involving 12 healthy males receiving 100 mg of spironolactone once daily for 15 days, peak serum concentrations of spironolactone were 72 ± 45 µg/L on day 1 and 80 ± 20 µg/L on day 15. The area under the curve (AUC) (0–24) values on day 15 were 231 ± 50 µg/L/h, and post-steady elimination half-life was 1.4 ± 0.5 hours.[27] Spironolactone has very high protein binding (more than 90%). Metabolism is by the liver; metabolites can be divided into two main categories: those in which the sulphur of the parent molecule is removed (canrenone) and those in which the sulphur is retained (7α- thiomethylspirolactone, 6β-hydroxy-7α-thiomethylspirolactone). About 25–30% of spironolactone is converted to canrenone.[28-30]

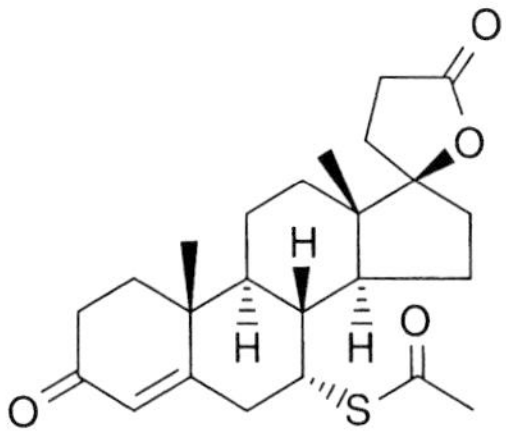

Fig. 6.2 Chemical stucture of spironolactone.

Canrenone has been long considered the major active metabolite of spironolactone. However, pharmacodynamic studies indicate that canrenone can only partly explain the action of spironolactone. Moreover, the recent advent of modern high performance liquid chromatographic techniques has shown that previously employed techniques were non-specific and possibly overestimated canrenone levels. It is now believed that both spironolactone and 7α- thiomethylspirolactone possess anti-mineralocorticoid activity and that these moieties may be mainly responsible for the activity of spironolactone.[31,32] Spironolactone has a plasma half-life of only 10 minutes, but canrenone has a plasma half-life of about 16 hours. The action of spironolactone is slow in onset and takes several days to develop. The metabolites are excreted primarily in the urine and secondarily in bile. It has been reported that 14–24% of spironolactone, canrenone or canrenoate is excreted in the urine within 5 days as measured by fluorescence assays, and 33% of an oral dose of potassium canrenoate within 4 days as measured by radioactivity analysis.[33]

Aspirin and other NSAIDs have been shown to attenuate the diuretic effect of spironolactone.[34] In 1962, Elliott was the first to suggest a possible antagonism of natriuretic effect of spironolactone when co-administered with aspirin.[35] This was later documented by others in animals and humans.[36,37] Acetylsalicylic acid 600 mg significantly reduced the urinary excretion and the fractional excretion of canrenone between 4 and 6 hours after administration of 50 mg spironolactone. There was a significant correlation between the reduction in canrenone excretion and the inhibition of the urinary electrolyte response.[38] Active secretion of canrenone by proximal renal tubule is via a transport mechanism shared by weak organic acids,[39] including metabolites of aspirin.[40] It may be concluded that competition for a common secretory mechanism in the renal tubule led to the reduced secretion and excretion of canrenone. The clinical significance of these interactions is uncertain. Aspirin does not appear to counteract the antihypertensive effect of spironolactone.[41]

In cirrhosis, the metabolism of spironolactone is impaired. The terminal half-lives of spironolactone and its metabolites including canrenone, 7α-thiomethylspirolactone and 6β-hydroxy-7α-thiomethylspirolactone are all increased in cirrhosis.[42]

In renal impairment the excretion of spironolactone and its metabolites is impaired. Spironolactone should be used with great caution or even avoided completely in severe renal impairment (GFR less than 10 mL/minute).

Pharmacodynamics

Aside from renal effects, spironolactone has been shown to act on various extra-renal and non-epithelial sites. Mineralocorticoid receptors have been detected in the colon, ureter, bladder, salivary glands, brain, heart and arterial system.[43–45] Some authors have reported aldosterone production in extra-adrenal tissues such as blood vessels, brain and heart.[46,47]

Heart In both animal models and in humans, spironolactone has been shown to prevent myocardial fibrosis and to reduce markers of fibrosis, as well as reducing left ventricular hypertrophy.[11,13,48–50] However, a low salt diet is as effective as aldosterone antagonism in preventing myocardial damage.[51] In rat models of primary and secondary aldosteronism, aldosterone antagonism with spironolactone has been shown to prevent myocardial fibrosis independent of BP.[11] Moreover, spironolactone decreased procollagen type III amino-terminal peptide (PIIINP), a marker of cardiac fibrosis in humans with congestive cardiac failure.[13] Sato et al. studied the combination of spironolactone with an ACE inhibitor and found that this combination produced greater reduction in left ventricle (LV) mass compared with ACE inhibitor alone.[49] In a further study they also demonstrated that the reduction in LV mass correlated with reduction in PIIINP levels.[48] In acute anterior myocardial infarction after revascularization, spironolactone along with ACE inhibitor was superior to ACE inhibitor alone in preventing post-infarct LV remodeling.[50] This benefit was associated with significant suppression of the trans-cardiac extraction of aldosterone measured at the aortic root and coronary sinus as well as suppression of plasma PIIINP.[50]

Blood vessels Spironolactone has been shown to improve vascular endothelial function in patients with heart failure.[52,53] The possible underlying mechanisms are enhanced endothelial nitric oxide bioactivity and inhibition of angiotensin I to angiotensin II conversion. Furthermore, in animal models, spironolactone inhibits angiogenesis.[54]

Brain In animal models, mineralocorticoid receptors (MR) in the central nervous system have been shown to play a role in mineralocorticoid hypertension as well as in the cardiovascular control of normotensive animals.[55–57] Moreover blockade of brain MR by spironolactone prevents sympathetic hyperactivity and improves cardiac function in rats post myocardial infarction.[58]

Steroidogenesis (Fig. 6.3, Tables 6.1 & 6.2)

Spironolactone inhibits adrenal and testicular cytochrome P450[59] and the terminal oxidases of several steroidogenic enzymes.[60–63] The effects of spironolactone and 7α- thiospironolactone (an intermediate in the activation pathway) on the adrenal cortex cause a decrease in ACTH-stimulated cortisol production as a result of the selective inhibition of 17α- hydroxylation.[64] Spironolactone is also an effective inducer of several hepatic drug metabolizing enzymes.[65,66]

Spironolactone has anti-androgenic effects and hence associated anti-acne effects.[67] Spironolactone antagonizes the effect of testosterone at target tissues in animals and in humans.[68–70] Neither spironolactone nor canrenoate K reduces prostatic 5α-reductase activity even in high concentrations,[71] indicating that the effect is unlikely to be mediated by inhibition of this enzyme and suggesting that the drugs may block the effect of androgens, particularly 5α- dihydrotestosterone (DHT), at their cytoplasmic receptors.[68,72]

Adverse effects

Several side effects of spironolactone are a consequence of its renal and extrarenal actions. Adverse effects are summarized in Table 6.3:

Renal impairment Spironolactone has been shown to worsen renal function in hypertensive and heart failure subjects. The risk factors are increasing age, increasing severity of heart failure, underlying renal impairment and diabetes mellitus.[73–75] In the RALES study involving 1663 patients with heart failure, during the first year of follow-up, the median creatinine concentration in the spironolactone group increased by approximately 0.05 to 0.10 mg per decilitre

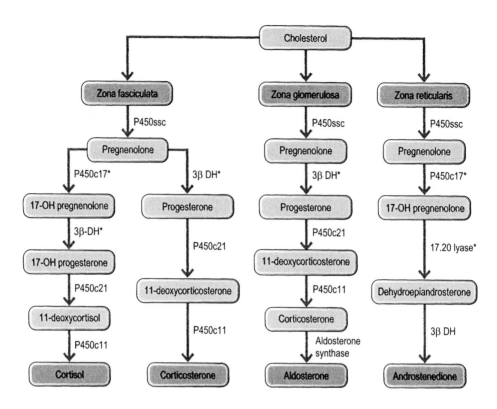

Fig. 6.3 The pathways of steroid biosynthesis and the effect of spironolactone. *(Adapted with permission from Dr King. http://isu.indstate.edu/mwking/steroid-hormones.html.)* P450ssc=P450 linked side chain cleaving enzyme; P450c17=17α-hydroxylase; 3β-DH=3β-dehydrogenase; P450c21= 21β-hydroxylase; P450c11=11β-hydroxylase. 17,20 lyase is the same as 17,20 desmolase in the testis. Yellow boxes=enzymes inhibited by spironolactone.

Table 6.1 Enzymes of steroid biosynthesis inhibited by spironolactone

17α-hydroxylase
17, 20 desmolase/17, 20 lyase
3β-dehydrogenase-isomerase

(Adapted from refs (59–62).)

Table 6.2 Hepatic microsomal drug metabolizing enzymes induced by spironolactone

Ethylmorphine N-demethylase
Aniline hydroxylase
NADPH oxidase
Cytochrome c reductase
NADPH cytochrome P-450 reductase
Cytochrome P-450 (CYP3A1)

(Adapted from refs (62,63).)

Table 6.3 Adverse effects of spironolactone

System	Side effects
Digestive	Gastric bleeding, ulceration, gastritis, diarrhoea, cramping, nausea, vomiting
Metabolic/endocrine	Hyperkalaemia, hyponatraemia, gynaecomastia, impotence, dysmenorrhoea, amenorrhoea, postmenopausal bleeding, deepening of voice, hirsutism, decrease in libido, carcinoma of breast has been reported (but cause–effect not proved)
Haematological	Agranulocytosis
Hypersensitivity	Fever, urticaria, rash, anaphylaxis, vasculitis
Nervous system/psychiatric	Mental confusion, ataxia, headache, drowsiness, lethargy
Liver/biliary	Mixed cholestatic/hepatocellular toxicity and one reported fatality
Renal	Renal dysfunction/failure

(Adapted from refs (18,26).)

(4–9 µmol/L). The median creatinine did not change in the placebo group. The differences between the two groups were significant ($p<0.001$).[18]

Electrolyte and acid–base disturbances Spironolactone has been shown to increase serum potassium levels in hypertensive and heart failure subjects.[74,75] In RALES the median potassium concentration increased significantly by 0.30 mmol/L compared with placebo ($p<0.001$). Serious hyperkalaemia occurred in 10 patients in the placebo group and 14 patients in the spironolactone group.[18] In a recent observational study in Canada, publication of the RALES study was associated with abrupt increases in the rate of prescriptions for spironolactone and this resulted in a marked increase in hyperkalaemia and renal failure-associated morbidity and mortality.[74] Closer laboratory monitoring and the more judicious use of spironolactone is required to reduce the occurrence of hyperkalaemia, as suggested previously.[75] However, 31% of the patients in this study had renal insufficiency and 46% had diabetes mellitus at baseline.[76] Spironolactone can also induce hyponatraemia, dehydration, hyperchloraemia and metabolic acidosis.[77]

Endocrine disorders Spironolactone lacks specificity for mineralocorticoid receptors and binds to both progesterone and dihydrotestosterone receptors. This can lead to various endocrine side effects that can limit the use of spironolactone. In females spironolactone can induce menstrual disturbances, breast enlargement and breast tenderness.[78]

In men spironolactone can induce gynaecomastia and impotence. In RALES gynaecomastia or breast pain was reported by 10% of the men in the spironolactone group and 1% of the men in the placebo group ($p<0.001$), causing more patients in the spironolactone group than in the placebo group to discontinue treatment, despite a mean spironolactone dose of 26 mg.[18]

Carcinogenesis In very high doses, spironolactone is carcinogenic in rats. There have been increased incidences of tumours of the testes, thyroid, liver, uterus as well as leukaemia in rats.[26] Breast cancer has been reported in five patients who had taken spironolactone for prolonged periods.[79]

Contraindications/cautions

Spironolactone can cause life-threatening hyperkalaemia. Therefore, spironolactone is contraindicated in hyperkalaemia and is relatively contraindicated in those at an increased risk of hyperkalaemia (Table 6.4).

The risk of hyperkalaemia is high in patients with diabetes mellitus, renal impairment, co-administration of other potassium-retaining medications (ACE inhibitor & ARBs) and in those receiving potassium supplements.[74,80] Other potential risk factors are increasing age and increasing severity of heart failure.[73]

Table 6.4 Contraindications of spironolactone

Anuria
Acute renal insufficiency
Significant renal impairment
Hyperkalaemia

Drug interactions (Table 6.5)

Table 6.5 Drug interactions with spironolactone

Drug	Interactions
ACE inhibitors	Hyperkalaemia
Non-steroidal anti-inflammatory drugs (NSAIDs)	↓ tubular secretion of canrenone (active metabolite of spironolactone) and hence ↓ diuretic, natriuretic, antihypertensive effects of spironolactone
Digoxin	↑ serum half-life, digitalis toxicity
Lithium	↓ renal clearance, lithium toxicity; best avoided
Corticosteriods, ACTH	Electrolyte depletion
Alcohol, barbiturates, narcotics	Orthostatic hypotension

Clinical use/outcome data/beneficial effects

Hypokalaemia Spironolactone is indicated for the treatment of hypokalaemia due to a variety of causes.[81,82]

Hypertension Spironolactone does not have a licence for hypertension in the UK; the license having been withdrawn because of (probably unfounded) concerns about carcinogenesis. The British Hypertension Society guidelines recommend spironolactone as a step 4 drug in the treatment algorithm for hypertension.[83] There are increasing data to suggest that around 10% of hypertensive subjects may have biochemical evidence for primary aldosteronism as suggested by the high aldosterone-to-renin ratio.[84,85] These subjects are more likely to have more severe and resistant hypertension.[86] Targeting these subjects with spironolactone has been shown to result in better BP control with fewer medications.[87] Moreover, various early randomized controlled trials also showed that spironolactone is an effective and safe antihypertensive.[88–90]

Primary hyperaldosteronism The response to a therapeutic trial of spironolactone may be useful in establishing the diagnosis of primary hyperaldosteronism. Spironolactone is also indicated in the pre-operative treatment of Conn's adenoma as well as for maintenance therapy in those who are unsuitable for surgery and those with hyperaldosteronism due to adrenal hyperplasia (idiopathic hyperaldosteronism) that does not lateralize to one adrenal. However, at present, there have been no randomized clinical trials published to determine the efficacy of spironolactone in primary hyperaldosteronism. Some have argued that spironolactone is effective in low renin hypertension and that aldosteronism is a misleading term.[91]

Secondary hyperaldosteronism

Congestive cardiac failure   Spironolactone is useful in the management of oedema and sodium retention along with other measures. Moreover, RALES evaluated the benefits of spironolactone in severe heart failure with decreased left-ventricular ejection fraction treated with standard therapy for heart failure; however, only a small proportion was taking β-blockers. A total of 822 patients were randomly assigned to receive spironolactone 25 mg daily, and 841 to receive placebo. The primary endpoint was death from all causes. The trial was discontinued early, after a mean follow-up period of 24 months, because an interim analysis determined that spironolactone was efficacious. There was a 31% reduction in the risk of death among patients in the spironolactone group, which was attributed to a lower risk of both death from progressive heart failure and of sudden death from cardiac causes. The frequency of hospitalization for worsening heart failure was 35% lower in the spironolactone group than in the placebo group. In addition, patients who received spironolactone had a significant improvement in the symptoms of heart failure, as assessed on the basis of the New York Heart Association (NYHA) functional class.[18] Hence, spironolactone is recommended for those patients already treated with diuretics, an ACE inhibitor and/or digoxin, who are in NYHA classes III and IV.[92]

Cirrhosis of liver   Secondary hyperaldosteronism and fluid retention are characteristics of decompensated liver disease. Spironolactone is indicated as a maintenance therapy along with dietary sodium restriction and bed rest.[93,94] Spironolactone is used in doses higher than in hypertension or heart failure, traditionally 100–200 mg daily, increased to 400 mg if required.

Nephrotic syndrome   Spironolactone has been shown to be useful in nephrotic syndrome in addition to other measures including the use of other diuretics and restriction of sodium and fluid intake. In a study on sodium-loaded nephrotic syndrome patients, spironolactone was shown to be useful in increasing the excretion of sodium.[95]

Miscellaneous uses

In view of its anti-androgen properties, spironolactone has been used in various clinical conditions including acne[96], rosacea and hirsutism, polycystic ovarian syndrome (PCOS),[97] and it has also been tried in carcinoma of prostate and benign prostatic hypertrophy.[98]

Potassium canrenoate

Potassium canrenoate is also known as canrenoate potassium or canrenoic acid potassium. Potassium canrenoate is an aldosterone antagonist with similar indications to those of spironolactone, but with the advantage that potassium canrenoate can be given parenterally as well as orally. The primary metabolite is canrenone. The chemical structure is described as monopotassium

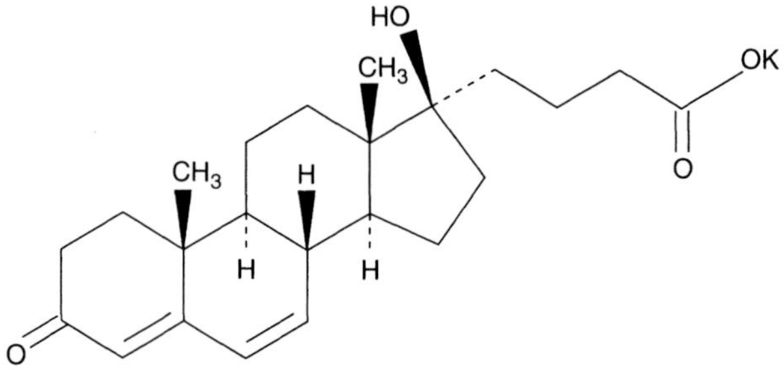

Fig. 6.4 Potassium canrenoate.

17-hydroxy-3-oxo-17 α-pegna-4,6-diene-21-carboxylate; the molecular formula is $C_{22}H_{29}KO_4$; molecular weight is 396.57. Potassium canrenoate is a pale yellow-white to yellow-brown crystalline powder. Its pH is 8.4 to 9.4.

Potassium canrenoate (Fig. 6.4) is metabolized primarily in the liver to canrenone, which is further metabolized to canrenoate ester glucuronide and hydroxycanrenone. Protein binding is significant. The primary route of elimination is by the kidneys and the secondary route is biliary/faecal.

In a study involving five healthy male volunteers, following a dose of IV potassium canrenoate 200 mg, the maximum plasma level of canrenone was 2066 ± 876 ng/mL after 29 ± 15 minutes. Total clearance was 4.2 ± 1.7 mL/minute/kg. Within 24 hours, 0.4 mg of canrenone was excreted by the kidney. The half-life of elimination was 4.9 ± 1.8 hours.[99]

Canrenoate has been given in doses of 50–600 mg daily (orally or intravenously) in one to three divided doses. The adverse effect profile is similar to that of spironolactone, although fewer endocrine side effects have been claimed.[100]

In animals, there have been reports of carcinogenicity. In 2-year studies in the rat, oral administration of potassium canrenoate was associated with myelocytic leukaemia and hepatic, thyroid, testicular and mammary tumours.[26]

There are very few clinical trial or outcome data with canrenoate. However, potassium canrenoate has been shown to be an effective antihypertensive agent in comparison with other usual medications.[101,102]

The combination of captopril plus canrenoate is well tolerated following acute myocardial infarction, and has a beneficial effect on diastolic and systolic LV parameters and may decrease post-MI remodelling.[103] Another study in acute myocardial infarction has shown that potassium canrenoate reduces post infarction collagen synthesis and progressive left ventricular dilation.[104] In rats potassium canrenoate reduces cardiac fibrosis.[105] Anti-arrhythmic activity in digoxin toxicity has been explored.[106]

In cirrhosis of the liver, potassium canrenoate has been shown to reduce portal pressures.[107] Potassium canrenoate has also been used in the treatment of cirrhotic ascites.[108]

Eplerenone

Eplerenone is a selective aldosterone receptor antagonist (SARA), with structural similarities to spironolactone, but with a lower incidence of androgenic and progestogenic side effects.

Chemistry

Eplerenone (Fig. 6.5) is also known as epoxymexrenone, CGP-30083 and SC-66110. The chemical structure of eplerenone is described as pregn-4-ene-7, 21-dicarboxylic acid, 9,11-epoxy-17-hydroxy-3-oxo-, γ-lactone, methyl ester, $(7\alpha,11\alpha,17\alpha)$-. The empirical formula is $C_{24}H_{30}O_6$ and the molecular weight 414.50.[109] Eplerenone is an odourless, white to off-white crystalline powder. Aqueous solubility is low and is essentially pH independent.

Mechanism of action (Table 6.6)

Eplerenone binds to the mineralocorticoid receptor and blocks the binding of aldosterone. Eplerenone selectively binds to mineralocorticoid receptors relative to glucocorticoid, progesterone and androgen receptors. To illustrate this phenomenon, de Gasparo et al. characterized binding affinities of eplerenone for various receptors both in vivo and in vitro.[110] In vitro studies have shown that the mineralocorticoid receptor affinity of eplerenone (IC 50=220 nM) (IC 50=inhibitory concentration 50%) was 15- to 20-fold less than that of spironolactone. However, eplerenone's affinity for androgen, progesterone and glucocorticoid receptors (IC50 >10 000nM) is 10- to 500-fold less than that of spironolactone. In vivo studies in rats have shown that eplerenone has 1 to 2 times the potency of spironolactone for binding to the mineralocorticoid receptor. But in rats and rabbits there was a three to 10-fold less affinity of eplerenone for androgen and progesterone receptors compared with spironolactone.[110,111] Eplerenone has decreased affinity for the aldosterone receptor in vitro, but has been shown to be at least as potent as spironolactone in vivo. This is because of its minimal (49%) protein binding compared to >90% protein binding of spironolactone. This allows a greater percentage of eplerenone to diffuse to the mineralocorticoid receptor.[112]

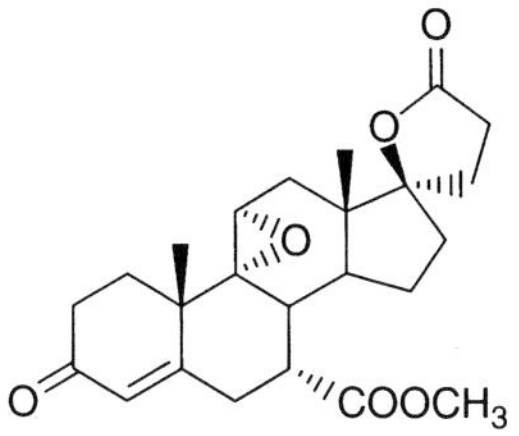

Fig. 6.5 Chemical structure of eplerenone.

Table 6.6 Relative receptor binding affinities of spironolactone and eplerenone (mean ± SE)

	Mineralocorticoid receptor (aldosterone=1)	Glucocorticoid receptor (dexamethasone=1)	Androgen receptor (methyltrienolone=1)	Progesterone receptor (progesterone=1)
Spironolactone	1.1×10^{-1} ± 36.4% (7)	1.8×10^{-3} ± 16.1% (4)	9.1×10^{-3} ± 16.5% (7)	7.0×10^{-3} ± 11.0% (5)
Eplerenone	7.5×10^{-2} ± 4.3% (3)	7.5×10^{-3} ± 9.5% (3)	1.1×10^{-5} ± 16.4% (4)	7.4×10^{-4} ± 16.8% (3)

(Adapted from ref. (111).)

Eplerenone has been shown to produce sustained increases in both plasma renin and serum aldosterone, consistent with inhibition of the negative regulatory feedback of aldosterone on renin secretion. However, the resulting increase in the circulating levels of plasma renin activity and aldosterone do not appear to overcome the effects of eplerenone.[113]

Pharmacokinetics (Table 6.7)

The pharmacokinetics of eplerenone have been studied both in animals[114] and humans.[115,116] Eplerenone has been shown to be readily absorbed after a single oral dose of 100 mg. Absorption does not seem to be affected by food.[114] The area under the plasma concentration curve (AUC) was 9537±3201 ng/mL/hour. The peak plasma concentration (C_{max}) obtained was 1721±290 ng/mL. The time to achieve maximum concentrations (T_{max}) of eplerenone was 1–2 hours with a terminal half-life ($T_{1/2}$) of 4–5 hours.[115] The plasma protein binding of eplerenone is about 50% and it is primarily bound to α1-acid glycoproteins. In vitro studies show that eplerenone is metabolized predominantly in liver by cytochrome P450 (CYP3A4 isoenzyme). Eplerenone is extensively metabolized with <1.7% of the dose excreted unchanged in urine and 0.8% in faeces. No active metabolites of eplerenone have been detected. Of the administered dose, about 66% was recovered in urine and 32% in faeces.[115]

The pharmacokinetics of eplerenone 100 mg/d is similar in males and females. The C_{max} and area-under-the-concentration curve (AUC) of eplerenone are increased 22% and 45%, respectively, in subjects ≥65 years compared with subjects 18–45 years old. The C_{max} and AUC are 19% and 26% lower, respectively, in blacks compared with whites. The C_{max} and AUC are increased in renal insufficiency, and eplerenone is not removed by haemodialysis. The C_{max} and AUC of eplerenone are increased 3.6% and 42%, respectively, in patients with Child-Pugh Class B hepatic impairment compared with normal subjects. Compared with the controls, in patients with stable heart failure, steady-state AUC and C_{max} increased by 38% and 30% respectively.[113]

Pharmacodynamics

Electrolytes, renal, blood vessels and heart   The mineralocorticoid antagonist actions of eplerenone have been shown in animal models. In the saline loaded adrenalectomized rat eplerenone dose-dependently reversed the effects of

Table 6.7 Pharmacokinetics of spironolactone and eplerenone in humans

Drug	Tmax (hours)	Cmax ng/ml	Food–drug interactions	Protein binding (%)	t½ (hours)	Elimination
Spironolactone	2.6–5.1	80–391	Yes*	90	1.4–16.5	Hepatic (53% urine, 20% faeces)
Eplerenone	1–2	1721	No[†]	49	4–5	Hepatic (66% urine, 32% faeces)

Tmax=time to maximum plasma concentration; t½=elimination half-life; AUC=area under the plasma concentration curve
[†]Documented in a dog model only
*Spironolactone bioavailability increases by 100% when taken with food
(Adapted from refs (112,114,115).)

aldosterone on urinary sodium and potassium.[117] Moreover, it has also been shown in the stroke-prone spontaneously hypertensive rat (SHR-SP) that eplerenone mimics the reno-protective effects of spironolactone. Treatment with eplerenone attenuated proteinuria and renal damage independently of systolic BP.[118,119] In another rat model that combined elevated BP, moderate salt intake and activation of the RAAS, eplerenone reduced vascular injury (medial fibrinoid necrosis in small coronary arteries and arterioles) and subsequently reduced myocardial necrosis.[120] A further study showed that eplerenone protected against maladaptive responses following myocardial infarction by reducing left-ventricular remodelling and reactive fibrosis.[121]

Clinical use including outcome data

Hypertension The efficacy of eplerenone has been assessed in numerous clinical trials either as monotherapy or concomitantly with other antihypertensive medications including ACE inhibitors, angiotensin II receptor antagonists, calcium channel blockers, β-blockers, and hydrochlorothiazide. At the time of FDA approval, about 3091 patients with hypertension in total had been tested with eplerenone.[113] Weinberger at al. randomized 417 patients with mild-to-moderate hypertension to eplerenone (in different doses), spironolactone or placebo.[122] The mean changes in both office systolic BP (SBP) and diastolic BP (DBP) and 24-hour ambulatory BPs were significantly greater for all doses of eplerenone compared with placebo. Furthermore, a dose–response effect was observed. On a molecular-weight basis, however, eplerenone was only 50–75% as potent as spironolactone. There were no antiandrogenic or progestational side effects with eplerenone. A double-blind study (n=499) comparing eplerenone and enalapril in mild-to-moderate hypertension showed similar blood-pressure reductions in both groups. Moreover, in patients with baseline microalbuminuria, a significantly greater reduction in urinary albumin-to-creatinine ratio (UACR) was observed with eplerenone than with enalapril.[123] In a study involving hypertensive subjects with type 2 diabetes mellitus and microalbuminuria (n=257), eplerenone was compared with enalapril or a combination of both. All three groups had similar reduction in BP. Combination therapy produced significantly greater reductions in UACR than either medication alone: eplerenone alone was superior to enalapril alone.[124] Eplerenone has also been shown to be effective in low-renin hypertension.[125] Eplerenone was more effective than losartan in African-American patients who are characterized by low-renin hypertension.[126] Eplerenone was as efficacious as amlodipine in reducing SBP, pulse pressure and vascular compliance assessed by pulse wave velocity. But eplerenone reduced microalbuminuria to a greater extent than did amlodipine.[127] Eplerenone was substantially better tolerated than amlodipine.[128] When added to ACE inhibitor or ARB eplerenone produced further significant reductions in BP compared with placebo.[129] As an add-on therapy to β-blockers eplerenone has also been effective in reducing both SBP and DBP.[130]

In the Effects of Eplerenone, Enalapril, and Eplerenone/Enalapril in Patients with Essential Hypertension and Left Ventricular Hypertrophy(4E- Left Ventricular Hypertrophy Study), the effects on left-ventricular hypertrophy associated with mild-to-moderate hypertension were evaluated in patients who received either eplerenone alone (n=50), enalapril alone (n=54), or a combination of the two agents (n=49). Over a 9-month follow-up period, BP reductions were similar across the three groups. Eplerenone was as effective as enalapril in left-ventricular regression (-14.5 ± 3.36 g vs. -19.7 ± 3.20 g) and mean reductions in left-ventricular mass were greater with combination therapy (-27.2 ± 3.39 g) than with eplerenone alone ($p=0.007$).[131] In animal studies it has been shown that eplerenone markedly attenuated glomerular hyperfiltration, sodium retention and hypertension associated with dietary induced obesity, indicating that aldosterone may play a role in the pathogenesis of obesity induced hypertension.[132]

Thus, from the available data it appears that the effect of eplerenone on BP is similar to that of ACE inhibitors and CCBs with perhaps the added advantage of conferring greater renoprotection. Eplerenone also seems to be effective in low-renin hypertension and in regressing left-ventricular hypertrophy. The drug is an effective add-on therapy for hypertension in patients on ACE inhibitors, ARBs, CCBs and β-blockers. However, the long-term efficacy of eplerenone needs to be tested in larger clinical trials.

Congestive heart failure post myocardial infarction   In the Eplerenone Post-acute myocardial infarction Heart failure Efficacy and SUrvival Study (EPHESUS) trial, eplerenone was shown to significantly reduce mortality and morbidity in post-acute myocardial infarction patients with systolic dysfunction.[133] EPHESUS was a multinational, multicentre, double-blind, randomized, placebo-controlled study in patients clinically stable 3–14 days after an acute myocardial infarction (MI) and who had left-ventricular dysfunction (as measured by left ventricular ejection fraction [LVEF]=40%) and with either diabetes or clinical evidence of congestive heart failure (CHF) (pulmonary congestion by examinations or chest X-ray or by a clinician-diagnosed audible S_3). Patients were allowed to receive standard post-MI drug therapy and to undergo revascularization by angioplasty or coronary-artery bypass graft surgery. EPHESUS randomized 6632 patients and the study population was primarily white (90%) and male (71%). The mean age was 64 years (range 22–94 years). The mean ejection fraction was 33%. The mean dose of eplerenone was 43 mg/day.

Patients were followed for an average of 16 months. The co-primary endpoints for EPHESUS were (1) the time to death from any cause, and (2) the time to first occurrence of either cardiovascular (CV) mortality (defined as sudden cardiac death or death due to progression of CHF, stroke, or other CV causes) or CV hospitalization (defined as hospitalization for progression of CHF, ventricular arrhythmias, acute myocardial infarction, or stroke). The primary endpoints were death from any cause and death from cardiovascular causes or hospitalization for cardiovascular events. The risk of death from any cause was reduced by 15% by eplerenone (hazard ratio equal to 0.85 (95% confidence interval) 0.75–0.96; $p=0.008$). The death from cardiovascular causes or hospitalization from cardiovascular events was reduced by 13% by eplerenone [hazard ratio 0.87 (95% confidence interval 0.79–0.95); $p= 0.002$]. The combined endpoints, including combined all-cause hospitalization and mortality, were driven primarily by CV mortality. Most CV deaths were attributed to sudden death, acute MI, and CHF. The time to first event for the co-primary endpoint of CV death or hospitalization as defined above, was also significantly longer in the eplerenone group.

Adverse effects (Tables 6.8 & 6.9)

From the available data, the overall rates of adverse events of eplerenone in hypertension and heart failure studies are similar to those of placebo.[113] Adverse events occur at a similar rate regardless of age, gender, or race.

Renal and electrolyte abnormalities In EPHESUS, adverse events that occurred more frequently with eplerenone were hyperkalaemia (3.4% vs. 2.0%) and increased creatinine (2.4% vs. 1.5%).[12] One of the most common adverse effects of eplerenone seen in clinical trials for hypertension was hyperkalaemia, the mean increase in serum potassium being dose-dependent.[113] The frequency and severity of hyperkalaemia increase in patients with renal insufficiency, diabetes mellitus and microalbuminuria. Patients with these conditions were often excluded from clinical trials of eplerenone in hypertension. Mild dose-dependent decreases in serum sodium have also been observed with eplerenone.[113]

Table 6.8 Changes in serum potassium with eplerenone in hypertension studies

Daily dosage (mg)	n	Mean change mEq/l	% >5.5 mEq/l
Placebo	194	0	1
25	97	0.08	0
50	245	0.14	0
100	193	0.09	1
200	139	0.19	1
400	104	0.36	8.7

(Adapted from ref. (113).)

Table 6.9 Rate (%) of adverse events occurring in hypertension studies in ≥1% of patients treated with eplerenone (25–400 mg)

	Eplerenone	Placebo
Metabolic		
Hypercholesterolaemia	1%	0%
Hyperglycaemia	1%	0%
Hyperkalaemia	2.7%	1.3%
Digestive		
Diarrhoea	2%	1%
Abdominal pain	1%	0%
Urinary		
Albuminuria	1%	0%
Respiratory		
Cough	2%	1%
Central nervous system		
Dizziness	3%	2%
Others		
Fatigue	2%	1%
Influenza-like symptoms	2%	1%

(Adapted from refs (112,113).)

Endocrine disturbances (Table 6.10)   The rate of sex-hormone-related adverse events in EPHESUS was similar to that of placebo. However, in studies of eplerenone in hypertension, there was a 1% incidence of either gynaecomastia or mastodynia in males and 0.6% incidence of abnormal vaginal bleeding in females compared to none reported in those on placebo. The rates increased slightly with increased duration of therapy.

Miscellaneous   Eplerenone increases serum alanine aminotransferase (ALT) and γ-glutamyl transpeptidase (GGT) in a dose-related manner.[113] Increases in uric acid to greater than 9 mg/dL were reported in 0.3% of patients administered eplerenone. Additional laboratory adverse events observed are mild dose-dependent increases in serum cholesterol and serum triglycerides.[113]

Drug interactions

There are only minimal data on drug interactions with eplerenone.[113] Eplerenone metabolism is predominantly mediated via CYP3A4. In pharmacokinetic studies, ketoconazole, a potent inhibitor of CYP3A4 induced a fivefold increase in the AUC of eplerenone, while less potent CYP3A4 inhibitors (erythromycin, amiodarone, diltiazem, saquinavir, verapamil, and fluconazole) induced a two-fold increase in the AUC of eplerenone. Hence, eplerenone use is contraindicated with strong inhibitors of CYP3A4 (see Table 6.11). Eplerenone dose should not exceed 25 mg when mild-to-moderate inhibitors of CYP3A4 are co-administered. Grapefruit juice caused a 25% increase in eplerenone exposure. Eplerenone can increase the AUC of digoxin by 16%. Combining eplerenone with ACE inhibitors and ARBs may increase the risk of hyperkalaemia and hence should be co-administered with caution. The risk is especially high in type 2 diabetes with microalbuminuria.[124] Patients receiving eplerenone should be informed not to use potassium supplements, salt substitutes containing potassium or contraindicated drugs without consulting the prescribing physician.

In the UK, eplerenone has been recently licensed for heart failure after recent myocardial infarction.[134] The contraindications for eplerenone are given in Tables 6.11 and 6.12.

Pregnancy and children

There are no adequate or well-controlled studies in pregnant women. The safety and effectiveness of eplerenone has not been established in paediatric patients. Embryo-fetal development studies in rats or rabbits did not show any teratogenic effects. However, no human fetal data are available.

Table 6.10 Rates of sex-hormone-related adverse events in EPHESUS

	Rates in males			Rates in females
	Gynaecomastia	*Mastodynia*	*Either*	*Abnormal vaginal bleeding*
Eplerenone	0.4%	0.1%	0.5%	0.4%
Placebo	0.5%	0.1%	0.6%	0.4%

(Adapted from refs (113,131).)

Table 6.11 Contraindications to eplerenone (licensed for post-myocardial infarction systolic dysfunction) in the UK

Hypersensitivity to eplerenone or any of the excipients
Patients with a serum potassium level of >5.0 mmol/L at initiation
Patients with moderate-to-severe renal insufficiency (creatinine clearance <50 mL/minute)
Patients with severe hepatic insufficiency (Child–Pugh class C)
Patients receiving potassium-sparing diuretics, potassium supplements or strong inhibitors of CYP 3A4 (e.g. itraconazole, ketaconazole, ritonavir, nelfinavir, clarithromycin, telithromycin)

(Adapted from ref. (134).)

Table 6.12 Contraindications to eplerenone for the treatment of hypertension (outside UK)

In all patients	In hypertension
Serum potassium >5.5 mEq/L at initiation	Type 2 diabetes with microalbuminuria
Creatinine clearance ≤30 mL/minute	Serum creatinine >2.0 mg/dL in males or >1.8 mg/dL in females
Concomitant use of potent CYP 3A4 inhibitors	Creatinine clearance <50 ml/minute
	Concomitant use of potassium supplements or potassium-sparing diuretics (amiloride, spironolactone or triamterene)

(Adapted from ref. (113).)

Elderly individuals

Due to age-related decreases in creatinine clearance, the incidence of laboratory-documented hyperkalaemia was increased in patients 65 and older in EPHESUS.

Carcinogenesis, mutagenesis, impairment of fertility

Statistically significant increases in benign thyroid tumours were observed after 2 years of eplerenone in both male and female rats. Repeat dose administration of eplerenone to rats increases the hepatic conjugation and clearance of thyroxin, which results in increased levels of TSH by a compensatory mechanism.

Male rats treated with eplerenone had decreased weights of seminal vesicles and epididymides and slightly decreased fertility. Dogs administered had dose-related prostate atrophy.

Overdosage

No cases of human overdosage with eplerenone have been reported. The most likely manifestations would be anticipated to be hypotension or hyperkalaemia. Eplerenone cannot be removed by haemodialysis, but it has been shown to bind extensively to charcoal. If symptomatic hypotension should occur, supportive treatment should be instituted. If hyperkalaemia develops, standard treatment should be initiated. Very high doses in animals have been shown to induce emesis, salivation, tremors, sedation and convulsions.[113]

CONCLUSION

The importance of aldosterone antagonists has greatly increased over the past 50 years since the discovery of aldosterone. Initially recognized primarily for their diuretic action, these agents are increasingly recognized for their various other important non-epithelial actions. The importance of providing more complete inhibition of aldosterone is becoming apparent as increasing evidence reveals its contribution towards various cardiovascular conditions including cardiac and vascular fibrosis, heart failure, hypertension, endothelial dysfunction, fibrinolysis and arrhythmia. Aldosterone antagonists have evolved and now play a vital role in the treatment of primary aldosteronism, hypertension, cardiac failure and cirrhosis of the liver. The more selective aldosterone antagonists, due to minimal androgenic and progestogenic side effects, have increased the attractiveness. However, there is clearly more to discover about aldosterone and research into this neuro-hormonal system needs to continue.

Acknowledgement

We thank Prof Gordon McInnes, Professor of Clinical Pharmacology, Division of Cardiovascular and Medical Sciences, Gardiner Institute, Western Infirmary, Glasgow for providing valuable references towards preparation of this chapter.

References

1. Gross JB, Imai M, Kokko JP. A functional comparison of the cortical collecting tubule and the distal convoluted tubule. *J Clin Invest* 1975;55:1284–1294.
2. Stone DK, Seldin DW, Kokko JP, Jacobson HR. Mineralocorticoid modulation of rabbit medullary collecting duct acidification. A sodium-independent effect. *J Clin Invest* 1983;72:77–83.
3. Schwartz GJ, Burg MB. Mineralocorticoid effects on cation transport by cortical collecting tubules in vitro. *Am J Physiol* 1978;235:F576–F585.
4. Endou H, Hosoyamada M. *Diuretics: potassium-retaining diuretics, aldosterone antagonists, 2nd edn.* London: Springer; 1995.
5. Binder HJ, McGlone F, Sandle GI. Effects of corticosteroid hormones on the electrophysiology of rat distal colon: implications for Na^+ and K^+ transport. *J Physiol* 1989;410:425–441.
6. Omland E, Mathisen O. Mechanism of ursodeoxycholic acid- and canrenoate-induced biliary bicarbonate secretion and the effect on glucose- and amino acid-induced cholestasis. *Scand J Gastroenterol* 1991;26:513–522.
7. Mori N, Yura K, Uozumi N, Sakai S. Effect of aldosterone antagonist on the DC potential in the endolymphatic sac. *Ann Otol Rhinol Laryngol* 1991;100:72–75.
8. Selye H. The general adaptation syndrome and the diseases of adaptation. *J Clin Endocrinol* 1946;6:117–230.
9. Schachter M. Aldosterone antagonism: new ideas, new drugs. *Br J Cardiol* 2002;9:533–537.
10. Brilla CG, Pick R, Tan LB, et al. Remodeling of the rat right and left ventricles in experimental hypertension. *Circ Res* 1990;67:1355–1364.
11. Brilla CG, Matsubara LS, Weber KT. Anti-aldosterone treatment and the prevention of myocardial fibrosis in primary and secondary hyperaldosteronism. *J Mol Cell Cardiol* 1993;25: 563–575.
12. Rocha R, Rudolph AE, Frierdich GE, et al. Aldosterone induces a vascular inflammatory phenotype in the rat heart. *Am J Physiol Heart Circ Physiol* 2002;283:H1802–H1810.
13. Zannad F, Alla F, Dousset B, et al. Limitation of excessive extracellular matrix turnover may contribute to survival benefit of spironolactone therapy in patients with congestive heart failure: insights from the randomized aldactone evaluation study (RALES). Rales Investigators. *Circulation* 2000;102:2700–2706.

14. Sato A, Funder JW, Saruta T. Involvement of aldosterone in left ventricular hypertrophy of patients with end-stage renal failure treated with hemodialysis. *Am J Hypertens* 1999;12: 867–873.

15. Duprez DA, Bauwens FR, De Buyzere ML, et al. Influence of arterial blood pressure and aldosterone on left ventricular hypertrophy in moderate essential hypertension. *Am J Cardiol* 1993;71:17A–20A.

16. Swedberg K, Eneroth P, Kjekshus J, Wilhelmsen L. Hormones regulating cardiovascular function in patients with severe congestive heart failure and their relation to mortality. CONSENSUS Trial Study Group. *Circulation* 1990;82:1730–1736.

17. Struthers AD. Aldosterone: cardiovascular assault. *Am Heart J* 2002;144:S2–S7.

18. Pitt B, Zannad F, Remme WJ, et al. The effect of spironolactone on morbidity and mortality in patients with severe heart failure. Randomized Aldactone Evaluation Study Investigators. *N Engl J Med* 1999;341:709–717.

19. McMurray JJ, Ostergren J, Swedberg K, et al. Effects of candesartan in patients with chronic heart failure and reduced left-ventricular systolic function taking angiotensin-converting-enzyme inhibitors: the CHARM-Added trial. *Lancet* 2003;362:767–771.

20. Farquharson CA, Struthers AD. Aldosterone induces acute endothelial dysfunction in vivo in humans: evidence for an aldosterone-induced vasculopathy. *Clin Sci (Lond)* 2002;103: 425–431.

21. Rizzoni D, Porteri E, Castellano M, et al. Vascular hypertrophy and remodeling in secondary hypertension. *Hypertension* 1996;28:785–790.

22. Oikawa T, Freeman M, Lo W, et al. Modulation of plasminogen activator inhibitor-1 in vivo: a new mechanism for the anti-fibrotic effect of renin-angiotensin inhibition. *Kidney Int* 1997;51:164–172.

23. Brown NJ, Kim KS, Chen YQ, et al. Synergistic effect of adrenal steroids and angiotensin II on plasminogen activator inhibitor-1 production. *J Clin Endocrinol Metab* 2000;85:336–344.

24. Vasan RS, Evans JC, Larson MG, et al. Serum aldosterone and the incidence of hypertension in nonhypertensive persons. *N Engl J Med* 2004;351:33–41.

25. Kagawa CM, Cella JA, Van Arman CG. Action of new steroids in blocking effects of aldosterone and deoxycorticosterone on salt. *Science* 1957;126:1015–1016.

26. Aldactone- Full US Prescribing Information Information can be accessed from *www.pfizer. com*

27. Gardiner P, Schrode K, Quinlan D, et al. Spironolactone metabolism: steady-state serum levels of the sulfur-containing metabolites. *J Clin Pharmacol* 1989;29:342–347.

28. Dahlof CG, Lundborg P, Persson BA, Regardh CG. Re-evaluation of the antimineralocorticoid effect of the spironolactone metabolite, canrenone, from plasma concentrations determined by a new high-pressure liquid-chromatographic method. *Drug Metab Dispos* 1979;7:103–107.

29. Merkus FW, Overdiek JW, Cilissen J, Zuidema J. Pharmacokinetics of spironolactone after a single dose: evaluation of the true canrenone serum concentrations during 24 hours. *Clin Exp Hypertens A* 1983;5:239–248.

30. Kojima K, Yamamoto K, Fujioka H, Kaneko H. Pharmacokinetics of spironolactone and potassium canrenoate in humans. *J Pharmacobiodyn* 1985;8:161–166.

31. Overdiek HW, Hermens WA, Merkus FW. New insights into the pharmacokinetics of spironolactone. *Clin Pharmacol Ther* 1985;38:469–474.

32. Overdiek HW, Merkus FW. The metabolism and biopharmaceutics of spironolactone in man. *Rev Drug Metab Drug Interact* 1987;5:273–302.

33. Sadee W, Dagcioglu M, Schroder R. Pharmacokinetics of spironolactone, canrenone and canrenoate-K in humans. *J Pharmacol Exp Ther* 1973;185:686–695.

34. Mirouze D, Zipser RD, Reynolds TB. Effect of inhibitors of prostaglandin synthesis on induced diuresis in cirrhosis. *Hepatology* 1983;3:50–55.

35. Elliott Jr. HC, Murdaugh Jr. HV. Effects of acetylsalicylic acid on excretion of endogenous metabolites by man. *Proc Soc Exp Biol Med* 1962;109:333–335.

36. Hofmann LM, Krupnick MI, Garcia HA. Interactions of spironolactone and hydrochlorothiazide with aspirin in the rat and dog. *J Pharmacol Exp Ther* 1972;180:1–5.

37. Tweeddale MG, Ogilvie RI. Antagonism of spironolactone-induced natriuresis by aspirin in man. *N Engl J Med* 1973;289:198–200.

38. Ramsay LE, Harrison IR, Shelton JR, Vose CW. Influence of acetylsalicylic acid on the renal handling of a spironolactone metabolite in healthy subjects. *Eur J Clin Pharmacol* 1976;10: 43–48.

39. Weiner IM, Mudge GH. Renal tubular mechanisms for excretion of organic acids and bases. *Am J Med* 1964;36:743–762.

40. Schachter D, Manis JG. Salicylate and salicyl conjugates: fluorimetric estimation, biosynthesis and renal excretion in man. *J Clin Invest* 1958;37:800–807.

41. Hollifield JW. Failure of aspirin to antagonize the antihypertensive effect of spironolactone in low-renin hypertension. *South Med J* 1976;69:1034–1036.

42. Sungaila I, Bartle WR, Walker SE, et al. Spironolactone pharmacokinetics and pharmacodynamics in patients with cirrhotic ascites. *Gastroenterology* 1992;102:1680–1685.

43. Lombes M, Farman N, Oblin ME, et al. Immunohistochemical localization of renal mineralocorticoid receptor by using an anti-idiotypic antibody that is an internal image of aldosterone. *Proc Natl Acad Sci U S A* 1990;87:1086–1088.

44. Grillo C, Vallee S, McEwen BS, De Nicola AF. Properties and distribution of binding sites for the mineralocorticoid receptor antagonist [3H]ZK 91587 in brain. *J Steroid Biochem* 1990;35:11–15.

45. Young M, Fullerton M, Dilley R, Funder J. Mineralocorticoids, hypertension, and cardiac fibrosis. *J Clin Invest* 1994;93:2578–2583.

46. Takeda Y, Yoneda T, Demura M, et al. Cardiac aldosterone production in genetically hypertensive rats. *Hypertension* 2000;36:495–500.

47. Takeda Y, Miyamori I, Yoneda T, et al. Production of aldosterone in isolated rat blood vessels. *Hypertension* 1995;25:170–173.

48. Sato A, Takane H, Saruta T. High serum level of procollagen type III amino-terminal peptide contributes to the efficacy of spironolactone and angiotensin-converting enzyme inhibitor therapy on left ventricular hypertrophy in essential hypertensive patients. *Hypertens Res* 2001;24:99–104.

49. Sato A, Suzuki Y, Saruta T. Effects of spironolactone and angiotensin-converting enzyme inhibitor on left ventricular hypertrophy in patients with essential hypertension. *Hypertens Res* 1999;22:17–22.

50. Hayashi M, Tsutamoto T, Wada A, et al. Immediate administration of mineralocorticoid receptor antagonist spironolactone prevents post-infarct left ventricular remodeling associated with suppression of a marker of myocardial collagen synthesis in patients with first anterior acute myocardial infarction. *Circulation* 2003;107:2559–2565.

51. Martinez DV, Rocha R, Matsumura M, et al. Cardiac damage prevention by eplerenone: comparison with low sodium diet or potassium loading. *Hypertension* 2002;39:614–618.

52. Macdonald JE, Kennedy N, Struthers AD. Effects of spironolactone on endothelial function, vascular angiotensin converting enzyme activity, and other prognostic markers in patients with mild heart failure already taking optimal treatment. *Heart* 2004;90:765–770.

53. Abiose AK, Mansoor GA, Barry M, et al. Effect of spironolactone on endothelial function in patients with congestive heart failure on conventional medical therapy. *Am J Cardiol* 2004;93:1564–1566.

54. Klauber N, Browne F, Anand-Apte B, D'Amato RJ. New activity of spironolactone. Inhibition of angiogenesis in vitro and in vivo. *Circulation* 1996;94:2566–2571.

55. van den Berg DT, de Kloet ER, van Dijken HH, de Jong W. Differential central effects of mineralocorticoid and glucocorticoid agonists and antagonists on blood pressure. *Endocrinology* 1990;126:118–124.

56. Rahmouni K, Barthelmebs M, Grima M, et al. Involvement of brain mineralocorticoid receptor in salt-enhanced hypertension in spontaneously hypertensive rats. *Hypertension* 2001;38:902–906.

57. Rahmouni K, Barthelmebs M, Grima M, et al. Brain mineralocorticoid receptor control of blood pressure and kidney function in normotensive rats. *Hypertension* 1999;33:1201–1206.

58. Huang BS, Leenen FH Blockade of brain mineralocorticoid receptors or Na+ channels prevents sympathetic hyperactivity and improves cardiac function in rats post-MI. *Am J Physiol Heart Circ Physiol* 2005;288:H2491–2497.

59. Menard RH, Guenthner TM, Kon H, Gillette JR. Studies on the destruction of adrenal and testicular cytochrome P-450 by spironolactone. Requirement for the 7alpha-thio group and evidence for the loss of the heme and apoproteins of cytochrome P-450. *J Biol Chem* 1979;254:1726–1733.

60. Hall PF. Role of cytochromes P-450 in the biosynthesis of steroid hormones. *Vitam Horm* 1985;42:315–368.

61. Serafini P, Lobo RA. The effects of spironolactone on adrenal steroidogenesis in hirsute women. *Fertil Steril* 1985;44:595–599.

62. Canosa LF, Ceballos NR. Effects of different steroid-biosynthesis inhibitors on the testicular steroidogenesis of the toad Bufo arenarum. *J Comp Physiol [B]* 2001;171:519–526.

63. Kossor DC, Kominami S, Takemori S, Colby HD. Destruction of testicular cytochrome P-450 by 7 alpha-thiospironolactone is catalyzed by the 17 alpha-hydroxylase. *J Steroid Biochem Mol Biol* 1992;42:421–424.

64. Rourke KA, Bergstrom JM, Larson IW, Colby HD. Mechanism of action of spironolactone on cortisol production by guinea pig adrenocortical cells. *Mol Cell Endocrinol* 1991;81:127–134.

65. Feller DR, Gerald MC. Interactions of spironolactone with hepatic microsomal drug-metabolizing enzyme systems. *Biochem Pharmacol* 1971;20:1991–2000.

66. Buck ML. The cytochrome P450 enzyme system and its effect on drug metabolism. *Pediatric Pharmacotherapy* 1997;3(5).
67. Price VH. Testosterone metabolism in the skin. A review of its function in androgenetic alopecia, acne vulgaris, and idiopathic hirsutism including recent studies with antiandrogens. *Arch Dermatol* 1975;111:1496–1502.
68. Steelman SL, Brooks JR, Morgan ER, Patanelli DJ. Anti-androgenic activity of spironolactone. *Steroids* 1969;14:449–450.
69. Baba S, Murai M, Jitsukawa S, et al. Antiandrogenic effects of spironolactone: hormonal and ultrastructural studies in dogs and men. *J Urol* 1978;119:375–380.
70. Walsh PC, Siiteri PK. Suppression of plasma androgens by spironolactone in castrated men with carcinoma of the prostate. *J Urol* 1975;114:254–256.
71. Corvol P, Michaud A, Menard J, et al. Antiandrogenic effect of spirolactones: mechanism of action. *Endocrinology* 1975;97:52–58.
72. Basinger GT, Gittes RF. Antiandrogenic effect of spironolactone in rats. *J Urol* 1974;111:77–80.
73. Svensson M, Gustafsson F, Galatius S, et al. Hyperkalaemia and impaired renal function in patients taking spironolactone for congestive heart failure: retrospective study. *BMJ* 2003;327:1141–1142.
74. Juurlink DN, Mamdani MM, Lee DS, et al. Rates of hyperkalemia after publication of the Randomized Aldactone Evaluation Study. *N Engl J Med* 2004;351:543–551.
75. Jeunemaitre X, Chatellier G, Kreft-Jais C, et al. Efficacy and tolerance of spironolactone in essential hypertension. *Am J Cardiol* 1987;60:820–825.
76. Bozkurt B, Agoston I, Knowlton AA. Complications of inappropriate use of spironolactone in heart failure: when an old medicine spirals out of new guidelines. *J Am Coll Cardiol* 2003;41: 211–214.
77. Greenblatt DJ, Koch-Weser J. Adverse reactions to spironolactone. A report from the Boston Collaborative Drug Surveillance Program. *Jama* 1973;225:40–43.
78. Hughes BR, Cunliffe WJ. Tolerance of spironolactone. *Br J Dermatol* 1988;118:687–691.
79. Loube SD, Quirk RA. Letter: Breast cancer associated with administration of spironolactone. *Lancet* 1975;1:1428–1429.
80. McMurray JJ, O'Meara E. Treatment of heart failure with spironolactone – trial and tribulations. *N Engl J Med* 2004;351:526–528.
81. Colussi G, Rombola G, De Ferrari ME, et al. Correction of hypokalemia with antialdosterone therapy in Gitelman's syndrome. *Am J Nephrol* 1994;14:127–135.
82. Lindeman RD. Hypokalemia: causes, consequences and correction. *Am J Med Sci* 1976;272: 5–17.
83. Williams B, Poulter NR, Brown MJ, et al. British Hypertension Society guidelines for hypertension management 2004 (BHS-IV): summary. *BMJ* 2004;328:634–640.
84. Mulatero P, Stowasser M, Loh KC, et al. Increased diagnosis of primary aldosteronism, including surgically correctable forms, in centers from five continents. *J Clin Endocrinol Metab* 2004;89:1045–1050.
85. Lim PO, Young WF, MacDonald TM. A review of the medical treatment of primary aldosteronism. *J Hypertens* 2001;19:353–361.
86. Calhoun DA, Nishizaka MK, Zaman MA, et al. Hyperaldosteronism among black and white subjects with resistant hypertension. *Hypertension* 2002;40:892–896.
87. Lim PO, Jung RT, MacDonald TM. Raised aldosterone to renin ratio predicts antihypertensive efficacy of spironolactone: a prospective cohort follow-up study. *Br J Clin Pharmacol* 1999;48:756–760.
88. Schersten B, Thulin T, Kuylenstierna J, et al. Clinical and biochemical effects of spironolactone administered once daily in primary hypertension. Multicenter Sweden study. *Hypertension* 1980;2:672–679.
89. Leary WP, Asmal AC, Williams PC, Marwick B. Aldactone and acebutolol in treatment of hypertension. *J Int Med Res* 1979;7:29–32.
90. Karlberg BE, Kagedal B, Tegler L, et al. Controlled treatment of primary hypertension with propranolol and spironolactone. A crossover study with special reference to initial plasma renin activity. *Am J Cardiol* 1976;37:642–649.
91. Padfield PL. Primary aldosteronism, a common entity? The myth persists. *J Hum Hypertens* 2002;16:159–162.
92. SIGN guidelines: Diagnosis and Treatment of Heart Failure due to Left Ventricular Systolic Dysfunction, 1999. Can be accessed from *www.sign.ac.uk*
93. Perez-Ayuso RM, Arroyo V, Planas R, et al. Randomized comparative study of efficacy of furosemide versus spironolactone in nonazotemic cirrhosis with ascites. Relationship between the diuretic response and the activity of the renin-aldosterone system. *Gastroenterology* 1983;84:961–968.
94. Alaniz C. Management of cirrhotic ascites. *Clin Pharm* 1989;8:645–654.

95. Shapiro MD, Hasbargen J, Hensen J, Schrier RW. Role of aldosterone in the sodium retention of patients with nephrotic syndrome. *Am J Nephrol* 1990;10:44–48.

96. Shaw JC, White LE. Long-term safety of spironolactone in acne: results of an 8-year followup study. *J Cutan Med Surg* 2002;6:541–545.

97. Sciarra F, Toscano V, Concolino G, Di Silverio F. Antiandrogens: clinical applications. *J Steroid Biochem Mol Biol* 1990;37:349–362.

98. Namer M. Clinical applications of antiandrogens. *J Steroid Biochem* 1988;31:719–729.

99. Krause W, Karras J, Seifert W. Pharmacokinetics of canrenone after oral administration of spironolactone and intravenous injection of canrenoate-K in healthy man. *Eur J Clin Pharmacol* 1983;25:449–453.

100. Traina M, Vizzini GB. [Controlled study of the effect of long-term administration of canrenoate potassium in cirrhotic ascites]. *Minerva Med* 1986;77:87–91.

101. Niutta E, Cusi D, Colombo R, et al. Antihypertensive effect of captopril, canrenoate potassium, and atenolol. Relations with red blood cell sodium transport and renin. *Am J Hypertens* 1988;1:364–371.

102. Glorioso N, Melis MG, Manunta P, et al. Different sensitivity to hydrochlorothiazide and to potassium-canrenoate among essential hypertensive patients. *Clin Exp Hypertens* 1993;15 (Suppl 1):187–196.

103. Di Pasquale P, Cannizzaro S, Giubilato A, et al. Additional beneficial effects of canrenoate in patients with anterior myocardial infarction on ACE-inhibitor treatment. A pilot study. *Ital Heart J* 2001;2:121–129.

104. Modena MG, Aveta P, Menozzi A, Rossi R. Aldosterone inhibition limits collagen synthesis and progressive left ventricular enlargement after anterior myocardial infarction. *Am Heart J* 2001;141:41–46.

105. Bos R, Mougenot N, Mediani O, et al. Potassium canrenoate, an aldosterone receptor antagonist, reduces isoprenaline-induced cardiac fibrosis in the rat. *J Pharmacol Exp Ther* 2004;309:1160–1166.

106. Yeh BK, Chiang BN, Sung PK. Antiarrhythmic activity of potassium canrenoate in man. *Am Heart J* 1976;92:308–314.

107. Koda M, Murawaki Y, Kawasaki H, Ikawa S. Effects of canrenoate potassium, an aldosterone antagonist on portal hemodynamics in patients with compensated liver cirrhosis. *Hepatogastroenterology* 1996;43:887–892.

108. Bernardi M, Laffi G, Salvagnini M, et al. Efficacy and safety of the stepped care medical treatment of ascites in liver cirrhosis: a randomized controlled clinical trial comparing two diets with different sodium content. *Liver* 1993;13:156–162.

109. Delyani JA, Rocha R, Cook CS, et al. Eplerenone: a selective aldosterone receptor antagonist (SARA). *Cardiovasc Drug Rev* 2001;19:185–200.

110. de Gasparo M, Joss U, Ramjoue HP, et al. Three new epoxy-spirolactone derivatives: characterization in vivo and in vitro. *J Pharmacol Exp Ther* 1987;240:650–656.

111. Roniker B. Eplerenone, a selective antagonist of the aldosterone receptor [abstract]. *Hypertension* 1997;30:995.

112. Coleman IC, Reddy P, Song CJ, et al. Eplerenone: The first aldosterone receptor antagonist for the treatment of hypertension. *Formulary* 2002;37:514–524.

113. Inspra Description. Information can be accessed from *http://www.fda.gov*

114. Cook CS, Zhang L, Fischer JS. Absorption and disposition of a selective aldosterone receptor antagonist, eplerenone, in the dog. *Pharm Res* 2000;17:1426–1431.

115. Tobert D, Karim A, Cook C, et al. SC-66110 (eplerenone): A selective antialdosterone antagonist: disposition kinetics in man and identification of its major CYP450 isoenzyme in its biotransformation. In: *American Association of Pharmaceutical Scientists*;1998.

116. Cook CS, Berry LM, Kim DH, et al. Involvement of CYP3A in the metabolism of eplerenone in humans and dogs: differential metabolism by CYP3A4 and CYP3A5. *Drug Metab Dispos* 2002;30:1344–1351.

117. Delyani J, Myles K, Funder J. Eplerenone (SC 66110), a highly selective aldosterone antagonist [abstract]. *Am J Hypertens* 1998;11:94A.

118. Rocha R, Chander PN, Khanna K, et al. Mineralocorticoid blockade reduces vascular injury in stroke-prone hypertensive rats. *Hypertension* 1998;31:451–458.

119. Rocha R, Chander PN, Zuckerman A, Stier Jr. CT. Role of mineralocorticoids in renal injury in stroke-prone hypertensive rats [abstract]. *Hypertension* 1998;32:598.

120. Rocha R, Stier Jr. CT, Kifor I, et al. Aldosterone: a mediator of myocardial necrosis and renal arteriopathy. *Endocrinology* 2000;141:3871–3878.

121. Delyani JA, Robinson EL, Rudolph AE. Effect of a selective aldosterone receptor antagonist in myocardial infarction. *Am J Physiol Heart Circ Physiol* 2001;281:H647–H654.

122. Weinberger MH, Roniker B, Krause SL, Weiss RJ. Eplerenone, a selective aldosterone blocker, in mild-to-moderate hypertension. *Am J Hypertens* 2002;15:709–716.

123. Burgess E, Niegowska J, Tan KW, et al. Antihypertensive effects of eplerenone and enalapril in patients with essential hypertension [abstract]. *Am J Hypertens* 2002;15 (Suppl 1):23A.

124. Epstein M, Buckalew V, Martinez F, et al. Antiproteinuric efficacy of eplerenone, enalapril and eplerenone/enalapril combination therapy in diabetic hypertensives with microalbuminuria [abstract]. *Am J Hypertens* 2002;15(Suppl 1):24A.

125. Weinberger M, MacDonald T, Conlin PR, et al. Comparison of eplerenone and losartan in patients with low-renin hypertension [abstract]. *Am J Hypertens* 2002;15(Suppl 1):24A.

126. Flack JM, Oparil S, Pratt JH, et al. Efficacy and tolerability of eplerenone and losartan in hypertensive black and white patients. *J Am Coll Cardiol* 2003;41:1148–1155.

127. White WB, Duprez D, St Hillaire R, et al. Effects of the selective aldosterone blocker eplerenone versus the calcium antagonist amlodipine in systolic hypertension. *Hypertension* 2003;41:1021–1026.

128. Hollenberg NK, Williams GH, Anderson R, et al. Symptoms and the distress they cause: comparison of an aldosterone antagonist and a calcium channel blocking agent in patients with systolic hypertension. *Arch Intern Med* 2003;163:1543–1548.

129. Krum H, Nolly H, Workman D, et al. Efficacy of eplerenone added to renin-angiotensin blockade in hypertensive patients. *Hypertension* 2002;40:117–123.

130. Van Mieghem W, Von Behren V, Balazovjech I, et al. Eplerenone is safe and effective as an add-on therapy in hypertensive patients uncontrolled with calcium channel blockers or beta blockers [abstract]. *Eur Heart J* 2002;23(Suppl):211.

131. Pitt B, Reichek N, Willenbrock R, et al. Effects of eplerenone, enalapril, and eplerenone/enalapril in patients with essential hypertension and left ventricular hypertrophy: the 4E-left ventricular hypertrophy study. *Circulation* 2003;108:1831–1838.

132. de Paula RB, da Silva AA, Hall JE. Aldosterone antagonism attenuates obesity-induced hypertension and glomerular hyperfiltration. *Hypertension* 2004;43:41–47.

133. Pitt B, Remme W, Zannad F, et al. Eplerenone, a selective aldosterone blocker, in patients with left ventricular dysfunction after myocardial infarction. *N Engl J Med* 2003;348: 1309–1321.

134. Inspra: *Summary of Product Characteristics*, UK, September 2004. Available in File, Pfizer, UK.

III

Centrally acting drugs

7 | Methyldopa and imidazoline agonists

Brian N.C. Prichard and Pieter A. van Zwieten

INTRODUCTION

Hypertension develops from the interaction of a variety of genetic and environmental influences; it is an important cardiovascular risk factor. Besides drug treatment to lower the blood pressure (BP) it is important to attend to other facets of the problem, which vary according to the individual patient, particularly lipid metabolism, glucose metabolism and the increasingly frequent association of obesity.

Various postulates have been made to explain an increase in BP. The importance of the sympathetic nervous system in the development of essential hypertension is well described; it is associated with increased sympathetic nerve activity,[1] and it is accentuated by physiological[2] and psychological stress.[3,4]

Control of the autonomic nervous system, modulated in the medulla oblongata, is pivotal in maintaining cardiovascular control. The autonomic nervous system regulates vascular tone mainly by variation in α-adrenergic-mediated vasoconstriction, while cardiac control is achieved by the balance of sympathetic-mediated β-adrenergic stimulation and parasympathetic vagal inhibition.[5] The sympathetic nervous system is influenced by efferent impulses that are processed by the limbic system and hypothalamus. Vagal afferents convey information on circulatory status to the nucleus tractus solitarii (NTS) from which impulses are relayed to the rostral ventrolateral medulla (RVLM). The NTS exerts a powerful inhibitory influence in the RVLM. Baroreceptor afferents, which sense increases in pressure, and volume receptor afferents, which sense increase in volume, terminate in the NTS. The NTS also receives input from chemoreceptors and is thus involved in the response to oxygen deprivation.

Sympathetic activation appears to have other adverse consequences in cardiovascular disease, besides directly increasing BP. Sympathetic-mediated vasoconstriction impairs glucose delivery to muscle, increasing insulin resistance and hyperinsulinaemia; post prandial clearance of lipids in the liver is reduced, predisposing to dyslipidaemia, both features of the metabolic syndrome (syndrome x). Subsequently diabetes may develop,[6] and atheroma in the coronary arteries and cerebral vessels is increased.[4,7,8] It is also probable that there is a trophic effect of sympathetic stimulation that contributes to the development of left ventricular hypertrophy.[8,9,10] Sympathetic-activated dys-rhythmias are also important in sudden death associated with heart failure and probably in hypertension. It has also been noted that the increase in sudden death peaks in the morning soon after waking and this is associated with an increase in sympathetic activity and a rise in BP. Increased catecholamine levels can result in hypokalaemia sufficient to contribute to the development of cardiac arrhythmias.[4,8,10] Even 50 years after the introduction of methyldopa, for a time the most widely prescribed drug in therapeutics,[11] there remain good reasons to expect that a drug that acts to decrease sympathetic activity will be a useful agent to lower BP.

The two early central inhibitors of sympathetic tone, methyldopa[12] and later clonidine,[13] suffered from the disadvantage of frequently resulting in sedation, and their general usage has greatly declined, except for methyldopa in pregnancy hypertension.[14–16] Subsequently, developments have been directed to find agents, such as moxonidine and rilmenidine,[17] with less of this problem; the current article, therefore, covers these drugs in more detail than the older agents.

CENTRAL RECEPTORS

Based on responses to various agonists and antagonists, the α-adrenergic receptors can be subdivided into two groups: α_1- and α_2-receptors.[18,19] The α_2-adrenergic postsynaptic receptors are the predominant α-receptors in the central nervous system (CNS), stimulation of which induces a fall in BP and bradycardia. Central α_2-receptors have been demonstrated in various parts of the brain. In the medulla oblongata there is a high concentration of α_2-receptors, most notably in the NTS.[20,21] The forebrain, where stimulation increases BP, and the spinal cord have been shown to possess α_2-receptors. Additionally, there are presynaptic α_2-receptors that mediate a reduction in transmitter release.[18]

Central α_1-receptors have been demonstrated by receptor blocking techniques,[19] and may be involved in mediating baroreceptor reflex function. Blockade of these receptors by prazosin may explain the relative lack of reflex tachycardia with this drug.[22]

Methyldopa, guanabenz and guanfacine (first-generation, centrally acting sympatholytics) act by stimulating central α_2-receptors, most probably in the NTS.[21] Baroreflexes are facilitated and inhibitory impulses to the RVLM are increased. Heart rate is reduced by facilitation of parasympathetic activity in the NTS. Initial suggestions for the different sites of action for the different classes of centrally acting agents (phenylethylamines and imidazolines) came from Ruffolo et al.[23,24,25] and Bousquet et al.,[26] although differences in the responses induced by these two groups of compounds were still thought to arise from effects on α_2-receptors. More definitive evidence for a new receptor arose from the observations of Bousquet et al.,[26] who examined the action of microinjection of clonidine and α-methylnoradrenaline into the RVLM. It was found that α-methylnoradrenaline, in contrast to clonidine, did not lower BP. Imidazoline binding sites in the RVLM were considered to be the explanation for these findings.

Two subtypes of imidazoline binding sites[27] can be distinguished in the bovine RVLM. I_1-binding sites are sensitive to clonidine and idazoxan, while I_2-binding sites found in mitochondria and possibly associated with mono-amine-oxidases are also sensitive to idazoxan, but in contrast are largely insensitive to clonidine.[28] I_1-receptors have also been identified in adrenomedulla chromaffin cells and the carotid body.[29] The various binding studies have been summarized.[29,30] The binding (k_1 values) at the I_1-imidazoline receptor and the α_2-receptor have been compared; the I_1-receptor selectivity, imidazoline I_1/alpha$_2$ ratio, was 32.6 for moxonidine, 29.5 for rilmenidine, 3.8 for clonidine and under 0.0007 for guanabenz. Besides high affinity imidazoline I_1-receptor sites,[29] low-affinity sites have also been described. These sites are unlikely to be important in the central regulation of BP because the dosage of drugs required to occupy these sites is far above therapeutic levels and the binding efficiency is unrelated to antihypertensive efficacy.[29] These findings were supported by the finding that the antihypertensive action of agents injected into the RVLM correlated with radioligand binding affinities at I_1, but not α_2 sites in membranes of the ventral medulla.[31–33]

ENDOGENOUS LIGAND

Based on its displacement of various ligands from the I_1-receptor, agmatine, a decarboxylated metabolite of aginine, has been proposed as the endogenous ligand for the imidazoline receptors.[34] However, the efficacy of the binding of agmatine for the I_1-receptor is relatively low, casting doubt on this concept.[28] Bousquet et al.[28] concluded that imidazoline receptors are not coupled to G proteins, the post receptor coupling being obscure. However, Ernsberger and colleagues have suggested that imidazoline receptors are linked to phosphatidylcholine-selective phospholipase via an unidentified G protein, and so to phosphatidylcholine diacylglyceride to protein kinase C.[29]

CHEMISTRY AND MECHANISM OF ACTION

Methyldopa

α-Methyldopa (α-methyl-dioxyphenylalanine) is an amino acid that was designed with the aim of inhibiting the enzyme dopa-decarboxylase and, hence, to impair the formation of noradrenaline. As other inhibitors of this enzyme do not lower BP, this is not thought to be the reason why methyldopa is an antihypertensive.[35] Only the l-isomer was decarboxylated and only the l-isomer lowered BP[36] and thus studies were performed with this isomer.

Methyldopa-dopa is converted to yield the metabolite α-Methyldopamine as a result of decarboxylation of the amino acid. The α-methyldopamine is then converted by hydroxylation in the β-position, to yield α-methy lnoradrenaline (see Fig. 7.1), now generally considered to be the active metabolite of α-methyldopa. α-Methylnoradrenaline stimulates the central α_2-adrenoceptors in the brain stem involved in the regulation of peripheral sympathetic activity. Stimulation of the central α_2-adrenoceptors explains the blood pressure lowering effect of α-methyldopa (a prodrug), through its active metabolite

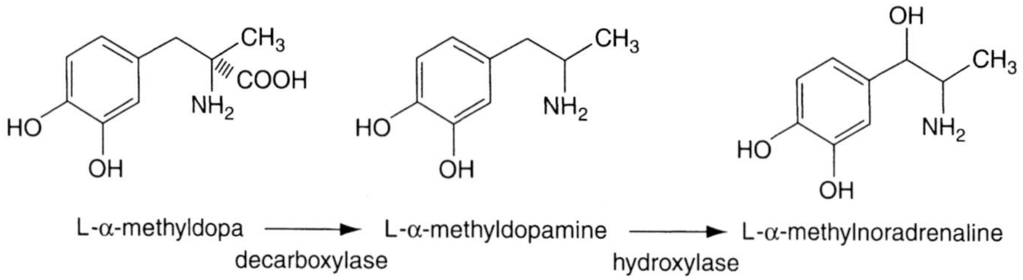

L-α-methyldopa ⟶ L-α-methyldopamine ⟶ L-α-methylnoradrenaline
　　　　　　　decarboxylase　　　　　　　　　hydroxylase

Fig. 7.1 Chemical structure of L-α-methyldopa and its metabolites: L-α-methyldopamine and L-α-methylnoradrenaline.

α-methylnoradrenaline. The central antihypertensive activity of α-methyldopa can be counteracted by α_2-adrenoceptor antagonists, such as yohimbine or rauwolscine.[37]

Day and Rand[38] postulated the false transmitter theory that α-methyldopa acted by being metabolized to α-methylnoradrenaline, which then functioned as a false transmitter when liberated at sympathetic nerve endings. However, in both the cat and the dog, α-methylnoradrenaline is approximately equipotent to noradrenaline,[39] while in human smooth muscle it is just slightly less potent than noradrenaline.[40] In addition, while acute administration of α-methyldopa reduces the function of sympathetic nerves, reducing the response of the cat nictating membrane to nerve stimulation,[41] with long-term treatment no effect is seen. It appears, therefore, that an effect on peripheral nerve function is not the reason for the antihypertensive effect of methyldopa.[42]

Henning and van Zwieten[43] observed that a small dose of methyldopa injected into the vertebral artery of the cat resulted in a fall in BP at doses that showed no effect when administered intravenously. Ingenito et al.[44] then reported that the administration of α-methyldopa to the vascularly isolated, perfused cat brain gave a fall in BP in the remainder of the animal, while Baum et al.[45] showed in renal hypertensive rats that methyldopa reduced sympathetic nerve traffic. Furthermore, the antihypertensive action is reduced by inhibition of transport of methyldopa across the blood–brain barrier using large doses of isoleucine.[46]

The administration of a centrally active dopa-decarboxylase inhibitor to inhibit the metabolism of methyldopa abolishes the antihypertensive effect, but this does not occur if the dopa-decarboxylase inhibitor is unable to penetrate the brain.[47] Some investigations in humans are in agreement, as peripheral decarboxylase inhibition with α-methylhydrazine does not influence the hypotensive response to methyldopa.[48] Inhibition of α-noradrenaline synthesis following the destruction of central adrenergic neurons by intraventricular 6-hydroxydopamine does prevent the hypotensive effect of α-methyldopa,[49] while intravenous 6-hydroxydopamine reduces, but does not prevent the hypotensive effect.[50,51] Finally, absence of peripheral effect of methyldopa is illustrated by the observation that after a dose of α-methyldopa that results in hypotension, the pressor response that is seen when the entire sympathetic outflow is stimulated is not reduced.[50]

The metabolism of α-methyldopa (a prodrug) to α-methylnoradrenaline, therefore, occurs in the brain.[47,52] The active moiety then stimulates the central α_2-adrenergic receptors, most likely in the nucleus tractus soltarii of the medulla.[11] The consequent fall in BP is blocked by central α-adrenoceptor blockade.[50,53]

Evidence of reduced sympathetic activity has been found in humans. The fall in BP after single doses of methyldopa has been found to correlate with the fall in plasma noradrenaline.[54] Methyldopa also reduces the 24-hour urinary excretion of noradrenaline in patients with essential hypertension. While methyldopa reduces renin, falls in renin do not correlate with reduction in BP;[55] methyldopa 500 mg and 1000 mg resulted in similar falls in renin while the reduction in BP was almost twice as great with the higher dose. However, a poor antihypertensive effect with methyldopa has been reported in some studies of low-renin hypertension.[56]

Clonidine and imidazolines

Clonidine is the prototype of imidazoline derivatives with central antihypertensive activity (Fig. 7.2). Clonidine stimulates α_2-adrenoceptors in the brain stem and thus reduces peripheral sympathetic activity and increases vagal tone.[57,58] The centrally induced antihypertensive effect of clonidine can be counteracted by α_2-adrenoceptor antagonists such as yohimbine or rauwolscine. Clonidine, in addition to activation of central α_2-adrenoceptors also stimulates imidazoline (type 1)-receptors in the RVLM. Stimulation of these I_1-receptors also causes peripheral sympathetic inhibition and a decrease in elevated BP (see below).

The original concept was that clonidine, like α-methyldopa, reduced central sympathetic activity and lowered BP solely by an action on central α_2-receptors,[57,58,59,60] with possibly some contribution from presynaptic α_2-receptors.[46,61] However, it appears that neither central nor peripheral presynaptic α_2-receptors are involved in the hypotensive effect of clonidine.[57] Clonidine still inhibits sympathetic nerve activity in animals whose hindbrain noradrenaline is depleted by reserpine or 6-hydroxydopamine, or when noradrenaline synthesis is inhibited by α-methyl-p-tyrosine.[62,63] Stimulation of peripheral sympathetic nerves in animals treated with clonidine results in the normal release of noradrenaline.[59,64] The absence of any effect from 6-hydroxydopamine or α-methyl-p-tyrosine is also evidence that the action of clonidine is not dependent on an intact noradrenaline synthesis pathway, i.e. it is an action of a direct stimulant, unlike methyldopa.[57]

Clonidine intravenously results in an initial pressor response in animals[64,65] and humans;[66] this is due to stimulation of peripheral postsynaptic α_2-receptors resulting in vasoconstriction.[19,65] While oral administration of increasing doses of clonidine gives a progressive dose-dependent fall in BP, this dose–response

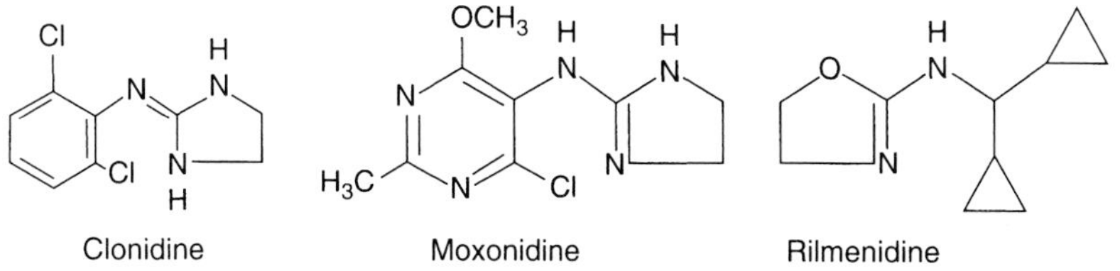

| Clonidine | Moxonidine | Rilmenidine |

Fig. 7.2 Chemical structure of clonidine, moxonidine and rilmenidine. Clonidine and moxonidine are imidazoline derivatives. Rilmenidine contains an oxazoline nucleus.

relationship is lost when plasma concentrations rise above 1.5 to 2 μg/L. At levels greater than 3 μg/L clonidine may then increase BP; presumably peripheral α-stimulation is then even more prominent.[67]

Evidence of reduced central sympathetic activity following clonidine is indicated by reduced plasma catecholamine levels,[68,69,70] which correlate with the fall in BP. This is seen with both single doses[54] and with chronic administration.[71] Additionally, sympathetic peroneal nerve activity is reduced.[72] The catecholamine response to standing and exercise is not inhibited by clonidine despite a lower level at baseline.[69]

The reduction of renin by clonidine has been reported to correlate with the reduction of BP after 1 day of treatment, but not thereafter.[73] Likewise responses following chronic treatment in low- and high-renin patients are similar.[73] A reduction in BP independent of falls in renin has been found in unilateral renal artery stenosis.[74] Guanfacine is also a central α2-stimulant drug, its action in animal experiments being blocked by phentolamine. This drug has selectivity for α2-adrenoceptors relative to α1-receptors 12 times that of clonidine; 1:3400 compared with 1:280.[75,76] Postsynaptic α2-stimulation, as with clonidine, is suggested by the initial rise in BP after intravenous administration.[75] Guanabenz is chemically closely related to clonidine, and the main antihypertensive effect is by stimulation of central α2-adrenoceptors.[77] Guanabenz also reduces the response to peripheral sympathetic nerve stimulation, and there is some evidence for an adrenergic neuron-blocking action (Table 7.1).[77]

Attempts have been made to develop imidazoline-receptor agonists that are more selective than clonidine, devoid of α-adrenoceptor stimulating activity. From this research two agents emerged for use in the treatment of hypertension, moxonidine and rilmenidine (Fig. 7.2). The imidazoline moiety in moxonidine is attached via an N-bridge to a pyrimidine nucleus. Strictly speaking, rilmenidine is not an imidazoline derivative, since its structure is based on an oxazoline nucleus.[78]

Several investigations have shown that moxonidine[30,32,79] and rilmenidine[80] act centrally to reduce BP. Only minute amounts of moxonidine[32,81] or rilmenidine[82] are required to reduce BP when directly injected into the RVLM in contrast to administration intravenously. Similar to clonidine,[83] moxonidine was first thought to reduce BP exclusively by a central α2 agonist effect.[79] However, imidazoline binds to sites that are not α2-receptors.[24,84] The RVLM is very sensitive to clonidine.[26] The BP reduction from clonidine analogues injected

Table 7.1 Central receptors stimulated by centrally acting antihypertensive agents

Compound	Receptors
α-methyldopa via α-methylnoradrenaline (norepinephrine)	α2
Guanfacine	α2
Guanabenz	α2
Clonidine	α2 + I1
Moxonidine	+I1 > α2
Rilmenidine	+I1 > α2

into the RVLM is related to the imidazoline structure rather than affinity for the α_2-receptors, whereas catecholamines and phenylethylamines are without effect.[26] The suggestion that the antihypertensive effect of imidazolines was not due to an α_2 action gave impetus to the development of compounds with less α_2 activity and thus the possibility of fewer problems with sedation and dry mouth, the major side effects of clonidine.[58] Stimulation of α_2-receptors in the locus coeruleus is responsible for the sedative action.[85]

While clonidine possesses little selectivity for the imidazoline receptor relative to the α_2-receptor, the oxazoline rilmenidine has 30-fold selectivity for the imidazoline I_1-receptor compared with the α_2-receptor;[86] findings similar to those with moxonidine.[87] Microinjection of the ligand for the I_1- and α_2-receptor, idazoxan, into the RVLM nucleus blocked the hypotensive effect of rilmenidine in the rat,[88] whereas the specific antagonist for the α_2-receptor, SKF 86466, had no effect. Microinjection of idazoxan also prevented the blood pressure lowering effect of intravenous clonidine in the rat.[89] Chan and Head[90] reported experiments in conscious rabbits where administration of efaroxan into the fourth ventricle was more effective than α-antagonism with 2-methoxyidazoxan in reversing the antihypertensive effect of intravenous rilmenidine and moxonidine. However, the two antagonists were equally effective in antagonizing the fall in BP due to clonidine. Unlike previous acute studies, Head and colleagues[91] reported studies in the rabbit in which 3 weeks of chronic administration of clonidine and moxonidine 1 mg/kg/day, and rilmenidine 5 mg/kg/day induced falls in mean arterial BP of 13 ± 3, 15 ± 2 and 13 ± 2 mmHg respectively, with no change in heart rate. Administration of efaroxan into the fourth ventricle on days 9 and 23 resulted in an average increase of mean arterial BP with moxonidine of 9.6 mmHg ($p < 0.05$), rilmenidine 9.9 mmHg ($p < 0.05$), and clonidine 14.7 mmHg ($p < 0.01$), while the administration of 2-methoxyidazoxan, an α_2-receptor antagonist, resulted in increases of mean arterial BP respectively of 0.8 mmHg (NS), 6.9 mmHg (NS), and 11.3 mmHg ($p < 0.05$). These findings confirm the importance of I_1-receptors in the action all three drugs, but also indicate that α_2-receptors play a part with clonidine. The concept that the antihypertensive action of clonidine was due to an effect on imidazoline I_1-receptors has been challenged and it is argued that the mode of action is α_2-receptor mediated.[92]

Similar to clonidine, as would be expected, a reduction in central adrenergic tone after moxonidine leads to falls in noradrenaline levels after single doses in normal volunteers,[93] in heart failure[94] and in hypertension;[95,96] in hypertension the changes in noradrenaline concentration correlated with the fall in BP.[95] Resting adrenaline levels fall,[93,95] although not significant in all studies.[96] Exercise noradrenaline levels are reduced by single doses of moxonidine 0.4 mg in normals,[93] in hypertensives[96] and in heart failure.[94,97,98] Results from animal studies with rilmenidine have not been confirmed in humans. In a recent double-blind study in 25 hypertensive patients, with an average age of 55 years, moxonidine significantly decreased muscle sympathetic nerve activity.[99]

Resting renin levels fall after single doses of moxonidine in hypertensive patients,[95,96] after exercise,[96] and non-significantly in heart failure.[94] Reductions in plasma renin by 58% after acute administration of rilmenidine,[100] and by 44% after repeated dosing have been reported,[101] while aldosterone levels were unchanged.[101]

The interest in I_1-receptors has led to the synthesis of various new compounds, including highly I_1-selective agents, such as AGN1924023, which are still at experimental, pre-clinical development. The imidazoline binding sites and their ligands have recently been reviewed.[78]

CLINICAL PHARMACOLOGY

Pharmacokinetics

Methyldopa

Bioavailability of methyldopa is about 25% with a range of 8–62%, indicating first-pass metabolism in the liver and gut wall.[48,102,103,104] Absorption is widely variable and incomplete.[105,106] Chronic administration (8 weeks) has been associated with an increase in absorption of methyldopa from 26 ($\pm$10.8)% to 33 ($\pm$8.9)% on day 56, as estimated from urinary secretion of methyldopa and its metabolites.[107] Food, particularly high protein, delays and reduces absorption.[108] There is no information on biliary excretion in humans, but it is minimal in the rat.[109] Absorption occurs probably at least partly by a stero-specific system, as only 8–13% of carbon-14 appeared in the urine after the administration of radio-labelled D-α-methyldopa.[104] Both ferrous sulphate and gluconate substantially inhibit absorption of methyldopa.[110] There are differences in the metabolites formed after oral and intravenous administration that also suggest first-pass metabolism.[105] Methyldopa-O-sulphate is found in small amounts after intravenous administration, about 40% after oral dosing.[105,111]

Methyldopa is widely distributed in the body. Animal studies reveal that it is taken up and stored in peripheral adrenergic neurons[112] and it penetrates the central nervous system.[52] Methyldopa does not show a correlation between antihypertensive effect and plasma concentration.[105] Peak levels of methyldopa occur between 2 and 6 hours after oral administration.[48,102,105] The plasma half-life is about 2 hours.[48,106] Chronic administration (8 weeks) has been reported to reduce half-life from 2.22 to 1.56 hours in normal volunteers.[107] The maximum effect on BP is, however, 6–10 hours after oral administration,[105,113] lasting up to 24 hours, which is consistent with the formation of an active metabolite.[36] The apparent volume of distribution averages 0.60 L/kg,[108] and about 10–15% of methyldopa is protein bound.[108]

Approximately 10% of a single dose of methyldopa is metabolized to α-methyldopa and then to α-methylnoradrenaline; this is excreted or further metabolized to the 3-methoxyderivative.[114,115,116] There are several other metabolites,[102,103,117] that are formed to a variable extent. The major urinary metabolite is the sulphate conjugate (methyldopa-O-sulphate), between 20 and 80% of the urinary excretion products being handled in this way. There is excretion of an approximately similar amount unchanged. Other excretion products include free and conjugated 3-0-methyl methyldopa (0–15%), α-methyldopamine and 3-0-methoxy-α-methyldopamine, up to 20% of the total, and small amounts of 3–4-dihydroxyphenylacetone. Renal clearance accounts for about two-thirds of the plasma clearance of methyldopa acutely.[104] Normal volunteer studies indicate that renal clearance of unmetabolized methyldopa increases from 62.7 mL/minute with acute administration to 99.3 mL/minute ($p < 0.01$) after 8 weeks.[107] Patients with renal impairment have an increased hypotensive response to methyldopa,[105] possibly due to increased levels of methyldopa-O-sulphate or of α-methyldopamine.[118]

There is excretion of methyldopa in breast milk; some is free, but most is conjugated and thus unlikely to affect the infant.[119,120] In infants born to mothers being treated with methyldopa, it takes several days for any methyldopa to be eliminated.[119]

Clonidine

Clonidine is very well absorbed; bioavailability from 70%[121] to 100% has been reported.[122] Absorption in hypertensive patients was similar to that in younger normotensive volunteers.[68] T_{max} is reached in about 1 hour.[121,122] A 6-month study revealed a reduction in oral bioavailability from 90% to about 65% with $T_{1/2}$.[123] The steady-state volume of distribution of clonidine was reported to be 2.1 L/kg^{-1};[121] clonidine is 20–40% protein bound.[124]

The half-life was initially reported as 7–11 hours when assessed by gas chromatography;[121,125] however, radio immunoassay techniques indicated a terminal half-life of 20–25 hours.[122] Steady state is reached in 4 days;[122] otherwise there is no evidence of accumulation.[68] In a study of five intravenous doses of clonidine from 75 μg to 275 μg in patients with essential hypertension, employing gas chromatography, it was found that with 275 μg, compared to a dose of 150 μg, the plasma time–concentration curve was no longer linearly related due to a decreased elimination constant.[125] Using more reliable radio immunoassay estimation, a linear relationship up to 300 μg was found.[126] There is a good correlation between the plasma concentration and inhibition of saliva flow or sedation score.[127]

An average of 62% (43–78%) of clonidine is excreted unchanged with $T_{1/2}$ of 20–25 hours.[122] As would be expected with predominantly renal excretion, elimination from the plasma is reduced with elevated creatinine levels, with a $T_{1/2}$ of 40 hours in severe renal failure.[124,128] A small proportion of clonidine is metabolized by two main pathways, hydroxylation of the phenyl ring to produce p-hydroxyclonidine and a cleavage of the imidazoline ring to produce dichlorophenylguanidine;[129,130] sulphate and glucuronide conjugates of the compounds are probably formed.[131] The metabolite p-hydroxyclonidine has some blood pressure lowering action following intrasternal injection in the anaesthetized rabbit.[130] Studies of carbon labelled clonidine indicate that about 65% of the radioactivity is recovered in the urine and 22% in the faeces.[131] Studies with transdermal patches of clonidine indicate that steady state is reached over 2 days;[132,133] levels remain steady for 11 days, and after patch removal elimination half-life is 14–26 hours.[133]

Moxonidine and rilmenidine

In many respects moxonidine and rilmenidine have a similar pharmacokinetic profile. Moxonidine has a high bioavailability approaching 90%. T_{max} is reached in about 1 hour and the volume of distribution is 1.83 L/kg.[134] Rilmenidine also has a high bioavailability (almost 100%); the maximum concentration is reached in under 2 hours and the volume of distribution is 5.1 L/kg.[135]

Moxonidine is eliminated mainly by the kidneys; about 50–60% of the dose is recovered in the urine.[136,137] The pharmacokinetics of moxonidine are not greatly affected by food; an insignificant reduction of C_{max} has been reported.[138] The half-life of moxonidine is about 2 hours,[134] although its duration of antihypertensive effect is much longer, perhaps indicating retention in the central nervous system. Experiments in eight hypertensive patients found that the maximum fall in BP with moxonidine was about 2–4 hours after the maximum blood concentration.[95] Normal volunteer studies demonstrated that rilmenidine is also mainly excreted by the kidneys, with about 65% of the dose of rilmenidine recovered in the urine as the parent drug; no metabolites were detected. The plasma half-life of rilmenidine is approximately 8 hours. There was dose linearity with 0.5, 1 or 2 mg and in most respects with 3 mg.[135] The pharmacokinetics in hypertensive patients were similar.[139]

Kirch et al.[140] studied the elimination of moxonidine in hypertensive or borderline hypertensive patients with various degrees of renal impairment. In patients with normal function ($n = 8$), average 41 years old (GFR > 90 mL/minute), moxonidine had a half-life ($T_{1/2}$) of 2.6 hours. In those patients with a GFR of 30–60 mL/minute, average age 56 years ($n = 8$), the $T_{1/2}$ was 3.5 hours, whereas in patients with a GFR of < 30 mL/minute, average age 61 years ($n = 8$), the $T_{1/2}$ was prolonged to 6.9 hours. Rilmenidine single-dose studies show a tendency for T_{max} and C_{max} to increase with worsening renal function, while the volume of distribution of rilmenidine tended to fall, with weak correlation with renal function. The elimination kinetics are related to the degree of renal impairment. $T_{1/2}$ with a GFR of 45–75 mL/minute ($n = 5$) was 18 ± 3 hours, 23 ± 6 hours with a GFR of 15–45 mL/minute ($n = 4$), and 34 ± 3 in patients with a GFR of 5–15 mL/minute ($n = 6$). A 20% reduction in apparent clearance was found in patients with hepatic insufficiency.[139] Increasing half-life of rilmenidine in renal failure was confirmed by Aparicio et al.[141]

Moxonidine in subjects aged over 65 years led to higher blood levels than those in volunteers under 40 years. Steady-state AUC was increased by 43%, but the increase in C_{max} of 20% was not statistically significant. Urinary excretion was increased by about 30% in the elderly, presumably due to reduced hepatic metabolism. It is not considered necessary to recommend a reduction in dosage in the elderly, in the absence of renal insufficiency.[142] Rilmenidine exhibits pharmacokinetic changes in elderly hypertensive subjects similar to those in renal impairment. C_{max} was increased and a slight decrease in the volume of distribution was seen. The AUC doubled, total clearance fell by 50%, while the $T_{1/2}$ was increased to 13 ± 1 hours in 16 subjects aged 81.9 ± 1.9 years (range 70–95). These patients had an estimated creatinine clearance of 51.3 ± 3.3 mL/minute (range 31–74 mL/minute).[139]

Moxonidine has been reported in breast milk at between 50 and 100% of the level found in the plasma.[143] Blood levels of digoxin, hydrochlorothiazide or glibenclamide are not affected by moxonidine.[134]

Haemodynamic effects

Methyldopa

Methyldopa intravenously reduces BP principally by reducing peripheral resistance. Cardiac output in both supine and erect positions does not change significantly.[144,145] Likewise, following short-term oral administration no change in the supine cardiac output accompanied the fall in BP.[146–149] Chamberlain and Howard[150] did not observe any fall in cardiac output from short-term oral dosage with 0.75–3 g of α-methyldopa daily; the fall in BP in the supine position was associated with reduced peripheral resistance. An increased fall in BP on standing and on exercise was associated with failure of peripheral resistance to increase. There was no evidence of an increase in venous pooling on standing as the normal fall of cardiac output on adopting the erect position was not increased with α-methyldopa. It should be noted that the BPs in many of these patients were relatively high even after treatment with α-methyldopa and thus these results may not be fully applicable to patients when BP is adequately controlled, although all except one patient showed at least some postural hypotension. When there is more adequate control of the BP, venous pooling may play some part, as a venodilator effect has been demonstrated after oral administration of α-methyldopa (2.0–5.0 g daily) for between 21 and 49 days.[151]

There is evidence that methyldopa increases blood volume,[148,152,153] but cardiopulmonary blood volume is unchanged, as is stroke volume.[148] As cardiac output is unchanged, despite afterload reduction due to reduced peripheral resistance and BP fall, and blood volume is increased, it is suggested that reduced sympathetic tone increases venous capacity so that venous return is maintained rather than increased.[148]

In contrast to other work, when Lund-Johansen[152] studied a series of 13 mild hypertensives before and after treatment with α-methyldopa (500–1500 mg/day, average 896 mg/day) for 1 year, he found that the fall in BP at rest, standing and on exercise was associated with a fall in cardiac output, no change in peripheral resistance being observed. There was no postural drop in BP; the supine and erect BPs with α-methyldopa averaged 139/88 mmHg and 150/93 mmHg respectively.

There is little effect on heart rate following intravenous administration,[144] whereas after oral administration there is a modest reduction, supine, standing and after exercise.[150,152] α-Methyldopa causes less of a fall in heart rate than that with the adrenergic neuron inhibitory drugs, bethanidine or guanethidine for a similar fall in BP.[154]

As might be expected with agents that inhibit α-adrenergic tone, higher doses of α-methyldopa used in the treatment of hypertension are associated with postural and exercise hypotension, but not to the degree seen with the sympathetic inhibiting drugs bethanidine and guanethidine.[154,155] The cardiovascular response to Valsalva's manoeuvre is also altered in a way characteristic of inhibition of vasoconstriction, such that overshoot is abolished[147,156] and during the effort phase the rise in BP is attenuated.[157]

Overall symptoms of postural or exertional hypotension are relatively unusual on α-methyldopa;[154,158] some studies have not reported these symptoms.[159] Excessive hypotension with methyldopa has been reported, particularly in patients under 55 years with elevated blood urea.[160] This study was unusual in that hypotension, often postural, occurred in over 10%; drowsiness and depression occurring in under 3%. Hypotension was more common in patients taking over 1 g a day, and most cases occurred within the first week of treatment, suggesting that the initial dose was too high.[160]

Meyer et al.[161] found a slight increase in cerebral flow in hypertensive patients with cerebrovascular disease despite a reduced BP after 2 weeks' administration of methyldopa. The administration of intravenous α-methyldopa has been found to reduce vascular resistance in the coronary circulation[145] and in the skin.[162]

Clonidine

Onesti et al.[163] reported that acute oral administration of clonidine reduced mean supine arterial pressure by 17% and cardiac output by 21%, while vascular resistance did not change significantly (+3%). Reduced venous return is indicated by a 2.3 mmHg fall in right atrial pressure,[164] and while Muir et al.[165] reported a non-significant fall in right atrial pressure in hypertensive patients after intravenous clonidine, there was a fall in cardiopulmonary blood volume from 494.9 to 417.3 mL/sq M ($p < 0.01$). Animal work indicates a shift of blood to capacitance vessels.[166] In the 45° tilt position after clonidine, compared with values in the same position before the drug, mean arterial pressure decreased 33%, cardiac output fell 15% and there was a reduction of 21% in vascular resistance.[163] These results were supported by other investigations[65,167] and by Brod et al.,[164] who also noted an average fall of 2.3 mmHg in superior vena cava and right atrial pressures.

The fall in supine BP with clonidine was associated with a moderate reduction in cardiac output and insignificant changes in vascular resistance, but clonidine inhibits the expected compensatory increase in arteriolar resistance in response to a fall in cardiac output. In the 45° tilt position, the antihypertensive effect of clonidine was associated with an inhibition of the increase of peripheral resistance that occurs in the absence of the drug. The studies of Onesti et al.[163] indicated that not only is the usual compensatory vasoconstriction of approximately 30%, which is associated with changes of posture,[168] largely abolished, but the drug in addition caused a moderate decrease in the cardiac output, which was already reduced by orthostatic change. Because of these simultaneous reductions in cardiac output and peripheral resistance, acute clonidine produced a considerable degree of postural hypotension;[163] however, these findings are not in accord with the relative absence of postural hypotension with chronic administration in the normal clinical use of clonidine. The concept of a contribution of reduced cardiac output and decrease in peripheral resistance contributing to the fall of BP from clonidine is supported by recent observations of the effect of intravenous clonidine on normal volunteers.[169]

In treatment of hypertension clonidine rarely results in exercise hypotension, compared with α-methyldopa or the adrenergic neuron inhibiting drugs.[170,171] Muir et al.[165] reported an acute study in six hypertensive patients who were studied when supine and two who were studied during walking exercise. Clonidine did not alter the percent increases of mean arterial pressure and of cardiac output which occurred during exercise. As clonidine did not change the percent decrease in peripheral resistance, it is suggested that this drug does not inhibit vasoconstriction in non-exercising parts of the body.

Lund-Johansen[167] described a study of the effects of 1 year's administration of clonidine on 13 hypertensive patients. Cardiac output supine and sitting was reduced by 13 and 12%, respectively, reductions in heart rate were similar (13 and 11%), while mean arterial pressure declined by 16 and 13%, respectively. In contrast to these significant changes, those observed in exercise cardiac index and heart rate were not significant, nor was the fall in mean arterial pressure significant at the highest work load (900 kpm). Both at rest and during exercise, falls in peripheral resistance were inconsistent.

Moxonidine and rilmenidine

The reduction of BP with single doses of moxonidine is the result of a reduced peripheral resistance, while cardiac output is maintained in normotensives[172] and hypertensives.[95,96] Haemodynamic changes after moxonidine and nifedipine are similar.[173] After moxonidine, ejection fraction at rest and on exercise has been found to increase.[174]

Single doses of moxonidine had no effect on pulmonary artery resistance.[96] However, after 4 weeks' administration of moxonidine there was a fall of pulmonary artery resistance similar to the fall in systemic resistance, while there was no change in pulmonary artery pressure.[173] Studies of peripheral blood flow after ischaemia indicate that flow is increased by moxonidine and that indicators of ischaemia are reduced.[175]

Peripheral blood flow was increased by moxonidine in hypertensive patients, as measured by the influence of 1 minute cooling on nail fold capillary blood flow. The administration of moxonidine 0.2 or 0.4 mg for 8 weeks increased flow from 0.65 mm/second to 1.13 mm/second ($p < 0.05$); the increase with diazapril (0.79 to 0.93 mm/second) was not significant.[176]

Mitrovic et al.[94] reported that single doses of moxonidine 0.4 mg reduced BP at rest and on exercise in heart failure patients. A small fall in cardiac output was seen 2 hours post drug, with no change at 3 hours, while stroke volume showed a small increase at 3 hours post drug. Exercise heart rate fell by 7 beats/minute, but cardiac output was unchanged and stroke volume tended to increase (NS). Motz et al.[97] described a 3-month study of moxonidine in heart failure ($n = 20$). Initially, the starting dose was 0.05 mg, but as contractility was not reduced the later starting dose was 0.1 mg, with the dosage increased to 0.2 mg and then 0.4 mg over 2 weeks. Seventeen patients completed the study, showing an improvement in ejection fraction, cardiac output and stroke volume.

Rilmenidine is associated with a dose-dependent fall in BP in normal volunteers and hypertensive patients.[177] Zannad et al.[178] administered single oral doses of rilmenidine, 25 μg/kg (1.4–2.4 mg) to eight untreated hypertensive patients (age 47–60 years). BP and peripheral resistance were reduced, while cardiac output, measured by thermodilution, was unchanged over the 10-hour observation period. In a further investigation, rilmenidine 1 mg was administered to patients with a supine diastolic BP of 95–104 mmHg ($n = 8$), and 1 mg b.d. to those with supine diastolic BP of 105–115 mmHg ($n = 6$). BP fell in both groups over the first 3 hours. Cardiac output fell acutely, but peripheral resistance increased. However, after 4 weeks' administration, the BP reduction was due to a fall in peripheral resistance; cardiac output was unchanged from baseline.[179]

McKaigue and Harron[180] reported a double-blind cross-over study in six male volunteers aged from 19 to 34 years, in which rilmenidine 2 mg exhibited a postural fall in BP. The supine BP before administration of rilmenidine 2 mg was 114/56 mmHg, and post drug administration was 99/51 mmHg; 3 minutes after standing BP was 118/69 mmHg before and 75/48 mmHg after rilmenidine. The rise in BP provoked by handgrip was reduced significantly. The bradycardic reponse to phenylephrine-induced increase in BP was enhanced, suggesting an increase in baroreceptor sensitivity with rilmenidine. Galley et al.[181] reported a fall in systolic BP after erect tilt in elderly patients of 5.3 ± 1.3 mmHg after 3 weeks of rilmenidine and of 6.7 ± 1.1 mmHg with methyldopa. However, at 6 weeks the rilmenidine patients showed no change on tilting ($+ 0.4 \pm 1.2$ mmHg), while methyldopa still resulted in a small fall of BP (6.4 ± 1.3 mmHg). Studies in 12 male hypertensive patients indicated that rilmenidine reduced the tachycardia associated with mental arithmetic, but not the increase in BP. Similarly the rise in BP on exercise was unaltered, while exercise tachycardia was reduced from 59 to 50 beats/minute.[182]

Oral treatment of hypertensive patients is associated with a small fall in heart rate with rilmenidine,[183,184,185] although this is inconsistent and may be less than that seen with clonidine.[186] Rilmenidine does not affect heart rate variability.[187]

Cardiovascular remodelling

The evidence that methyldopa reduces left-ventricular hypertrophy in humans is modest, although it has been demonstrated in the spontaneous hypertensive rat (SHR). A reduction of left ventricular mass (LVM) of 26.12 ± 35.09 g in 10 patients treated for 1 year has been reported,[188] and a reduction in combined posterior wall (PW) and intraventricular septal thickness (IVST) after 3 months methyldopa has also been described ($n = 17$).[189] In 23 hypertensive subjects treated with clonidine for 1 year, Timio et al.[190] found significant reductions in IVST, PWT and left-ventricular mass index (LVMI). However, while transdermal clonidine failed to regress left ventricular hypertrophy (LVH) in contrast to indapamide,[191] a similar reversal of LVH was found with clonidine ($n = 10$) and nifedipine ($n = 11$).[192] The large Veterans study[193] did not find any reduction in LVM at 1 year with clonidine, diltiazem or clonidine and prazosin, in contrast with a reduction in LVM with hydrochlorothiazide (42.9 g/m^2), captopril (38.7 g/m^2) and atenolol (28.1 g/m^2).

Moxonidine given for 6 months reduced LVH,[194] while, more recently, a 9-month study of 20 patients, dose titrated (0.2, 0.4, 0.6 mg) according to the BP response, also showed a reduction of LVH.[195] Trimarco et al.[196] reported a 1-year study in 23 patients demonstrating a reduction of LVH after rilmenidine 1 or 2 mg; this has been confirmed in a recent large study of rilmenidine.[197] A comparative 1-year trial of rilmenidine 1 or 2 mg ($n = 35$) and nifedipine SR, 20 mg b.d. ($n = 58$) resulted in reductions in LVM, 22.1 ± 23.3 g/m^2 and 26.9 ± 29.5 g/m^2, respectively, both highly significant differences from baseline ($p < 0.001$), but no difference between treatments.[198] Finally, a 3-month study found that rilmenidine 1 mg, perindopril 4 mg and nifedipine SR 20 mg daily, reversed LVM to a similar degree.[199]

Motz et al.[200] found an improvement in coronary flow reserve in hypertensive patients after 6–9 months of treatment with moxonidine 0.4 to 0.8 mg. The maximum coronary flow with dipyridamole increased from a baseline of 190 ± 90 mL/minute/100 g to 278 ± 94 mL/minute/g ($p < 0.05$), after moxonidine, which was withdrawn one week prior to the measurements. Trimarco et al.[196] reported an improvement in brachial artery compliance with rilmenidine from 0.92 ± 0.06 to 1.16 ± 0.08 cm^4/dyne ($p < 0.05$); the change persisted for 1 month after drug withdrawal.

Effects on other organs/systems: side effects

Central nervous system

The most common factor limiting dosage with methyldopa is tiredness,[158] which is seen more frequently than with other drugs.[155] Prichard et al.[154] reported tiredness in 75% of patients on methyldopa, 10% on bethanidine and 17% on guanethidine. A general impairment of mental activity may be seen.[201] Dreams may be affected,[154,158] and depression has been described in 5–10% of patients.[154,158,159,202,203]

While many of the above studies used large doses, in a double-blind study, more moderate doses (250 mg t.d.s) of methyldopa were shown to impair psychomotor tests.[204] In a recent double-blind study, methyldopa (250 mg or 500 mg, average 405 mg daily) along with five other antihypertensives, atenolol, metoprolol, hydrochlorothiazide, enalapril and verapamil, all produced small treatment effects in four of seven cognitive performance tests. Metoprolol and methyldopa reduced manual dexterity. In contrast, all treatments favourably affected performance in tests requiring working memory.[205] Fewer central nervous system side effects have been reported in hospital in-patients, where sedation might be less noticeable.[160]

The reported incidence of impotence has varied between 2%[158] and 25%.[206] Single doses and long-term administration of methyldopa 750–1000 mg has been found to elevate prolactin levels,[207] which could be responsible for the rare side effect of galactorrhoea described in women.[208,209] Methyldopa may increase prolactin concentration by reducing hypothalmic dopamine, a potential prolactin inhibitory factor.[207] Reduced dopamine may also be responsible for Parkinsonian side effects that have been reported with methyldopa.[209–211]

Clonidine dose dependently results in drowsiness, tiredness, dry mouth and constipation in the majority of patients.[212–217] These symptoms diminish with time,[212,216–219] and, therefore, whenever possible, it is best to increase the dose of the drug gradually at intervals of at least 2 weeks in order to increase its acceptance. Sedation is the most commonly troublesome side effect. A recent study confirmed the decline in psychomotor performance and cognition measures from clonidine, whereas nicardipine was without effect.[220] Clonidine may worsen sleep apnoea.[221]

Normal volunteer experiments indicated slight sedation with sensitive laboratory tests after moxonidine, but this was less than that seen with clonidine,[172] while no effect was observed in hypertensive patients in single dose studies.[95] Moxonidine 0.4 mg did not adversely affect performance in choice reaction time, digital vigilance tests and immediate word recall in contrast to lorazepam (2 mg) or diazepam (10 mg), though there was evidence of an interaction between moxonidine and lorazepam.[222] No untoward effect on various driving skills was found in hypertensive patients treated with moxonidine 0.2 or 0.4 mg daily.[223] An experimental sustained release preparation of moxonidine (1.5 mg o.d.) had a marginal effect on performance after the first dose, but by 1 week and 4 weeks results were not different from those with placebo.[224]

Open studies suggest an incidence of somnolence of around 8% with moxonidine,[225,226] while controlled studies indicated a 7.3% incidence of somnolence or asthenia with moxonidine ($n = 742$) against 3.8% with placebo ($n = 339$).[225,226] Schwartz and Kandziora[227] reported dry mouth in 12.9% initially, but at 3 months the rate had reduced to 2.6% and at 12 months the incidence was

2.1%. Lassitude (4.8%) also occurred early, but disappeared by 3 months. When moxonidine ($n = 718$) was compared with comparitor drugs ($n = 776$), the incidence of somnolence or asthenia was 5.3% and 4.0% respectively. Schacter et al.[226] reported a decline in somnolence from 24% in 1–4 week studies, to 10.1% with studies of 4 weeks to 6 months and down to 3.6% in studies over 6 months.

Mahieux[228] reviewed studies of rilmenidine and vigilance. Utilizing visual analogue scales, double-blind studies using rilmenidine 0.5–3.0 mg in normal volunteers found that rilmenidine 1 mg was not different from placebo. Results from experiments in normal volunteers also revealed that there was no difference seen in reaction times to an audio-visual stimulus and critical flicker fusion tests between rilmenidine, 1 or 2 mg, and placebo.[228,229] Saccadic eye movements were not impaired by rilmenidine 1 mg, unlike clonidine (150 μg), and auditory evoked responses of the electroencephalogram indicated less interference from rilmenidine than with clonidine and lorazepam.[230] Rapid eye movement sleep is less affected by rilmenidine than by clonidine.[228]

Renal effects

Onesti et al.[144] observed an insignificant decline in renal blood flow following intravenous α-methyldopa in the supine position (8%), while glomerular filtration rate fell by 13% ($p < 0.05$). There was a relatively greater fall in arterial BP and, therefore, calculated renal vascular resistance was reduced. Short-term oral administration of methyldopa resulted in a fall in renal vascular resistance, while renal blood flow and glomerular filtration were unchanged.[146,231] Mohammed et al.[232] confirmed these findings in patients with diminished renal function.

Significant increases of serum creatinine, even in patients with advanced renal impairment, do not occur with clonidine.[170,215,219] Several investigations[163,164,212] report that intravenous or oral administration of clonidine lowered BP in both normotensive and hypertensive subjects in the supine, sitting and 45° tilt positions, but did not reduce renal blood flow or glomerular filtration rate, i.e. indicating a fall in renal vascular resistance. Onesti et al.[215] confirmed these findings in four out of seven hypertensive patients who had advanced renal impairment with glomerular filtration rates between 9 and 23 mL/minute/1.7 m² prior to administration of clonidine. The use of clonidine in hypertension tends to preserve renal blood flow and glomerular filtration, similar to findings with α-methyldopa.[216] However, the acute administration of clonidine has been reported to cause retention of sodium and water[163,212] and chronic treatment with clonidine alone can increase weight.[212,213] While there may be some retention of sodium acutely associated with weight gain, natriuresis in 3 or 4 days has been reported.[233]

Moxonidine at a dose (0.2 mg) which is sufficient to reduce BP did not have any diuretic or natriuretic effect in subjects on a low salt intake.[234] Normal volunteer experiments showed rilmenidine 1 mg did not increase urine volume, sodium or other electrolyte loss.[235] Similarly, rilmenidine 1 mg daily for 1 month in mild hypertensive patients ($n = 10$) did not change effective renal blood, plasma flow and glomerular filtration; BP fell and renal vascular resistance declined from 8191 ± 402 to 6893 ± 333 dynes/second/cm^{-5} ($p < 0.002$).[185]

Renal insufficiency increases the $T_{1/2}$ of moxonidine and rilmenidine. BP fell by 9.5/9.4 mmHg 24 hours post dose with moxonidine in patients with normal renal function ($n = 8$) after 7 days' treatment. Where glomerular filtration rate (GFR) was between 30 and 60 mL/minute ($n = 8$), a fall of 8.1/6.9 mmHg was seen, while in the group with GFR of less than 30 mL/minute ($n = 8$), the fall was 14.3/10.6 mmHg.[140] Moxonidine was as well tolerated as nitrendipine as add-on therapy, in hypertensive patients with advanced renal failure, in a 24-week study.[236] The increase in serum creatinine 12.7 ± 49.2 µmol with moxonidine 0.3 mg ($n = 89$) was less than with nitrendipine 20 mg ($n = 82$), 43.3 ± 71.3 µmol ($p < 0.05$).

A surveillance of high-risk patients for 1 year revealed a small rise in creatinine levels with rilmenidine from 89.6 to 91.3 µmol/L ($p < 0.01$), but in the subset with renal impairment a fall ($n = 328$) from 126.2 ± 19.7 to 117.0 ± 25.4 µmol/L was observed ($p = 0.001$).[237] Lins et al.[238] described a 6-month open study of rilmenidine 1 mg or 1 mg b.d. in 17 patients with a creatinine clearance of 35 ± 4 mL (range 12–58); 12 patients completed 6 months' treatment. At 4½ months supine BP was reduced by 12.4/10.4 mmHg, compared to baseline, but at 6 months the reduction was 12.3/6.1 mmHg as pressures increased in three patients.

Airways

In a double-blind study in 12 asthmatic subjects neither rilmenidine (1 mg), nor clonidine (150 µg) affected baseline FEV_1 compared with placebo. Histamine challenge had an effect after clonidine (a 40% decrease in FEV_1; $p < 0.01$ vs. placebo), more than the 31% decrease with rilmenidine ($p < 0.05$), which in turn was greater than the decrease with placebo (22%; $p < 0.01$).[239] However, asthma has not featured in clinical reports with these agents.

In a further study of asthmatics, there was no difference in the concentration of methacholine required to induce a 20% fall in FEV_1 after clonidine or placebo.[240] In high concentrations clonidine, but not guanfacine, inhibits histamine release from human basophils and mast cells.[241] Clonidine does not affect the respiratory response to CO_2 in normal volunteers or influence the depressive effect of morphine.[242]

Moxonidine did not affect histamine responses in asthmatic subjects.[243] Lung function was not influenced by moxonidine 0.2 or 0.4 mg in hypertensive patients with chronic obstructive pulmonary disease.[244]

Skin

Methyldopa may cause various skin rashes including urticaria, seborrhoeic dermatitis, eczema,[245,246] particularly in patients with previous skin problems.[246] Lichenoid reactions may occur,[247,248,249] and these may ulcerate.[250] Methyldopa may be responsible for ulceration of the oral mucous membrane; oral lichen planus and other reactions have been described.[251] Methyldopa-treated patients have positive anti-nuclear antibodies with an incidence of 14–18% and methyldopa-induced lupus has been reported.[252]

Gastrointestinal

Weight gain is reported in 64% of methyldopa-treated individuals.[158] Diarrhoea is seen in 4%[158] to 8%[154] of methyldopa-treated patients, but is much less frequent than with guanethidine. Diarrhoea is associated with dilation of the small intestine and malabsorption has been reported,[253] with one case of colitis and hepatitis (see below).[254]

Dry mouth caused by clonidine can be relieved by measures that increase salivary secretion, for instance the application of lemon juice on the tongue, sucking citrus sweets, etc. Drinking large amounts of water may result in inconvenient frequent diuresis and is usually ineffective. Constipation is usually minor; however, one instance of paralytic ileus has been reported, relieved within 24 hours of stopping the drug.[212]

There is an increase in the incidence of dry mouth with both moxonidine and rilmenidine, but this is less than with clonidine. Moxonidine 0.2 mg in normal volunteers reduced saliva flow to a lesser extent than that with clonidine at the same dose.[172] Other investigations showed single doses of 0.25 mg moxonidine in hypertensive patients were without effect on salivary secretion.[95]

The incidence of dry mouth in controlled studies was 8.9% with moxonidine and 2.3% with placebo.[226] Schacter et al.[226] also reported a decline in incidence of dry mouth with duration of administration; 31.4% in 1–4 week studies ($n = 121$), 14.4% in studies of 4 weeks to 6 months ($n = 377$), and 10.4% in studies over 6 months ($n = 530$).

Liver

Drug-induced thiamine-mediated liver injury may be hepatic, cholestatic or have mixed features.[255] An incidence of about 6% of minor abnormalities of liver chemistry has been reported in patients treated with methyldopa,[256] with serious reactions in about 0.19%.[257] Rarely, methyldopa may lead to an illness clinically and histologically similar to viral hepatitis. The onset has been reported from 1 week to 1 year after starting the drug,[256,258,259] but may occur after up to 5 years' exposure.[260] The histological picture may be that of chronic aggressive hepatitis.[258,259,260]

When methyldopa was in widespread use in the treatment of hypertension, it was found to be the cause of almost one-quarter of cases of active chronic hepatitis.[261] Methyldopa is still frequently used in the management of hypertension in pregnancy and may be responsible for liver damage.[262] Most cases make a clinical recovery when methyldopa is stopped. The cases occurring soon after methyldopa was started resolved more rapidly than those developing after a long period of drug administration.[260] Acute submassive hepatic necrosis has been reported.[263] There have been rare cases of fatal progression of liver injury.[264,265,266] In one of two patients with subacute hepatic necrosis, in a total series of seven with liver injury in spite of corticosteroids, there was progressive hepatic failure. Post-mortem histology revealed continuing necrosis with changes of postnecrotic cirrhosis.[259]

Inadvertent re-administration of methyldopa has led to a dramatic recurrence of symptoms, supporting suggestions that a hypersensitivity mechanism is responsible,[259,267] but desensitization may occur as the reaction may be less marked on re-exposure.[256] The basis for methyldopa liver damage is not clear; a drug metabolite protein complex may act as a hapten and a genetic predisposition has been implicated.[260] Women have a higher incidence.[268] Another possible mechanism is that reactive metabolites reduce glutathiamine reserve and thus make the liver more subject to damage.[269]

Methyldopa is a rare cause of cholestatic jaundice without any evidence of hepatocellular damage.[258,270,271] A case of acute severe colitis in association with hepatitis after methyldopa, subsiding when the drug was stopped, recurring with re-challenge, has been described, suggesting drug allergy because of the association with fever, skin rash and eosinophilia.[254]

The use of methyldopa may be associated with a febrile reaction, occasionally marked in 1–2% of patients, usually within 1–3 weeks of starting treatment. It appears to be associated with depressed metabolism of methyldopa.[272] While fever may occur with hepatic dysfunction, it is associated with hepatocellular damage in only about one-third of cases.[264]

Hormone levels

Methyldopa, clonidine, moxonidine and rilmenidine all reduce catecholamine and renin levels (see above) and reductions in aldosterone levels have been observed. Clonidine in both low-renin and high-renin patients reduces 24-hour urinary aldosterone after 5 days[273] and 4 weeks' treatment.[73] Niarchos et al.[274] found that responders to clonidine showed a fall in 24-hour aldosterone, whereas in non-responders, levels were elevated. Reductions in resting angiotensin II and aldosterone levels after moxonidine were not significant in hypertensive patients.[96] Aldosterone levels in heart failure fell at rest, but changes were non-significant on exercise,[94] while levels of angiotensin, resting and on exercise fell after single doses of moxonidine.[94] Atrial natriuretic failure (ANF) at rest was unchanged, but on exercise a 23% fall was seen in hypertensive patients;[96] changes in heart failure were not significant.[94]

An increase in growth hormone has been reported with methyldopa[275] and clonidine.[275,276] However, in adolescents on chronic treatment no effect on resting or exercising growth hormone levels was observed.[277] A transient increase in growth hormone has been seen with 0.3 mg moxonidine 0.3 mg[278] and rilmenidine 2 mg.[279]

Clonidine did not affect thyroid hormone levels in hyperthyroidism, but did reduce catecholamines.[280] Thyroid-stimulating hormone, prolactin, gonadotropins and adrenocorticotrophic hormones were unchanged with moxonidine.[278] Methyldopa may cause impotence associated with increased prolactin levels and two cases of amenorrhoea and galactorrhoea have been reported.[275] Rilmenidine 1 mg o.d. 0.5 b.d. for 12 weeks did not affect prolactin levels.[281]

Glucose

Increasing levels of obesity are likely to cause a rise in the incidence of the metabolic syndrome[282,283] with its associated increase in mortality.[284] Although the exact mechanism is not clear[283] it is apparent that the metabolic syndrome, obesity, insulin resistance, are associated with increased sympathetic nerve activity. There is increased sympathetic nerve activity affecting the kidneys and skeletal muscle, whether or not BP is elevated. Sympathetic nerve activity to the heart is reduced in normotensive individuals with obesity, but is normal or increased in obese patients with hypertension.[285] It has been suggested that elevated sympathetic activity may lead to an insulin resistance syndrome, by the activation of adrenergic α_1-receptors in adipocytes.[286] It has been suggested, therefore, that centrally acting drugs that reduce sympathetic activity would be a logical choice for blood pressure control in patients with the metabolic syndrome or overt diabetes.[285,286]

Animal and clinical investigations have confirmed that centrally acting drugs have beneficial influences in the metabolic syndrome. Rosen et al.[287] utilized moxonidine, while Pénicaud et al.[288] employed rilmenidine in insulin clamp experiments and found that the development of insulin resistance and hypertension was prevented in Wistar rats fed a high fructose diet. Moxonidine reduced fasting plasma insulin and improved glucose tolerance in the obese SHR, while equihypotensive doses of methyldopa and hydralazine worsened glucose tolerance.[289]

Improved fasting glucose and glucose clearance have been found with clonidine compared with placebo in type II diabetes.[290] Moxonidine was reported to reduce blood sugar, with the fall significantly correlating to pretreatment fasting blood glucose level[291] (R = -0.698 $p < 0.0001$). However, with a higher dose of moxonidine, 0.4 mg b.d., no effect was seen, possibly owing to a peripheral α_2-agonist effect.[291] Similarily, Pillion et al.,[237] in their study of high-risk patients treated with rilmenidine, found no change in blood glucose overall, but in the diabetic subset ($n = 393$) glucose fell from 7.0 ± 1.6 to 6.6 ± 1.5 mmol/L ($p < 0.001$).

Improved insulin sensitivity was reported in overweight hypertensive patients with the use of moxonidine.[292] Rilmenidine also reduces blood sugar in women with the metabolic syndrome.[293] Type 2 diabetics showed a fall in glucose and triglyceride, and reduction in insulin resistance with moxonidine compared with metoprolol,[294] similar to a previous comparison of rilmenidine and methyldopa.[281]

Comparisons with amlodipine have revealed more favourable changes in glucose metabolism in obese hypertensives with moxonidine[295] and with rilmenidine in hypertensive patients with the metabolic syndrome.[296] Bauduceau et al.[297] in a small study reported similar reductions in microalbuminaemia with rilmenidine and captopril.

Blood

Methyldopa is associated with a high incidence of positive Coomb's test. In a series of 202 patients, this reaction was found to be dose-dependent: 9% at less than 1 g, 19% between 1 g and 2 g, and 36% when patients were given over 2 g a day.[298] However, autoimmune haemolytic anaemia, of the warm antibody type (IgG), is unusual and is not enhanced or inhibited by methyldopa or its metabolites in vitro.[299] The antibody receptor appears to be part of the Rh antigen complex.[300] Acute antibodies against red blood cells have been found in 10–20% of patients taking methyldopa for over 4 months.[301] Only a minority of these haemolyse. Anaemia occurs in only about 0.02% of patients receiving α-methyldopa (most at 1 g or less a day),[302] but is possibly more frequent in women.[268] The prognosis is good, recovery is rapid when methyldopa is stopped and steroids are given. In a 30-patient series, two died while still anaemic, one with multiple pulmonary emboli possibly due to haemolysis, and one from duodenal ulceration possibly exacerbated by prednisolone.[298]

Rarely, reversible leucopenia[303] or thrombocytopenia may occur.[304,305] Agranulocytosis has been reported.[306] A positive reaction for antinuclear factor has been reported in about 15% of patients treated with methyldopa.[307]

Clonidine inhibits noradrenaline-induced platelet aggregation, rilmenidine has a lesser effect and moxonidine is ineffective. This could be taken to indicate that the effect is mediated by an atypical non-adrenoceptor imidazoline binding site.[308]

Lipids

Methyldopa has been considered lipid neutral,[309] although in a 6-week study of hypertensives it has been reported to reduce HDL-cholesterol (HDL-C) and give a 10% increase in the ratio of total : HDL-cholesterol.[310] A 6-month study of hypertensives with doses of methyldopa from 500 to 2500 mg a day resulted in increases in triglyceride with no effect on LDL-C in patients with normal cholesterol levels, while in patients with hypercholesterolaemia triglycerides were not increased and LDL-C levels were reduced.[311]

Early studies with clonidine indicated decreases in total cholesterol, LDL-C and triglycerides, with no change or slight increases in HDL-C.[312] In a 16-week parallel group study of clonidine (8 weeks at 0.1 mg t.d.s., then 8 weeks at 0.2 mg t.d.s.), in 27 hypertensive patients, clonidine resulted in a reduction in HDL-C compared with placebo-treated patients, but not compared with baseline, while total cholesterol, LDL-C and triglycerides were not affected.[312] In the Veterans Comparative study, clonidine had no long-term adverse effect on lipid profiles.[313]

Löw-Kröger and Rosenthal[314] reported a large post-marketing surveillance study; 3 months of moxonidine 0.2 to 0.6 mg per day had no effect on glucose, triglycerides or cholesterol levels. Similarly, a more recent study of moxonidine 0.4 mg for 8 weeks in hypertensives did not find any effect on lipid profile.[315] A small study of moxonidine 0.2 mg daily for 6 weeks in hypertensive patients with hyperlipidaemia [Fredricksen 2B] revealed significant reduction of cholesterol (10%), LDL-C (10%), with non-significant improvements in HDL-C and triglycerides.[316]

Scemama et al.[317] reported an 8-week double-blind study of rilmenidine ($n = 24$) 1 or 2 mg, and captopril ($n = 24$) 25 or 50 mg in hypertensive patients and found no changes in total cholesterol, LDL-C, HDL-C, triglycerides or apolipoproteins. However, the 12-week UKWP study[281] ($n = 66$) reported a small fall in total cholesterol from 6.54 to 6.36 mmol ($p < 0.05$) and in LDL cholesterol from 4.49 to 4.18 ($p < 0.01$); changes in triglycerides and HDL-C were not significant. The large surveillance study of rilmenidine for 1 year ($n = 2635$) with 60% ($n = 1591$) over 60 years old, reported by Pillion et al.[237] revealed a small effect on the total cholesterol: a fall from 6.0 ± 0.9 to 5.8 ± 0.9 mmol ($p < 0.001$) with a larger fall in patients with dyslipidaemia ($n = 1007$) of 6.7 ± 0.8 to 6.2 ± 0.8 mmol ($p = 0.0001$). The corresponding figures for triglycerides were 1.5 ± 0.4 to 1.4 ± 0.4 ($p < 0.001$) and 1.7 ± 0.8 to 1.6 ± 0.8 ($p < 0.001$) respectively. In a recent study, rilmenidine, 1 mg for 12 weeks, was reported to increase HDL-C by 0.19 mmol ($p > 0.05$).[293]

Other laboratory parameters

In their large study, Pillion et al.[237] did not find any change in urate or potassium levels with rilmenidine. A small rise in urate (330 to 350 mmol) was reported in a previous study with rilmenidine ($n = 65$).[281]

Pressor reactions and withdrawal

Intravenous methyldopa has been reported to give a pressor response in a patient who had no evidence of phaeochromocytoma, judged by normal vanilmandelic acid excretion.[318] There have been two isolated cases of rebound hypertension following abrupt withdrawal of methyldopa.[319,320]

If clonidine is abruptly stopped the patient may experience within 8–24 hours an exaggerated elevation of BP, tachycardia, palpitation, sweating and anxiety,[321,322] associated with elevations of urinary and plasma catecholamines;[321,323] plasma renin is unchanged.[323] The withdrawal syndrome has been treated with intravenous phentolamine and propranolol,[321] intravenous labetalol[324] or by oral thymoxamine and propranolol.[325] Intravenous clonidine, 300 μg,[326] or oral clonidine also provides effective treatment, but the onset of action is slower after oral administration.[171]

While a beta-blocker with an α-blocking drug may be useful to control the tachycardia associated with clonidine withdrawal, a β-blocker alone is dangerous. This was illustrated by a case report where administration of the non-selective β-blocker timolol during clonidine withdrawal resulted in a catastrophic rise in BP.[327]

The frequency of the withdrawal syndrome is difficult to assess. The syndrome was not reported in several cross-over studies of clonidine compared with placebo or other antihypertensive drugs.[214,321,328] In a prospective study in 20 patients who were not receiving a diuretic, clonidine was stopped in hospital after 3 days' treatment (average dose 500 μg daily) and after 30 days (average dose 620 μg daily). In neither case was an overshoot seen, although noradrenaline levels increased above baseline and reached the upper limit of normal.[329] However, Goldberg et al.[325] found an acute rise of BP in nine of 15 patients. Pressure increased 12 hours after withdrawal and in those patients taking 600 μg/day or more reached a peak within 24 hours of the last dose. In one of three patients on 900 μg/day, a gradual reduction in dosage over 3 days still resulted in a marked increase in BP. It was not clear in this study whether or not patients were receiving a diuretic. In a further report,[330] all three patients showing a pressor response on withdrawal of clonidine were receiving a diuretic. In another study of 14 patients on clonidine 900 μg alone, only one patient had no exercise BP increase when clonidine was withdrawn.[323]

The hyperadrenergic state with clonidine withdrawal may result in major cardiovascular events. Ventricular tachycardia that was suppressed by intravenous phentolamine,[331] and myocardial infarction[332] have been reported.

Pressor responses can be avoided if clonidine is gradually discontinued over 1–2 weeks. Patients should be advised against stopping the drug abruptly; they should always have spare tablets. If clonidine cannot be discontinued gradually, as before surgery, an oral dose should be given as close as possible to surgical intervention and a supply of intravenous medication should be available.[171]

Severe vomiting has been reported to follow abrupt withdrawal of clonidine; this can be relieved by parenteral administration.[333]

The rate of rise of BP in the 3 days after moxonidine and clonidine were stopped was studied by Plänitz[334] in a randomized cross-over study. The 6% increase of systolic BP at the end of the 1st day after moxonidine was stopped was significantly less than the 14% increase after clonidine withdrawal ($p < 0.01$). Webster & Koch[335] cited unpublished data of Kaan, where the frequency of a fall of BP of over 5 mmHg on treatment together with a rise of pressure of 5 mmHg above baseline on withdrawal of treatment was assessed in placebo-controlled studies. This phenomenon was observed in 2/113 (1.8%) patients after moxonidine was stopped and in none after placebo. In reports with various comparator drugs, the occurrence was found to be 10/489 with moxonidine (2.0%) and in 6/401 (1.5%) patients with comparator drugs. These observations must be regarded as tentative, as the studies were not designed to assess the presence of withdrawal hypertension.

OVERDOSAGE

Reports of overdosage with moxonidine and rilmenidine have not been identified. There are several reports with methyldopa and a considerable literature with clonidine.[336,337]

Methyldopa

Underlying depression may be exacerbated, especially at the start of treatment by methyldopa[338] and this may, therefore, be a factor in deliberate overdosage. Tiredness, the most common side effect from the use of methyldopa, is increased, leading to coma following overdosage. Nausea, weakness, dizziness, bradycardia and hypotension are frequent. BP is likely to fall further on standing as methyldopa in large doses interferes with the cardiovascular response to gravity.[154] Paradoxically, large amounts of methyldopa may have a hypertensive effect due to peripheral α_2 stimulation.[339]

Clonidine

Klein-Schwartz[340] reported a 7-year survey, up to December 31st 1999, of exposure to clonidine in children under the age of 19 in the database of American centres. There were 10 060 reported experiences. Symptoms were encountered in 60% (6042) of cases, and were minor in 39% (of the total). Most common were lethargy (80%), bradycardia (17%), hypotension (15%) and respiratory depression (5%); there was one death in a 23-month-old.[340]

Life-threatening manifestations include coma, bradycardia, hypotension and apnoea.[337] Central nervous system changes occur within 1 hour, cardiovascular effects occur later. Hypertension, due to peripheral α_2 stimulation, has been reported in about 25% (range 19–48%) of cases;[337] peak BPs of around 240/125 mmHg have been reported.

DRUG INTERACTIONS

Methyldopa

Since methyldopa may cause depression, this drug should probably be avoided in depressed patients. Methyldopa does not appear to interact with mianserin,[341] but has been reported to provoke lithium toxicity.[342] Schizophrenic patients given chlorpromazine in combination with methyldopa experienced falls of BP and orthostatic dizziness. The combination of methyldopa and haloperidol has resulted in somnolence and dizziness, and two cases of dementia have been reported with the combination.[343]

Ferrous sulphate and ferrous gluconate reduce the absorption of methyldopa from 29.1% to 7.9% and decrease 'free' methyldopa excreted as a sulphate. Two weeks' administration of ferrous sulphate was found to increase BP in four out of five hypertensive patients receiving methyldopa treatment.[110]

Clonidine

Intravenous clonidine reduces the dose requirement of anaesthetics. This has been demonstrated in a double-blind study where, in the absence of clonidine, 5.50 mg/kg of thiopental was required to produce a loss of the lash reflex; whereas after 2.5 µg/kg and 5.0 µg/kg of clonidine, the required dose of thiopental was 4.15 mg/kg and 3.48 mg/kg, respectively.[344] Similarly, clonidine has been shown to reduce requirements of fentanyl[345] and propofol.[346] Clonidine has also been found to enhance analgesia from pentazocine[347] and to reduce the amount of isoflurane, alfentanil and midazolam required.[348,349] Clonidine attenuates the increased sympathetic activity induced by ketamine[350] and the mydriasis caused by rapid increases in desflurane concentration.[351] A double-blind study demonstrated that the tricyclic anti-depressant desipramine reversed the antihypertensive effect of clonidine in four out of five patients.[352] However, in another study, neither amitriptyline nor imipramine interfered with BP control from clonidine in 10 out of 11 patients.[171]

Complete AV block and hypertension has been reported in patients receiving verapamil after the addition of clonidine.[353] No untoward effects were observed with the combination of the dihydropyridine calcium channel blocker, nifedipine, in patients with hypertension; there was a useful additive antihypertensive effect.[96] Beta-blockers are likely to enhance rises of BP when clonidine is withdrawn, thus the combination is best avoided (see below).

Moxonidine and rilmenidine

There is little information on interactions with moxonidine or rilmenidine. The blood levels of digoxin, hydrochlorothiazide or glibenclamide are not affected by moxonidine.[134]

CLINICAL USE

Methyldopa

The antihypertensive effect of methyldopa was first observed by Oates et al.[354] Methyldopa is similar in efficacy to adrenergic neurone inhibitory drugs.[154,155,158] Prichard et al.,[154] in an individualized dose within-patient study ($n = 30$), found α-methyldopa gave similar control to that with the adrenergic neurone inhibitory drugs, bethanidine and guanethidine, although six patients could not tolerate α-methyldopa. There was less orthostatic effect with methyldopa and thus better control of supine BP for similar standing BPs. A further study confirmed that α-methyldopa produced control of the standing BP similar to that with bethanidine and propranolol.[355]

The Boston Collaborative Drug Surveillance Program of in-patients reported adverse reactions in 14% of 1067 methyldopa recipients, mainly hypotension (10.3% of the 1067), often postural. Drowsiness occurred in 2.4%, depression in 0.5%.[160] Chronic out-patient studies reported postural or post-exercise dizziness as an occurrence relatively frequently, 29% and 37% respectively,[154] but less often than with the adrenergic neurone blocking drugs that were in widespread use in the 1960s. Similarly, tiredness is a very frequent occurrence with methyldopa; a frequency of 75% has been reported.[154] Croog et al.[356] reported a large quality-of-life survey ($n = 626$), in which withdrawals because of adverse reactions occurred in 20% with methyldopa, 13% with propranolol and 8% with captopril. Similarly, overall assessment of quality of life was best with captopril and worst with methyldopa. A more recent quality-of-life assessment found the combination of isradipine and captopril was superior to methyldopa with captopril, or to methyldopa or isradipine alone.[357]

Commonly methyldopa 250 mg two to three times daily was the starting dose, although others used smaller doses (e.g. 125 mg b.d.) to minimize initial side effects, particularly if other antihypertensives were being given, unless BP was unduly high. Increments of 250 mg per dose may be made. Some physicians limit doses to 2 g/day; others have employed higher doses, e.g. 6 g/day.[203] Similar control of BP to that with three times daily dosing may be achieved by a single dose of methyldopa at bedtime.[358] Methyldopa combines well with diuretics,[359] and a diuretic should be added if side effects such as sedation occur, and is usually added if a daily dosage of 2 g is reached. In the EWPHE study, methyldopa was added in 35% of the cases on active treatment, hydrochlorothiazide and triamterene.[360] A combination of hydrochlorothiazide, enalapril and methyldopa has been reported[361] (see below). It has recently been advocated for the acute control of BP in Africans.[362] Methyldopa combines well with β-blocking drugs.[363] Tolerance is not uncommon, but it can usually be overcome by increasing the dose.[159] Side effects tend to become less when BP control is maintained.[154]

In the double-blind EWPHE study in patients aged over 60 years, diuretic, with methyldopa added in 35% of patients, gave falls in BP over the 7-year trial period averaging 19–23/5–10 mmHg compared with placebo, with a 27% ($p = 0.037$) reduction in cardiovascular mortality (intention to treat), 30% ($p = 0.023$) per protocol.[360] Dry mouth and diarrhoea were associated with methyldopa administration, and active treatment was associated with an increase in creatinine, urate, gout and mild hypokalaemia.[364] In a 15-year survival study of patients treated with methyldopa, mortality of those older than 60 years of age was similar to that of the general population; however, in patients younger than 50 years, mortality was higher than in the general population.[365]

Methyldopa has been widely used to lower BP in pregnancy; maternal morbidity and perinatal mortality are reduced. No detrimental fetal effects have been observed,[366] and methyldopa is still regarded as the drug of choice for hypertension in pregnancy.[367]

Clonidine

Intravenous clonidine lowers BP rapidly and has been assessed in hypertensive emergencies.[164,171,216] After rapid intravenous injection, within 1 minute there is an increase in pressure of between 5 and 20 mmHg, which lasts between

30 seconds and 5 minutes. The antihypertensive effect starts within 5–10 minutes of administration, peaks within 1 hour and may last for several hours.[164,171] After intramuscular or subcutaneous injection the initial pressor response is not seen.[216] The increase in BP can also be largely avoided if the intravenous injection is given slowly over 5–10 minutes or if a 5 mg intravenous injection of the α-blocker phentolamine is given prior to the clonidine.[171] A convenient initial dose of clonidine is 300 μg, and subsequent intravenous or intramuscular injections of 150–300 μg can be given every 1–6 hours.[215] A total daily dose of 5–6 mg has been used without untoward effects.[215] Injections of larger doses, 2–3 mg, can cause dangerously prolonged hypertensive reactions. It has been strongly advised that these doses should not be used to treat accelerated hypertension or other types of hypertensive emergencies or urgencies.[216] Intravenous clonidine does not lower pressure adequately in a sufficiently high proportion of patients and, therefore, it is not the drug of choice for use in acute hypertensive emergencies. Repeated oral dosage with clonidine has been used for rapid BP control.[368]

Clonidine is principally used for the chronic treatment of hypertension; some have suggested that it is a more effective antihypertensive agent than α-methyldopa,[214,216] while in contrast, others suggest clonidine rarely controls BP unless it is used with a diuretic.[212,213,216,218] In a study in 559 patients with mild or moderate hypertension treated with low-dose clonidine, 75 μg twice daily, 54.2% responded (a reduction of diastolic pressure to 90 mmHg or less, or a fall of 10 mmHg or more) to clonidine and 41.5% to placebo. In the nonresponders, the combination of chlorthalidone (15 mg) plus clonidine controlled 69% and chlorthalidone plus placebo only 34.7%.[369] Eight patients of those treated with clonidine alone ($n = 233$) were withdrawn due to side effects, three were withdrawn from clonidine plus chlorthalidone ($n = 184$), one from placebo ($n = 70$) and one from placebo plus chlorthalidone ($n = 72$).[369] There have been some studies that have reported a larger proportion of patients controlled with transdermal clonidine; however, other studies suggest a similar efficacy to that of oral clonidine.[70]

Oral administration lowers BP in 30–60 minutes, with peak effect at 2–4 hours and a duration of action of approximately 6–12 hours.[163,212,218,370] The initial dose of clonidine is usually 0.1 mg twice daily with variation between 75 μg and 6 mg/day.[170,212,213,214,216] Administration of clonidine in the evening more effectively suppresses the morning elevation of BP seen in treated hypertensive patients.[371] It is postulated that this may be important in reducing catastrophic cardiovascular events that occur within the first hour of awakening.[371,372]

A transdermal preparation of clonidine that can be given once a week has been produced.[70] This formulation can be used in renal failure[373] and a 5-year study has been reported ($n = 102$), in combination with a diuretic in one-third of the patients.[374]

Clonidine is frequently given in combination with a diuretic, with which as many as 80% of patients may be controlled.[216,217] The combination is useful in the elderly.[375] It combines well with a diuretic in low dosage, 75 μg twice daily (see above).[369] Clonidine, as it reduces heart rate, can be combined with a direct-acting vasodilator, such as minoxidil or hydralazine. Clonidine has been used in combination with β-blocking agents. Vanholder et al.[376] found that the combination of treatment with clonidine plus propranolol gave a fall in BP at 1 year of 11%/13% while with the β_1-selective atenolol, the combination gave a fall of 17%/19%. However, β-blocking agents enhance any pressor withdrawal reaction, and thus the combination is not advised.[363] The combination of transdermal clonidine with a variety of agents has been reported, including nifedipine-GITS,[377] sustained release diltiazem,[378] or enalapril.[379]

Moxonidine and rilmenidine

Two open 1-year studies of moxonidine hypertension have been reported.[227,380] In the larger study ($n = 185$ completing 1 year) 24% were controlled with 0.1 mg b.d., 45% 0.2 mg b.d., 25% 0.3 mg b.d., while the remaining 6% had hydrochlorothiazide (12.5 or 25 mg) added.[380] In a recent open study moxonidine lowered the BP in 112 obese hypertensive patients, 25 of whom had type 2 diabetes; there was a slight reduction in creatinine clearance.[381]

A study with rilmenidine had 269 patients who completed 1 year; 87 were controlled with 1 mg daily, 63 with 2 mg, while 90 received a diuretic in addition and 29 required a vasodilator added as one-third drug for BP control, i.e. to achieve a diastolic BP of 90 mmHg or less. The fall in systolic BP in these various groups was 30–32 mmHg in those over 65 years and 21–22 mmHg in those aged less than 65 years.[382] Subsequently, in one of the largest studies reported, of 15 963 patients completing a 1-year open study,[383] 60% were controlled by monotherapy with rilmenidine 1 mg, 25% with 2 mg, and the remainder had additional drugs to control BP. BP reduction was similar in those below age 40 years and those above 80 years.

Pillion et al.[237] reported a 1-year multicentre open study of rilmenidine 1 mg or 1 mg b.d. if diastolic BP remained above 90 mmHg in 2635 high-risk patients, 1591 of whom were aged over 60 years.[383] Baseline supine diastolic pressures were >90 mmHg and <115 mmHg. At 12 weeks a second drug could be chosen if diastolic BP was still >90 mmHg. In patients with diabetes ($n = 393$), renal insufficiency ($n = 328$), or dyslipidaemia ($n = 1007$) about 50% were controlled by rilmenidine 1 mg and 20–23% by 1 mg twice daily. In patients with angina ($n = 301$) or chronic heart failure ($n = 84$), only 37% and 36% were controlled by 1 mg daily and about 35% of these patients required the addition of one or more other antihypertensive drugs. After 1 year, 58% had 'normalized' BPs with rilmenidine 1 mg, 21% with 2 mg daily and 15% with a combination treatment. The control in the various high-risk groups overall was 94%, including the 60.3% of patients who were aged over 60 years. Dry mouth was recorded in 5.6% on monotherapy and 6.1% on combination treatment; 2.7% and 3.4%, respectively, experienced drowsiness, with 3.1% and 8.5% having asthenia, and 2.3% and 5.5% patients, respectively, complaining of dizziness. A small increase in serum creatinine occurred, 89.6 to 91.3 µmol/L ($p < 0.001$) in the general population, while patients with renal failure showed a fall, 126.2 to 117 µmol/L ($p = 0.001$). Blood glucose was unchanged overall, but in diabetics fell from 7.0 to 6.6 mmol/L ($p < 0.001$). Cholesterol fell from 6.0 to 5.8 µmol/L ($p < 0.001$) in the general population and 6.7 to 6.2 µmol/L ($p < 0.001$) in the dyslipidaemics. Many of these changes probably reflected regression to the mean. Potassium and urate levels were unchanged.

In a meta-analysis of pooled results from controlled trials comparing moxonidine with various established antihypertensives,[384] age did not influence response. Below the age of 50 years BP fell by 18.1/10.5 mmHg ($n = 209$), between 50 and 60 years by 20.0/11.5 mmHg ($n = 248$) and in those over 60 years by 21.1/11.6 mmHg ($n = 257$). Examining 24-hour BPs from double-blind studies against enalapril, BP falls after 8 weeks' treatment, corrected for placebo, showed a 4.8 mmHg fall with moxonidine from 0.2 mg daily, 9.4 mmHg with 0.4 mg daily and 10.3 mmHg with moxonidine 0.6 mg daily.[385] In a 4-week parallel group study of rilmenidine 1 mg daily, BPs were reduced to < 160/90 mmHg in 61% of the rilmenidine patients and in 23% of those treated with placebo ($p < 0.001$).[184]

Sides et al.[225] and Schachter et al.[226] have reviewed placebo-controlled ($n = 339$) studies with moxonidine ($n = 742$) to assess its side effect profile. Somnolence and asthenia occurred in 7.3% on moxonidine, 3.8% on placebo, while the incidence of dry mouth was 8.9% and 2.3% respectively. Other possible side effects were similar on moxonidine and placebo; one or more events were mentioned by 38.7% on moxonidine and 30.8% on placebo.[225] Age did not affect the results.[226]

Side effects in controlled studies where moxonidine ($n = 718$) was compared with other antihypertensive drugs ($n = 776$) have also been reviewed.[225,226] Somnolence or asthenia had an incidence of 5.3% with moxonidine, 4.0% on the various comparator drugs. The incidence of dry mouth at 7.8% and 3.4% confirmed findings from placebo-controlled studies. The occurrence of one or more events was 29.2% on moxonidine and 30.9% on the comparator drug.

In a placebo-controlled study the incidence of dry mouth after 2 weeks of rilmenidine 1 mg b.d. was over 30% and one-tenth of that level on placebo; however, increased incidence had subsided after 4 weeks of treatment. Drowsiness was not reported.[184]

Frei et al.[386] described a parallel group in a placebo-controlled factorial trial of moxonidine and hydrochlorothiazide. Defining control as a diastolic pressure of < 90 mmHg and/or a fall of 10 mmHg, each of the drugs achieved this in 70%, whereas the combination had an 88% response rate. Adverse events were seen with placebo in 22% of patients, in 40% with moxonidine, in 35% with hydrochlorothiazide, and in 33% with the combination. Headache (7.3%) was most frequent on placebo and dry mouth (20%) on moxonidine.

TOPIC[387] was a parallel group study in patients not responding to open label moxonidine (0.2 or 0.4 mg). Amlodipine 5 mg ($n = 81$) produced a trough fall of sitting diastolic BP of 7.3 mmHg, significantly more than that with enalapril 10 mg ($n = 82$), 4.8 mmHg ($p = 0.016$) and hydrochlorothiazide 12.5 mg ($n = 90$), 3.2 mmHg ($p = 0.001$). The standing systolic BPs followed a similar pattern.

In open studies, a diuretic has been used with moxonidine[227,380] and dihydralazine[382] or various antihypertensives[237] were employed in combination with rilmenidine. Some of the double-blind comparative trials versus various antihypertensive drugs have employed a diuretic added to each treatment arm, to assist BP control, e.g. rilmenidine versus methyldopa,[281] or versus atenolol.[388]

In a recent open study in 14 elderly patients[389] employing ambulatory BP measurements, moxonidine 0.2 mg or 0.4 mg for 6 weeks was used as a treatment where two or more agents had not controlled BP. Average daytime BP fell from baseline 169.2/91.6 mmHg by 15.4/7.4 mmHg ($p = 0.003/0.017$), and night-time BP from baseline of 151.1/77.9 mmHg by 9.3/3.2 mmHg ($p = 0.05$/N.S.).

COMPARATIVE STUDIES

Comparisons between centrally acting drugs

Methyldopa and clonidine
Connolly et al.[390] in an open cross-over study of titrated clonidine and methyldopa to achieve a supine diastolic BP of less than 100 mmHg. BP control was similar, with an average daily dose of clonidine 1.33 mg, methyldopa 4150 mg. Dry mouth was more frequent on clonidine; the frequency of sedation was similar in both treatments.

The addition of methyldopa or clonidine to chlorthalidone in patients with moderately severe or severe hypertension has been reported to give similar falls in BP. Sitting BP fell from 176/116 mmHg to 163/107 mmHg with 3 weeks of chlorthalidone. In the combination phase, each drug was given for 12 weeks, the combination phases being separated by 2 weeks of chlorthalidine plus placebo. The addition of methyldopa (250 mg t.d.s.) reduced BP to 145/96 mmHg, and the addition of clonidine (0.15 mg t.d.s.) reduced BP to 143/92 mmHg. Side effects were seen in 23 of the 41 patients who completed the study on each combination. Sedation occurred in 32% on the clonidine combination and in 22% on the methyldopa combination; the figures for dizziness were 10% and 24% respectively.[217]

Methyldopa and rilmenidine
Moxonidine has not been directly compared with methyldopa. A parallel group study compared rilmenidine ($n = 78$) 1 mg o.d. or 1 mg b.d. with methyldopa ($n = 79$) 250 mg b.d. or 500 mg b.d. After 8 weeks' monotherapy average supine BPs were 151/91 mmHg on rilmenidine, 152/91 mmHg on methyldopa. Hydrochlorothiazide was then added if the diastolic BP was 90 mmHg or more, i.e. in 29% of the rilmenidine and 35% of the methyldopa patients. Drug-related withdrawal, side effects, weakness, orthostatic dizziness and drowsiness were more frequent on methyldopa. Methyldopa resulted in a small but significant fall in systolic BP (some 6 mmHg) on standing, unlike rilmenidine.[281] Spontaneously volunteered side effects totalled 46 on rilmenidine, 76 on methyldopa. There was a lower incidence of several side effects with rilmenidine compared with methyldopa: headaches occurred in six and 15, weakness in zero and seven, daytime drowsiness in four and 16, orthostatic dizziness in two and 11, and dry mouth in 11 and 18 cases, respectively.[281] In a further report, a quality of life survey in these patients revealed no significant difference between methyldopa and rilmenidine. There was the same trend for improvement in psychological wellbeing with rilmenidine, whereas methyldopa patients had increased depression and cognitive impairment.[391]

Galley et al.[181] utilized the same dosage as in the above study[281] in patients aged over 70 years. BP control was again similar on rilmenidine and methyldopa. Moderate dry mouth was noted in 15% with both drugs. After withdrawal of treatment, BPs in the methyldopa group reached baseline levels in 2 days ($p < 0.05$ vs. rilmenidine), whereas with rilmenidine readings remained below baseline at 1 week after the drug withdrawal.

Methyldopa and other centrally acting drugs

In a retrospective analysis, BP up to 3 years was lower with reserpine, compared to methyldopa in combination with a diuretic. Drowsiness and sleep disturbances were significantly less frequent on methyldopa (10% on over 1000 mg a day) than with reserpine (57% over 0.25 mg a day).[392] Systolic BP in an open randomized study was reported to be lowered significantly more by guanfacine than by methyldopa.[393]

Clonidine vs. moxonidine or rilmenidine

Plänitz[334] described a double-blind cross-over study of moxonidine and clonidine in 20 younger patients aged 24–54 years (average 40 years). BP control was similar. At the end of the study BP rose significantly more rapidly in those patients who had clonidine ($n = 10$) as their second treatment. The total number of patients who complained of any side effects on clonidine was 85%, mostly tiredness (60%) and dry mouth (75%), and on moxonidine 30% ($p = 0.003$), where tiredness occurred in 15%, and 20% had dry mouth. Plänitz[394] reported a further double-blind parallel study, in older patients (up to age 88 years, average 58 years). Moxonidine gave a fall in BP from 177/100 mmHg to 151/87 mmHg in the 115 patients who completed the 6 weeks active treatment phase with moxonidine. Clonidine reduced BP from 176/99 to 147/87 mmHg in the 27 patients who completed. There were two patients who had dry mouth and were withdrawn from moxonidine, while the clonidine group had three patients where side effects led to treatment withdrawal; the overall incidence of side effects was 30% and 53%, respectively.

Fillastre et al.[183] reported a large trial of rilmenidine ($n = 162$) versus clonidine ($n = 171$). The fall in BP was similar in each arm, 19/12 mmHg and 19/13 mmHg, respectively. Side effects necessitated withdrawal in 17 patients on clonidine, but none on rilmenidine ($p < 0.01$). Dry mouth ($p < 0.001$), drowsiness ($p < 0.01$) and constipation ($p < 0.01$), were 2–3 times more frequent with clonidine. Similar results were obtained in a smaller study.[186]

Moxonidine and rilmenidine

One published 8-week double-blind study compared moxonidine 0.2 mg b.d. (patients aged 22–75 years, average age 56 years, $n = 69$) and rilmenidine 1 mg o.d. (patients aged 20–74 years, average 54 years, $n = 72$). BP control was similar, with supine BPs falling from 168.9/102.7 mmHg to 150.7/94.4 mmHg with moxonidine, and from 170.7/103.2 mmHg to 153.9/96.6 mmHg with rilmenidine.[314]

Centrally acting drugs and other antihypertensives

α_1-blockade

In a small study, trimazosin (up to 800 mg) or methyldopa (up to 2000 mg/day) added to polythiazide gave similar falls of BP.[395] Similarly α_1-blockade with prazosin and clonidine had equivalent antihypertensive effects; prazosin was better tolerated, notably because of drowsiness and dry mouth with clonidine.[396] In an open cross-over non-randomized study in 30 patients a similar antihypertensive effect was found with prazosin and moxonidine.[397]

Veterans comparative study

This was a major parallel group double-blind comparative study.[398,399] Success, defined as control of diastolic BP to less than 90 mmHg at the end of titration and a level of less than 95 mmHg at the end of 1 year's treatment, was achieved by 62% of those patients treated with clonidine ($n = 170$); diltiazem, 72% ($n = 185$); atenolol, 60% ($n = 178$); hydrochlorothiazide, 55% ($n = 188$); prazosin, 54% ($n = 188$); captopril, 50% ($n = 188$) and placebo, 31% ($n = 187$).

Clonidine had a high response rate in whites and less in blacks where diltiazem controlled most patients. In the South Eastern US (stroke belt), sodium intake is higher, potassium lower, and the response rate to clonidine was 43%, whereas it was 69% in the remainder of the US.[400] Likewise, response rates to hydrochlorothiazide, atenolol and captopril were worse in the 'stroke belt', whereas no difference was seen with diltiazem or prazosin.[400] Clonidine and diltiazem showed consistent responses regardless of renin levels. The response to atenolol was intermediate in low renin and good in high renin, while hydrochlorothiazide and prazosin were best in low- and medium-renin patients.[401] Body mass did not appear to influence the response to clonidine or other drugs.[402]

All drugs except prazosin reduced heart rate at 2 years; atenolol had the greatest effect, 10.3 beats/min ($p < 0.0001$), compared with clonidine 2.8 beats/min ($p = 0.0669$).[403] Pulse pressure (placebo corrected) at the end of titration was reduced by clonidine (6.7 mmHg) and hydrochlorothiazide (6.2 mmHg) ($p < 0.001$) more than with captopril, diltiazem and atenolol. At 1 year, the greatest effect was seen with hydrochlorothiazide (8.6 mmHg), the least with captopril (4.1 mmHg) and atenolol (4.1 mmHg) ($p < 0.001$), while clonidine (6.3 mmHg), diltiazem (5.5 mmHg) and prazosin (5.0 mmHg) were intermediate.[404] No difference in urine protein excretion was found between the various drugs.[405]

Hydrochlorothiazide produced the greatest reduction in left atrial size, a fall of 4.6 mm ($p < 0.002$) at 2 years compared with atenolol (1.9 mm, $p < 0.07$); the effects with other drugs were not significant.[406] Patients with adequate control of BP on captopril, hydrochlorothiazide and atenolol after 1 year showed a reduction in LV mass; clonidine, diltiazem and prazosin did not.[193]

Only clonidine and prazosin had more side effects than placebo during the titration phase. For clonidine versus placebo, side effects were dry mouth 57% vs. 6%, sleepiness 30% vs. 6%, fatigue 17% vs. 8% and non-postural dizziness 8% vs. 5%, respectively.[398]

Calcium antagonists

In a double-blind study, transdermal clonidine reduced BP from 148/95 to 139/84 mmHg after dose titration and 135/86 mmHg after 8 weeks; corresponding figures for verapramil SR were 156/96, 144/85 and 148/88 mmHg, respectively. Compliance was better with clonidine; adverse events and quality of life assessment gave similar results.[407]

Wolf[408] reported a multicentre parallel group double-blind study of nifedipine sustained release ($n = 113$, 20 mg o.d. in 52.7%, 20 mg b.d. in 47.3%) and moxonidine ($n = 116$, 0.2 mg o.d. in 57.3%, 0.2 mg b.d. in 42.7%). The falls in BP from placebo baseline after 26 weeks were similar, 27.8/19.0 and 23.8/16.3 mmHg, respectively. Side effects were seen in 28% of patients on moxonidine, and in 37.2% of nifedipine patients. One patient, because of dry mouth and tiredness, was withdrawn from moxonidine. In the moxonidine group, dry mouth (8.6% of patients), headache (8.6%), vasodilation (4.4%) and dizziness (2.6%) were observed. A 4-week haemodynamic, single blind study also showed that nifedipine and moxonidine gave similar BP control.[173]

A parallel group study compared nifedipine retard 20 mg b.d. ($n = 32$) with rilmenidine 1 or 2 mg ($n = 24$). BP fell by 22.1/17.1 and 16.5/14.2 mmHg respectively after 1 year's treatment. Seven patients withdrew from rilmenidine because of lack of efficacy and one because of unspecified adverse events, while with nifedipine one patient was withdrawn for lack of efficacy, two for unspecified adverse events[198]

Angiotensin converting enzyme inhibitors: captopril and enalapril

In a randomized single blind study, ramipril 5 mg o.d. ($n = 13$) was compared with methyldopa 250 mg b.d. ($n = 14$) for 8 weeks. BP falls were similar with monotherapy or when the drugs were combined with furosemide. No side effects were reported.[409]

A double-blind parallel group study of clonidine transdermal ($n = 39$) equivalent to 0.2 mg/day was performed against oral captopril ($n = 41$), average dose 122.9 mg daily. BPs fell with clonidine from 146.3/95.4 mmHg at baseline, to 134.7/85.1 mmHg at the end of titration, and after 8 weeks BP averaged 132.9/85.2 mmHg ($n = 22$). The corresponding figures for patients treated with captopril were 143.0/96.1 mmHg, 134.8/87.1 mmHg and 131.2/82.5 mmHg ($n = 16$) respectively. In black patients, the responses to clonidine were greater than with captopril. Four patients had treatment withdrawn because of side effects with clonidine, and one with captopril because of an urticarial reaction.[410]

Kraft & Vetter[411] compared moxonidine 0.2 mg b.d. ($n = 13$) and captopril 25 mg b.d. ($n = 10$) in a double-blind study with ambulatory BP recordings. After 4 weeks' single blind placebo baseline, 24-hour BPs with moxonidine fell by 4.9/7.3 mmHg, and with captopril by 5.7/4.4 mmHg. Other studies comparing moxonidine and captopril have found similar antihypertensive efficacy.[412,413]

Several studies have compared enalapril and moxonidine. Moxonidine 0.2–0.4 mg daily ($n = 22$) and enalapril 10–20 mg daily ($n = 19$) were each given for 8 weeks in a parallel group study.[414] Supine BP fell from 164/99 mmHg on placebo to 145/87 mmHg with moxonidine, and from 164/101 mmHg to 140/85 mmHg with enalapril. No difference in the overall incidence of side effects was seen. The incidence of dry mouth, 23% and 26%, or drowsiness (18% and 21% on moxonidine and enalapril, respectively) was similar.

Kuppers et al.[415] reported a double-blind parallel group comparison of moxonidine ($n = 47$) 0.2 mg o.d. for 2 weeks, followed by 0.4 mg o.d. for 6 weeks with enalapril ($n = 47$) 5 mg o.d. for 2 weeks and 10 mg o.d. for 6 weeks, and placebo ($n = 45$). In each group 36 patients had 24-hour ambulatory BPs measured. The fall from placebo baseline was 13.8/10.1 mmHg on moxonidine, 14.0/12.6 mmHg on enalapril, and 2.5/1.1 mmHg on placebo. The whole group showed falls in clinic BPs of 19.5/12.3 mmHg on moxonidine, 18.9/11.8 mmHg on enalapril, and 4.6/4.7 mmHg placebo. The trough to peak ratio for systolic/diastolic BP was 0.74/0.65 and 0.77/0.58 for moxonidine and enalapril respectively. The reduction on enalapril was similar regardless of baseline levels; 18.5/11.6 mmHg with baseline diastolic pressure 100 mmHg or less, and 17.9/11.7 mmHg with baseline diastolic BP above 100 mmHg, whereas the moxonidine-treated patients suggested a greater response with the higher baseline level, 11.3/8.8 mmHg and 22.6/13.7 mmHg respectively (personal communication). Side effects were reported in 29% on placebo, 36% on moxonidine, and 32% on enalapril; no patients stopping treatment because of adverse reactions.

In a further study, placebo ($n = 50$), moxonidine ($n = 51$) 0.2 mg, after 2 weeks increased to 0.6 mg, was compared with enalapril ($n = 53$) 5 mg, increased to 20 mg after 2 weeks, again for a total of 8 weeks. Twenty-four-hour BPs showed reduction of 25.8/9.9 mmHg with moxonidine, 25.4/10.4 mmHg with enalapril, and 2.5/0.5 mmHg with placebo. Dry mouth occurred in nine patients on moxonidine, in one placebo, and in none on enalapril. Adverse effects totalled 22, 11 and 17, respectively; there were no drug-related withdrawals.[416] Prichard et al.[385] briefly reported a further study where moxonidine 0.2 mg was compared with enalapril 5 mg; again falls in BP at these doses were similar.

Scemama et al.[317] described an 8-week double-blind parallel group study in uncomplicated hypercholesteraemic hypertensive patients treated with rilmenidine 1 mg o.d. to 1 mg b.d. compared with captopril 25 to 50 mg b.d. Supine BPs fell from an average of 163/99 mmHg to 143/85 mmHg with rilmenidine, with falls of 169/100 mmHg to 146/85 mmHg in the captopril group. Blood lipids were not affected. In a recent 12-week randomized open, blinded end-point study, rilmenidine 1 mg reduced ambulatory BPs by 11.9/7.7 mmHg, similar to that with lisinopril (11.0/6.7 mmHg); in both cases significant ($p < 0.001$). Rilmenidine reduced ambulatory heart rate by 3.6 bpm, lisinopril did not (difference $p < 0.002$).[293]

β-blockade

Prichard et al.[355] reported a variable dose comparative-within-patient study with approximately two-thirds of the patients also receiving a diuretic. While supine diastolic pressures (130/80 mmHg) were significantly lower with propranolol (average dose 825 mg) compared to methyldopa (141/85 mmHg) at an average dose of 2055 mg, the contrary was true for standing systolic pressures: 129/88 mmHg and 120/85 mmHg, respectively. In a further comparison of methyldopa and propranolol, while BP control was similar, the incidence of cold extremities was less with methyldopa.[417] A comparative study found low-dose oxprenolol (80 mg/day) to be less effective than methyldopa (500 mg/day) added to a diuretic in subjects aged 65–80 years,[418] whereas metoprolol (50 mg b.d.) achieved BP control similar to that with methyldopa (500 mg b.d.), but was better tolerated.[419]

Leonetti and colleagues[361] reported a double-blind parallel group study in 120 patients comparing the triple regimen of hydrochlorothiazide, propranolol and hydralazine with hydrochlorothiazide, enalapril and methyldopa. BP control was similar but only 3.4% of patients were withdrawn from the latter regimen because of adverse drug reactions compared with 10% with the former. Hypokalaemia in the enalapril group (four cases) was less frequent than in the propranolol group (19 cases).

A variable dose, cross-over study of clonidine, propranolol and placebo, 3 months on each treatment, resulted in similar control of the BP with active treatment. Heart rate was reduced by both drugs, propranolol more than clonidine, compared with placebo. More central side effects were seen with clonidine.[420]

After a single blind washout, moxonidine ($n = 25$) (0.2 mg or 0.2 mg b.d.) was compared with atenolol ($n = 28$) (50 or 100 mg o.d.) in an 8-week parallel group double-blind trial study. Sitting BPs fell by 19/14 mmHg with moxonidine, and by 22/15 mmHg with atenolol; various side effects were reported in six patients on moxonidine, nine on atenolol.[421]

In a multicentre double-blind parallel group study ($n = 90$), 8 weeks on rilmenidine 1 mg, increased to 2 mg (in 23%) if diastolic pressure remained above 90 mmHg, resulted in a fall of BP of 18/13 mmHg. Atenolol 50 mg, titrated to 100 mg daily in 33%, reduced BP by 21/15 mmHg. If diastolic BP remained above 90 mmHg hydrochlorothiazide 25 mg daily was added: in 12% on rilmenidine, and in 16% on atenolol. After 13 weeks, supine BP had fallen from placebo baseline by 21/14 mmHg on rilmenidine and 23/17 mmHg on atenolol. Asthenia, drowsiness and insomnia were more frequent at week 4 on atenolol, but not at other times in the trial. At the end of the study (week 13) HDL-cholesterol showed a small (0.2 mmol/L; $p = 0.008$) fall on atenolol, LDL-cholesterol exhibited a small fall (0.3 mmol/L; $p = 0.04$) with rilmenidine. Other lipid parameters and glucose were not changed.[388] A small ($n = 12$) double-blind cross-over study, utilizing the same dosage regimen of rilmenidine (1–2 mg) and atenolol (50–100 mg), performed primarily for autonomic and mental testing in hypertensive patients, found similar results.[182]

Diuretics

In a double-blind cross-over study ($n = 20$), methyldopa and hydrochlorothiazide resulted in similar control of the BP. However, side effects were more frequent with methyldopa.[359]

In a parallel group double-blind study of 8 weeks' active treatment, BPs on hydrochlorothiazide 25 or 50 mg ($n = 34$) fell from 167.3/103.3 mmHg on placebo to 151.4/92.1 mmHg and from 160.1/103 mmHg on placebo to 147.6/91.9 mmHg with moxonidine ($n = 28$). The incidence of side effects was similar.[422] Fiorentini et al.[423] compared rilmenidine 1 mg ($n = 114$) with hydrochlorothiazide 25 mg ($n = 116$) in an 8-week parallel group study. Four weeks' monotherapy gave average falls of supine BP of 16/10 mmHg and 15/9 mmHg, respectively. In each group 57% were controlled to DBP ≤90 mmHg. The addition of hydrochlorothiazide to rilmenidine controlled a further 14.5% to ≤90 mmHg, 19.5% when rilmenidine was added to hydrochlorothiazide. Pelemans et al.,[424] described an 8-week, double-blind study in elderly patients (aged 64 to 93 years) with hydrochlorothiazide (n = 42, 25–50 mg) and rilmenidine (n = 46, 1–2 mg). The falls in BP were similar from 172/101 mmHg baseline to 155/87 mmHg, and 167/101 mmHg to 154/89 mmHg with hydrochlorothiazide and rilmenidine, respectively. There were 14 spontaneous complaints of side effects in the rilmenidine group, 8 in the hydrochlorothiazide group, including 4 patients with drowsiness or tiredness with rilmenidine but none on hydrochlorothiazide. Direct questioning revealed a significant occurrance of mild transient dry mouth at week 6, and daytime drowsiness at weeks 4 and 6 with rilmenidine. Asymptomatic postural falls in systolic BP, over 20 mmHg, were found in 6 patients on hydrochlorothiazide and 5 patients on rilmenidine. Smaller studies have found similar levels of BP control with rilmenidine and hydrochlorothiazide.[185,425]

Other uses: heart failure

The recently reported MOXCON study[426] may be taken to indicate that centrally acting hypotensives should be avoided or only used with caution in heart failure. Sympathetic inhibition, however, is a well established approach to the treatment of heart failure,[427,428] both ACE inhibitors and β-blockers having been convincingly shown to improve prognosis.

Manolis et al.[429] studied the effect of a bolus of methyldopa 750 mg in six patients with NYHA grade IV heart failure. At 4–6 hours after the bolus pulmonary wedge pressure fell by 48% (33 ± 6 to 17 ± 2 mmHg, $p < 0.05$), stroke volume increased by 39%, vascular resistance fell by 15%, heart rate was reduced from 97 ± 7 to 76 ± 3 bpm (all $p < 0.05$). Methyldopa was then given as an infusion, 1–2 mg/min, and the improvements were maintained. Small short-term studies have also shown that clonidine improves central haemodynamics in heart failure, reduces noradrenaline levels and improves exercise tolerance.[428,430] In a longer study, clonidine 75 µg or 150 µg twice daily, improved exercise tolerance and ejection fraction after 5 months' treatment.[430] Similarly, in a 3-month study in heart failure with moxonidine titrated over 2 weeks to 0.4 mg/day, there was an increase in cardiac output, stroke volume and left-ventricular ejection fraction after 2 weeks and 3 months of treatment.[97]

In patients with heart failure plasma noradrenaline levels are reduced by moxonidine, dose dependently up to 0.3 mg b.d.,[431] or up to 1.5 mg b.d. with a sustained release preparation.[98,432] However, when a large study (MOXCON) was performed in heart failure, with titration up to 1.5 mg b.d. sustained release moxonidine, added to conventional therapy, an excess of deaths in moxonidine-treated patients led to premature closure of the study.[426]

In MOXCON the dose of moxonidine employed was several-fold higher than that used in hypertension or in earlier heart failure investigations. The MOXCON results need not be regarded as a contraindication for moxonidine in the treatment of hypertension, with usual dosages, in patients with evidence of heart failure. Floras[433] discussed possible reasons for the MOXCON findings. The reduction in noradrenaline levels and sympathetic outflow at the dosage of moxonidine 1.5 mg b.d.[98] may have resulted in levels insufficient to support cardiac output, leading to progressive pump failure. While normal dosages of moxonidine are not associated with an overshoot in sympathetic outflow,[334] at 1.5 mg b.d. there was a rebound of 275% accompanied by an increase in heart rate and premature beats.[98] It is possible that short periods of non-adherence might have contributed to the increase in mortality on moxonidine in MOXCON.[433]

Other uses of clonidine

Clonidine has been tried for varied clinical indications besides hypotension, with varying degree of success.

Cardiovascular

Clonidine causes a reduction in hypoadrenergic orthostatic hypotension, although to a lesser extent than with dihydroergotamine.[434] There have been reports that clonidine increases exercise tolerance in patients with angina[435] and reduces ST elevation in acute myocardial infarction.[436] Clonidine has been used as a test for phaeochromocytoma, patients with essential hypertension showing suppression of noradrenaline and adrenaline levels, whereas patients with phaeochromocytoma do not suppress.[437]

Operative use

Clonidine has been shown to reduce the dose of propofol and thiopental required for anaesthesia (see interactions). Clonidine can also be used as the sole analgesic agent for epidural anaesthesia.[438] Clonidine reduces the sympathetic response to surgery,[439] the incidence of intra-operative episodes of myocardial ischaemia in patients having vascular surgery,[440,441] and recently in a double-blind study it has been found to significantly reduce perioperative mortality ($p = 0.035$) for up to 2 years, from 29% to 15% (RR 0.43).[441]

Neurological and psychiatric uses

Clonidine can be used as a prophylactic in migraine at a dosage of 50–150 μg daily, but even at this dose, sedation and dry mouth may be a problem.[442] Clonidine suppresses the symptoms of the restless legs syndrome[443,444] and Tourette's syndrome.[445]

Clonidine has been used in varied neuropsychiatric disorders,[446] in acute mania,[447] in nicotine withdrawal,[448] in alcohol withdrawal[449] (where clonidine has been found superior to diazepam)[450] and in opiate withdrawal, although clonidine is less effective than tramadol.[451]

Menopausal symptoms

Clonidine reduces post menopausal flushes[452] and also those associated with tamoxifen for breast cancer.[453]

Gastrointestinal uses

Clonidine has been reported to be as effective as prednisolone and more effective than sulfasalazine in ulcerative colitis in reducing bloody diarrhoea and improving endoscopic, histological and radiological features.[454] Clonidine has been found to reduce diarrhoea in patients where this is due to autonomic neuropathy in diabetes.[455] Clonidine improves gastric emptying in patients with diabetic gastroparesis,[456,457] improves gall bladder contraction in insulin-treated diabetics and prolongs small bowel transit time.[458]

Glaucoma

Clonidine locally applied to the eye reduces intraocular pressure in open angle glaucoma.[459]

CONCLUSIONS

Central inhibition of sympathetic vasoconstrictor tone represents a logical approach to the treatment of hypertension. Classically, this was achieved by methyldopa, which is converted within the brain to α-methylnoradrenaline, which in turn lowers BP by stimulation of central α_2-receptors. At one time methyldopa was the most widely prescribed antihypertensive. Clonidine, like methyldopa, inhibits central sympathetic tone. Clonidine was initially considered to exert its action exclusively via central α_2-receptors, as experimentally, effects were inhibited by α_2-blocking drugs. The problem with both of these antihypertensives is the high incidence of central nervous system side effects, most notably sedation. This was responsible for the progressive decline in the use of centrally active antihypertensive agents; other agents such as guanfacine, guanabenz had the same disadvantage and failed to become established.

It was later found that clonidine also stimulated imidazoline I_1-receptors in the rostral ventrolateral medulla in the brain stem and inhibition of I_1-receptor stimulation, as with α_2-blockade, also inhibited the antihypertensive effect. As a central α_2 action appears to be responsible for the sedative effect, this opened the possibility of developing agents with more selectivity for imidazoline I_1-receptors compared to α_2-receptor binding. Whereas clonidine has low selectivity for the imidazoline I_1-receptor compared with α_2-receptor, the newer compounds rilmendine and moxonidine are much more selective. As predicted from the lesser contribution from α_2 stimulation to the antihypertensive effect of moxonidine and rilmenidine, these agents have a lower incidence of sedation than clonidine or methyldopa.

Many studies have been performed comparing the centrally acting drugs with examples from the major classes of antihypertensive drugs. Centrally acting agents have similar antihypertensive efficacy and the newer agents, moxonidine and rilmenidine, largely because of the lower incidence of α_2-mediated adverse reactions, have a relatively favourable side effect profile. There are no outcome studies except the EWHPE study[360] in the elderly where methyldopa was added to a diuretic in elderly patients where necessary; survival was improved compared with placebo.

Most patients with hypertension require two or more drugs to give fully satisfactory blood pressure control. The centrally acting antihypertensives represent a useful group of agents to help to achieve satisfactory BP control.

Acknowledgements

We are most grateful to Mrs H. Hannam and Mr B. R. Graham for assistance in the preparation of this chapter.

References

1. Mary DASG, Stoker JB. The activity of single vasoconstrictor nerve units in hypertension. *Acta Physiol Scand* 2003;177:367–376.
2. Mancia G, di Rienzo M, Parati G, et al. Sympathetic activity, blood pressure variability and end organ damage in hypertension. *J Hum Hypertens* 1997;11(Suppl 1):S3–S8.
3. Pickering TG. The effects of environmental and lifestyle factors on blood pressure and the intermediary role of the sympathetic nervous system. *J Human Hypertens* 1997;11(Suppl 1):S9–S18.
4. Ernsberger P, Koletsky RJ, Friedman JE. Contribution of sympathetic nervous system overactivity to cardiovascular and metabolic disease. *Rev Contemp Pharmacother* 1998;9:411–428.
5. van Zwieten PA. Centrally acting antihypertensives: a renaissance of interest. Mechanisms and haemodynamics. *J Hypertens* 1997;15(Suppl 1):S3–S8.

6. Reaven GM. Role of insulin resistance in human disease (syndrome X): an expanded definition. *Ann Rev Med* 1993;44:121–131.
7. Julius S. Sympathetic hyperactivity and coronary risk in hypertension (Corcoran Lecture). *Hypertens* 1993;21:866–893.
8. Esler M. The sympathetic nervous system and hypertension. *Am J Hypertens* 2000;13:99S–105S.
9. Bobik A, Dilley R, Kanellakis P. Sympatho-adrenal mechanisms regulating cardiovascular hypertrophy in primary hypertension: a role for rilmenidine? *J Hypertens* 1998;16(Suppl 3): S51–S55.
10. Esler M. High blood pressure management: potential benefits of I_1 agents. *J Hypertens* 1998;16(Suppl 3):S19–S24.
11. Frohlich ED. Methyldopa – mechanisms and treatment 25 years later. *Arch Intern Med* 1980;140:954–959.
12. Reid JL, Elliott HL. Methyldopa. In: Birkenhäger WH, Reid JL, Series eds. *Handbook of hypertension Vol. II. Clinical pharmacology of antihypertensive drugs.* Doyle AE, ed. Amsterdam: Elsevier; 1988:103–124.
13. Jarrott B. Clonidine and related compounds. In: Birkenhäger WH, Reid JL, Series eds. *Handbook of hypertension Vol. II. Clinical pharmacology of antihypertensive drugs.* Doyle AE, ed. Amsterdam: Elsevier; 1988:125–186.
14. Barron WM, Lindheimer MD. Management of hypertension during pregnancy. In: Laragh JH, Brenner BM, eds. *Hypertension, pathophysiology, diagnosis and management. 2nd edn.* Raven Press Ltd, New York; 1995:2427–2450.
15. Khedun SM, Moodley J, Naicker T, et al. Drug management of hypertensive disorders of pregnancy. *Pharmacol Ther* 1977;74:221–258.
16. Borghi C, Esposit DD, Cassani A, et al. The treatment of hypertension in pregnancy. *J Hypertens* 2002;20(Suppl 2):S52–S56.
17. Prichard BNC, Graham BR. I_1-imidazoline agonists, general clinical pharmacology of imidazoline receptors. *Drugs & Aging* 2000;2:133–159.
18. Langer SZ, Duval N, Massingham R. Pharmacologic and therapeutic significance of alpha-adrenoceptor subtypes. *J Cardiovasc Pharmacol* 1985;7(Suppl 8):S1–S8.
19. van Zwieten PA, Jie K, Van Brummelen P. Post synaptic α_1 and α_2 adrenoceptor changes in hypertension. *J Cardiovasc Pharmacol* 1987;10(Suppl 4):S68.
20. Gillis RA, Gatti PJ, Quest JA. Mechanism of the antihypertensive effect of alpha$_2$-agonists. *J Cardiovasc Pharmacol* 1985;7(Suppl 8):S38–S44.
21. Ernsberger P, Collins LA, Graves ME, et al. Imidazoline I_1 receptors in the ventrolateral medulla and their role in cardiorespiratory control. In: Trouth CO, Millis RM, Kiwell-Schone H, et al., eds. *Ventral Brainstem Mechanisms and Control Functions.* New York: Marcel Dekker; 1995:319–358.
22. Huchet AM, Doursout MF, Chelly J, et al. Possible role of central α_1-adrenoceptors in the control of the autonomic nervous system in normotensive and spontaneously hypertensive rats. *Eur J Pharmacol* 1982;85:239–242.
23. Ruffolo RR, Fowble JW, Miller DD, et al. Binding of [^{3}H]dihydroazapetine to alpha adrenoceptor related proteins from rat vas deferens. *Proc Nat'l Acad Sci USA* 1976;73:2730–2734.
24. Ruffolo RR, Turowski BS, Patil PN. Lack of cross desensitisation between structurally dissimilar α-adrenoceptor agonists. *J Pharm Pharmacol* 1977;29:378–380.
25. Ruffolo RR, Rice PJ, Patil PN, et al. Differences in the applicability of the Easson-Stenman hypothesis to the α_1- and α_2-adrenergic effects of phenylethylamines and imidazoles. *Eur J Pharmacol* 1983;86:471–475.
26. Bousquet P, Feldman J, Schwartz J. Central cardiovascular effects of alpha adrenergic drugs. Differences between catecholamines and imidazolines. *J Pharmacol Exp Ther* 1984;253:232–236.
27. Ernsberger P, Meeley MP, Mann JJ, et al. Clonidine binds to imidazole binding sites as well as alpha$_2$-adrenoceptors in the ventrolateral medulla. *Eur J Pharmacol* 1987;134:1–13.
28. Bousquet P, Dontenwill M, Greney H, et al. I_1-imidazoline receptors: an update. *J Hypertens* 1998;16(Suppl 3):S1–S5.
29. Ernsberger P. The I_1-imidazoline receptor agonist moxonidine: molecular, cellular and organismic actions. *Rev Contemp Pharmacother* 1998;9:441–462.
30. Ziegler D, Haxhiu MA, Kaan EC, et al. Pharmacology of moxonidine, an I_1-imidazoline receptor agonist. *J Cardiovasc Pharmacol* 1996;27(Suppl 3):S26–S37.
31. Ernsberger P, Giuliano R, Willette RN, et al. Role of imidazole receptors in the vasodepressor response to clonidine analogs in the rostral ventrolateral medulla. *J Pharmacol Exp Ther* 1990;253:408–418.
32. Haxhiu MA, Dreshaf I, Schafer SG, et al. Selective antihypertensive action of moxonidine is mediated mainly by I_1-imidazoline receptors in the rostral ventrolateral medulla. *J Cardiovasc Pharmacol* 1994;24(Suppl 1):S1–S8.

33. Buccafusco JJ, Lapp CA, Westbrooks KL, et al. Role of medullary I$_1$-imidazoline and α_2-adrenergic receptors in the antihypertensive responses evoked by central administration of clonidine analogs in conscious spontaneously hypertensive rats. *J Pharmcol Exp Ther* 1995;273:1162–1171.

34. Li G, Regunathan S, Barrow C, et al. Agmantine: an endogenous clonidine-displacing substance in the brain. *Science* 1994;263:966–969.

35. Levine RJ, Sjoerdsma A. Dissociation of the decarboyxylase-inhibiting and norepinephrine-depleting effects of α-methyldopa, α-ethyldopa, 4-bromo-3-hydroxy-benzyloxymine and relation substance. *J Pharmacol Exp Ther* 1964;146:42–47.

36. Gillespie L, Oates JA, Crout JR, et al. Clinical and chemical studies with α-methyldopa, in patients with hypertension. *Circulation* 1962;25:281–291.

37. van Zwieten PA. Basic pharmacology of alpha-adrenoceptor antagonists and hybrid drugs. *J Hypertens* 1986;(Suppl 6):S3–S11.

38. Day MD, Rand MJ. A hypothesis for the mode of action of α-methyldopa, in relieving hypertension. *J Pharmacy Pharmacol* 1963;15:221–224.

39. Trinker RF. The significance of the relative potencies of noradrenaline and α-methyl-noradrenaline for the mode of action of α-methyldopa. *J Pharmacy Pharmacol* 1971;23:306–308.

40. Coupar IM, Turner P. Relative potencies of some false transmitters on isolated human smooth muscle. *Brit J Pharmacol* 1970;38:463P–464P.

41. Day MD, Rand MJ. Some observations on the pharmacology of α-methyldopa. *Brit J Pharmacol* 1964;22:72–86.

42. Haefely W, Hurlimann A, Thoenen H. Adrenergic transmitter changes and response to sympathetic nerve stimulation after differing pre-treatment with α-methyldopa. *Brit J Pharmacol* 1967;31:105–109.

43. Henning M, van Zwieten PA. Central hypotensive effect of α-methyldopa. *J Pharmacy Pharmacol* 1968;20:409–417.

44. Ingenito AJ, Barrett JP, Procita L. A centrally mediated peripheral hypotensive effect of α-methyldopa. *J Pharmacol Exp Ther* 1970;175:593–599.

45. Baum T, Shropshire AT, Varner LL. Contribution of the central nervous system to the action of several antihypertensive agents (methyldopa, hydralazine and guanethidine). *J Pharmacol Exp Ther* 1972;182:135–144.

46. Bobik A, Jennings G, Jackman G, et al. Evidence for a predominantly central hypotensive effect of alpha-methyldopa in humans. *Hypertension* 1986;8:16–23.

47. Henning A, Rubenson A. Evidence for the hypotensive action of methyldopa is mediated by central actions of methyl-noradrenaline. *J Pharmacy Pharmacol* 1971;23:407–411.

48. Sjoerdsma A, Vendsalu A, Engelman K. Studies of the metabolism and mechanism of action of methyldopa. *Circulation* 1963;28:492–502.

49. Uretsky NJ, Iversen LL. Effects of 6-hydroxydopamine on catecholamine containing neurones in the rat brain. *J Neurochem* 1970;17:269–278.

50. Finch L, Haeusler G. Further evidence for a central hypotensive action of α-methyldopa in both the rat and the cat. *Br J Pharmacol* 1973;47:217–228.

51. Korner PI, Head GA, Bobik A, et al. Central and peripheral autonomic mechanisms involved in the circulatory actions of methyldopa. *Hypertension* 1984;6(5 pt 2):II63–II70.

52. Carlsson A, Lindqvist M. In-vivo decarboxylation of α-methyldopa, and α-methyl metatyrosine. *Acta Physiologica Scandinavika* 1962;54:87–94.

53. Heise A, Kroneberg G. α-Sympathetic receptor stimulation in the brain and hypotensive activity of α-methyldopa. *Eur J Pharmacol* 1972;17:315–317.

54. Struthers AD, Brown MJ, Adams EF, et al. The plasma noradrenaline and growth hormone response to alpha-methyldopa and clonidine in hypertensive subjects. *Br J Clin Pharmacol* 1985;19:311–317.

55. Leonetti G, Terzoli L, Morgananti A, et al. Relation between the hypotensive and renin-suppressing activities of alpha-methyldopa in hypertensive patients. *Am J Cardiol* 1977;40:762–767.

56. Weidmann P, Hirsch D, Maxwell MH, et al. Plasma renin and blood pressure during treatment with methyldopa. *Am J Cardiol* 1974;34:671–676.

57. Prichard BNC, Owens CWI, Tuckman J. Clinical features of adrenergic agonists and antagonists. In: Szekeres L, (ed.), *Handbook of experimental pharmacology, Vol 54*, part 2. Berlin: Springer-Verlag; 1981:559–697.

58. van Zwieten PA, Thoolen JMC, Timmermans PBMWM. The hypotensive activity and side-effects of α-methyldopa, clonidine and guanfacine. *II28-Hypertension* 1984;6(Suppl 2): II28–II33.

59. Hoefke W, Kobinger W. Pharmacological effects of 2-(2,6-dichlorophenylamino)-2-imidazoline hydrochloride, a new, antihypertensie substance. *Arzneimittelforschung* 1966; 16(8):1038–1050.

60. Schmitt H. The pharmacology of clonidine and related products. *Handbook of experimental pharmacology, Vol XXXIX.* Berlin: Springer-Verlag; 1977:299–396.
61. Starke K, Altmann KP. Inhibition of adrenergic neurotransmission by clonidine: an action on prejunctional receptors. *Neuropharmacology* 1973;12:339–347.
62. Hauesler G. Studies on the possible contribution of a peripheral presynaptic action of clonidine and dopamine to their vascular effects under in vivo conditions. *Naunyn Schmiedebergs Arch Pharmacol* 1976;295:191–202.
63. Finch L. The central hypotensive action of clonidine and BAY 1470 in cats and rats. *Clin Sci Mol Med* 1975;48:273S–276S.
64. Rand MJ, Wilson J. Mechanisms of the pressor and depressor actions of ST 155 (2(2,6-Dichlorophenylamine-)-2-imidazoline hydrochloride, catapres). *Eur J Pharmaco* 1968; l 3:27–33.
65. Houston MC. Clonidine hydrochloride: review of pharmacologic and clinical aspects. *Prog Cardiovas Dis* 1981;23:337.
66. Rudd P, Blaschke TF. Antihypertensive drugs and the drug therapy of hypertension. In: Gilman AG, Goodison LS, Rall TW, et al., eds. *The pharmacological basis of therapeutics, 7th edn.* New York: Macmillan; 1985:784–805.
67. Frisk-Holmberg M, Paalzow L, Wibell L. Relationship between the cardiovascular effects and steady-state kinetics of clonidine in hypertension: demonstration of a therapeutic window in man. *Eur J Clin Pharmacol* 1984;26:309–313.
68. Wing LMH, Reid JL, Davies DS, et al. Pharmacokinetic and concentration-effect relationships of clonidine in essential hypertension. *Eur J Clin Pharmacol* 1977;12:463–469.
69. Bravo EL. Effects of clonidine on sympathetic function. *Chest* 1983;83:369–371.
70. Langley MS, Heel RC. Transdermal clonidine: A preliminary review of its pharmaco-dynamic properties, and therapeutic efficacy. *Drugs* 1988;35:123–142.
71. Golub MS, Thananopavarn C, Eggena P, et al. Hormonal and hemodynamic effects of short- and long-term clonidine therapy in patients with mild-to-moderate hypertension. *Chest* 1983;83(2 suppl):377–379.
72. Wallin BG, Frisk-Holmberg M. The antihypertensive mechanism of clonidine in man: evidence against a generalized reduction of sympathetic nerve activity. *Hypertension* 1981;3:340–346.
73. Weber MA, Drayer JIM, Hubbell FA. Effects on the renin-angiotensin system of agents acting at central and peripheral adrenergic receptors. *Chest* 1983;83:374–377.
74. Mathias CJ, Wilkinson AH, Pike FA, et al. Clonidine in unilateral renal artery stenosis and unilateral renal parenchymal disease – similar antihypertensive but different renin suppressive effects. *J Hypertens* 1983;1(Suppl 2):123–125.
75. Sorkin EM, Heel RC. Guanfacine: A review of its pharmacodynamic and pharmacokinetic properties and therapeutic efficacy in the treatment of hypertension. *Drugs* 1986;31:301–336.
76. Mosqueda-Garcia R. Guanfacine: A second generation alpha$_2$ adrenergic blocker. *Am J Med Sci* 1990;299:73–76.
77. Holmes B, Brogden RN, Heel RC, et al. Guanabenz: A review of its pharmaco-dynamic properties and therapeutic efficacy in hypertension. *Drugs* 1983;26:212–229.
78. Dardonville C, Rozas I. Imidazoline binding sites and their ligands: an overview of the different chemical structures. *Med Res Revs* 2004;24:639–661.
79. Armah BI, Hofferber E, Stenzel W. General pharmacology of the novel centrally acting antihypertensive agent moxonidine. *Drug Research* 1988;38:1426–1434.
80. van Zwieten PA. Pharmacology of the alpha 2-adrenoceptor agonist rilmenidine. *Am J Cardiol* 1988;61(7):6D–14D.
81. Ernsberger P, Haxhiu MA. The I$_1$-imidazoline binding site is a functional receptor mediating vasodepression via the ventral medulla. *Am J Physiol* 1997;273:R1572–R1579.
82. Head GA, Burke SL, Chan CKS. Site and receptors involved in the sympathoinhibitory actions of rilmenidine. *J Hypertens* 1998;16(Suppl 3):S7–S12.
83. Cheung DG, Burris JF, Graettinger WF, et al. Clonidine. In: Messerli FH, ed. *Cardiovascular drug therapy, 2nd edn.* USA: WB Saunders Co.; 1996, pp. 622–628.
84. Karppanen H, Paakkari I, Paakkari P, et al. Possible involvement of central histamine H2-receptors in the hypotensive effect of clonidine. *Nature* 1976;259(5544):587–588.
85. De Sarro GB, Ascioti C, Froio F, et al. Evidence that locus coeruleus is the site where clonidine and drugs acting at α$_1$-and α2-adrenoceptors affect sleep and arousal mechanisms. *Br J Pharmacol* 1987;90:675–685.
86. Bricca G, Dontenwill M, Molines A, et al. Rilmenidine selectivity for imidazoline receptors in human brain. *Eur J Pharmacol* 1989;163:373–377.
87. Ernsberger P, Damon TH, Graff LM, et al. Moxonidine, a centrally acting antihypertensive agent, is a selective ligand for I$_1$-imidazoline sites. *J Pharm Exp Ther* 1993;264:172–182.
88. Gomez RE, Ernsberger P, Feinland G, et al. Rilmenidine lowers arterial pressure via imidazole receptors in brainstem C1 area. *Eur J Pharmacol* 1991;95:181–191.

89. Punnen S, Urbanski R, Krieger AJ, et al. Ventrolateral medullary pressor area: site of hypotensive action of clonidine. *Brain Res* 1987;422:336–346.
90. Chan CKS, Head GA. Relative importance of central imidazoline receptors for the antihypertensive effects of moxonidine and rilmenidine. *J Hypertens* 1996;14:855–864.
91. Parkin ML, Godwin SJ, Head GA. Importance of imidazoline-preferring receptors in the cardiovascular actions of chronically administered moxonidine, rilmenidine and clonidine in conscious rabbits. *J Hypertens* 2003;21(1):167–178.
92. Guyenet PG. Is the hypotensive effect of clonidine and related drugs due to imidazoline binding sites? *Am J Physiol* 1997;l 273:R1580–R1584.
93. Wenzel RR, Mitchell A, Siffert W, et al. The I_1-imidazoline agonist moxonidine decreases sympathetic tone under physical and mental stress. *Br J Clin Pharmacol* 2003;57:545–551.
94. Mitrovic V, Strasser R, Walenta R, et al. Haemodynamic and neurohormonal effects of a single oral dose of the imidazoline I_1 receptor agonist moxonidine in patients with idiopathic dilated cardiomyopathy and heart failure. *Eur J Clin Res* 1996;8:149–161.
95. Kirch H, Hutt H-J, Plänitz V. Pharmacodynamic action and pharmacokinetics of moxonidine after single oral administration in hypertensive patients. *J Clin Pharmacol* 1990;30:1088–1095.
96. Mitrovic V, Patyna WD, Hüting J, et al. Hemodynamic and neurohormonal effects of moxonidine in patients with essential hypertension. *Cardiovasc Drugs Ther* 1991;5:967–972.
97. Motz W, Scheler S, Möx B. The potential clinical application of moxonidine in congestive heart failure. *Rev Contemp Pharmacother* 1998;9:473–479.
98. Swedberg K, Bristow MR, Cohn JN, et al. Effects of sustained release moxonidine, an imidazoline agonist, on plasma norepinephrine in patients with chronic heart failure. *Circulation* 2002;105:1797–1803.
99. Wenzel RR, Spieker L, Qui S, et al. I1-imidazoline agonist moxonidine decreases sympathetic nerve activity and blood pressure in hypertensives. *Hypertension* 1998;32:1022–1027.
100. De Broe ME, Verpooten G, Thomas JR. Renal effects of oxaminozoline (S3341), on renal function (abstract). First International Symposium on Oxaminozoline. *Heidelberg* 1986.
101. Zech P, Pozet N. Effects of a new alpha-2 agonist, oxaminozoline (S3341), on renal function. First International Symposium on Oxaminozoline. *Heidelberg* 1986.
102. Prescott LF, Buhs RP, Beattie JO, et al. Combined clinical and metabolic study of the effects of alpha-methyldopa on hypertensive patients. *Circulation* 1966;34:308–321.
103. Au WYM, Dring LG, Grahame-Smith D, et al. The metabolism of ^{14}C-labelled α-methyldopa in normal and hypertensive human subjects. *Biochem J* 1972;9:1–10.
104. Kwan KC, Foltz EL, Breault GO, et al. Pharmacokinetics of methyldopa in man. *J Pharmacol Exp Ther* 1976;198:264–277.
105. Saavedra JA, Reid JL, Jordan W, et al. Plasma concentration of alpha methyldopa and sulphate conjugate after oral administration of methyldopa hydrochloride ethyl ester. *Eur J Clin Pharmacol* 1975;8:381–386.
106. Barnett AJ, Bobik A, Carson V, et al. Pharmacokinetics of methyldopa. Plasma levels following single intravenous, oral and multiple oral dosage in normotensive and hypertensive subjects. *Clin Exp Pharmacol Physiol* 1977;14:331–339.
107. Campbell NRC, Patrick W. Increases in methyldopa absorption and renal excretion after multiple doses. *J Clin Pharmacol 19*, 1992;32:450–454.
108. Myhre E, Rugstad HE, Hansen T. Clinical pharmacokinetics of methyldopa. *Clin Pharmacokinetics* 1982;7:221–233.
109. Porter CC, Titus DC. Distribution and metabolism of methyldopa in the rat. *J Pharmacol Exp Ther* 1963;139:77–87.
110. Campbell N, Paddock MD, Sundaram MD. Alteration of methyldopa absorption, metabolism, and blood pressure control caused by ferrous sulfate and ferrous gluconate. *Clin Pharmacol Ther* 1988;43:381–386.
111. Stenbaek O, Myhre E, Rugstad HE, et al. Pharmacokinetics of methyldopa in healthy man. *Eur J Clin Pharm* 1977;12:117–123.
112. Muscholl E, Maitre L. Release of sympathetic stimulation of α-methylnoradrenaline stored in the heart after administration of α-methyldopa. *Experientia* 1963;19:658–659.
113. Wright JM, Orozco-Gonzalez M, Polak G, et al. Duration of effect of single daily dose of methyldopa therapy. *Brit J Clin Pharmacol* 1982;13:847–884.
114. Muscholl E, Rahn KH. Über den Nachweis und die Bedeutung von α-Methylnoradrenalin im Harn von Hypertonikern bei Verabreichung von α-Methyldopa. *Pharmacol Clin* 1968; I:19–29.
115. Stott A, Robinson R, Smith P. Total metadrenaline excretion in patients treated with methyldopa. *Lancet* 1963;1:266–267.
116. Muscholl E, Rahn KH. Nachweis von α-Methylnoradrenalin in Harn von Hypertonikern während einer Behandlung mit α-Methyldopa. *Klin Wochenschr* 1966;44:1412–1413.

117. Buhs RP, Beck JL, Speth OC, et al. The metabolism of methyldopa in hypertensive human subjects. *J Pharmacol Ther* 1964;143:205–214.
118. Verbeeck RK, Branch RA, Wilkinson GR. Drug metabolites in renal failure: Pharmacokinetics and clinical implications. *Clin Pharmacokinetics* 1981;6:329–334.
119. Jones HMR, Cummings AJ, Setchell KDR, Lawson AM. A study of the disposition of α-methyldopa in newborn infants following its administration to the mother for the treatment of hypertension during pregnancy. *Br J Clin Pharmacol* 1979;8:433–440.
120. White WB, Andreoli JW, Cohn RD. Alpha-methyldopa disposition in mothers with hypertension and in their breast-fed infants. *Clin Pharmacol Ther* 1985;37:387–390.
121. Davies DS, Wing LMH, Reid JL, et al. Pharmacokinetics and concentration-effect relationship of intravenous and oral clonidine. *Clin Pharmacol Ther* 1977;21:593–601.
122. Arndts D, Doevendans J, Kirsten R, et al. New aspects of the pharmacokinetics and pharmacodynamics of clonidine in man. *Eur J Clin Pharmacol* 1983;24:21–30.
123. Frisk-Holmberg M, Paalzow L, Edlund PO. Clonidine kinetics in man – evidence of dose-dependency and changed pharmacokinetics during chronic therapy. *Br J Clin Pharmacol* 1981;12:653–658.
124. Hulter HN, Licht JH, Ilnicki LP, Singh S. Clinical efficacy and pharmacokinetics of clonidine in hemodialysis and renal insufficiency. *J Lab Clin Med* 1979;94:223–231.
125. Frisk-Holmberg M, Edlund PO, Paalzow L. Pharmacokinetics of clonidine and its relation to the hypotensive effect in patients. *Br J Pharmacol* 1978;6:227–232.
126. Anavekar SN, Jarrott B, Toscano M, et al. Pharmacokinetic and pharmacodynamic studies of oral clonidine in normotensive subjects. *Eur J Clin Pharmacol* 1982;23:1–5.
127. Dollery CT, Davies DS, Draffan GH, et al. Clinical pharmacology and pharmacokinetics of clonidine. *Clin Pharmacol Ther* 1976;19:11–17.
128. Lowenthal DT, Affrime MB, Meyer A, et al. Pharmacokinetics and pharmacodynamics of clonidine in varying states of renal function. *Chest* 1983;83(Suppl):386–390.
129. Darda S, Förster H-J, Stähle H. Metabolischer Abbau von Clonidin. *Arzneimittelforschung* 1978;28:255–259.
130. Hoefke W, Darda S, Gaida W. The influence of metabolic degradation on the blood pressure lowering effect of clonidine in rabbits after different routes of administration. *Arzneim Forsch* 1985;35:401.
131. Rehbinder D, Deckers W. Untersuchungen zur Pharmakokinetik und zum Metabolismus des 2-(2,6-Dichlorphenylamino)-2-imidazolin-hydrochlorid (St 155). *Arzneimittelforschung* 1969;19:169–176.
132. Arndts D, Arndts K. Pharmacokinetics and pharmacodynamics of transdermally administered clonidine. *Eur J Clin Pharmacol* 1984;26:79–85.
133. MacGregor TR, Matzek KM, Keirns JJ, et al. Pharmacokinetics of transdermally delivered clonidine. *Clin Pharmacol Ther* 1985;38:278–284.
134. Weimann HJ, Rudolph M. Clinical pharmacokinetics of moxonidine. *J Cardiovasc Pharmacol* 1992;20(Suppl 4):S37–S41.
135. Genissel P, Bromet N, Fourtillan JB, et al. Pharmacokinetics of rilmenidine in healthy subjects. *Am J Cardio* 1988;61:47D–53D.
136. Theodor R, Weimann H-J, Weber W, Michaelis K. Absolute bioavailability of moxonidine. *Eur J Drug Metab Pharmacokinet* 1991;16:153–159.
137. He MM, Abraham TL, Lindsay TJ, et al. Metabolism and disposition of the antihypertensive agent moxonidine in humans. *Drug Metab Disposition* 2003;31:334–342.
138. Theodor RA, Weimann H-J, Weber W, et al. Influence of food on the oral bioavailability of moxonidine. *Eur J Drug Metab Pharmacokinet* 1992;17:61–66.
139. Singlas E, Ehrhardt JD, Zech P, et al. Pharmacokinetics of rilmenidine. *Am J Cardiol* 1988;61:54D–59D.
140. Kirch H, Hutt H-J, Plänitz V. The influence of renal function on clinical pharmacokinetics of moxonidine. *Clin Pharmacokinet* 1988;15:245–253.
141. Aparicio M, Dratwa M, El Esper N, et al. Pharmacokinetics of rilmenidine in patients with chronic renal insufficiency and in hemodialysis patients. *Am J Cardiol* 1994;74:43A–50A.
142. Theodor RA, Weimann H-J, Müller M, et al. Age-related effects on the pharmacokinetics of moxonidine. *Eur J Clin Res* 1996;8:63–74.
143. Klink F. Clinical investigation of the passage of moxonidine from the maternal blood stream to the breast milk in patients with hypertension. *Beiersdorf AG Study* 1990 No. 200:029- 5895-2228-52.
144. Onesti G, Brest AN, Novack P, et al. Pharmacodynamic effects of α-methyldopa in hypertensive subjects. *Am Heart J* 1964;67:32–38.
145. Cohen A, Maxmen JS, Ragheb M, et al. Effects of alpha-methyldopa on the myocardial blood flow, utilizing the coincidence counting method. *J Clin Pharmacol* 1967;7:77–83.

146. Sannerstedt R, Varnauskas E, Werko L. Haemodynamic effects of methyldopa (Aldomet) at rest and during exercise in patients with arterial hypertension. *Acta Medica Scandinavika* 1962;171:75–82.

147. Dollery CT, Harrington M, Hodge JV. Haemodynamic studies with methyldopa: effect on cardiac output and response to pressor amines. *Br Heart J* 1963;25:670–676.

148. Safar ME, London BM, Levenson JA, et al. Effect of alpha-methyldopa on cardiac output in hypertension. *Clinical Pharmacology and Therapeutics* 1979;25:266–272.

149. Mancia G, Ferrari A, Gregorini L, et al. Methyldopa and neural control of circulation in essential hypertension. *Am J Cardiol* 1980;45(6):1237–1243.

150. Chamberlain DA, Howard J. Guanethidine and methyldopa: A haemodynamic study. *Br Heart J* 1964;26:528–536.

151. Mason DT, Braunwald L. Effects of guanethidine, reserpine, and methyldopa on reflex venous and arterial constriction in man. *J Clin Invest* 1964;43:1449–1463.

152. Lund-Johansen P. Haemodynamic changes in long term α-methyldopa therapy of essential hypertension. *Acta Medica Scandinavika* 1972;192:221.

153. Finnerty FA Jr, Davidov M, Mroczek WJ, Gavrilovich L. Influence of extracellular fluid volume on response to antihypertensive drugs. *Circ Res* 1970;27(1):71–82.

154. Prichard BNC, Johnston AW, Hill ID, Rosenheim ML. Bethanidine, guanethidine and methyldopa in treatment of hypertension: A within-patient comparison. *BMJ* 1968;1:135–144.

155. Oates JA, Seligmann AW, Clark MA, et al. The relative efficacy of guanethidine, methyldopa and pargyline as antihypertensive agents. *N Engl J Med* 1965;273:729–734.

156. Wilson WR, Fisher FD, Kirkendall WM. The acute hemodynamic effects of α-methyldopa in man. *J Chronic Dis* 1961;15:907–913.

157. Prichard BNC, Gillam PMS, Graham BR. Beta receptor antagonism in hypertension: Comparison with the effect of adrenergic neurone inhibition on cardiovascular responses. *Int J Clin Pharmacol* 1970;4:131.

158. Johnson P, Kitchin AH, Lowther CP, Turner RW. Treatment of hypertension with methyldopa. *BMJ* 1966;1:133–137.

159. Smirk H. Hypotensive action of methyldopa. *BMJ* 1963;1:146–151.

160. Lawson DH, Gloss D, Jick H. Adverse reactions to methyldopa with particular reference to hypotension. *Am Heart J* 1978;96:572–579.

161. Meyer JS, Sawada T, Kitamura A, et al. Cerebral blood flow after control of hypertension in stroke. *Neurology* 1968;18:772–781.

162. Mendlowitz M, Naftchi NE, Wolf RL, et al. The effects of guanethidine and of alpha methyldopa on the digital circulation in hypertension. *Am Heart J* 1965;69:731–739.

163. Onesti G, Schwartz AB, Kim KE, et al. Pharmacodynamic effects of a new antihypertensive drug, catapres (ST 155). *Circulation* 1969;39:219–228.

164. Brod J, Horbach L, Just H, et al. Acute effects of clonidine on central and peripheral haemodynamics and plasma renin activity. *Eur J Clin Pharmacol* 1972;4:107–114.

165. Muir AL, Burton JL, Lawrie DM. Circulatory effects at rest and exercise on clonidine; an imidazoline derivative with hypotensive properties. *Lancet* 1969;II:181–185.

166. Nayler WG, Price JM, Swann JB, et al. Effect of the hypotensive drug ST 155 (catapres) on the heart and peripheral circulation. *J Pharmacol Exp Ther* 1968;164:45–59.

167. Lund-Johansen P. Hemodynamic changes at rest and during exercise in long-term clonidine therapy of essential hypertension. *Acta Med Scand* 1974;195:111–115.

168. Tuckman J, Shillingford JP. The effect of different degrees of tilt on cardiac output, heart rate and blood pressure in normal man. *Br Heart J* 1966;28:32–39.

169. Mitchell A, Bührmann S, Opazo S, et al. Clonidine lowers blood pressure by reducing vascular resistance and cardiac output in young, healthy males. *Cardiovasc Drugs Ther* 2005;19:49–55.

170. MacDougall AI, Addis GJ, Mackay N, et al. Treatment of hypertension with clonidine. *BMJ* 1970;III:440–442.

171. Raftos J, Bauer GE, Lewis RG, et al. Clonidine in the treatment of severe hypertension; trial carried out in, 1968–1972. *Med J Australia* 1973;1:786–793.

172. MacPhee GJA, Howier CA, Elliott HL, et al. A comparison of the haemodynamic and behavioural effects of moxonidine and clonidine in normotensive subjects. *Br J Clin Pharmaco* 1992;33:261–267.

173. Hüting J, Mitrovic V, Bahavar H, et al. Vergleich der Wirkungen von Moxonidin und Nifedipin auf die linksventrikuläre Funktion bei Monotherapie der essentiellen Hypertonie. *Herz Kreislauf* 1992;24:132–137.

174. Klepzig H, Spingler A, Hör G, et al. Akuter und chronischer einfluss von Moxonidin auf Blutdruck und linksventriculäre. Function in Ruhe und unter Belastung. In: Hayduk K, Stumpe CO, eds. *Ein neues Therapieprinzip zur Behandlung der Hypertonie.* Stuttgart: Schattauer; 1992:23–30.

175. Mitrovic V, Patyna WD, Yahya H, et al. Einfluss des Imidazol-rezeptoragonisten Moxonidin auf die zentrale und periphere Hämodynamik bei patienten mit essentieller Hypertonie. Interlaken. *Joint Meeting Swiss and German Society of Cardiology* 1994.

176. Martina B, Surber C, Jakobi C, et al. Effect of moxonidine and cilazapril on microcirculation as assessed by finger nailfold capillaroscopy in mild-to-moderate hypertension. *Angiology* 1998;49:897–901.

177. Dollery CT, Davies DS, Duchier J, et al. Dose and concentration-effect relations for rilmenidine. *Am J Cardio* 1988;l 61:60D–66D.

178. Zannad F, Aliot E, Florentin J, et al. Hemodynamic and electrophysiologic effects of a new alpha$_2$-adrenoceptor agonist, rilmenidine, for systemic hypertension. *Am J Cardiol* 1988;61:67D–71D.

179. N'Guyen van Cao AN, Levy B, Slama R. Noninvasive study of cardiac structure and function after rilmenidine for essential hypertension. *Am J Cardiol* 1988;61:72D–75D.

180. McKaigue JP, Harron DWG. The effects of rilmenidine on tests of autonomic function in humans. *Clin Pharmacol Ther* 1992;52:511–517.

181. Galley P, Manciet G, Hessel JL, et al. Antihypertensive efficacy and acceptability of rilmenidine in elderly hypertensive patients. *Am J Cardiol* 1988;61:86D–90D.

182. Panfilov V, Morris AD, Donnelly R, et al. Comparative effects of rilmenidine and atenolol on tests of autonomic function and mental and dynamic exercise in patients with essential hypertension. *J Cardiovasc Pharmacol* 1995;26(Suppl 2):S44–S47.

183. Fillastre J-P, Letac B, Galinier F, et al. A multicenter double-blind comparative study of rilmenidine and clonidine in 333 hypertensive patients. *Am J Cardiol* 1988;l 61:81D–85D.

184. Ostermann G, Brisgand B, Schmitt J, et al. Efficacy and acceptability of rilmenidine for mild to moderate systemic hypertension. *Am J Cardiol* 1988;61:76D–80D.

185. Licata G, Scaglione R, Guillet C, et al. Double-blind controlled study of rilmenidine versus hydrochlorothiazide in mild hypertension: clinical and renal haemodynamic evaluation. *J Human Hypertens* 1993;7:153–157.

186. Velasco M, Soltero I, Sukerman M, et al. Double-blind, randomised study of the efficacy, tolerance and rebound effects of the antihypertensive drug rilmenidine: comparative evaluation with clonidine. *Curr Ther Res* 1993;54:202–207.

187. Eryonucu B, Ulgen MS, Bilge M, et al. The chronic effect of rilmenidine on heart rate variability in patients with mild hypertension. *Angiology* 2002;53:199–204.

188. Fernandez PG, Snedden W, Kim BK, Lee CC. A novel therapeutic approach for reversal of left ventricular hypertrophy and blood pressure control in hypertensive patients treated with alpha-methyldopa or propranolol. *Can J Physiol Pharmacol* 1985;63:304–308.

189. Feldstein CA, Olivieri AO, Porto Sabaris R. Comparison between the effects of urapidil and methyldopa on left ventricular hypertrophy and haemodynamics in humans. *Drugs* 1988;35 (Suppl 6):90–97.

190. Timio M, Venanzi S, Gentili M, et al. Reversal of left ventricular hypertrophy after one-year treatment with clonidine: relationship between echocardiographic findings, blood pressure, and urinary catecholamines. *J Cardiovasc Pharmacol* 1987;10(Suppl 12):S142–S146.

191. Tan SA, Berk LS, Tan LG. Indapamide regresses, but transdermal clonidine does not regress, left ventricular hypertrophy in hypertensive diabetic patients. *Am J Cardiol* 1996;77:20B–22B.

192. Kleine P, Meissner E, von Bruchhausen V, Brückner S. Effects of clonidine and nifedipine on left ventricular hypertrophy and muscle mass in hypertensive patients. *J Cardiovasc Pharmacol* 1987;10(suppl 12):S180–S186.

193. Gottdiener JS, Reda DJ, Massie BM, et al. Effect of single-drug therapy on reduction of left ventricular mass in mild to moderate hypertension. *Circulation* 1997;95:2007–2014.

194. Eichstädt H, Richter W, Bäder W, et al. Demonstration of hypertrophy regression with magnetic resonance tomography under the new adrenergic inhibitor moxonidine. *Cardiovasc Drugs Ther* 1989;3(Suppl 2):583–587.

195. Haczynski J, Spring A, Przewlocka-Kosmala M, Flasinski J. Effect of moxonidine on left ventricular hypertrophy in hypertensive patients. *J Clin Basic Cardiol* 2001;4:61–65.

196. Trimarco B, Rosiello G, Sarno D, et al. Effects of one-year treatment with rilmenidine on systemic hypertension-induced left ventricular hypertrophy in hypertensive patients. *Am J Cardiol* 1994;74:36A–42A.

197. Farsang C, Lengyel M, Borbás S, et al. VERITAS investigators. Value of rilmenidine therapy and its combination with perindopril on blood pressure and left ventricular hypertrophy in patients with essential hypertension (VERITAS). *Curr Med Res Opin* 2003;19:205–217.

198. Sadowski Z, Szwed H, Koch-Wocial H, et al. Regression of left ventricular hypertrophy in hypertensive patients after 1 year of treatment with rilmenidine: a double-blind, randomised, controlled (versus nifedipine) study. *J Hypertens* 1998;16(Suppl 3):S55–S62.

199. Koldas L, Ayan F, Ikitimur B. Short-term effects of rilmenidine on left ventricular hypertrophy and systolic and diastolic function in patients with essential hypertension: comparison with an angiotensin converting enzyme inhibitor and a calcium antagonist. *Jpn Heart J* 2003;44:693–704.

200. Motz W, Vogt M, Scheler S, Strauer BE. Hypertensive coronary microcirculation – effects of the imidazoline-receptor-agonist moxonidine. *Cardiovasc Risk Factors* 1995; 5(Suppl 1):28–32.

201. Adler S. Methyldopa-induced decrease in mental activity. *JAMA* 1974;230:1428–1429.

202. Dollery CT, Harrington M. Methyldopa in hypertension – clinical and pharmacological studies. *Lancet* 1962;1:759–763.

203. Hamilton M, Kopelman H. Treatment of severe hypertension with methyldopa. *BMJ* 1963;1:151.

204. Johnson B, Hoch K, Errichetti A, Johnson J. Effects of methyldopa on psychometric performance. *J Clin Pharmacol* 1990;30:1102–1105.

205. Muldoon MF, Waldstein SR, Ryan CM, et al. Effects of six antihypertensive medications on cognitive performance. *J Hypertens* 2002;20:1643–1652.

206. Newman RJ, Salerno HR. Letter: Sexual dysfunction due to methyldopa. *BMJ* 1974;4:106.

207. Steiner J, Cassar J, Mashiter K, et al. Effects of methyldopa on prolactin and growth hormone. *BMJ* 1976;1:1186–1188.

208. Pettinger WA, Horwitz D, Sjoersdma A. Lactation due to methyldopa. *BMJ* 1963;1:1460.

209. Vaidya RA, Vaidya AB, Van Woert MH, Kase NG. Galactorrhoea and Parkinson-like syndrome: an adverse effect of α-methyldopa. *Metabolism* 1970;19:1068–1070.

210. Groden BM. Parkinsonism occurring with methyldopa treatment. *BMJ* 1963;1:1001.

211. Peaston MJT. Parkinsonism associated with alpha-methyldopa therapy. *BMJ* 1964;2:168.

212. Davidov M, Kakaviatos N, Finnerty FA Jr. The antihypertensive effects of an imidazoline compound. *Clin Pharmacol Ther* 1967;8:810–816.

213. Gifford RW Jnr. Clonidine in the management of mild hypertension in twenty-two patients. *Cleveland Clin Q* 1969;36:173–182.

214. Amery A, Verstraete M, Bossaert H, Verstreken G. Hypotensive action and side effects of clonidine - chlorthalidone and methyldopa - chlorthalidone in treatment of hypertension. *BMJ* 1970;IV:392–395.

215. Onesti G, Bock KD, Heimsoth V, et al. Clonidine, a new antihypertensive agent. *Am J Cardiol* 1971;28:74–83.

216. Onesti G, Schwartz AB, Kim KE, et al. Antihypertensive effect of clonidine. *Circ Res* 1971;28 (Suppl 2):53–69.

217. Mroczek WJ, Davidov M, Finnerty FA. Prolonged treatment with clonidine: comparative antihypertensive effects alone and with a diuretic agent. *Am J Cardiol* 1972;30:536–541.

218. Smet G, Hoobler SW, Sanbar S, et al. Clinical observations on a new antihypertensive drug 2-(2,6-dichlorphenylamine)-2-imidazoline hydrochloride. *Am Heart J* 1969;77:473–478.

219. Hoobler SW, Sagastume E. Clonidine hydrochloride in the treatment of hypertension. *Am J Cardiol* 1971;28:67–73.

220. Denolle T, Sassano HA, Allain H, et al. Effects of nicardapine and clonidine on cognitive functions and electroencephalography in hypertensive patients. *Fund Clin Pharmacol* 2002;16:527–535.

221. Roberge RJ, Kimball ET, Rossi J, Warren J. Clonidine and sleep apnea syndrome interaction: antagonism with yohimbine. *J Emerg Med* 1998;16:727–730.

222. Grahnen A, Wiemann H-J, Wesnes K, et al. Acute cognitive effects following addition of single doses of lorazepam to moxonidine/placebo maintenance treatment. *J Hypertens* 1996;14(Suppl 1):S228.

223. Schmidt U, Frerick H, Kraft K, et al. Hypertension: a possible risk in road traffic. *J Cardiovasc Pharmacol* 1992;20(Suppl 4):S50–S56.

224. Kemme MJB, Post JP, Schoemaker C, et al. Central nervous system effects of moxonidine experimental sustained release formulation in patients with mild to moderate essential hypertension. *J Clin Pharmacol* 2003;55:518–525.

225. Sides GD, Leschinger MI, Walenta R, McNay JL Jnr. The tolerability and adverse event profile of moxonidine. *Rev Contemp Pharmacother* 1998;9:491–499.

226. Schachter M, Luszick J, Jager B, et al. Safety and tolerability of moxonidine in the treatment of hypertension. *Drug Safety* 1998;19:191–203.

227. Schwartz VW, Kandziora J. Langzeiterfahrungen mit Moxonidin, einem neuen Antihypertensivum. *Fortschrite der Medizin* 1990;108:64–70.

228. Mahieux F. Rilmenidine and vigilance. Review of clinical studies. *Am J Med* 1989;87(3C): 67S–72S.

229. Weerasuriya K, Shaw E, Turner P. Preliminary clinical pharmacological studies of S3341, a new hypotensive agent, and comparison with clonidine in normal males. *Eur J Clin Pharmacol* 1984;27:281–286.

230. Harron DWG, Hasson B, Regan M, et al. Effects of rilmenidine and clonidine on the electroencephalogram, saccadic eye movements and psychomotor function. *J Cardiovasc Pharmacol* 1995;26:S48–S54.

231. Morin Y, Turmel L, Fortier J. Methyldopa. Clinical studies in arterial hypertension. *Am J Med Sci* 1989;248:633, 19647-19660.

232. Mohammed S, Hanenson IB, Magenheim HG, Gaffney TE. The effects of alpha-methyldopa on renal function in hypertensive patients. *Am Heart J* 1968;76:21–27.

233. Houston MC. Clonidine hydrochloride. *Southern Med J* 1982;75:713–721.

234. Fliser D, Wiecek A, Ritz E. Renal hemodynamics. *Cardiovascular Risk Factors* 1995;5(Suppl 1): S40–S44.

235. Leary WP. Renal excretory actions of antihypertensive agents. Effects of rilmenidine. *Am J Med* 1989;87(Suppl 3C):63S–66S.

236. Vonend O, Marsalek P, Russ H, et al. Moxonidine treatment of hypertensive patients with advanced renal failure. *J Hypertens* 2003;21:1709–1717.

237. Pillion H, Fevrier B, Codis P, et al. Long term control of blood pressure by rilmenidine in high-risk populations. *Am J Cardiol* 1994;74:58A–65A.

238. Lins RL, Daelemans R, Dratwa M, et al. Acceptability of rilmenidine and long-term surveillance of plasma concentrations in hypertensive patients with renal insufficiency. *Am J Med* 1989;87(Suppl 3C):41S–45S.

239. Xuan ATD, Lockhart A. Bronchial effects of alpha$_2$-adrenoceptor agonists and of other antihypertensive agents in asthma. *Am J Med* 1989;87(Suppl 3C):34S–37S.

240. Foxworth JW, Reisz GR, Pyszcynski DR, Knudson SM. Oral clonidine in patients with asthma: no significant effect on airway reactivity. *Eur J Clin Pharmacol* 1995;48: 19–22.

241. Lindgren BR, Grundstrom N, Andersson RG. Comparison of the effects of clonidine and guanfacine on the histamine liberation from human mast cells and basophils and on the human bronchial smooth muscle activity. *Arzneimittelforschung* 1987;37:551–553.

242. Bailey PL, Sperry RJ, Johnson GK, et al. Respiratory effects of clonidine alone, and combined with morphine, in humans. *Anesthesiology* 1991;74(1):43–48.

243. Wilkens H, Wilkens H, Hecht M, et al. *Effect of moxonidine, an alpha$_2$ adrenergic agonist, on histamine-induced bronchial constriction and ventilatory and occlusion responses to carbon dioxide in asthmatics.* Joint Meeting of the Societas Europaea Physiologiae Clinicae Respiratorine (SEP-SEPCR), London, September 9–14, 1990.

244. Feuring M, Cassel W, Thun B, et al. *Moxonidine in patients with arterial hypertension and chronic obstructive pulmonary disease.* 1999, Unpublished observations.

245. Peterkin GA, Khan SA. Iatrogenic skin disease. *Practitioner* 1969;202(207):117–126.

246. Church R. Eczema provoked by methyl dopa. *Br J Dermatol* 1974;91:373–378.

247. Stevenson CJ. Lichenoid eruptions due to methyldopa. *Br J Dermatol* 1971;85:600.

248. Burry JN, Kirk J. Lichenoid drug reaction from methyldopa. *Br J Dermatol* 1974;91:475–476.

249. Holt PJ, Navaratnam A. Lichenoid eruption due to methyldopa. *BMJ* 1974;3:234.

250. Burry JN. Ulcerative lichenoid eruption from methyldopa. *Arch Dermatol* 1976;112:880 (case report).

251. Hay KD, Reade PC. Methyldopa as a cause of oral mucous membrane reactions. *Br Dent J* 1978;145:195–203.

252. Price EJ, Venables PJW. Drug-induced lupus. *Drug Safety* 1995;12:283–290.

253. Shneerson JM, Gazzard BG. Reversible malabsorption caused by methyldopa. *BMJ* 1977;2:1456.

254. Bonkowsky HL, Brisbane J. Colitis and hepatitis caused by methyldopa. *Med J Australia* 1976;2:1602–1603.

255. Liu ZX, Kaplowitz N. Immune-mediated drug-induced liver disease. *Clin Liver Dis* 2002;6:755–774.

256. Elkington SG, Schreiber WM, Conn HO. Hepatic injury caused by 1-alpha-methyldopa. *Circulation* 1969;40:589–595.

257. Cacace LG, Cohen M. Alpha-methyldopa (Aldomet) hepatitis. A report of six cases and review of the literature. *Drug Intelligence* 1976;10:144–152.

258. Toghill PJ, Smith PG, Benton P, et al. Methyldopa liver damage. *BMJ* 1974;3:545–548.

259. Thomas E, Rosenthal WS, Zapiach L, et al. Spectrum of methyldopa liver injury. *Am J Gastroenterol* 1977;68:125–133.

260. Sotaniemi EA, Hokkanen OT, Ahokas JT, Ahlqvist J. Hepatic injury and drug metabolism in patients with alpha-methyldopa-induced liver damage. *Eur J Clin Pharmacol* 1977;12: 429–435.

261. Goldstein GB, Lam KC, Mistilis SP. Drug-induced active chronic hepatitis. *Digestive Dis* 1973;18:177–184.

262. Thomas LA, Cardwell MS. Acute reactive hepatitis in pregnancy induced by alpha-methyldopa. *Obstet Gynecol* 1997;90:658–659.

263. Schweitzer IL, Peters RL. Acute submassive hepatic necrosis due to methyldopa. *Gastroenterol* 1974;66:1203–1211.
264. Rodman JS, Deutsch DJ, Gutman SL. Methyldopa hepatitis. A report of six cases and review of the literature. *Am J Med* 1976;60:941–948.
265. Hoyumpa AM, Connell AM. Methyldopa hepatitis. *Digestive Dis* 1973;18:213–222.
266. Rehman OU, Keith TA, Gall EA. Methyldopa-induced submassive hepatic necrosis. *J Am Med Assoc* 1973;224:1390–1392.
267. Maddrey WC, Boitnott JK. Severe hepatitis from methyldopa. *Gastroenterol* 1975;68:351–360.
268. Furhoff AK. Adverse reactions with methyldopa – a decade's reports. *Acta Medica Scandinavika* 1978;203:425–428.
269. Arranto AJ, Sotaniemi EA. Morphologic alterations in patients with alpha-methyldopa-induced liver damage after short-and-long-term exposure. Scand J Gastrolenterol 16:853–863.
270. Hoffbrand BI, Fry W, Bunton GL. Cholestatic jaundice due to methyldopa. *BMJ* 1974;3:559.
271. Moses A, Zahger D, Amir G. Cholestatic liver injury after prolonged exposure to methyldopa. *Digestion* 1989;42:57.
272. Valnes K, Hillestad L, Hansen T, Arnold E. Alpha-methyldopa and drug fever. A study of the metabolism of alpha-methyldopa in patients and normal subjects. *Acta Med Scand* 1978;204(1–2):21–25.
273. Weber MA, Case DB, Baer L, et al. Renin and aldosterone suppression in the antihypertesive action of clonidine. *Am J Cardiol* 1976;38:825–830.
274. Niarchos AP, Baer L, Radichevich I. Role of renin and aldosterone suppression in the antihypertensive mechanism of clonidine. *Am J Med* 1978;65:614–618.
275. Brass EP. Effects of antihypertensive drugs on endocrine function. *Drugs* 1984;27:447–458.
276. Grossman A, Weerasuriya K, Al-Damlugi S, et al. Alpha 2-adrenoceptor agonists stimulate growth hormone secretion but have not acute effects on plasma cortisol under basal conditions. *Horm Res* 1987;25:65–71.
277. Falkner B, Onesti G, Moshang Jr. T, Lowenthal DT. Growth hormone release in hypertensive adolescents treated with clonidine. *J Clin Pharmacol* 1981;21:31–36.
278. Mill G, Gödde-Salz E, Heidemann HT, et al. Effects of a new alpha$_2$-adrenergic agonist moxonidine on anterior pituitary hormone secretion in comparison to clonidine and GHRH. *Acta Endocrinol* 1989;120(Suppl 1):80–84.
279. Kuhn JM, Wolf LM. The effects of oxaminozoline (S3341), on the hypothalamo-pituitary axis in the healthy subject. *First International Symposium on Oxaminozoline*, 1986, Heidelberg.
280. Herman VS, Joffe BI, Kalk WJ, et al. Clinical and biochemical responses to nadolol and clonidine in hyperthyroidism. *J Clin Pharmacol* 1989;29:1117–1120.
281. UKWP. UK Working Party on Rilmendine. Rilmenidine in mild to moderate essential hypertension. A double-blind, randomised, parallel-group, multicenter comparison with methyldopa in 157 patients. *Curr Ther Res* 1990;47:194–211.
282. Balkau B. Epidemiology of the metabolic syndrome and the RISC study. *Eur Heart J* 2005; 7(Suppl D):D6–D9.
283. Eckel RH, Grundy SM. The metabolic syndrome. *Lancet* 2005;365:1415–1428.
284. Standl E. Aetiology and consequences of the metabolic syndrome. *Eur Heart J* 2005;7(Suppl D):D10–D13.
285. Esler M, Rumantir M, Wiesner G, et al. Sympathetic nervous system and insulin resistance: from obesity to diabetes. *Am J Hypertens* 2001;14:304S–309S.
286. McCarty MF. Elevated sympathetic activity may promote insulin resistance syndrome by activating alpha-1 adrenergic receptors on adipocytes. *Medical Hypotheses* 2004;62:830–838.
287. Rosen P, Ohly P, Gleichmann H. Experimental benefit of moxonidine on glucose metabolism and insulin secretion in the fructose-fed rat. *J Hypertens* 1997;15(Suppl 1): S31–S38.
288. Pénicaud L, Berthault MF, Morin J, et al. Rilmenidine normalizes fructose-induced insulin resistance and hypertension in rats. *J Hypertens* 1998;16(Suppl 3):S45–S49.
289. Velliquette RA, Ernsberger P. Contrasting metabolic effects of antihypertensive agents. *J Pharmacol Exp Ther* 2003;307:1104–1111.
290. Giugliano D, Acampora R, Marfella R, et al. Hemodynamic and metabolic dependent diabetes mellitus. *Am J Hypertens* 1998;11:184–189.
291. Kaan EC, Brückner R, Frohly P, et al. Effects of agmantine and moxonidine on glucose metabolism: an integrated approach towards pathophysiological mechanisms in cardiovascular metabolic disorders. *Cardiovasc Risk Factors* 1995;5(Suppl 1):19–27.
292. Haenni A, Lithell H. Moxonidine improves insulin sensitivity in insulin resistant hypertensives. *J Hypertens* 1999;17(suppl 3):S29–S35.
293. Anichkov DA, Shostak NA, Schastnaya OV. Comparison of rilmenidine and lisinopril on ambulatory blood pressure and plasma lipid and glucose levels in hypertensive women with metabolic syndrome. *Curr Med Res Op* 2005;21:113–119.

294. Jacob S, Klimm H-J, Rett K, et al. Effects of moxonidine vs. metoprolol on blood pressure and metabolic control in hypertensive subjects with type 2 diabetes. *Exp Clin Endocrinol Diabetes* 2004;112:315–322.

295. Sanjuliani AF, Genelhu de Abreu V, Ueleres Braga J, et al. Effects of moxonidine on the sympathetic nervous system, blood pressure, plasma renin activity, plasma aldosterone, leptin, and metabolic profile in obese hypertensive patients. *J Clin Basic Cardiol* 2004;7:19–25.

296. De Luca N, Izzo R, Fontana D, et al. Haemodynamic and metabolic effects of rilmenidine in hypertensive patients with metabolic syndrome X. A double-blind parallel study versus amlodipine. *J Hypertens* 2000;18:1515–1522.

297. Bauduceau B, Mayaudon H, Dupuy O. Rilmendine in the hypertensive type-2 diabetic: a controlled pilot study versus captopril. *J Cardiovasc Risk* 2000;7:57–61.

298. Carstairs KC, Breckenridge A, Dollery CT, et al. Incidence of a positive direct Coombs Test in patients on α-methyldopa. *Lancet* 1966;2:133–135.

299. Lobuglio AF, Jandl JH. The nature of alpha-methyldopa red-cell antibody. *N Engl J Med* 1967;276:658–665.

300. Masouredis SP, Sudora E. Ultra-structural mapping of methyldopa and anti-D IgG erythrocyte antigen receptors. *J Clin Invest* 1975;55:771–782.

301. Murphy WG, Kelton JG. Methyldopa-induced autoantibodies against red blood cells. *Blood Rev* 1988;2(1):36–42.

302. Worlledge SM, Carstairs KC, Dacie JV. Autoimmune haemolytic anaemia associated with α-methyldopa therapy. *Lance* 1966;2:135–139.

303. Clark KG. Case history: haemolysis and agranulocytosis complicating treatment with methyldopa (case report). *BMJ* 1967;4:94.

304. Benraad AH, Schoenaker AH. Thrombopenia after use of methyldopa. *Lance* 1965;2:292.

305. Marcus GJ, Stevenson M, Brown T. Alpha-methyldopa induced immune thrombocytopenia. *Am J Clin Pathol* 1975;64:113–115.

306. van der Klauw MM, Wilson JH, Stricker BH. Drug-associated agranulocytosis. *20 years of reporting in the Netherlands (1974–1994).* 1998;57:206–211.

307. Breckenridge A, Dollery CT, Worlledge SM, et al. Positive direct Coombs' Tests and antinuclear factor in patients treated with methyldopa. *Lancet* 1967;2:1265–1268.

308. Pinthong D, Songsermsakul P, Rattanachamnong P, Kendall DA. The effects of imidazoline agents on the aggregation of human platelets. *J Pharm Pharmacol* 2004;56(2):213–220.

309. Leren P. Lipid effects of antihypertensive drugs. *Clin Exp Hypertens A* 1990;12:761–768.

310. Leon AS, Agre J, McNally C, et al. Blood lipid effects of antihypertensive therapy: a double-blind comparison of the effects of methyldopa and propranolol. *J Clin Pharmacol* 1984;24:209–217.

311. Dujovne CA, DeCoursey S, Krehbiel P, et al. Serum lipids in normo- and hyperlipidemics after methyldopa and propranolol. *Clin Pharmacol Ther* 1984;36:157–162.

312. Houston MC, Burger C, Taylor Hays J, et al. The effects of clonidine hydrochloride versus atenolol monotherapy on serum lipids, lipid subfractions, and apolipoproteins in mild hypertension. *Am Heart J* 1990;120:172.

313. Lakshman MR, Reda DJ, Materson BJ, et al. Diuretics and beta-blockers do not have adverse effects at 1 year on plasma lipid and lipoprotein profiles in men with hypertension. Department of Veteran Affairs Cooperative Study Group on Antihypertensive Agents. *Arch Intern Med* 1999;159:541–542.

314. Löw-Kröger A, Rosenthal J. Antihypertensive Therapie mit moxonidine: Bestätigung des imidazolinrezeptoragonisten in der breiten anwendug. *Herz/Kreisl* 1994;26:206–211.

315. Elisaf MS, Petris C, Bairaktari E, et al. The effect of moxonidine on plasma lipid profile and on LDL subclass distribution. *J Human Hypertens* 1999;13:781–785.

316. Lumb PJ, McMahon Z, Chik Z, Wierzbicki AS. Effect of moxonidine on lipid subfractions in patients with hypertension. *Int J Clin Pract* 2004;58:465–468.

317. Scemama M, Février B, Beucler I, Dairou F. Lipid profile and antihypertensive efficacy in hyperlipidemic hypertensive patients: comparison of rilmenidine and captopril. *J Cardiovasc Pharmacol* 1995;26(Suppl 2):S34–S39.

318. Levine RJ, Strauch BS. Hypertensive responses to methyldopa. *N Engl J Med* 1966;275:946–948.

319. Burden AC, Alexander CP. Rebound hypertension after acute methyldopa withdrawal. *BMJ* 1976;1(6017):1056–1057.

320. Frewin DB, Penhall RK. Rebound hypertension after sudden discontinuation of methyldopa therapy. *Med J Aust* 1977;1:659.

321. Hunyor SN, Hansson L, Harrison TS, Hoobler SW. Effects of clonidine withdrawal: possible mechanisms and suggestions for management. *BMJ* 1973;II:209–211.

322. Sarlis NJ, Caticha O, Anderson JL, et al. Hyperadrenergic state following acute withdrawal from clonidine used at supratherapeutic doses. *Clin Auton Res* 1996;6(2):115–117.

323. Geyskes GG, Boer P, Dorhout Mees EJ. Clonidine withdrawal: mechanism and frequency of rebound hypertension. *Br J Clin Pharmacol* 1979;7:55–62.

324. Brown JJ, Agabiti Rosei E, Lever AF, et al. Emergency treatment of hypertension crisis following clonidine withdrawal (letter). *BMJ* 1976;I:1147.

325. Goldberg AD, Raftery EB, Wilkinson PR. The over-shoot phenomenon on withdrawal of clonidine therapy. *Postgrad Med J* 1976;52(Suppl 7):128–134.

326. Tuckman J. Unpublished, cited by 57.

327. Bailey RR, Neale TJ. Rapid clonidine withdrawal with blood pressure overshoot exaggerated by beta-blockade. *BMJ* 1976;1:9.

328. Mroczek WJ, Leibel BA, Finnerty Jr. FA. Comparison of clonidine and methyldopa in hypertensive patients receiving a diuretic. A double-blind crossover study. *Am J Cardiol* 1972;29:712–717.

329. Whitsett TL, Chrysant SG, Dillard BL, Anton AH. Abrupt cessation of clonidine administration: a prospective study. *Am J Cardiol* 1978;41:1285–1290.

330. Strauss FG, Franklin SS, Lewin AJ, et al. Withdrawal of antihypertensive therapy: hypertensive crisis in renovascular hypertension. *JAMA* 1977;238:1734–1736.

331. Nakagawa S, Yamamoto Y, Koiwaya Y. Ventricular tachycardia induced by clonidine withdrawal. *Br Heart J* 1985;53:654–658.

332. Simic J, Kishineff S, Goldberg R, Gifford W. Acute myocardial infarction as a complication of clonidine withdrawal. *J Emerg Med* 2003;25:399–402, Erratum 2004;26:491.

333. Hopkirk JAC, Simpson NB, Fitzgerald WR. Vomiting with clonidine withdrawal. *BMJ* 1975; III:435.

334. Plänitz V. Crossover comparison of moxonidine and clonidine in mild to moderate hypertension. *Eur J Clin Pharmacol* 1984;27:147–152.

335. Webster J, Koch HF. Aspects of tolerability of centrally acting antihypertensive drugs. *J Cardiovasc Pharmacol* 1996;26(Suppl 3):S49–S54.

336. Zarafis J, Lip GY, Ferner RE. Poisoning with antihypertensive drugs: methyldopa and clonidine. *J Hum Hypertens* 1995;9:787–790.

337. Seger DL. Clonidine toxicity revisited. *Clin Toxicol* 2002;40:145–155.

338. Bant W. Methyldopa and depression (letter). *BMJ* 1973;4:553.

339. Engelman K. Side-effects of sympatholytic antihypertensive drugs. *Hypertension* 1988;11 (Suppl II):II30–II33.

340. Klein-Schwartz W. Trends and toxic effect 1978s from pediatric clonidine exposures. *Arch Pediatr Adolesc Med* 2002;156:392–396.

341. Elliott HL, McLean K, Sumner DJ, Reid JL. Absence of an effect of mianserin on the actions of clonidine or methyldopa in hypertensive patients. *Eur J Clin Pharmacol* 1983;24:15–19.

342. Byrd GJ. Lithium carbonate and methyldopa: apparent interaction in man. *Clin Toxicol* 1977;11:1–4.

343. Markowitz JS, Wells BG, Carson WH. Interactions between antipsychotic and antihypertensive drugs. *Ann Pharmacother* 1995;29:603–609.

344. Leslie K, Mooney PH, Silbert BS. Effect of intravenous clonidine on the dose of thiopental required to induce anesthesia. *Anesth Analg* 1992;75:530–535.

345. Ghignone M, Quintin L, Duke PC, et al. Effects of clonidine on narcotic requirements and hemodynamic response during induction of fentanyl anesthesia and endotracheal intubation. *Anesthesiol* 1986;64:36–42.

346. Guglielminotti J, Descraques C, Petitmaire S, et al. Effects of premedication on dose requirements for propofol: comparison of clonidine and hydroxyzine. *Br J Anaesth* 1998;80:733–736.

347. Gordon NC, Heller PH, Levine JD. Enhancement of pentazocine analgesia by clonidine. *Pain* 1992;48:167–169.

348. Quintin L, Bouillac X, Butin E, et al. Clonidine for major vascular surgery in hypertensive patients: a double-blind, controlled, randomised study. *Anesth Analg* 1996;83:687–695.

349. Laisalmi M, Koivusalo AM, Valta P, et al. Clonidine provides opioid-sparing effect, stable hemodynamics, and renal integrity during laparoscopic cholecystectomy. *Surg Endosc* 2001;15:1331–1335.

350. Taittonen MT, Kirvela OA, Aantaa R, Kanto JH. The effect of clonidine or midazolam premedication on perioperative responses during ketamine anesthesia. *Anesth Analg* 1998;87:161–167.

351. Daniel M, Larson MD, Eger EI, et al. Fentanyl, clonidine and repeated increases in desflurane concentration, but not nitrous oxide or esmolol, block the transient mydriasis caused by rapid increases in desflurane concentration. *Anesth Analg* 1995;81: 372–378.

352. Briant RH, Reid JL, Dollery CT. Interaction between clonidine and desipramine in man. *BMJ* 1973;1:522–523.

353. Jaffe R, Livshits T, Bursztyn M. Adverse interaction between clonidine and verapamil. *Ann Pharmacother* 1994;28(7):881–883.

354. Oates JA, Gillespie L, Udenfriend S, Sjoerdsma A. Decarboxylase inhibition and blood pressure reduction by alpha-methyl-3,-4,-dihydroxy-DL-phenylanine. *Science* 1960;131:1890–1891.

355. Prichard BNC, Boakes AJ, Graham BR. A within patient comparison of bethanidine, methyldopa and propranolol in the treatment of hypertension. *Clin Sci Mol Med* 1976;51 (Suppl 3):567s–570s.

356. Croog SH, Levine S, Testa MA, et al. The effects of antihypertensive therapy on the quality of life. *N Engl J Med* 1986;314:1657–1664.

357. Yodfat Y, Bar-On D, Amir M, Cristal N. Quality of life in normotensives compared to hypertensive men treated with isradipine or methyldopa as monotherapy or in combination with captopril: the LOMIR-MCT-IL study. *J Human Hypertens* 1996;10:117–122.

358. Wright JM, McLeod PJ, McCullough W. Antihypertensive efficacy of a single bedtime dose of methyldopa. *Clin Pharm Ther* 1976;20:733–737.

359. Colwill JM, Dutton AM, Morrissey J, YU PN. Alpha-methyldopa and hydrochlorothiazide. *N Engl J Med* 1964;271:696–703.

360. Amery A, Birkenhager W, Brixko P, et al. Mortality and morbidity results from the European Working Party on High Blood Pressure in the Elderly Trial. *Lancet* 1985;1: 1349–1354.

361. Leonetti C, Cuspidi C, Sampieri L, et al. Evaluation of the efficacy and safety of enalapril plus hydrochlorothiazide plus methyldopa vs standard triple therapy in the treatment of moderate to severe hypertension: results from a multicentre study. *J Human Hypertens* 1990;4:5–11.

362. Ofor OO. Oral enalapril – hydrochlorothiazide – methyldopa as first line treatment for severe hypertension in Nigerians. *Trop Doct* 2004;34:32–33.

363. Cruickshank JM, Prichard BNC. *Beta-blockers in clinical practice, 2nd edn.* New York: Churchill Livingstone; 1994:1–1204.

364. Fletcher A, Amery A, Birkenhager W, et al. Risks and benefits in the trial of the European Working Party on High Blood Pressure in the Elderly. *J Hypertens* 1991;9:225–230.

365. Dollery CT, Hartley K, Bulpitt PF, et al. Fifteen-year survival of patients beginning treatment with methyldopa between 1962 and 1966. *Hypertension* 1984; 8(Suppl II):82–92.

366. Lowe SA, Rubin PC. The pharmacological management of hypertension in pregnancy. *J Hypertens* 1992;10:201.

367. Lindheimer MD. Hypertension in pregnancy. *Hypertension* 1993;22:127.

368. Cohen IM, Katz MA. Oral clonidine loading for rapid control of hypertension. *Clin Pharmacol Ther* 1978;24:11–15.

369. CLOBASS Study Group. Low-dose clonidine administration in the treatment of mild to moderate essential hypertension: results from a double-blind placebo-controlled study (CLOBASS). *J Hypertens* 1990;8:539–546.

370. Ng J, Phelan EL, McGregor DD, et al. Properties of catepres, a new hypotensive drug: a preliminary report. *NZ Med J* 1967;66:864–870.

371. Hashimoto J, Chonan K, Aoki Y, et al. Therapeutic effects of evening administration of guanabenz and clonidine on morning hypertension: evaluation using home-based blood pressure measurements. *J Hypertens* 2003;21:805–811.

372. Head GA. Therapeutic effects of evening administration of guanabenz and clonidine on morning hypertension. *J Hypertens* 2003;21:701–703.

373. Lowenthal DT, Saris SD, Paran E, Cristal N. The use of transdermal clonidine in the hypertensive patient with chronic renal failure. *Clin Nephrol* 1993;39:37–42.

374. Breidthardt J, Schumacher H, Mehlburger L. Long-term (5 year) experience with transdermal clonidine in the treatment of mild to moderate hypertension. *Clin Auton Res* 1993;3(6):385–390.

375. Thananopavarn C, Golub MS, Sambhi P. Clonidine in the elderly hypertensive. *Chest* 1983;83(Suppl):410–411.

376. Vanholder R, Lameire N, Ringoir S. Long-term experience with the combination of clonidine and beta-adrenoceptor blocking agents in hypertension. *Eur J Clin Pharmacol* 1985;28:125–130.

377. Houston MC, Hays L. Transdermal clonidine as an adjunct to nifedipine-GITS therapy in patients with mild-to-moderate hypertension. *Am Heart J* 1993;126:918–923.

378. Lueg MC, Herron J, Zellner S. Transdermal clonidine as an adjunct to sustained release diltiazem in the treatment of mild-to-moderate hypertension. *Clin Ther* 1991;13: 471–481.

379. Weidler D, Wallin JD, Cook E, et al. Transdermal clonidine as an adjunct to enalapril: an evaluation of efficacy and patient compliance. *J Clin Pharmacol* 1992;32:444–449.

380. Trieb G, Jäger B, Hughes PR, et al. Long-term evaluation of the antihypertensive efficacy and tolerability of the orally-acting imidazoline I_1 receptor agonist moxonidine in patients with mild to moderate essential hypertension. *Eur J Clin Res* 1995;7:227–240.

381. Abellán, Leal M, Hernánanedez-Menáarguez F, et al. Efficacy of moxonidine in the treatment of hypertension in obese, noncontrolled hypertensive patients. *Kidney International* 2005; 67(Suppl 93):S20–S24.

382. Beau B, Mahieux F, Paraire M, et al. Efficacy and safety of rilmenidine for arterial hypertension. *Am J Cardiol* 1988;61:95D–102D.

383. Luccioni R. Evaluation pharmaco-épidémiologique de la rilmenidine chez 18 235 hypertendus. *La Presse Médicale* 1995;24:1857–1864.

384. Kaan EC. Unpublished observations.

385. Prichard BNC, Küster LJ, Hughes PR, et al. Dose relation of blood pressure reduction with moxonidine: findings from three placebo- and active-controlled randomised studies. *J Clin Basic Cardiol* 2003;6:49–51.

386. Frei M, Küster L, Gardosch von Krosigk P-P, et al. Moxonidine and hydrochlorothiazide in combination: a synergistic antihypertensive effect. *J Cardiovasc Pharmacol* 1994;24(Suppl 1): S25–S28.

387. Waters J, Ashford J, Jäger B, Wonnacott S. Verboom CN for the TOPIC Investigators. Use of moxonidine as initial therapy and in combination in the treatment of essential hypertension – results of the TOPIC (Trial of Physiotens in Combination) study. *J Clin Basic Cardiol* 1999;2:219–224.

388. Dallochio M, Gosse P, Fillastre JP, et al. La rilmenidine, un nouvel antihypertenseur dans la traitement de premiere intention de l'hypertension arterielle essentielle. *Presse Med* 1991;20:1265–1271.

389. Martin U, Hill C, O'Mahoney DO. Use of moxonidine in elderly patients with resistant hypertension. *J Clin Pharm Ther* 2005;30:433–437.

390. Connolly ME, Briant RH, George CF, Dollory CT. A crossover comparison of clonidine and methyldopa in hypertension. *Eur J Clin Pharmacol* 1972;4:222–227.

391. Fletcher AE, Beevers DG, Dollery CT, et al. The effects of two centrally-acting antihypertensive drugs on the quality of life. *Eur J Clin Pharmacol* 1991;41:397–400.

392. Applegate WB, Carper ER, Sherman EK, et al. Comparison of the use of reserpine versus alpha-methyldopa for second step treatment hypertension in the elderly. *J Am Geriatr Soc* 1985;33:109–115.

393. Viskoper RJ, Laszt A, Paran E, et al. Low dose guanfacine and methyldopa in mild essential hypertension. *Netherlands J Med* 1987;31:58–65.

394. Plänitz V. Comparison of moxonidine and clonidine HC1 in treating patients with hypertension. *J Clin Pharmaco* 1987;l 27:46–51.

395. Moyer RR. A double-blind study of trimazosin and methyldopa in hypertensive patients receiving polythiazide. *Am Heart J* 1983;106:1250–1253.

396. Kirkendall WM, Hammond JJ, Thomas JC, et al. Prazosin and clonidine for moderately severe hypertension. *JAMA* 1978;240:2553–2556.

397. Plänitz V. Intraindividual comparison of moxonidine and prazosin in hypertensive patients. *Eur J Clin Pharmacol* 1986;29:645–650.

398. Materson BJ, Reda DJ, Cushman WC, et al. Single-drug therapy for hypertension in men. A comparison of six antihypertensive agents with placebo. *N Engl J Med* 1993;328: 914–921.

399. Materson BJ, Cushman WC, Reda DJ. Department of Veteran affairs single-drug therapy of hypertension study. Revised figures and new data. *Am J Hypertens* 1995;8:189–192.

400. Cushman WC, Reda DJ, Perry HM, et al. Regional and racial differences in response to antihypertensive medication use in a randomised controlled trial of men with hypertension in the United States. *Arch Intern Med* 2000;160:825–831.

401. Preston RA, Materson BJ, Reda DJ, et al. Age-race subgroup compared with renin profile as predictors of blood pressure response to antihypertensive therapy. *JAMA* 1998;280:1168–1172.

402. Materson BJ, Williams DW, Reda DJ, et al. Response to six classes of antihypertensive medications by body mass index in a randomised controlled trial. *J Clin Hypertens* 2003;5:197–201.

403. Materson BJ, Reda DJ, Williams DW. Effects of antihypertensive single-drug therapy on heart rate. *Am J Hypertens* 1999;12:9S–11S.

404. Cushman WC, Materson BJ, Williams DW, Reda DJ. Pulse pressure changes with six classes of antihypertensive agents in a randomised, controlled trial. *Hypertension* 2001;38: 953–967.

405. Preston RA, Materson BJ, Reda DJ, et al. Proteinuria in mild to moderate hypertension: results of the VAcooperative study of six antihypertensive agents and placebo. *Clin Nephrol* 1997;47:310–315.

406. Gottdiener JS, Reda DJ, Williams DW, et al. Effect of single-dose therapy on reduction of left atrial size in mild to moderate hypertension. *Circulation* 1998;98:140–148.

407. Burris JF, Papademetrioli V, Wallin JD, et al. Therapeutic adherence in the elderly: transdermal clonidine compared to oral verapamil for hypertension. *Am J Med* 1991;91(Suppl 1A):22s–28s.

408. Wolf R. The treatment of hypertensive patients with a calcium antagonist or moxonidine: a comparison. *J Cardiovasc Pharmacol* 1992;20(Suppl 4):S42–S44.

409. Kundu SC, Vakil HB. Ramipril and methyldopa compared in patients with mild to moderate hypertension. *Clin Ther* 1990;12:393–397.

410. McMahon FG, Jain AK, Vargas R, Fillingim J. A double blind comparison of transdermal clonidine and oral captopril in essential hypertension. *Clin Ther* 1990;12:88–100.

411. Kraft K, Vetter H. Twenty-four-hour blood pressure profiles in patients with mild-to-moderate hypertension: moxonidine versus captopril. *J Cardiovasc Pharmacol* 1994;24:S29–S33.

412. Lotti G, Gianrossi R. Moxonidine vs. captopril in minor to intermediate hypertension. Double-blind study of effectiveness and tolerance. *Fortschr Med* 1993;111:429–432.

413. Ollivier JP, Christen MO, Schäfer SG. Moxonidine: a second generation of centrally acting drug, an appraisal of clinical experience. *J Cardiovasc Pharmacol* 1992;20:S31–S36.

414. Schäfers RF, Löw-Kröger A, Philipp Th. Wirksamkeit und Verträglichkeit des neuen zentralwirksamen antihypertensivums moxonidine im vergleich zu enalapril. *Neiren-und Hochdruckdrankheiten* 1994;23:S221–S224.

415. Kuppers HE, Jager BA, Luszick JH, et al. Placebo-controlled comparison of the efficacy and tolerability of once-daily moxonidine and enalapril in mild-to-moderate essential hypertension. *J Hypertens* 1997;15:93–97.

416. Prichard BNC, Jäger BA, Luszick JH, et al. Placebo-controlled comparison of the efficacy and tolerability of once-daily moxonidine and enalapril in mild to moderate essential hypertension. *Blood Pressure* 2002;11:166–172.

417. Vandenburg MJ, Cooper WD, Woollard ML, et al. Reduced peripheral vascular symptoms in elderly patients treated with α-methyldopa – a comparison with propranolol. *Eur J Clin Pharmacol* 1984;26:325–329.

418. Traub YM. Comparison of oxprenolol vs methyldopa as second-line antihypertensive agents in the elderly. *Arch Intern Med* 1988;148:77–80.

419. Karachalios GN. A comparative study of metoprolol and methyldopa in the treatment of hypertension. *Int J Clin Pharm Ther Tox* 1983;21:476–478.

420. Wilkinson PR, Raftery EB. A comparative trial of clonidine, propranolol and placebo in the treatment of moderate hypertension. *Br J Clin Pharmacol* 1977;4:289–294.

421. Prichard BNC, Simmons R, Rooks MJ, et al. A double-blind comparison of moxonidine and atenolol in the management of patients with mild-to-moderate hypertension. *J Cardiovasc Pharmacol* 1992;20(suppl 4):S45–S49.

422. Larrat V. Efficacy and tolerance of moxonidine in comparison with a standard therapy with hydrochlorothiazide. *Hamburg: Beiersdorf-Lilly GmbH* 1990;200:029–28–54.

423. Fiorentini C, Guillet C, Guazzi M. Etude multicentrique en double aveugle comparant la rilmenidine 1mg et l'hydrochlorothiazide 25mg chez 244 patients. *Arch Mal Coeur* 1989;82:39–46.

424. Pelemans W, Vergaeghe J, Creytens G, et al. Efficacy and safety of rilmendine in elderly patients – comparison with hydrochlorothiazide. *Am J Cardiol* 1994;74:51A–57A.

425. de Divitis O, Di Somma S, Liguori V, et al. Effort blood pressure control in the course of antihypertensive treatment. *Am J Med* 1989;87(3C):46S–56S.

426. Cohn JN, Pfeffer MA, Rouleau J, et al. Adverse mortality effect of central sympathetic inhibition with sustained-release moxonidine in patients with heart failure (MOXCON). *Eur J Heart Fail* 2003;5:659–667.

427. Gavras I, Manolis AJ, Gavras H. The economics of therapeutic advances. *Arch Intern Med* 1999;159:2634–2636.

428. Gavras I, Manolis AJ, Gavras H. The alpha$_2$-adrenergic receptors in hypertension and heart failure: experimental and clinical studies. *J Hypertens* 2001;19:2115–2124.

429. Manolis AS, Varriale P, Nobile J. Short-term hemodynamic effects of intravenous methyldopa in patients with congestive heart failure. *Pharmacotherapy* 1987;7:216–222.

430. Manolis AS, Olympios C, Sifkaki C, et al. Chronic sympathetic suppression in the treatment of chronic congestive heart failure. *Clin Exp Hypertens* 1998;20:717–731.

431. Swedberg K, Bergh C-H, Dickstein K, et al. The effects of moxonidine, a novel imidazoline, on plasma norepinephrine in patients with congestive heart failure. *J Am Coll Cardiol* 2000;35:398–404.

432. Dickstein K, Monhenke C, Aarsland T, et al. The effects of chronic, sustained release moxonidine therapy on clinical and neurohumoral status in patients with heart failure. *Int J Cardiol* 2000;75:167–176.

433. Floras JS. The "unsympathetic" nervous system of heart failure. *Circulation* 2002;105:1753–1755.

434. Victor RG, Talman WT. Comparative effects of clonidine and dihydroergotamine on venomotor tone and orthostatic tolerance in patients with severe hypoadrenergic orthostatic hypotension. *Am J Med* 2002;112:361–368.

435. Thomas MG, Quiroz AC, Rice JC, et al. Antianginal effects of clonidine. *J Cardiovasc Pharmacol* 1986;8:S69–S75.

436. Zochowski RJ, Lada W. Intravenous clonidine treatment in acute myocardial infarction (with comparison to a nitroglycerin-treated and control group). *J Cardiovasc Pharmacol* 1986;8(Suppl 3):S41–S45.

437. Bachmann AW, Gordon RD. Clonidine suppression test reliably differentiates phaeochromocytoma from essential hypertension. *Clin Exp Pharmocol Physiol* 1991;18:275–277.

438. De Kock M, Wiederkher P, Laghmiche A, Scholtes JL. Epidural clonidine used as the sole analgesic agent during and after abdominal surgery. A dose-response study. *Anesthesiol* 1997;86:285–292.

439. Dorman T, Clarkson K, Rosenfeld BA, et al. Effects of clonidine on prolonged postoperative sympathetic response. *Crit Care Med* 1997;26:1293.

440. Stühmeier K-D, Mainzer B, Cierpka J, et al. Small, oral dose of clonidine reduces the incidence of intraoperative myocardial ischemia in patients having vascular surgery. *Anesthesiol* 1996;85:706–712.

441. Wallace AW, Galindez D, Salahieh A, et al. Effect of clonidine on cardiovascular morbidity and mortality after noncardiac surgery. *Anesthesiol* 2004;101:284–293.

442. Brogden RN, Pinder RM, Sawyer PR, et al. Low-dose clonidine: a review of its therapeutic efficacy in migraine prophylaxis. *Drugs* 1975;10:357–365.

443. O'Keefe ST. Restless legs syndrome. A review. *Arch Intern Med* 1996;156:243–248.

444. Wagner ML, Walters AS, Coleman EG, et al. Randomized, double-blind, placebo-controlled study of clonidine in restless legs syndrome. *Sleep* 1996;19:52–58.

445. Leckmann JF, Detlor J, Harcherik DR, et al. Short- and long-term treatment of Tourette's syndrome with clonidine: a clinical perspective. *Neurology* 1985;35:343–351.

446. Bond WS. Psychiatric indications for clonidine: The neuropharmacologic and clinical basis. *J Clin Psychopharmacol* 1986;6:81–87.

447. Zubenko GS, Cohen BM, Lipinski Jr. JF, Jonas JM. Clonidine in the treatment of mania and mixed bipolar disorder. *Am J Psychiatry* 1984;141:1617–1618.

448. Gourlay SG, Stead LF, Benowitz NL. Clonidine for smoking cessation. *Update of Cochrane Database Syst Rev* 2004, CD 000058 Rev.

449. Bayard M, McIntyre J, Hill KR, Woodside J. Alcohol withdrawal syndrome. *Am Fam Physician* 2004;69:1443–1450.

450. Dobrydnjov I, Axelsson K, Berggren L, et al. Intrathecal and oral clonidine as prophylaxis for postoperative alcohol withdrawal syndrome: a randomised double-blind study. *Anesth Analg* 2004;98:738–744.

451. Sobey PW, Parran Jr. TV, Grey SF, et al. The use of tramadol for acute heroin withdrawal: a comparison with clonidine. *J Addict Dis* 2003;22:1–4.

452. Clayden JR, Bell JW, Pollard P. Menopausal flushing: double-blind trial of a non-hormonal medication. *BMJ* 1974;1:409–412.

453. Pandya KJ, Raubertus RF, Flynn PJ, et al. Oral clonidine in postmenopausal patients with breast cancer experiencing tamoxifen-induced hot flushes: a University of Rochester Cancer Center Community Clinical Oncology Program study. *Ann Intern Med* 2000;132:788–793.

454. Lechin F, van der Dijs B, Insausti CL, et al. Treatment of ulcerative colitis with clonidine. *J Clin Pharmacol* 1985;25:219–226.

455. Fedorak RN, Field M, Chang EB. Treatment of diabetic diarrhea with clonidine. *Ann Intern Med* 1985;102:197–199.

456. Rosa-E-Silva L, Troncon LEA, Oliveira RB, et al. Treatment of diabetic gastroparesis with oral clonidine. *Aliment Pharmacol Ther* 1995;9:179–183.

457. Huilgol V, Evans J, Hellman RS, Soergel KH. Acute effect of clonidine on gastric emptying in patients with diabetic gastropathy and controls. *Pharmacol Ther* 2002;16:945–950.

458. Morali GA, Braverman DZ, Lissi J, et al. Effect of clonidine on gallbladder contraction and small bowel transit time in insulin-treated diabetics. *Am J Gastroenterol* 1991;86:995–999.

459. Harrison R, Kaufmann CS. Clonidine: effects of a topically administered solution on intraocular pressure and blood pressure in open-angle glaucoma. *Arch Ophthalmol* 1977;95:1368–1373.

IV

Vasodilator drugs

8 | α-blocking drugs

Peter A. Meredith

INTRODUCTION

Increased total peripheral vascular resistance is the most consistent haemodynamic change that characterizes essential hypertension. Since the discovery of α- and β-adrenoceptors nearly 60 years ago,[1] the impact both of stimulation and blockade these receptors have on the circulatory system has become apparent. It is clear that α-adrenoceptors play a role not only in the physiological regulation of peripheral vascular resistance, but also in the genesis of hypertension.[2] Although hypertension is considered to be a complex syndrome of multiple haemodynamic, neuroendocrine and metabolic abnormalities, it is also widely accepted that the sympathetic nervous system plays a role in the initiation and maintenance of the increased peripheral vascular resistance which is characteristic of established essential hypertension.[3,4] Increases in arteriolar and venous tone, and, hence, blood pressure (BP), are mediated by noradrenaline released from sympathetic nerve terminals and acting at α_1-adrenoceptors located postjunctionally in the BP wall (Fig. 8.1).[5,6] Thus, in the treatment of hypertension, selective α_1-blockers interfere directly with sympathetically-mediated vasoconstrictor mechanisms and thereby promote a reduction in BP.

CLASSIFICATION

The first α-blockers were developed during the 1960s and were originally thought to be direct-acting vasodilators. It was subsequently demonstrated that the effects of phenoxybenzamine and phentolamine were mediated by relatively selective blockade of α_1-adrenoceptors. However, these agents have significant effects on α_2-adrenoceptors and efficacy is limited by modest supine blood-pressure reductions and the development of pharmacological tolerance and unacceptable side effects, such as orthostatic hypertension and tachycardia.[7,8] Therefore, these relatively non-selective α_1-adrenoceptor blockers are no longer used in the treatment of hypertension. Further developments led to the identification of several agents, particularly the quinazoline derivatives,

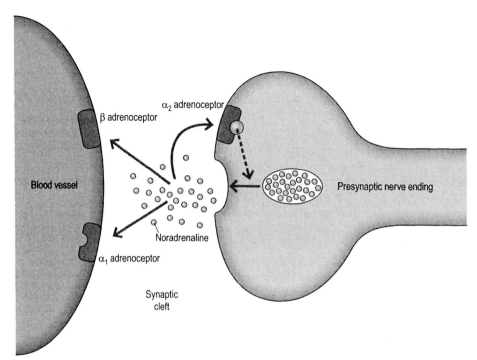

Fig. 8.1 A diagrammatic representation of the pre- and postjunctional α-adrenoceptors in the neuroeffector junction.

which are selective for the post-synaptic α_1-adrenoceptor. The particular advantage of selective α_1-adrenoceptor blockers, compared with non-selective agents, is that there is no interference with the negative feedback control mechanism mediated via the prejunctional α_2-adrenoceptor (Fig. 8.1). Catecholamine 'spill over', which occurs as a consequence of pre-synaptic α_2-adrenoceptor blockade, is significantly reduced and the risk of reflex cardio-acceleration during chronic treatment is attenuated. It is reasonable to suggest that selective α-blockers fulfil the required basic criteria for an effective antihypertensive agent since they reduce peripheral vascular resistance without interfering with myocardial contractility or exercise tolerance.[9–11]

MECHANISM OF ACTION

Over the last 30 years there has been extensive research into the pharmacology of α_1-adrenoceptors, leading to identification of both α_1- and α_2-adrenoceptor subtypes. These were originally defined pharmacologically by functional and binding studies. Subsequently the receptors were also isolated and identified using cloning methods.[12] The study of α-adrenoceptors was revolutionized by the techniques of molecular biology, which established the present system of classification: α_1A-adrenoceptor subtype (cloned $\alpha(1c)$ and redesignated $\alpha(1a/c)$), α_1B-adrenoceptor subtype (cloned $\alpha(1b)$) and α_1D-adrenoceptor subtype (cloned $\alpha(1d)$ and redesignated $\alpha(1a/d)$). It has not proved easy to establish the distribution of these α_1-adrenoceptor subtypes in the various organs and tissues, or to define the functional response mediated by each in the different species studied. Nevertheless, it seems that the α_1A-adrenoceptor subtype is implicated more in the maintenance of basal vascular tone and of arterial BP in conscious animals, and the α_1B-adrenoceptor subtype participates more in responses to exogenous agonists. The expression of the α_1B-adrenoceptor subtype can be modified in pathological situations and particular attention has been paid to the regulation of expression of this receptor.

Since the α_1-adrenoceptor was identified as the type that mediates the contraction of smooth muscle, including that of the prostate, and the existence of subtypes of the receptor, this receptor has been considered to be of potential clinical relevance with respect to specific receptor blockade in vascular tissue and the prostate. However, despite extensive characterization of cloned and native receptors in many tissues[13] it is still difficult to ascribe clinical significance to each type of α_1-adrenoceptor. There is some in vitro evidence to suggest that tamsulosin has a higher affinity for the α_1-adrenoceptors in the prostate than in the aorta.[14] Direct in vitro comparative studies suggest that all available agents have a similar affinity for the α_1A-adrenoceptor subtype.[14] Despite this, the received wisdom is that α_1-blockers that are efficacious in hypertension (prazosin, doxazosin, terazosin) are more likely than tamsulosin to impair physiological BP control in normotensives with lower urinary tract symptoms (LUTS). Tamsulosin does not reduce elevated BP in comparison with placebo and has little effect on orthostatic BP control. It should also be appreciated that clinical selectivity and cardiovascular safety are also defined by aspects of the treatment regimen including dose, dosage interval, formulation, and the titration schedule following treatment initiation.

As tamsulosin is licensed exclusively for the treatment of prostatic obstruction and LUTS, it will not be considered further in this chapter.

PHARMACOKINETICS/METABOLISM

Prazosin

Prazosin, the prototype quinazoline α-blocker (Fig. 8.2), is a short-acting agent that requires multiple daily dosing (unless administered as a modified release formulation). When administered orally, prazosin is rapidly extensively absorbed but, with significant first-pass metabolism; the mean bioavailability ranges from 45% to 70%.[15] Prazosin is extensively metabolized by the liver with the major route of metabolism being O-demethylation followed by conjugation. Total body clearance of prazosin is relatively high with a short (2–3 hours) elimination half-life.

Terazosin

Structurally terazosin differs from prazosin only in that the furane ring of the terazosin molecule is saturated (Fig. 8.2). This small structural change results in a very large increase in the water solubility of terazosin when compared with prazosin. Despite the increase in solubility, terazosin is readily absorbed from the gastrointestinal tract, but the absorption rate is somewhat slower than that of prazosin.[16] Terazosin undergoes extensive hepatic metabolism and the major route of elimination is via the biliary tract. The metabolism of terazosin involves hydrolysis of the amide linkage to yield the free piperazine derivative.[16] Small amounts of the unchanged drug are excreted in urine.

Doxazosin

Although doxazosin is a quinazoline derivative, it is structurally distinct when compared with terazosin and prazosin (Fig. 8.2). Doxazosin also has disposition characteristics that differ from those of terazosin and prazosin. The oral absorption of doxazosin is relatively consistent, with bioavailability ranging from 62% to 69%.[17] Peak plasma concentrations of doxazosin are achieved between 3 and 4 hours post dose, with mean peak plasma concentrations increasing proportionally across the oral dose range from 1 mg to 16 mg in both normal volunteers and patients.[17–19] Doxazosin undergoes extensive biotransformation and the major route of metabolism appears to involve O-demethylation of the quinazoline substitute in a manner similar to that observed with prazosin.[19] The 6 and 7-O desmethyl metabolites comprise 16% and 17% of an oral dose respectively. Less than 10% of an orally administered dose of doxazosin is excreted in the urine and the main route of elimination is via the faeces. The plasma clearance of doxazosin is low when compared with prazosin and this translates into an elimination half-life in the range 10–14 hours. The elimination half-life of doxazosin does not appear to be influenced by age[17,20] or renal dysfunction.[21]

PHARMACODYNAMICS

The pharmacokinetic characteristics of α_1-adrenoceptor blockers are of importance, as the antihypertensive effect of these agents appears to be related to the circulating drug concentrations. In the case of both prazosin and doxazosin,

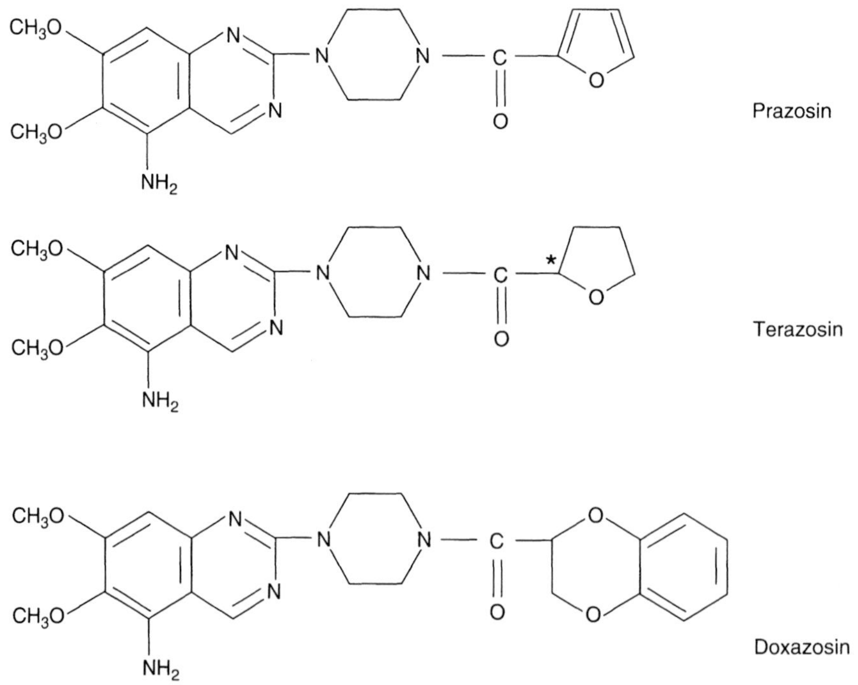

Fig. 8.2 Chemical structures of the selective quinazoline derivative α_1-adrenoceptor antagonists.

a simple direct linear relationship between plasma drug concentrations and the decrease in BP is not immediately apparent.[22,23] However, once allowance has been made for the temporal discrepancy between the concentration and effect profiles, it is possible to relate the circulating drug concentrations of both prazosin and doxazosin to the fall in BP based upon a linear relationship.[22,23] These relationships are apparent in both normotensive and hypertensive subjects and in elderly individuals.[24] Studies in hypertensive patients indicate that there is a systematic reduction in the slope of the relationship between drug concentration and antihypertensive effect in translation from acute to steady-state therapy.[22,23] The change in responsiveness is apparent within 1 week of initiating therapy and thereafter there was no further significant reduction in responsiveness. This suggests that this change in responsiveness should not be considered to be evidence of continuing tachyphylaxis and that there is no evidence of progressive development of 'tolerance'.

α₁-adrenoceptor antagonist in the treatment of hypertension

α_1-adrenoceptor antagonists lower BP through a reduction in peripheral vascular resistance without significant effects on heart rate, cardiac output or central haemodynamics.[25,26] Overall the evidence suggests that long-term treatment with specific α_1-adrenoceptor antagonists produces a reduction in BP comparable to that of all the other major classes of antihypertensive agents, such as diuretics, β-blockers, calcium-channel blockers and angiotensin converting enzyme (ACE) inhibitors.[27] α_1-adrenoceptor antagonists offer a potential advantage in that effectiveness in terms of blood pressure reduction appears to be relatively independent of age, race and renal function. In addition antihypertensive benefits have also been demonstrated in patients with concomitant illnesses, such as type 2 diabetes mellitus and chronic obstructive airways disease.

First-line therapy

As discussed previously, comparative clinical studies of the antihypertensive efficacy of α_1-adrenoceptor antagonists have shown that responses are similar to those of other antihypertensive drugs and, until comparatively recently, were considered by most major hypertension guidelines to be suitable for first line therapy. For example, the Treatment of Mild Hypertension Study (TOMHS) was a randomized, placebo-controlled, parallel group study in 910 patients with mild hypertension, who were treated for 4 years with representative agents from the major antihypertensive drug classes, including doxazosin.[28] All participants, including those on placebo, also underwent intense lifestyle modification consisting of weight loss, dietary sodium and alcohol reduction, and increased physical activity. All participants were free of clinical cardiovascular disease at entry and all the drugs used in TOMHS were well tolerated. At 48 months the calcium channel blocker amlodipine demonstrated the best persistence, with 83% of patients remaining on their initially prescribed treatment. Seventy-eight per cent remained on the β-blocker acebutolol and among those taking doxazosin, chlorthalidone or enalapril, approximately two-thirds continued on each of those therapies. Lifestyle changes alone plus placebo lowered systolic BP by 9 mmHg and the addition of the active drugs increased the reduction by a mean value of 6.8 mmHg. There were no major differences in BP lowering when comparing the five drugs, but there were potentially significant differences between the agents with respect to tolerability and metabolic side effects.

Combination therapy

All current national and international guidelines for the treatment of hypertension acknowledge the requirement for tight or optimal BP control, and recognize that this frequently requires combinations of antihypertensive drugs, particularly in high-risk patients. α_1-adrenoceptor antagonists are considered to be useful agents in designing rational combination regimens, in that there is no theoretical reason why these agents may not be combined with any of the other major classes of antihypertensive drugs. Indeed, α_1-adrenoceptor antagonists may have a role in regimens used for patients with renal impairment or with metabolic problems (particularly disorders of lipids and glucose metabolism) where other agents would be relatively contraindicated. In clinical trials α_1-adrenoceptor antagonists have been successfully added to β-blockers, diuretics, calcium antagonists and ACE inhibitors in patients with hypertension inadequately controlled by these agents. In most patients combination therapy achieved significant decreases in sitting and/or standing BP without compromising tolerability.[29–32] The usefulness and effectiveness of doxazosin as a general 'add-on' therapy was specifically studied in a randomized, double-blind, placebo-controlled study in patients with inadequately controlled BP.[33] The patients received doxazosin or placebo along with their original agent or two antihypertensive medications, predominantly calcium antagonist and ACE inhibitors. After a titration and 4-week maintenance period the doxazosin group experienced clinically and statistically significant decreases in both sitting and standing systolic and diastolic BP. The target reduction in sitting diastolic pressure (< 90 mmHg in addition to >10 mmHg improvement from baseline) was achieved by significantly more patients administered doxazosin than those given placebo ($p < 0.05$). In addition, the doxazosin group showed statistically significant reductions in total cholesterol and LDL cholesterol. A similar, but larger study demonstrated the incremental benefits of the controlled-release doxazosin gastrointestinal therapeutic system (GITS), compared with placebo, in reducing BP in patients who were poorly controlled at baseline despite antihypertensive therapy with one or two agents from the five major antihypertensive drug classes.[34]

ADVERSE EVENTS/CONTRAINDICATIONS

Cardiovascular effects

Since the introduction of the prototype selective α_1-adrenoceptor antagonist prazosin, it has been recognized that these agents occasionally provoke a 'first-dose effect' with symptomatic orthostatic hypertension and possible syncope, accompanied by tachycardia and palpitations. This well-recognized complication could often be attributed to the use of unnecessarily high starting doses, particularly in patients who were salt-volume depleted or were also receiving other antihypertensive treatments, such as thiazide diuretics and β-blockers. This side effect may be minimized by initiating treatment with the recommended low doses of the drugs at night and subsequent up-titration to therapeutic doses. The problem also appears to be minimized by the use of newer agents with more gradual onset of effect and longer duration of action. This is supported by the findings of the TOMHS study where the incidence of syncope with doxazosin was identical to that of the other drug groups.[28]

Effects on other systems

As discussed previously, α_1-adrenoceptor antagonists are well recognized as having effects on the genito-urinary system and have a positive therapeutic role in the relief of obstructive urinary symptoms in males with LUTS. However, this predictable pharmacological effect may occasionally lead to urinary incontinence in females.

In addition, there is evidence that male sexual dysfunction occurs less frequently with α_1-adrenoceptor antagonists than with most other types of antihypertensive agent. This observation was formally confirmed in the TOMHS study,[28] where after 4 years' treatment, the incidence of male participants reporting difficulty achieving erection was statistically lower in the doxazosin group when compared with placebo and all of the other active treatments. Whilst there is no evidence to suggest that this effect can be harnessed therapeutically, it may be postulated that α_1-adrenoceptor antagonists have a beneficial effect in combination treatment regimens where the other components of the regimen have a deleterious effect on sexual function.

Metabolic effects

Risk factors for coronary heart disease are highly prevalent in the general population; clustering of metabolic disorders, such as elevated lipids, insulin resistance and glucose intolerance, is common in patients with hypertension. For example, in the San Antonio Heart Study, which included 287 hypertensive patients, about 50% had type 2 diabetes or impaired glucose tolerance and only 15% were free of glucose intolerance, lipid disorder and obesity.[35]

Many studies have demonstrated a small, but potentially beneficial effect, of α_1-adrenoceptor antagonist on glucose and lipid metabolism. α-blockers are the only class of antihypertensive drug that have been shown consistently to have beneficial effects on plasma lipid profiles with reductions in total and LDL cholesterol and small increases in HDL cholesterol. In the TOMHS study[28] doxazosin was associated with significant increases in HDL:total cholesterol ratio when compared with placebo ($p<0.01$) and compared with antihypertensive therapy with β-blocker, calcium channel blocker and thiazide diuretic ($p<0.01$).

The beneficial effects of α_1-blockade on lipids and lipoproteins are paralleled by a beneficial effect on insulin responsiveness, leading to increased peripheral glucose uptake. Thus, selective α_1-adrenoceptor antagonists may be particularly well suited for the treatment of patients with type II diabetes and glucose intolerance.[36,37] This contention is supported by the TOMHS study[28] where fasting insulin (used as a measure of insulin resistance) was lower in all drug groups when compared to placebo, but the lowest level of fasting insulin was observed with doxazosin. It has also been observed that doxazosin treatment in patients with coronary heart disease resulted in a significant dose-dependent increase in tissue plasminogen activator (t-PA) resulting in a net increase in fibrinolytic potential.[38]

Whether or not these positive metabolic effects influence outcome remains uncertain. In this regard, the premature cessation of the doxazosin arm of the ALLHAT trial (see later) might be construed as an important, but missed opportunity, because there is now little or no likelihood of formally assessing the benefits attributable to improved insulin/glucose and lipid metabolism associated with specific α_1-adrenoceptor blockade. The selective α_1-adrenoceptor antagonists are theoretically particularly useful in the treatment of hypertension as non-specific tissue or organ toxicity has been identified and there are no co-morbid conditions that constitute contraindications.

Drug interactions

Drug interactions with α_1-adrenoceptor blocker are largely confined to the increased risk of an excessive hypotensive response when added to existing antihypertensive treatment regimens. There is anecdotal evidence to suggest that this risk is increased in patients who are sodium depleted as a result of diuretic therapy. Pharmacokinetic studies indicate that verapamil significantly increases the apparent oral bioavailability and peak concentrations of both prazosin and terazosin,[39,40] increasing the potential for a marked additive hypotensive response particularly when adding the α_1-adrenoceptor blockers to existing verapamil therapy.

CLINICAL USE INCLUDING OUTCOME DATA

Doxazosin gastrointestinal therapeutic system (GITS)

In the last 10 years the only new development of any note with respect to α_1-adrenoceptor antagonists has been the introduction of doxazosin GITS. Superficially, this might be considered to be a simple line extension product. However, there is a sound rationale underlying the development. As discussed previously, with some of the α_1-adrenoceptor antagonists, and with doxazosin in particular, a relationship has been established between the antihypertensive effect and the plasma drug-concentration–time profiles.[23] Thus, it would be anticipated that a modified pharmacokinetic profile with doxazosin could provide a more desirable clinical effect profile. Doxazosin GITS utilizes an osmotic pump formulation, which consists of a two-layer core of drug substance and osmotic polymer surrounded by a semi-permeable membrane. The outer membrane contains a small laser-drilled hole. When swallowed, the tablet absorbs water from the gut through the semi-permeable membrane. The drug-containing core layer forms a suspension that is then extruded through the laser-drilled hole at a constant rate by expansion of the polymer core layer (Fig. 8.3). Unlike other modified-release formulations, osmotic pump formulations provide drug delivery for around 12–16 hours in a 'zero order' fashion, which is analogous to a constant rate drug infusion. This results in a smooth and consistent plasma drug concentration–time profile. The comparative pharmacokinetic profiles of the immediate-release and GITS formulations of doxazosin are illustrated in Figure 8.4.[41] The discrepancies between the profiles at

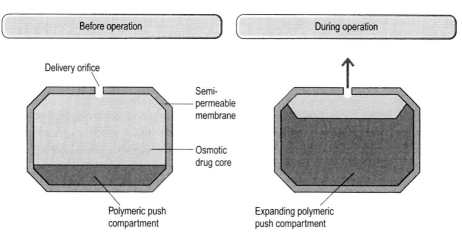

Fig. 8.3 A diagrammatic representation of the gastrointestinal therapeutic system (GITS) formulation of doxazosin.

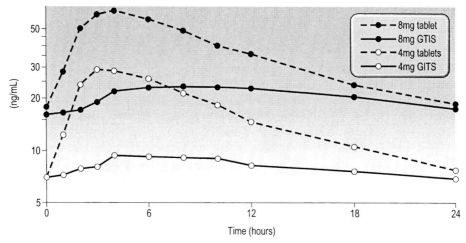

Fig. 8.4 The steady-state pharmacokinetic profiles of standard and gastrointestinal therapeutic system (GITS) formulation doxazosin.

steady-state are immediately apparent. Although both formulations achieve the same trough concentrations at the end of the steady-state dosing interval, the plasma concentration profile of doxazosin GITS is much more uniform. This is characterized by a reduction in peak concentrations with the GITS formulation and a delay in the time to achieve peak concentrations. The relative bioavailability of doxazosin GITS is approximately 60% when compared with instant release doxazosin and the maximum plasma concentration and the area under the concentration–time curve were increased by 31% and 18% respectively when administered with a high-fat meal.[41] In normal volunteers no clinically significant differences were apparent in the disposition of doxazosin GITS in young and elderly subjects.[41]

It was anticipated that the more favourable pharmacokinetic characteristics of doxazosin GITS would translate into potential benefit by way of a more sustained and consistent blood pressure lowering effect and by minimizing the need for dose titration upon initiation of therapy. The evidence from a series of clinical studies suggests that these theoretical benefits based upon pharmacokinetics are apparent.

In a study in hypertensive patients, using ambulatory BP monitoring, open-label doxazosin GITS (4 mg) daily for 6 weeks significantly reduced systolic and diastolic BP when compared with baseline, throughout a 24-hour period.[42] The antihypertensive effect was sustained consistently over the full dosage interval, preserving the normal 24-hour BP rhythm profile, with no significant changes in 24-hour, daytime or night-time heart rate. It might reasonably be anticipated that a smoother and consistent pharmacological effect would translate into a more favourable tolerability profile with similar clinical efficacy. Studies in both hypertension and LUTS support this hypothesis. In hypertension, an integrated analysis of two multicentre, double-blind, parallel-group studies evaluated the antihypertensive efficacy and tolerability of doxazosin GITS 4 or 8 mg daily vs. doxazosin immediate-release 1–8 mg and placebo.[43] The achieved BP reductions after 12 weeks' treatment were similar with no significant difference in trough BP at the end of the dosage interval. Similar results were apparent for the primary outcome measure of these trials with 64% of patients with doxazosin GITS and 68% with doxazosin immediate-release achieving target BP at trough. Despite similarities in the antihypertensive efficacy, differences were apparent between the two formulations. With doxazosin GITS the majority of patients (61%) were receiving the initial 4 mg dose at the end of the study, while in contrast, with immediate-release doxazosin, doses were in general evenly divided between the 2, 4 and 8 mg. This study and complementary studies in patients with LUTS provide evidence that when compared with the immediate-release form of doxazosin, treatments with the GITS formulation may be initiated at a higher therapeutic dose. This has been reinforced by two further studies, the first of which was a randomized, double-blind, three-way, cross-over, placebo-controlled comparison of 1 mg doxazosin immediate-release vs. doxazosin GITS 4 mg.[44] The study was performed in normotensive subjects with a mean age of 53 years. The study focused upon the orthostatic change in BP and heart rate after standing for 2 minutes. The maximum changes in the haemodynamic parameters over 24 hours were assessed along with the changes at the time of peak drug concentration. No significant differences were apparent for the orthostatic changes in systolic and diastolic BP and heart rate, either at the time of peak concentration or for the maximum changes during the 24-hour period.

A further study is relevant to the treatment of hypertension, particularly as sub-optimal compliance characterized by dosage emissions is frequently observed in this relatively asymptomatic condition.[45] The study involved 60 hypertensive patients previously treated with doxazosin 2 mg immediate-release, who were randomized in a double-blind fashion to parallel groups receiving either doxazosin 2 mg immediate-release or 4 mg GITS.[46] After 14 days' treatment, the achieved clinic BP did not differ between the two groups and at this point the dosage regimen was interrupted for 2 days with renewed drug ingestion on the 3rd day. Orthostatic tolerance tests were performed after renewed drug intake and the results of the maximum difference in BP between erect and supine position showed marked and significant differences between the formulations, with a substantial orthostatic effect in the doxazosin immediate-release patient group. These differences in blood pressure response were mirrored in the reported symptomatic responses of the patients, which are shown in Figure 8.5. It is apparent that the incidence of individually perceived orthostatic symptoms was statistically significantly higher with doxazosin immediate-release. Patients were also monitored with ambulatory BP monitoring during the 24-hour period after renewed drug intake. The summarizing mean profiles are illustrated in Figure 8.6 and two features warrant consideration. First, immediately before resumption of dosing, BP is significantly lower in the doxazosin GITS group compared with those on the immediate-release formulation. This suggests that, unlike immediate-release doxazosin,

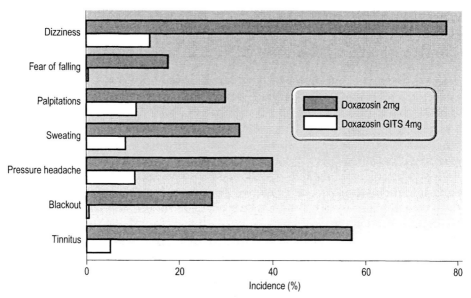

Fig. 8.5 The incidence of orthostatic symptoms after resumption of treatment with the standard and GITS formulations of doxazosin.

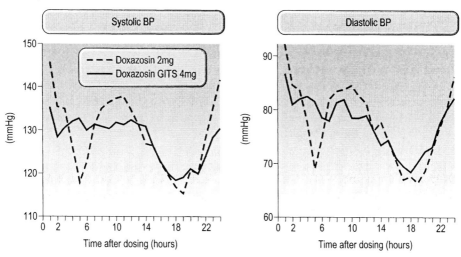

Fig. 8.6 Ambulatory blood pressure profiles following resumption of treatment after 2 days of dosage omission – comparison of standard and GITS formulations of doxazosin.

a residual benefit from treatment before the interruption in dosing is sustained with doxazosin GITS. This potential beneficial difference is also apparent 24 hours later at the end of the dosage interval. Secondly, it should be noted that a pronounced dose-related fall in BP is apparent 4–5 hours after ingestion with doxazosin immediate-release and overall blood pressure variability over the 24-hour monitoring period is much less marked with doxazosin GITS than with the immediate-release formulation.

Overall the evidence is reasonably compelling that the GITS formulation of doxazosin does produce a more favourable pharmacokinetic profile and that this translates into clinical benefit by way of a sustained and consistent pharmacodynamic effect avoiding the requirement for protracted dose titration upon initiating therapy and improved tolerability profile.

Cardiovascular outcomes

There are reasonable theoretical grounds to anticipate that α_1-adrenoceptor blockade should be associated with a significant reduction in cardiovascular events. This would be anticipated since these agents have been shown to be as effective as all the other major classes of antihypertensives in reducing BP. Furthermore there is a rationale to anticipate that α_1-blockers might offer selective benefit. Cardiovascular events occur more commonly in the morning than at other times of the day, and the diurnal BP variation also shows a peak early in the morning.[47–49] As discussed previously it is generally accepted that the sympathetic nervous system plays a major role in the regulation of BP changes and, therefore, an increase in α-adrenergic activity might be one of the major determinants of this morning BP surge.[50] The Hypertension and Lipid Trial (HALT) study revealed that the BP reduction with doxazosin was most pronounced in the morning period.[51,52] There is evidence that the morning BP surge, particularly that dependent on α-adrenergic activity, is closely associated with advanced silent cerebrovascular disease in hypertensive elderly individuals.[53]

Despite the theoretical benefits of α_1-blockade there is a relative paucity of data to support the benefit of these agents in reducing cardiovascular events. The results of a meta-analysis[54] indicate that treatment based upon α_1-adrenoceptor blockers is as effective as treatment based upon most types of antihypertensive drugs in regression of left-ventricular hypertrophy, which is often considered to be a valid surrogate, or intermediate endpoint for assessing the benefits of antihypertensive treatment. Furthermore, studies with doxazosin suggest that not only is there a significant reduction in left-ventricular mass index during 6-months therapy, but also that left-ventricular systolic and diastolic function are improved.[55]

Based upon the potential advantages associated with α_1-adrenoceptor blockade and doxazosin in particular, the ALLHAT study was designed to evaluate whether the newer antihypertensive agent was superior to standard therapy in reducing coronary events.[56] ALLHAT was a large outcome trial comparing amlodipine, lisinopril and doxazosin with the diuretic chlorthalidone. In early 2000, the doxazosin arm of ALLHAT was curtailed prematurely by the investigators due to concern related to specific outcome measures. At the time of cessation of this arm of the study, the overall result for the primary endpoint of fatal and non-fatal myocardial infarction was essentially identical in the comparison of doxazosin and chlorthalidone (Fig. 8.7). There was also no significant difference between the treatment groups with respect to all-cause mortality.[57,58] However, for the secondary endpoints there were significant ($p<0.001$) increases in combined cardiovascular disease and stroke events in patients randomized to doxazosin when compared with those assigned to chlorthalidone. Specifically, participants randomized to doxazosin experienced an 80% higher risk of heart failure (Fig. 8.8). It is interesting to note that the incidence of the heart failure endpoint at the time of termination of the doxazosin arm of the study, although somewhat higher, was not substantially different from that with lisinopril and amlodipine; yet, despite this, the investigators recommended termination of the doxazosin treatment arm.

The findings of ALLHAT have been the subject of considerable debate and the justification of the early termination of the doxazosin arm has been questioned. The investigators have argued that the rationale underlying the conduct of ALLHAT was to establish whether newer agents offered superiority when compared to established therapy. They considered that it would be highly

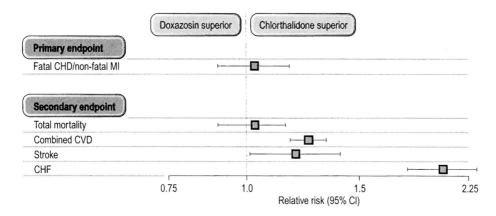

Fig. 8.7 Primary and secondary outcome measures from the ALLHAT study. Comparison of doxazosin and chlorthalidone.

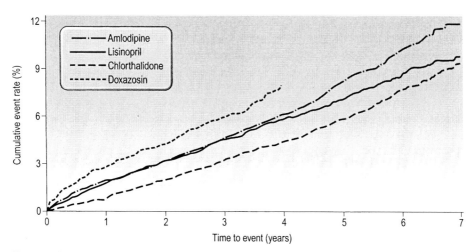

Fig. 8.8 Incidence of new onset heart failure in all treatment arms of the ALLHAT study.

unlikely that continuation of the study with doxazosin over the planned period of follow-up would result in a positive benefit for doxazosin and that the negative findings for the secondary outcomes were sufficient justification for early termination. Whilst this is not an unreasonable position, a number of issues warrant consideration. Of these the most important is that at the time of discontinuation the systolic BP levels were about 3 mmHg higher among those patients randomized to doxazosin compared with those randomized to chlorthalidone. Thus, despite seemingly inferior blood pressure control with doxazosin, there was no difference in the primary endpoint of the trial. It is important to acknowledge the impact on cardiovascular events of small blood-pressure differences, particularly in high-risk patients. Based upon the findings of the Hypertension Optimal Treatment (HOT) trial[59] and the United Kingdom Prospective Diabetes Study (UKPDS),[60] it can be argued that the 3 mmHg difference in systolic BP between the doxazosin- and chlorthalidone-treated patients could potentially explain most of the differences in stroke and heart failure between these two patient groups.[61]

There has also been much concern about the prognostic significance and the accuracy of the heart failure endpoint in ALLHAT.[62,63] The design of the study was such that patients were randomized to the four treatments immediately following cessation of previously prescribed therapy. It has been suggested that chlorthalidone, which causes a natriuresis and diuresis, and can treat or potentially mask heart failure symptoms, would result in fewer treatments or hospitalizations for heart failure when compared, in particular, with a drug such as doxazosin, which has the potential to cause sodium retention and peripheral oedema. The relatively high rates of the 'heart failure' endpoint in ALLHAT and the apparent lack of difference in mortality led to questions about whether this endpoint genuinely did represent heart failure.[61] To address this issue the ALLHAT HF Validation Study was designed to validate and elucidate the significance of heart failure events in ALLHAT.[64] An independent review of source documentation showed a high degree of agreement with the heart failure diagnosis assigned by site physicians and confirmed the higher risk of heart failure associated with first-step therapy using amlodipine, lisinopril or doxazosin, compared with chlorthalidone, at least in patients hospitalized for heart failure.

To date, ALLHAT is the only outcome study that provides any evidence regarding the cardiovascular outcomes associated with antihypertensive therapy with an α_1-adrenoceptor antagonist. However, in the Anglo Scandinavian Cardiac Outcomes Trial (ASCOT) the treatment algorithm utilized doxazosin GITS as the third agent to be introduced in both treatment arms when BP was poorly controlled. Around 50% of all patients received doxazosin GITS in ASCOT and, whilst it is difficult to draw definitive conclusions, there was no evidence of a deleterious effect on cardiovascular outcomes associated with doxazosin.[65,66]

CONCLUSIONS

With respect to the use of the selective quinazoline derivative α_1-adrenoceptor antagonist in the treatment of hypertension, no specific tissue or organ toxicity has been identified and there are no co-morbid conditions that constitute contraindications. The evidence favouring intensive BP control has clearly identified the requirement for combination drug treatment if lower BP targets are to be achieved. Furthermore, findings that patients with high levels of absolute cardiovascular risk, for example, those with diabetes mellitus or with concomitant hypercholesterolaemia, benefit most from antihypertensive treatment, indicate that an α_1-adrenoceptor antagonist may be particularly suitable in antihypertensive treatment regimens by virtue of its favourable metabolic profile. However, it is difficult to ignore the results of ALLHAT such that doxazosin, and probably all α_1-adrenoceptor antagonists, should no longer be considered as first-line agents for the treatment of hypertension, but should be regarded as a potential add-on therapy for the achievement of tight BP control.

References

1. Ahlquist RP. A study of the adrenotropic responses. *Am J Physiol* 1948;153:586–600.
2. Lund-Johansen P. Central haemodynamics in essential hypertension at rest and during exercise: a 20-year follow-up study. *Hypertens* 1989;7(Suppl):S52–S55.
3. De Quattro V, Miura Y. Neurogenic factors in human hypertension: mechanism or myth? *Am J Med* 1973;55:362–378.
4. Philipp T. Sympathetic nervous systems in essential hypertension: activity and reactivity. In: Meddeke M, Holzgreve H, eds. *New aspects of hypertension: adrenoceptors.* Berlin: Springer-Verlag; 1986:91–102.
5. Van Sweiten PA, Timmermans PBMWM, Van Brummelen P. Role of alpha adrenoceptors in hypertension and in antihypertensive drug treatment. *Am J Med* 1984;7(Suppl 4A): 17–25.
6. Reid JL. Alpha-adrenoceptors in hypertension. In: Kobinger W, Ahlquist RP, eds. *Alpha and beta adrenoceptors and the cardiovascular system.* Amsterdam: Excerpta Medica; 1984: 161–171.
7. Stokes GS, Marwood JF. Review of the use of alpha-adrenoceptor antagonists in hypertension. Methods Find Exp. *Clin Pharmacol* 1984;6:197–204.
8. Kelback H, Fransden H, Hilsted J, et al. Effects of alpha-adrenoceptor and of combined sympathetic and parasympathetic blockade on cardiac performance and vascular resistance. *Br J Clin Pharmacol* 1992;33:473–476.
9. Lund-Johansen P. Haemodynamic changes at rest and during exercise in long term prazosin therapy for essential hypertension. *Postgrad Med J* 1975;58(Suppl):45–52.
10. Lund-Johansen P, Omvik P, Haugland H. Acute and chronic haemodynamic effects of doxazosin in hypertension at rest and during exercise. *Br J Clin Pharmacol* 1986;21 (Suppl 1):45S–54S.
11. Hernandez RH, Armas de Hernandez MJ, Armas Padilla MC, et al. Doxazosin in the treatment of arterial hypertension: its effects on exercise and spirometry. *Curr Ther Res* 1998;43:610(Suppl. 1):45S–54S.
12. Civantos Calzada B, Aleixandre de Artinano A. Alpha-adrenoceptor subtypes. *Pharmacological Research* 2001;44:195–208.
13. Hieble JP, Ruffolo RRJ. Recent advances in the identification of alpha$_1$- and alpha$_2$-adrenoceptor subtypes: Therapeutic implications. *Exp Opin Invest Drugs* 1997;6:367–387.
14. Pool JL, Kirby RS. Clinical significance of alpha1-adrenoceptor selectivity in the management of benign prostatic hyperplasia. *Int Urol Nephrol* 2001;33:407–412.
15. Vincent J, Meredith PA, Reid JL, Elliott HL, Rubin PC. Prazosin. *Clin Pharmacokinet* 1985;10:144–154.
16. Sonders RC. Pharmacokinetics of terazosin. *Am J Med* 1986;80:20–24.
17. Elliott HL, Meredith PA, Vincent J, Reid J.L. The clinical pharmacology of doxazosin. *Br J Clin Pharmacol* 1986;21:S1 27S–31S.
18. Cubeddu LX, Fuenmayor N, Caplan N, Ferry D. Clinical pharmacology of doxazosin in patients with essential hypertension. *Clin Pharmacol Ther* 1987;41:439–449.
19. Frick MH, Halttunen P, Himanen P, et al. A long-term double-blind comparison of doxazosin and atenolol in patients with mild to moderate essential hypertension. *Br J Clin Pharmacol* 1986;21(Suppl 1):55S–62S.
20. Vincent J, Meredith PA, Elliott HL, Reid JL. The pharmacokinetics of doxazosin in elderly normotensives. *Br J Clin Pharmacol* 1986;21:521–524.

21. Carlson RV, Bailey RR, Begg EJ, et al. Pharmacokinetics and effect on blood pressure of doxazosin in normal subjects and patients with renal failure. *Clin Pharmacol Ther* 1986;40:561–566.

22. Elliott H.L, Donnelly R, Meredith P.A, Reid J.L. Predictability of antihypertensive responsiveness. Alpha adrenoceptor antagonism during prazosin treatment. *Clin Pharmacol Ther* 1989;46:576–583.

23. Meredith PA, Elliott HL, Kelman AW, et al. Pharmacokinetic and pharmacodynamic modelling of the alpha adrenoceptor antagonist doxazosin. *Xenobiotica* 1988;18:1293–1294.

24. Donnelly R, Meredith PA, Elliott HL. Pharmacokinetic-pharmacodynamic relationships of alpha adrenoceptor antagonists. *Clin Pharmacokinet* 1989;17:264–274.

25. Lund-Johansen P. Hemodynamic changes at rest and during exercise in long-term prazosin therapy for essential hypertension. *Postgrad. Med. J.* 1975;58(Suppl):45–52.

26. Lund-Johansen P, Omvik P, Haugland H. Acute and chronic haemodynamic effects of doxazosin in hypertension at rest and during exercise. *Br J Clin Pharmacol* 1986;21(Suppl. 1): 45S–54S.

27. Elliott HL. The case for alpha$_1$-adrenoceptor antagonists as first-line antihypertensive agents. *J Human Hypertens* 1991;5:309–311.

28. Neaton JD, Grimm JRH, Prineas RJ, et al. Treatment of mild hypertension study. Final results. *JAMA* 1993;270:713–724.

29. Brown MJ, Dickerson JEC. Alpha-blockade and calcium antagonism: an effective and well-tolerated combination for the treatment of resistant hypertension. *J Hypertens* 1995;13:701–707.

30. Brown MJ, Dickerson JEC. Synergism between alpha I blockade and angiotensin converting enzyme inhibition in essential hypertension. *J Hypertens* 1991;(Suppl 6):362–363.

31. Stokes GS, Gain JM, Mahony JF, et al. Long-term use of prazosin in combination or alone for treating hypertension. *Med J Aust* 1977;2(Suppl 1):13–16.

32. Elliott HL, McLean K, Sumner DJ, et al. Immediate cardiovascular responses to oral prazosin - effects of concurrent beta-blockers. *Clin Pharmacol Ther* 1981;29:303–309.

33. Black HR, Sollins JS, Garofalo JL. The additional of doxazosin to the therapeutic regimen of hypertensive patients inadequately controlled with other antihypertensive medications: A randomised, placebo-controlled study. *Am J Hypertens* 2000;13:468–474.

34. Black HR, Keck M, Meredith P, et al. Controlled-release doxazosin as combination therapy in hypertension: the GATES study. *J Clin Hypertens* 2006;8:159–166.

35. Mitchell BD, Stern MP, Haffner SM, et al. Risk factors for cardiovascular mortality in Mexican Americans and non-Hispanic whites. San Antonio Heart Study. *Am J Epidemiol* 1990;131:423–433.

36. Lithell HO. Effect of antihypertensive drugs on insulin, glucose, and lipid metabolism. *Diabetes Care* 1991;14:203–209.

37. Giorda C, Appendino M, Mason MG, et al. Alpha-1 blocker doxazosin improves peripheral insulin sensitivity in diabetic hypertensive patients. *Metabolism* 1995;44:673–676.

38. Zehetgruber M, Christ G, Gabriel H, et al. Effect of antihypertensive treatment with doxazosin on insulin sensitivity and fibrinolytic parameters. *Thromb Haemost* 1998;79:378–382.

39. Elliott HL, Meredith PA, Campbell L, Reid JL. The combination of prazosin and verapamil in the treatment of essential hypertension. *Clin Pharmacol Ther* 1988;43:554–560.

40. Lenz ML, Pool JL, Laddu AR, et al. Combined terazosin and verapamil therapy in essential hypertension. Hemodynamic and pharmacokinetic interactions. *Am J Hypertens* 1995;8:133–145.

41. Chung M, Vashi V, Puente J, et al. Clinical pharmacokinetics of doxazosin in a controlled-release gastrointestinal therapeutic system (GITS) formulation. *Br J Clin Pharmacol* 1999;48:678–687.

42. Lemmer B, Nold G. Effect of doxazosin GITS on 24-hour blood pressure profile in patients with stage 1 to stage 2 primary hypertension. *Blood Press Monit* 2003;8:119–125.

43. Lund-Johansen P, Kirby RS. Effect of doxazosin GITS on blood pressure in hypertensive and normotensive patients: a review of hypertension and BPH studies. *Blood Pressure* 2003; 1(Suppl):5–13.

44. Meredith PA, Koren A, Creanga D. A placebo-controlled comparison of first-dose effects of doxazosin GITS 4 mg and doxazosin standard 1 mg on blood pressure and heart rate in normotensive men. *J Clin Pharmacol* (in press).

45. Meredith PA. Therapeutic implications of drug "holidays". *Eur Heart J* 1996;17(Suppl A): 21–24.

46. Gotzen R. Vorteile der neuen Formulierung Doxazosin PP in der antihypertensiven Therapie: Orthostase - Toleranz im Vergleich zum herkömmlichen Doxazosin. *Perfusion* 1998;11:485–492.

47. Muller JE. Circadian variation in cardiovascular events. *Am J Hypertens* 1999;12(Suppl 1): 35S–42S.

48. White WB. Cardiovascular risk and therapeutic intervention for the early morning surge in blood pressure and heart rate. *Blood Press Monit* 2001;6:63–72.

49. Meredith PA, Perloff D, Mancia G, Pickering T. Blood pressure variability and its implications for antihypertensive therapy. *Blood Pressure* 1995;4:5–11.

50. Panza JA, Epstein SE, Quyyumi AA. Circadian variation in vascular tone and its relation to alpha-sympathetic vasoconstrictor activity. *N Engl J Med* 1991;325:986–990.

51. Pickering TG, Levenstein M. Hypertension and Lipid Trial Study Group and Walmsley P. Nighttime dosing of doxazosin has peak effect on morning ambulatory blood pressure. Results of the HALT Study. *Am J Hypertens* 1994;7:844–847.

52. Pickering TG, Levenstein M. Hypertension and Lipid Trial Study Group and Walmsley P. Differential effects of doxazosin on clinic and ambulatory pressure according to age, gender, and presence of white coat hypertension. Results of the HALT Study. *Am J Hypertens* 1994;7:848–852.

53. Kario K, Pickering TG, Hoshide S, et al. Morning blood pressure surge and hypertensive cerebrovascular disease: role of the alpha adrenergic sympathetic nervous system. *Am J Hypertens* 2004;17:668–675.

54. Jennings GL, Wong J. Assessment of hypertensive organ damage. In: Hansson L, Birkenhager WH, eds. *Handbook of hypertension, Vol 18*. Amsterdam: Elsevier; 1997.

55. Agabati-Rosei E, Miuiesan ML, Eizzoni D, et al. Reduction of left ventricular hypertrophy after long term antihypertensive treatment with doxazosin. *J Hum Hypertens* 1992;6:9–15.

56. Davis BR, Cutler JA, Gordon DJ, et al. Rationale and design for the Antihypertensive and Lipid Lowering Treatment to Prevent Heart Attack Trial (ALLHAT). ALLHAT Research Group. *Am J Hypertens* 1996;9:342–360.

57. ALLHAT Investigators. Major cardiovascular events in hypertensive patients randomized to doxazosin vs chlorthalidone: the Antihypertensive and Lipid-Lowering Treatment to Prevent Heart Attack Trial (ALLHAT). *JAMA* 2000;283:1967–1975.

58. Antihypertensive and Lipid-Lowering Treatment to Prevent Heart Attack Trial Collaborative Research Group. Diuretic versus alpha-blocker as first-step antihypertensive therapy: final results from the Antihypertensive and Lipid-Lowering Treatment to Prevent Heart Attack Trial (ALLHAT). *Hypertension* 2003;42:239–246.

59. Hansson L, Zanchetti AZ, Carruthers SG, et al; for the HOT Study Group. Effects of intensive blood-pressure lowering and low-dose aspirin in patients with hypertension: principal results of the Hypertension Optimal Treatment (HOT) randomised trial. *Lancet* 1998;351: 1755–1762.

60. United Kingdom Prospective Diabetes Study Group. Tight blood pressure control and risk of macrovascular and microvascular complications in type 2 diabetes: UKPDS 38. *BMJ* 1998;317:703–713.

61. Poulter N, Williams B. Doxazosin for the management of hypertension: implications of the findings of the ALLHAT trial. *Am J Hypertens* 2001;14:1170–1172.

62. Weber MA. The ALLHAT report: a case of information and misinformation. *J Clin Hypertens* 2003;5:9–13.

63. Messerli FH. ALLHAT, or the soft science of the secondary endpoint. *Ann Intern Med* 2003;139:777–780.

64. Einhorn PT, Davis BR, Massie BM, et al. ALLHAT Collaborative Research Group. The Antihypertensive and Lipid Lowering Treatment to Prevent Heart Attack Trial (ALLHAT) Heart Failure Validation Study: diagnosis and prognosis. *Am Heart J* 2007;153:42–53.

65. Dahlof B, Sever PS, Poulter NR, et al. ASCOT Investigators. Prevention of cardiovascular events with an antihypertensive regimen of amlodipine adding perindopril as required versus atenolol adding bendroflumethiazide as required, in the Anglo-Scandinavian Cardiac Outcomes Trial-Blood Pressure Lowering Arm (ASCOT-BPLA): a multicentre randomised controlled trial. *Lancet* 2005;366:895–906.

66. Poulter NR, Chang CL, Dahlof B, et al; for the ASCOT Investigators. The effects of doxazosin on blood pressure of subjects with treated but uncontrolled hypertension: evidence from the ASCOT trial. *J Human Hypertens* 2005;19:S23.

9 | Calcium channel blockers

Henry L. Elliott

INTRODUCTION

The antihypertensive efficacy of calcium channel blockers (CCBs) is well-recognized in routine clinical practice and there is now a considerable volume of evidence (from clinical outcome trials) that treatment with long-acting CCBs significantly reduces cardiovascular (CV) morbidity and mortality. This evidence of benefit has been derived in both 'primary' and 'secondary' prevention studies, in comparative studies of different antihypertensive drugs, and in different patient groups representing the whole spectrum of CV risk.

The term 'calcium channel blockers' is frequently applied as if CCBs constituted a homogeneous group in which all agents can be considered to be therapeutically equivalent, on the simplistic basis that they all share the same fundamental mechanism of action. This is a serious misconception. The positive clinical trial results cannot be generalized indiscriminately to all CCBs, but instead can only be applied to those few agents with closely similar clinical pharmacological and therapeutic profiles.

CLASSIFICATION/CHEMISTRY

The most widely used classification, and the most useful for clinical practice, reflects the chemical and structural differences between the different prototype agents: diltiazem, verapamil and nifedipine (Table 9.1). Nifedipine is the prototype for the dihydropyridine group, which has become, numerically, the most important group, while diltiazem and verapamil remain the most important representatives of their respective, relatively small, individual classes.

MECHANISM OF ACTION

Physiology

Calcium ions are involved fundamentally in a wide range of intra-cellular processes, including the release of neurotransmitters and hormones. In the

Table 9.1 Classification of calcium channel blockers (based on chemical structures: selected examples)

Dihydropyridines	Phenylalkylamines
Amlodipine	Verapamil
Felodipine	**Benzothiazepines**
Isradipine	Diltiazem
Lacidipine	
Lercanidipine	
Manidipine	
Nifedipine	
Nimodipine	
Nitrendipine	
Nisoldipine	

cardiovascular system, increased intra-cellular calcium concentrations trigger the actin-myocin interaction and the resultant contraction of myocardial cells and vascular smooth muscle cells. In the heart, calcium ions are also necessary for the pacemaker activity of the sinus node and for conduction through the atrio-ventricular node.

The concentration of intra-cellular calcium ions, under resting conditions, is far lower than that of the extra-cellular concentration. This concentration gradient is regulated by three pathways of which the 'voltage-operated' and 'receptor-operated' channels are the most important. Control of the entry of calcium ions and, thereby, control of the relative intra- and extra-cellular calcium ion concentrations in the cardiovascular system resides primarily with the 'voltage-operated' calcium channels. At least six different types of these channels have been identified in mammalian cells. However, according to present knowledge, it appears that functions within the CV system are mainly dependent upon the long-lasting L-type channel (which is the principal target of all currently available CCBs) and, to a lesser extent, the transient T-type channel.

Pharmacology

Interference with the entry of calcium ions (i.e. calcium channel blockade) and thereby interference with vascular smooth muscle contractility, i.e. vaso-relaxation/arterial vasodilatation are the most obvious consequences of calcium channel blocking drugs. The overall pattern of the therapeutic response to an individual CCB, however, is determined by the net result from the combination of:

(i) the arterial vasodilator effect
(ii) the direct effects on cardiac conduction and contractility
(iii) the indirect consequences of reflex activation of the sympathetic nervous system (SNS).

(*Note:* The extent of the activation of the SNS is a direct consequence of the rate of onset of the vasodilator effect.)

In pharmacological terms, the detailed impact on the CV system of each CCB is determined by its impact on the differential distribution and differential 'gating' thresholds of L- and T-Type calcium channels which, in turn, reflect

Table 9.2 Indicative cardiovascular profiles of different calcium channel blockers

	Nifedipine	Diltiazem	Verapamil
Peripheral vasodilatation	+++	++	++
Heart rate	~0*	− −	− −
Cardiac effects			
a) AV conduction	~0*	− −	− −
b) Contractility	~0*	− −	− −

*Only if long-acting GITS formulation

the differing abilities of each different CCB to penetrate to different tissues and different calcium channels. In pharmacokinetic terms, the rate of drug delivery into the systemic circulation is the defining factor.

In clinical terms, the most obvious differences between the three major classes of CCB relate to the relative differences of their effects on the arterial system and the heart (Table 9.2). These can be summarized as follows: arterial vasodilatation is the predominant feature of the dihydropyridine group, e.g. nifedipine/amlodipine; in contrast, with diltiazem and verapamil, there is a mixed picture of arterial vasodilatation and reduced cardiac activity with negative chronotropic and dromotropic effects. This 'reduced' cardiac activity is summarized in terms of reduced heart rate (the term 'rate-limiting' is often applied to these drugs), slowing of Atrio-ventricular (AV) conduction and anti-arrhythmic properties, and reduced cardiac contractility (Table 9.2).

Less well recognized, but arguably of greater practical importance, are the clinically relevant differences between different drugs within the dihydropyridine group. These relate to the rate of onset of action, the duration of action, and the magnitude and intensity of the reflex activation of the sympathetic (adrenergic) nervous system (see Pharmacodynamics).

PHARMACOKINETICS/METABOLISM

In contrast to their chemical and pharmacological diversity, there is a remarkable similarity in the pharmacokinetic characteristics of the three prototype CCBs in their original formulations (Table 9.3). In summary, diltiazem, nifedipine and verapamil are all subject to extensive, first-pass pre-systemic (hepatic) metabolism and rapid clearance. As a consequence, oral bioavailabilities are comparatively low; the apparent oral clearances are subject to wide inter- and

Table 9.3 Comparative pharmacokinetic characteristics of prototype calcium channel blockers

	Nifedipine	Verapamil	Diltiazem
Bioavailability (%)	30–60	10–30	30–60
Elimination half-life (hours)	3–5	3–7	3–6
Dosing schedule	t.i.d.	b.d./t.i.d.	b.d./t.i.d.

intra-individual variability; and elimination half-lives are relatively short. In practical terms, each of these drugs (in their original formulations) requires to be administered at least twice or three times daily to achieve any degree of consistency in the steady-state plasma drug-concentration–time profiles.

The synthesis of newer CCBs has resulted mainly in an expansion of the dihydropyridine group. Many of these agents have pharmacokinetic character-istics similar to those of nifedipine and, despite claims to the contrary, closely similar pharmacodynamic profiles. However, some agents, most notably amlo-dipine, have significant and important pharmacokinetic differences (Table 9.4). Although amlodipine undergoes extensive hepatic metabolism, there is no sig-nificant first-pass component, absorption from the gastrointestinal (GI) tract is gradual, oral bioavailability is relatively high, clearance is relatively slow and the elimination half-life is prolonged (approximately 40 hours). There also are so-called 'lipophilic' dihydropyridine derivatives, e.g. lacidipine and lercanidi-pine (Table 9.4), which again have extensive pre-systemic metabolism, rela-tively low bioavailability and relatively short plasma half-lives: but these agents have high volumes of distribution, which have been attributed to their membrane-binding characteristics which, in turn, extend the duration of action despite rapid drug elimination from plasma.

More recent CCB developments have had a more pragmatic focus on reduc-ing the fluctuations in the plasma drug concentrations and prolonging the duration of action. Such pharmaceutical manipulation is only relevant when there is a direct pharmacokinetic-pharmacodynamic relationship, i.e. the thera-peutic response profile is directly related to the drug-concentration–time pro-file. These concentration–effect relationships have now been established for most CCBs, particularly through studies of the antihypertensive response, and there is now a considerable volume of evidence that the magnitude and duration of the pharmacological/therapeutic response correlates directly with the drug-concentration–time profile. Thus, the essential rationale for development of modified release pharmaceutical formulations is to sustain the circulating drug-concentration profiles. The usual goal of these modified release formulations is the production of a steady-state, plasma drug-concentration–time profile, which is consistently sustained throughout 24 hours following once daily dosing. This goal has not been achieved with equal suc-cess with all such modified release formulations (despite the claims of some pharmaceutical companies!), but there are two successful formulations, which appear to be particularly worthy of note: nifedipine GITS and verapamil

Table 9.4 Comparative pharmacokinetic characteristics of selected 'modern' dihydropyridine calcium channel blockers

	Amlodipine	Nifedipine GITS	Felodipine	Lacidipine
Time to peak (hours)	6–12	5–10	3–7	1–3
'Apparent' half-life (hours)	35–50	16–22	10–15	3–8
Oral bioavailability (%)	65–80	30–60	15–35	5–15
Extensive first pass Metabolism	No	Yes	Yes	Yes

COER. The gastrointestinal therapeutic system (GITS) is a specialized osmotic pump formulation, which produces a plasma drug-concentration–time profile for nifedipine, which is relatively smooth and consistent throughout each 24-hour period (Table 9.4). The controlled onset extended release (COER) formulation of verapamil also utilizes osmotic pump technology, but with a further encapsulation: this formulation is deliberately designed to produce sustained and consistent therapeutic drug levels throughout the daytime period, but relatively low levels during the overnight period.

PHARMACODYNAMICS

The development of modified-release formulations for the majority of CCBs is a clear reflection of the direct relationship between the time profile of the therapeutic (antihypertensive) response and the underlying plasma (blood) drug-concentration–time profile. This fundamental consideration is often ignored.

Antihypertensive effect

The principal pharmacodynamic response to blockade of the L-type calcium channel is arterial vasodilatation and, thereby, blood pressure reduction. The magnitude and duration of the blood pressure lowering effect (and of other pharmacological effects) across each 24 hours is a reflection of a direct concentration–effect (pharmacokinetic–pharmacodynamic) relationship. This is most obvious under steady-state conditions when drug concentrations are relatively stable and without wide fluctuations. However, the net pharmacological response becomes more complex when there are rapid and wide fluctuations in the drug-concentration–time profile because the rapid onset of a pronounced vasodilator effect provokes a reflex activation of the sympathetic nervous system, which manifests most obviously as an increase in heart rate. Thus, 'rate of delivery' of drug into the systemic circulation is an important determinant of the overall, resultant pharmacodynamic profile. These pharmacological principles, and their important pharmacodynamic/therapeutic consequences, were clearly illustrated in an elegant study by Kleinbloesem et al. (1987).[1]

In this cross-over study, nifedipine was administered intravenously to a group of normal, healthy volunteers by two different infusion regimens: either by a rapid bolus followed by an exponential infusion (rapid infusion) or by a slow, constant rate infusion (slow infusion). Closely similar plasma nifedipine concentrations were attained across the period of 4–10 hours after the start of the two different infusion regimens (top panel, Fig. 9.1). However, the patterns of the heart rate and blood pressure (BP) responses were significantly different. Following the rapid infusion, there was a marked increase in heart rate but only a negligible blood pressure reduction: in contrast, with the slow infusion, there was no discernible increase in heart rate, but there was a significant blood pressure reduction (middle and lower panels, Fig. 9.1). Since the achieved plasma drug concentrations were essentially the same, the difference in the pattern of the haemodynamic responses was attributable to the rate of change (increase) in the drug concentrations. To complete the experiment,

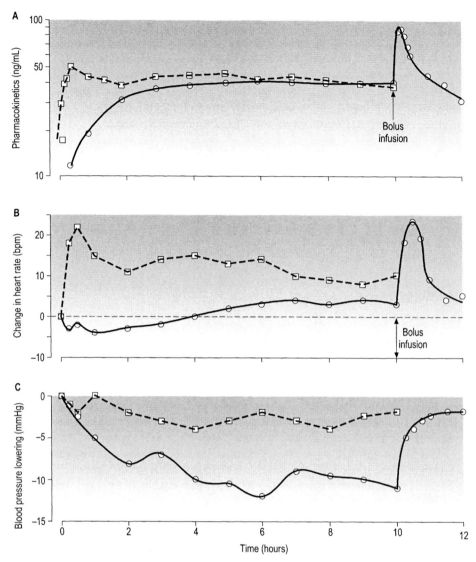

Fig. 9.1 A comparison of the drug-concentration profiles (upper panel), heart rate responses (middle panel) and blood pressure responses (lower panel) following nifedipine administered intravenously as a rapid bolus followed by an exponential infusion (□) or a continuous slow infusion. (○) *(Adapted from ref. (1).)*

a rapid intravenous bolus dose of nifedipine was superimposed at the end of the slow infusion: there was an almost immediate increase in heart rate and loss of the blood pressure-lowering effect.

In summary, rapid increases in nifedipine concentrations lead to a rapid vasodilator response, which provokes a reflex activation of the sympathetic (adrenergic) nervous system, a significant increase in heart rate (and cardiac output) and no effective blood pressure reduction. In contrast, the slow attainment of smoothly maintained nifedipine concentrations leads to a correspondingly gradual and sustained vasodilator effect and antihypertensive response, with little or no reflex sympathetic activation or cardio-acceleration.

Other pharmacological effects

As discussed for dihydropyridine CCBs, the pattern of the haemodynamic and related pharmacological effects is intimately linked to the rate of drug delivery. A wide range of other non-haemodynamic properties have been explored in the experimental setting: these include interference with the development of new atherosclerotic lesions, preservation/improvement of endothelial function, anti-oxidant activity, etc. In some of the clinical studies there is evidence consistent with the concepts derived from the experimental studies and suggestive evidence of benefits beyond the haemodynamic. In large-scale clinical outcome trials (ALLHAT and INSIGHT, for example), renal function (estimated GFR) was better preserved by a long-acting CCB compared with a thiazide diuretic; also in INSIGHT, markers for the progression of atherosclerotic disease in both the coronary and carotid arteries were significantly more retarded/blunted with the CCB despite comparable levels of clinic blood pressure control. The ultimate clinical relevance of these 'benefits beyond BP control' remains to be clearly established.

ADVERSE EFFECTS/CONTRAINDICATIONS

Dihydropyridine group

The most common adverse effects are pharmacologically predictable. With the early, short-acting, rapid-onset agents (e.g. nifedipine in its original capsule formulation) the rapid onset of vasodilatation is frequently associated with headache, flushing and tachycardia/palpitations. With the long-acting agents the tolerability profile is much more favourable with a much lower incidence of overt vasodilator effects: however, peripheral (ankle) oedema is reported in approximately 5–10% of patients, with clear dose-related frequency. For illustrative purposes, the rates of adverse effects reported in two comparative clinical outcome trials (INSIGHT and ASCOT) are summarized in Tables 9.5 and 9.6.

Table 9.5 Comparison of adverse events with amlodipine and atenolol in ASCOT

	Amlodipine-based (%)	Atenolol-based
Peripheral oedema	23	6
Cough	19	8
Joint swelling	14	3
Dizziness	12	16
Fatigue	8	16
Chest pain	8	9
Vertigo	7	8
Dyspnoea	6	10
Erectile dysfunction	6	7

Adverse events with an incidence of more than 5% and a statistically significant difference of more than 1% between treatment groups
(Adapted from ref. (14).)

Table 9.6 Comparison of symptomatic adverse events in INSIGHT

	Nifedipine GITS	Coamilozide
Peripheral oedema	28	4
Headache	12	9
Dizziness	8	10
Depression	4	6
Peripheral vascular disease	3	6

Adverse events with an incidence of more than 5% and a statistically significant difference of more than 1% between treatments
(Adapted from ref. (6).)

Diltiazem and verapamil

Vasodilator-related effects are also observed, albeit with lower incidences than with the dihydropyridines. Occasionally, bradycardia, AV conduction abnormalities and reduced cardiac contractility are seen: these also are dose related. Constipation is a recognized complication of verapamil treatment.

DRUG INTERACTIONS

Pharmacokinetic interactions

All CCBs undergo extensive hepatic metabolism and, potentially at least, there is the prospect of interactions related to effects on drug metabolism. This is particularly relevant for verapamil and diltiazem, which both inhibit hepatic enzyme activity. This creates the potential for not only a range of pharmacokinetic drug interactions, but also auto-inhibition of the clearance rate of the index drug, such that steady-state half-lives are significantly longer than single-dose half-lives. Because CCBs are most likely to be prescribed for patients with cardiovascular disorders, interactions of clinical relevance are most likely to occur with other cardiovascular drugs.

Digoxin
There is a well-recognized interaction with verapamil whereby the steady-state plasma digoxin concentrations are increased by 40–90% as a result of decreased clearance, both renal and non-renal. The exact mechanism remains unclear.

Ciclosporin
Co-administration with either verapamil or diltiazem leads to significant increases in ciclosporin concentrations as a consequence of reduced clearance. In some circumstances this interaction can be 'harnessed' to permit the deliberate use of smaller doses of ciclosporin.

Grapefruit juice
This affects some CCBs, most notably felodipine, whereby felodipine concentrations are significantly increased as a result of reduced clearance secondary to specific inhibition of the activity of hepatic cytochrome P450 3A4.

Pharmacodynamic interactions

In clinical practice, the combination of a dihydropyridine CCB with a β-blocker is illustrative of a positive pharmacodynamic interaction that enhances the overall therapeutic effect. Any tendency for the CCB to provoke a reflex increase heart rate is attenuated by the β-blocker and the tendency for the β-blocker to interfere with the peripheral circulation is countered by the vaso-dilator effect of the CCB.

Almost the converse of this is the negative pharmacodynamic interaction between verapamil (and diltiazem) and a β-blocker, which leads to a contraindi-cation for such a combination because of the additive, negative cardiac effects: reduced heart rate, slowed cardiac conduction and impaired myocardial contractility.

CLINICAL USE/OUTCOME DATA

Despite chemical diversity, and pharmacological differences, all CCBs are effective antihypertensive agents because calcium channel blockade opposes the mechanisms underlying the relative vasoconstriction and increased periph-eral vascular resistance of established essential hypertension. Nevertheless, there are clinically relevant differences not only between the dihydropyridine group and diltiazem/verapamil, but also within the dihydropyridine group where the once-daily, gradual-onset, long-acting drugs and formulations have the most favourable therapeutic profiles. Furthermore, the clinical outcome evidence in favour of CCBs in hypertension is heavily dependent upon the evidence derived from studies involving the long-acting dihydropyridines, amlodipine and nifedipine GITS.

General considerations

The benefits of antihypertensive drug treatment in patients with mild-to-moderate hypertension, in terms of reducing cardiovascular (CV) morbidity and mortality, were established about 10–20 years ago through a series of pla-cebo-controlled clinical trials. The accumulated evidence from these clinical trials was distilled in the well-known meta-analysis of Collins and McMahon (1994)[2] (Fig. 9.2). This analysis calculated that modest reductions in BP by about 6 mmHg in diastolic BP, for example, were associated with reductions of 38% in stroke (CVA) events and 16% in CHD events. However, none of the trials incorporated within the meta-analysis involved a CCB as a primary treatment.

Following upon the widespread acceptance that BP reduction by drug treatment is beneficial, clinical trials were then designed to address specific treatment issues, e.g. isolated systolic hypertension, overall cardiovascular risk and concomitant risk factors and, importantly for CCBs, the strength of the evi-dence supporting the use of a particular drug or drug class. In turn, some of the most recent clinical trials have focused on the relative efficacy of different types of antihypertensive drug treatment. Thus, the evidence base establishing the place of CCBs in current antihypertensive treatment has been derived from clinical trials undertaken within the past 10 years.

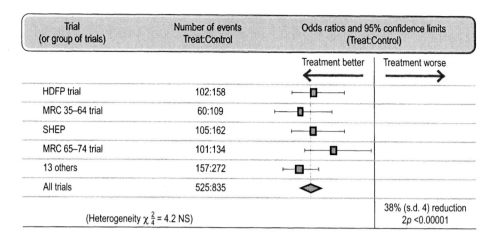

Fig. 9.2 Reductions in stroke (upper panel) and in coronary heart disease (lower panel) from a meta-analysis of the results from a total of 17 controlled, clinical outcome trials. *(Adapted from ref. (2).)*

Clinical trial evidence with calcium channel blockers

The results of the recent, most important CCB clinical outcome trials are briefly summarized as follows:

SYST-EUR (1997)

This was the first appropriately randomized intervention trial to show that antihypertensive treatment with a CCB (nitrendipine) significantly reduced CV morbidity and mortality.[3] In effect, this was the last major placebo-controlled clinical outcome trial in patients with isolated systolic hypertension. The trial was terminated early because of the substantial benefits in the active treatment group. These benefits with a CCB-based treatment were similar to those obtained in the earlier SHEP study (1991) that employed 'conventional' antihypertensive treatment based upon the diuretic, chlorthalidone (followed by the β-blocker, atenolol).

In summary, antihypertensive treatment based on a CCB led to significant reductions in fatal and non-fatal stroke (by 42%) and in all CV endpoints (by 31%). Although it failed to achieve conventional statistical significance, there was also a 30% reduction in myocardial infarction. These results were consistent with those obtained with 'conventional' antihypertensive drug treatment.

HOT (1998)

The Hypertension Optimal Treatment study is unique because it was not a placebo or treatment comparison, but instead its primary objective was the assessment of different levels of blood pressure control targeted to levels of ≤90, ≤85, and ≤80 mmHg for diastolic BP.[4] Treatment was based on felodipine (modified release) with other agents added to achieve the blood pressure targets. Ultimately, the blood pressure levels achieved in the three groups averaged respectively 145/85, 143/83 and 141/81 mmHg. Although there were only small differences in achieved BP between the three groups, better blood pressure control was associated with a progressive decline in all major CV events. This trend was significant for fatal and non-fatal myocardial infarction, and particularly in the sub-group of high-risk patients with diabetes mellitus.

In summary, the greater the reduction in BP with a CCB-based treatment, the greater the outcome benefits.

STOP-2 (1999)

This study in elderly hypertensive patients compared 'old' and 'new' types of antihypertensive drugs, i.e. treatment based on β-blockers (including atenolol) or diuretics, particularly hydrochlorothiazide plus amiloride, versus ACE inhibitors and CCBs, particularly felodipine and isradipine.[5] The overall conclusions were that the blood pressure reductions and the CV benefits were comparable for the two treatment approaches, although the study had only limited discriminatory power.

Again, a CCB-based regimen is equally as effective as a 'conventional' treatment regimen, i.e. no evidence of poorer outcomes or harmful consequences.

INSIGHT (2000)

This is one of the most important CCB trials insofar as treatment based on a 'modern', appropriately-formulated, long-acting, once-daily CCB (nifedipine GITS) was compared with a 'reference' antihypertensive agent, hydrochlorothiazide plus amiloride (coamilozide).[6] Control of BP in a total of about 6000 high-risk hypertensive patients was equivalent in both treatment groups, according to conventional clinic blood pressure measurements, and the rates for CV events were also equivalent.

This study clearly confirmed the safety and efficacy of a treatment based on a CCB as a primary prevention antihypertensive treatment, with outcome benefits similar to those seen with a 'reference' agent, the diuretic coamilozide.

NORDIL (2000)

The CCB in this trial was diltiazem, but the overall results and conclusions are consistent with those obtained in other recent clinical outcome trials with different dihydropyridine CCBs.[7] There was no statistically significant difference in terms of the primary endpoint (a composite of fatal and non-fatal stroke myocardial infarction and CV mortality), but for the secondary endpoint of stroke itself there was a 20% better outcome with the CCB.

Thus, the overall conclusion was that treatment based on a CCB was equally as effective as treatment based on a diuretic and/or a β-blocker.

ALLHAT (2002)

This is the larges-ever trial of the drug treatment of patients with hypertension. It was designed to compare four different types of initial treatment randomly assigned to more than 40 000 patients: amlodipine (CCB), chlorthalidone (diuretic), doxazosin (selective α_1-blocker) and lisinopril (ACE inhibitor).[8] Thereafter, using a slightly unusual selection of drugs, further drug treatments were added to achieve blood pressure control. The doxazosin arm was terminated prematurely because of significantly poorer results for heart failure and stroke, relative to chlorthalidone, which was the reference treatment. For the formal primary endpoint of fatal and non-fatal myocardial infarction and coronary heart disease events, there were no statistically significant differences between the other three treatments: the event rates were 11.5, 11.4 and 11.3%, respectively, for chlorthalidone, lisinopril and amlodipine. Unfortunately, despite the huge volume of data, very few definitive conclusions about differential treatment effects can be drawn from ALLHAT, because of imperfections in the concept, design, conduct, results and analysis of the trial. The most important factor confounding the interpretation of the results was that there were significant differences in blood pressure control: for example, achieved BP was significantly lower in the chlorthalidone group (for systolic BP, by 1 mmHg vs. the amlodipine group and by 2 mmHg vs. the lisinopril group). For the sub-group of African-American patients, this blood pressure difference increased to 4 mmHg for chlorthalidone vs. lisinopril, in association with a 40% reduction in stroke. However, it remains uncertain whether the outcome benefit is attributable to the superior stroke-prevention properties of chlorthalidone, or simply to the better blood pressure control achieved in that patient group.

In brief summary, the salient findings in ALLHAT are that blood pressure reduction is of primary importance for reducing CV morbidity and mortality and, in turn, that the CCB amlodipine as an initial treatment is equal in effectiveness to the 'reference' diuretic, chlorthalidone in reducing CV events. As a side issue, but one of considerable current importance, ALLHAT also identified that the development of type 2 diabetes might be a long-term problem with chlorthalidone, particularly relative to the long-term effect of the ACE inhibitor, lisinopril.

INVEST (2003)

As with NORDIL, this large trial involved a non-dihydropyridine CCB: verapamil.[9] The conclusions were similar to those of NORDIL and contribute to the body of evidence that antihypertensive treatment based on a CCB is at least equivalent to other types of antihypertensive treatment regimens. Thus, 22 576 patients with hypertension and coronary artery disease received either a CCB-based treatment or a β-blocker-based treatment (other agents, particularly the ACE inhibitor, trandolapril and the diuretic, hydrochlorothiazide, respectively, were added for blood pressure control).

In summary, a treatment strategy based upon a CCB (with added trandola-pril) was as clinically effective as a strategy based upon a β-blocker/thiazide combination.

VALUE (2004)

Conceptually, the Valsartan Antihypertensive Long-term Use Evaluation was a very ambitious project (perhaps over-ambitious!).[10] It was designed to test the hypothesis that, for equivalent blood pressure control in high-risk hypertensive patients, the angiotensin II receptor antagonist valsartan would reduce cardiac morbidity and mortality to a greater extent than the CCB amlodipine. Unfortu-nately, blood pressure control was not equivalent: especially during the first 6 months of treatment, blood pressure control was significantly better with amlodipine. Consequently, the outcome trends also favoured amlodipine, including a statistically significantly greater reduction (by 9%) in fatal and non-fatal myocardial infarction.

In an attempt to 'rescue' the original hypothesis, a further statistical analysis was undertaken to match patients for achieved BP (and other characteristics).[11] This post-hoc analysis concluded that, overall, both treatments were equivalent for preventing cardiac events (there was even an advantage for valsartan in a significantly lower rate of hospitalization for heart failure).

In summary, despite the statistical manipulations, it must again be con-cluded that the effectiveness of the blood pressure reduction determines the magnitude of the outcome benefits and that there is no evidence that a CCB is infe-rior to another type of antihypertensive drug treatment. From the post-hoc analy-sis, it might be further concluded that satisfactory blood pressure control should be attained as quickly as is reasonably possible (within 6 months of starting treatment).

ACTION (2004)

This is a clinical trial of patients with chronic stable angina, but it is directly rel-evant for the use of CCBs in hypertension for the following reasons: 52% of the 7665 patients were hypertensive (>140/90 mmHg) at baseline; the outcome benefits were particularly apparent in the hypertensive sub-group and, with the study designed in the light of the controversy of the early 1990s, the safety of CCBs was confirmed in high-risk hypertensive patients with known coronary artery disease.[12,13]

In summary, treatment with nifedipine GITS reduced BP by 6.6/3.6 mmHg in the hypertensive sub-group and was associated with a significant 13% reduction in the composite endpoint of all-cause mortality, myocardial infarc-tion, refractory angina, heart failure, stroke and revascularization interventions. Of particular note, was the 38% reduction in new heart failure.

ASCOT (2005)

The Anglo-Scandinavian Cardiac Outcomes Trial involved 19 257 patients, mean age 63 years, with hypertension and at least three other CV risk fac-tors.[14,15] The trial was statistically powered in terms of a reduction in the pri-mary endpoint of CHD events and involved two different types of treatment modality: antihypertensive drug treatment ('new' versus 'old' drugs) in combination with lipid-lowering treatment (statin versus placebo).

The 'new' treatment was based on amlodipine followed by perindopril and compared with 'old' antihypertensive treatment based on atenolol followed by bendroflumethiazide. Ultimately, 86% of patients in the amlodipine group and 91% in the atenolol group were on combination treatment: in effect, therefore, ASCOT compared amlodipine *plus* perindopril against atenolol *plus* bendroflumethiazide.

The following are the salient results from ASCOT:

(a) Because the totality of the outcome evidence was significantly better in the amlodipine group (Table 9.7), the trial was stopped prematurely. For this reason (probably), the achieved 10% reduction in the specified primary endpoint (fatal coronary heart disease and non-fatal myocardial infarction) fell short of statistical significance.
(b) There was a significant blood pressure difference in the course of the trial, by an overall average of 2.7/1.7 mmHg, in favour of the amlodipine group. This difference was most marked during the first 6 months of the trial.
(c) There were significantly fewer cases, by 33%, of new-onset type 2 diabetes mellitus in the amlodipine/perindopril group.
(d) The combination of a statin with antihypertensive drug treatment was associated with clear and significant additional benefits. By way of illustration, at the most extreme, the 'new' combined treatment strategy effectively halved the rate of CV events: 48% fewer CHD events and 48% fewer stroke events with amlodipine plus perindopril plus atorvastatin, relative to the 'old' strategy of atenolol plus bendroflumethiazide (plus placebo).

Other clinical trial evidence

In addition to the major outcome trials, there has been a plethora of other clinical studies exploring surrogate or intermediate CV endpoints. Studies of microalbuminuria and renal function in diabetic nephropathy have been

Table 9.7 Outcome evidence in ASCOT

	Amlodipine-based	Atenolol-based	RRR	Significance
	Rate per 1000 patients		%	p-value
Primary endpoint				
Non-fatal myocardial infarction	8.2	9.1	−10	n.s.
Secondary endpoints				
Non-fatal myocardial infarction (excluding fatal coronary heart disease)	7.4	8.5	−13	<0.05
Total coronary heart disease	14.6	16.8	−13	<0.01
Total cardiovascular events/ procedures	27.4	32.8	−16	<0.0001
All-cause mortality	13.9	15.5	−11	<0.05
Cardiovascular mortality	4.9	6.5	−24	<0.001
All stroke	6.2	8.1	−23	<0.0005
All heart failure	2.5	3.0	−16	n.s.

(Adapted from ref. (14).)

particularly numerous but there have been many other studies exploring anti-atherosclerotic properties, effects on endothelial function, etc. CCBs have featured in many such studies and the results with modern long-acting agents have been comparable to those with other agents. Overall, the results indicate that the greatest benefit is attributable to rigorous control of BP and that additional blood pressure reduction contributes more than any postulated differential drug effect.

CONCLUSIONS

That CCBs are effective antihypertensive drugs is not in doubt: arguably, CCBs are the most effective blood pressure-lowering drugs available at the present time. Despite this antihypertensive efficacy, the debate of the 1990s sought to suggest that CCBs might be less effective for reducing CV morbidity and mortality (in fact, that they might be positively harmful/dangerous). The concerns and controversies surrounding the safety and efficacy of CCBs in the 1990s should now be consigned to history, along with the short- and intermediate-acting CCBs, whose shortcomings contributed to the creation of the debate. There is now clear evidence that *modern*, long-acting CCBs are safe and effective antihypertensive drugs that achieve CV benefits, which are at least equivalent to those of other types of antihypertensive drugs.

Whilst recognizing that there are weaknesses and unanswered questions within the available evidence, the recent clinical outcome trials have established the safety and efficacy of CCBs for the routine management of hypertension. In conjunction with their clinical pharmacological characteristics, the evidence from clinical outcome trials and the results from other clinical trials addressing surrogate or intermediate endpoints, the 'best-qualified' CCBs for routine antihypertensive treatment appear to be amlodipine and nifedipine GITS. In specific types of patient, modified release formulations of either verapamil or diltiazem also have important clinical roles.

In line with the 'ABCD rule' guiding the routine use of antihypertensive drugs, there is clear evidence that CCBs should now be considered to be appropriate first-line agents, particularly in older (over 55 years) hypertensive patients.[16] However, with the increasing evidence that the magnitude of the blood pressure reduction and the attainment of 'tight' blood pressure control determine patient outcomes (rather than the pharmacological properties of any individual drug or drug class), there is an obvious move towards antihypertensive drug-treatment combinations. Since more than 50% of patients will require at least two antihypertensive drugs to achieve good blood pressure control, the choice of the first drug has become relatively unimportant. Instead, the emphasis is on the (relatively) rapid establishment of blood pressure control using a combination of drugs. In terms of the clinical-outcome evidence allied to the awareness of possible adverse, long-term metabolic effects, particularly type 2 diabetes, the most appropriate antihypertensive treatment appears to be the combination of a long-acting CCB and an ACE inhibitor. The evidence from ASCOT, in particular, highlights the requirement for combination treatments. This was noted earlier in NORDIL in which more than 50% of patients defaulted from their original assigned treatment: thus, it might be construed that the 'best' outcomes are associated with combination treatments, which include a CCB.

233

In summary, therefore, the evidence, in terms of volume, consistency and quality, seems to indicate that amlodipine and nifedipine GITS are the 'best qualified' CCBs for routine use in the modern management of hypertension across the whole spectrum of hypertensive patients and cardiovascular risk.

References

1. Kleinbloesem CH, van Brummelen P, van de Linde JA, et al. Nifedipine: kinetics and dynamics in healthy subjects. *Clin Pharm Ther* 1984;35:742–749.
2. Collins R, McMahon S. Blood pressure, antihypertensive drug treatment and the risks of stroke and coronary heart disease. *Br Med Bull* 1994;50:272–298.
3. Staessen JA, Fagard R, Thijs L, et al. Randomised double-blind comparison of placebo and active treatments for older patients with isolated systolic hypertension (Syst-Eur). *Lancet* 1997;350:757–764.
4. Hansson L, Zanchetti A, Carruthers SG, et al. Effects of intensive blood pressure lowering and low-dose aspirin in patients with hypertension: principal results of the Hypertension Optimal Treatment (HOT) trial. *Lancet* 1998;351:1755–1762.
5. Hansson L, Lindholm LH, Ekbom T, et al. Randomised trial of old and new antihypertensive drugs in elderly patients: cardiovascular morbidity and mortality in the Swedish Trial in Old Patients with Hypertension-2 study. *Lancet* 1999;354:1751–1756.
6. Brown M, Palmer C, Castaigne A, et al. Morbidity and mortality in patients randomised to double-blind treatment with a long-acting calcium channel blocker or diuretic in the International Nifedipine GITS study: Intervention as a Goal in Hypertension Treatment (INSIGHT). *Lancet* 2000;356:366–372.
7. Hansson L, Hedner T, Lund-Johanson P, et al. Randomised trial of effects of calcium antagonists compared with diuretics and beta-blockers on cardiovascular morbidity and mortality in hypertension: the Nordic Diltiazem (NORDIL) study. *Lancet* 2000;356:359–365.
8. The ALLHAT Officers and Coordinators for the ALLHAT Collaborative Research Group. Major outcomes in high-risk hypertensive patients randomised to angiotensin converting enzyme inhibitor or calcium channel blocker vs diuretic: The antihypertensive and lipid-lowering treatment to prevent heart attack trial (ALLHAT). *JAMA* 2002;288:2981–2997.
9. Pepine CJ, Handberg EM, Cooper-DeHoff RM, et al. A calcium antagonist vs. a non-calcium antagonist hypertension treatment strategy for patients with coronary artery disease: the International Verapamil-Trandolapril Study (INVEST): a randomised controlled trial. *JAMA* 2003;290:2805–2816.
10. Julius S, Kjeldsen SE, Weber M, et al. Outcomes in hypertensive patients at high cardiovascular risk treated with regimens based on valsartan or amlodipine: the VALUE randomised trial. *Lancet* 2004;363:2022–2031.
11. Weber MA, Julius S, Kjeldsen SE, et al. Blood pressure dependent and independent effects of antihypertensive treatment on clinical events in the VALUE trial. *Lancet* 2004;363:2049–2051.
12. Poole-Wilson PA, Lubsen J, Kirwan B-A, et al. Effect of long-acting nifedipine on mortality and cardiovascular morbidity in patients with stable angina requiring treatment (ACTION trial): randomised controlled trial. *Lancet* 2004;364:849–857.
13. Lubsen J, Wagener G, Kirwan B-A, et al. Effect of long-acting nifedipine on mortality and cardiovascular morbidity in patients with symptomatic stable angina and hypertension: the ACTION trial. *J Hypertens* 2005;23:641–648.
14. Dahlöf B, Sever PS, Poulter NR for the ASCOT investigators. Prevention of cardiovascular events with an antihypertensive regimen of amlodipine adding perindopril as required versus atenolol adding bendroflumethiazide as required, in the Anglo-Scandinavian Cardiac Outcomes Trial-Blood Pressure Lowering Arm (ASCOT-BPLA): a multicentre randomised controlled trial. *Lancet* 2005;366:895–906.
15. Poulter NR, Wedel H, Dahlöf B for the ASCOT investigators. Role of blood pressure and other variables in the differential cardiovascular event rates noted in the Anglo-Scandinavian Cardiac Outcomes Trial-Blood Pressure Lowering Arm (ASCOT-BPLA). *Lancet* 2005;366: 907–913.
16. Williams B, Poulter N, Brown M, et al. Guidelines for management of hypertension: report of the fourth working party of the British Hypertension Society 2004-BHS-IV. *J Human Hypertens* 2004;18:139–185.

10 | Potent vasodilators

Gordon T. McInnes

INTRODUCTION

Over the past three decades, antihypertensive drug therapy has made a tremendous impact on morbidity and mortality from cardiovascular disease. Nevertheless, despite the introduction of newer modalities for treatment, improvement in cardiovascular outcomes appears to have stalled. End-stage renal disease and congestive heart failure, both related to hypertension, continue to increase unabated. Since rigorous control of blood pressure (BP) is needed to maximally improve outcome and few patients achieve this with first-choice therapy, a wide selection of antihypertensive agents is desirable.

Most antihypertensive drugs lower BP through reduction of peripheral vascular resistance. In some cases, this effect is indirect as a result of actions upon neural or humoral control systems. Other drugs have direct actions upon vascular smooth muscle.

Among the most effective antihypertensive drugs are those that inhibit sympathetic activity. This may be achieved at practically any anatomic level of adrenergic function. For these compounds to maintain effectiveness over time, however, for the most part use in combination with a diuretic is necessary.

The term vasodilator was originally reserved for direct-acting vascular smooth muscle relaxants. Individual vasodilators may act upon resistance vessels, large arteries or venous capacitance vessels.

Differential actions at these sites play a major role in the haemodynamic profile of the drugs (Table 10.1).[1,2] A predominant action upon the resistance vessels causes an immediate fall in BP, activation of baroreceptor reflexes and increased cardiac output.[3,4] Orthostatic hypotension is not seen. By contrast, relaxation in the venous capacitance vessels causes a reduction of venous return to the heart and a fall in cardiac output associated with a fall in BP.[5] Cardiovascular baroreceptors are again activated.

Changes in the patterns of the large arterial waveform resulting from large arterial relaxation and dilatation of resistance vessels may have important consequences for the development of atheroma. These changes may not be

Table 10.1 Correlation of relative activity of vasodilator drugs in resistance and capacitance vessels with circulatory effects

	Arterioselective	Non-selective	Venoselective
Cardiac output	↓↑	↑	↓ (upright)
Arterial pressure	↓	↓	↓ (greater upright)
Central venous pressure	No change	No change	↓
Pulmonary artery pressure	↑		↓

reflected in BP measured conventionally in the brachial artery.[6] Therefore, it seems possible that different types of vasodilators may have differential consequences for cardiovascular morbidity, although there are no endpoint data to define a particularly favourable pattern.

There are other consequences of vasodilator therapy apart from activation of the sympathetic nervous system. Parasympathetic withdrawal contributes to the cardiac response.[7] Renin and aldosterone levels are usually increased, partly as a result of increased sympathetic activity and partly as a result of decreased renal arterial perfusion pressure.[8] Agents that have a predominant action upon resistance vessels produce oedema by increased capillary hydrostatic pressure resulting in disturbance of the Starling equilibrium. This is not seen with venodilator drugs.

Every direct-acting smooth muscle vasodilator and most adrenergic inhibitors induce compensatory sodium and water retention and extracellular fluid volume expansion following reduction of arterial pressure.[9–11] To maintain persistent and steady contraction of fluid volume, concomitant diuretic therapy is needed. A thiazide is generally the best choice for patients with relatively normal renal function because duration of action is greater than that of a loop diuretic. The diuretic enhances antihypertensive action by maintaining constriction of the extracellular and intracellular compartments.

ROLE OF VASODILATORS IN HYPERTENSION

The heterogeneous action of vasodilators is reflected in the different indications for usage. Because of the availability of newer, better tolerated drugs, in most developed countries use is restricted to management of patients with severe hypertension not readily controlled with other agents, parenteral treatment of hypertensive emergencies, and in hypertension of pregnancy.

Whereas use of vasodilators has decreased drastically in favour of newer agents with different mechanisms of action, these agents continue to be used widely around the world. No doubt, this is related to the availability of generic formulations of vasodilators and lower cost.

MECHANISM OF ACTION AND PHARMACOKINETICS

Adrenergic inhibitors

Central adrenergic efferent impulses pass through major cardiovascular control centres in the hypothalamus, medulla and other subcortical areas of the spinal cord to synapse with second neurones located in the sympathetic ganglia at the thoracolumbar level of the spinal column. These most distal neurones are stimulated at the ganglion level by the release of acetylcholine from the terminals of the central neurones, thereby propagating the peripheral outflow of adrenergic impulses. Neural impulses, passing distally via the adrenergic neurones, reach the heart or blood vessels, where noradrenaline (norepinephrine) is released from nerve terminals. Noradrenaline (norepinephrine) stimulates the effector organ – heart, venule or arteriole – by attachment to specific binding sites, α- or β-adrenergic receptors.

Noradrenaline (norepinephrine) is the major neurotransmitter released from post-ganglionic nerve terminals. Synthesis of noradrenaline (norepinephrine) begins with the essential amino acid, L-tyrosine and proceeds via various intermediates including dopamine. Noradrenaline (norepinephrine) is the major neurotransmitter and is mostly responsible for adrenergic stimulation. It is found in the axon sheath and is stored in the nerve terminal in vesicles that release noradrenaline (norepinephrine) on nerve stimulation. Noradrenaline (norepinephrine) is metabolized within the nerve terminal by monoamine oxidase in the mitochondria.

With the arrival of the adrenergic impulse at the post-ganglionic nerve terminal, there is release of free noradrenaline (norepinephrine). The neurotransmitter may bind to myocardial and/or vascular smooth muscle receptors, producing the adrenergic cardiovascular response. Noradrenaline (norepinephrine) may also be taken up by the nerve terminal (re-uptake) for conservation and later release or may be acted upon by the extraneuronal enzymatic system to form metabolites or circulate freely within the vascular system.

Binding of noradrenaline (norepinephrine) at the respective receptor may result in several possible processes. Stimulation of the β-adrenergic receptor will produce vasoconstriction of the arteriole and venule. Stimulation of the α-adrenergic receptor will promote peripheral vasodilatation and increase heart rate, myocardial contractility and myocardial metabolism.

There are many loci at which antihypertensive agents may inhibit the adrenergic nerve stimulus, including efferent sensory pathways from the heart, vessels and mechanoreceptors; centrally, at the ganglion level; or at the nerve terminal. Certain antihypertensive agents may also inhibit noradrenaline (norepinephrine) biosynthesis or block its action at the adrenergic receptor.

Ganglion blocking drugs

When the adrenergic pre-ganglionic impulse arrives at the ganglia, acetylcholine is released from the nerve terminals, crosses the synaptic gap, and stimulates the post-ganglionic axons. The physiochemical action at the axon membrane is complex but involves alteration of permeability. Thus, when acetylcholine attaches to the axon membrane, transmembrane ion flux is permitted, by which potassium ions move extracellularly and sodium ions intracellularly. When the depolarization process reaches the optimal rate, transmission of the neural impulse to the post-ganglionic neurone continues.[12]

Ganglion blockers act by occupying receptor sites on the post-ganglionic axon to stabilize the membrane against acetylcholine stimulation. These drugs have no effect on pre-ganglionic acetylcholine release, cholinesterase activity, post-ganglionic neuronal catecholamine release, or vascular smooth muscle contractility.[12–14]

Adrenergic transmission to the heart and vessels is impaired, with the result that heart rate, myocardial contractility and total peripheral resistance are reduced. The fall in arterial pressure and vascular resistance is not as great in the supine as in the upright position because the adrenergic venomotor effect is enhanced by the gravitational effect of pooling blood when the patient is upright.

Examples include hexamethonium, pentolinium, mecamylamine, pempidine, chlorisondamine and trimetaphan. At equivalent doses, chlorisondamine, mecamylamine and pentolinium are equally effective in reducing arterial pressure.[15] The only widely used agent in this class, trimetaphan, is excreted by glomerular filtration and active secretion; 30% is unchanged in urine.

Post-ganglionic adrenergic inhibitors

When acetylcholine stimulates the post-ganglionic axon at the ganglionic level, the impulse is propagated and cumulates in the release of noradrenaline (norepinephrine) at the nerve terminal with stimulation of adrenergic receptors in the vascular smooth muscle membrane. The impulse can be interrupted pharmacologically by a variety of mechanisms, including depletion of neurohumoral stores at the nerve terminal, prevention of noradrenaline (norepinephrine) uptake by the nerve terminal, inhibition of catecholamine biosynthesis, and therapeutic introduction of false neurotransmitters that block the adrenergic receptors on vascular smooth muscle.

Rawolfia alkaloids   Reserpine and more than 20 related compounds deplete the myocardium, blood vessels, adrenergic nerve terminals, adrenal medulla and brain of catecholamines and serotonin.[16,17] By depleting the nerve terminal of noradrenaline (norepinephrine) stores and inhibiting noradrenaline (norepinephrine) re-uptake, adrenergic transmission is altered so that vascular resistance falls. With prolonged treatment, persistent arterial hypotension is associated with slight decreases in renal blood flow and glomerular filtration rate. This may be related to the reduction in cardiac output or a venodilator effect similar to that of ganglion blocking drugs.[16,18]

Reserpine has oral bioavailability of 30%. Plasma half-life is prolonged (1–2 weeks). Plasma protein binding is 96%.

Adrenergic neurone-blocking agents   These agents interfere with adrenergic neurotransmission at the post-ganglionic nerve terminals. Like reserpine, there is depletion of catecholamine stores in nerve terminals, blood vessels and the myocardium but, unlike reserpine, there is little effect on catecholamine stores in the adrenal glands or brain. With catecholamine depletion and impairment of chemical neurotransmission, denervation supersensitivity of effector cells is achieved.[19,20]

After ingestion, there is a transient pressor phase associated with increased heart rate and cardiac output related to catecholamine release. A prolonged period of cardiac, vascular and nerve terminal catecholamine depletion follows, associated with progressive reduction in systemic and pulmonary arterial pressure. The arterial pressure reduction, brought about through interference in chemical neurotransmission, can be explained by reduction in vascular resistance. Hypotension is less marked in the supine posture or with agents that simultaneously contract or prevent re-expansion of plasma volume.[9–11]

Guanethidine has oral absorption of 50–60% despite undergoing quite extensive pre-systemic metabolism (30–40%). Plasma half-life is 2–8 days and protein binding is less than 10%. Metabolism is in the liver.

Bethanidine has complete oral absorption and undergoes no significant pre-systemic metabolism. Plasma half-life is 8–15 hours. Plasma protein binding is less than 10%. Bethanidine is excreted unchanged in the urine.

Debrisoquine has oral absorption of less than 85%. There is no pre-systemic metabolism and half-life is 10–26 hours. Protein binding is 25%.

Metabolism is subject to genetic polymorphism via the P450 isoenzyme, P450 II DI. Some 92% of Caucasians are extensive metabolizers and 8% have poor metabolizer phenotypes. Plasma concentrations are several-fold higher in poor metabolizers. Debrisoquine is used as a prototype drug for oxidative polymorphism which affects the metabolism of 20–30 other drugs.

After single oral doses (20 mg), antihypertensive efficacy is usually only evident in poor metabolizers and lasts up to 8 hours. Debrisoquine 40 mg causes detectable falls in standing BP in extensive metabolizers lasting up to 8 hours, and on lying and standing BP for up to 48 hours in poor metabolizers. Cardiac output falls initially, but returns to normal during chronic administration, probably because of salt and water retention.

Bretylium was withdrawn as an antihypertensive agent because of incomplete and variable absorption after oral administration, rapid occurrence of tolerance and high rate of side effects. This drug is unsuitable for long-term use.

Monoamine oxidase inhibitors   Examples include pargyline, tranylcypromine, phenylzine and iproniazid. Pargyline was introduced primarily as an antihypertensive agent. Only a relatively few hypertensive individuals were studied and results were not striking. One report claimed marked reduction in arterial pressure and vascular resistance, with moderate impairment of glomerular filtration.[21]

Veratrium alkaloids   These agents influence the responsiveness of vagal efferent nerve fibres in the coronary sinus, left ventricle, and carotid sinus so that any pressure will result in altered nerve traffic. The stimulus is interpreted in the medullary vasomotor centre as reflecting a higher pressure than actually exists, as a result of an induced delay in the vagal repolarization process.

The altered input to the cerebral vasomotor centres results in a reflexive fall in BP and heart rate; the latter response may be abolished by atropine. Because adrenergic function is not blocked, but only reset at a different pressure level, the usual postural and adrenergic reflexive responses are not altered. The result is a significant fall in peripheral resistance with little change in cardiac output despite marked bradycardia. Cerebral and renal blood flow and glomerular filtration rate remain normal unless the hypotensive response is excessive.

Direct-acting vascular smooth muscle relaxants

Agents in this class act by decreasing arteriolar resistance. Mechanisms of action are variable, although the final common pathway is vascular smooth muscle relaxation (Fig. 10.1).

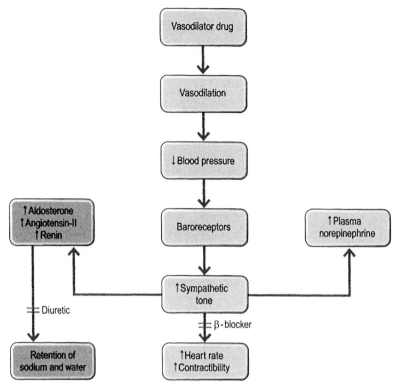

Fig. 10.1 Reflex mechanisms triggered by vasodilation induced by vasodilator drugs.

Hydralazine

Hydralazine is a dilator of resistance vessels and has little action on venous beds.[2,22] After intravenous administration hydralazine has slow onset of action over 15–20 minutes. BP fall is accompanied by baroreceptor-mediated sympathetic activation, with tachycardia and sweating. After oral administration, onset of action is gradual and duration of action is prolonged. The peak effect is seen 30–120 minutes after dosing. Higher doses do not increase the peak BP reduction but prolong the duration of action.

The precise mode of action is unknown but hydralazine causes activation of guanylate cyclase and accumulation of cyclic guanosine monophosphate (GMP).[23] By altering cellular calcium metabolism, hydralazine interferes with the movement of calcium that is responsible for initiating or maintaining the contractile state of vascular smooth muscle. Accumulation of cyclic GMP stimulates cyclic GMP-dependent protein kinase. This eventually leads to dephosphorylation of the light chain of myosin, which is thought to be involved in the contractile process in the phosphorylated form. Preferential dilation of arterioles (versus veins) minimizes postural hypotension, promotes increased cardiac output and tends to lower diastolic more than systolic BP. Blood flow increases in coronary, cerebral and renal vascular beds.

In addition, a component of action is dependent on the presence of intact endothelium. In vitro incubation of red cells with hydralazine gives rise to nitric oxide generation.[24,25] Thus, hydralazine may cause release of nitric oxide from the vascular endothelium. Hydralazine also stimulates the renin–angiotensin–

aldosterone (RAAS) system. This, together with a compensatory increase in heart rate and contractility, tends to counteract the antihypertensive effect.

Hydralazine is rapidly and completely (100%) absorbed from the gastrointestinal tract after oral administration.[22] The time to maximum serum concentration is 1–2 hours. Biotransformation commences in the gut wall and during first-pass through the liver (pre-systemic metabolism 65–90%).[22] The liver is the major site of metabolism of hydralazine. Of the administered dose, 80% is excreted in the urine almost entirely as metabolites. The major metabolic pathways are N-acetylation and hydroxylation with subsequent glucuronidation. Biotransformation is impaired in uraemia.[22] Plasma half-life is 2–4 hours.[22] The half-life of antihypertensive action is much longer than the plasma half-life.[22] Plasma protein binding is 87%.

The acetylation pathway is subject to genetic polymorphism. Elimination is more rapid in 'fast acetylators' than in 'slow acetylators'. 'Slow acetylators' have almost twice the plasma concentration of that in 'fast acetylators'. N-acetylation is significantly involved in first-pass metabolism. Acetylation phenotype has little effect on metabolism after parenteral administration. During the initial period, serum hydralazine concentrations correlate with antihypertensive effects.[22] This leads to greater antihypertensive effect and greater risk of a lupus syndrome in 'slow acetylators'.

Endralazine

Endralazine is a vasodilator chemically similar to hydralazine. Acetylation is not a major route of metabolism and, therefore, response is not related to acetylator phenotype.[26,27]

Minoxidil

Treatment is associated with dilatation of resistance vessels.[28] There is little or no action on the venous bed. Minoxidil acts by activation of adenosine triphosphate (ATP)-sensitive potassium channels in arterial smooth muscle.[29,30] As a result, the smooth muscle membrane is hyperpolarized and calcium influx through voltage-gated calcium channels is inhibited. Cytosolic calcium concentration is reduced.

Oral absorption is 100%. Plasma half-life is 2.8–4.2 hours and plasma protein binding is negligible. Minoxidil is extensively metabolized in the liver along four pathways: glucuronidation (67%), hydroxylation (25%), sulphation and conversion to an uncharacterized polar compound.[31] The sulphated metabolite is pharmacologically active and probably accounts for much of the activity of the parent drug.

Diazoxide

Diazoxide is a non-natriuretic thiazide congener that is an extremely potent vasodilator,[32,33] acting on resistance vessels and without effect on the venous bed.[34] The mode of action is opening of ATP-sensitive potassium channels in vascular smooth muscle cells.[34]

Oral absorption is 85–95%. Plasma half-life is 28 hours. Over 90% of diazoxide is protein bound. Elimination is primarily by glomerular filtration. About 20% is metabolized in the liver to non-active hydroxymethyl and carboxy metabolites.

Sodium nitroprusside

Sodium nitroprusside is administered as a slow intravenous infusion to produce a rapidly reversible decrease in BP.[35,36] The mode of action is to increase GMP within vascular smooth muscle activating vasorelaxation. This effect is probably mediated by non-enzymatic degradation of nitric oxide. The result is activation of vascular smooth muscle soluble guanylate cyclase with generation of cyclic adenosine monophosphate (AMP).[37]

Sodium nitroprusside is mainly excreted through the kidney. Clearance is extremely rapid. Half-life for BP lowering is 32–40 seconds. The antihypertensive effect is potentiated in renal failure but, since a dose-titration regimen is employed, adjustment of dose is unnecessary. The drug is metabolized non-enzymatically to cyanide, which reacts with thiosulphates to form thiocyanate, which is also excreted through the kidney.[38] The metabolic products of sodium nitroprusside are not active in the cardiovascular system.

Potassium channel agonists

The recognition that minoxidil and diazoxide acted through smooth muscle potassium channels increased interest in other agents with a similar mode of action and which may not give rise to the same serious side effects.[29,39,40] Hyperpolarization of the vascular smooth muscle membrane inhibits the opening of voltage-operated calcium channels and increases excretion of calcium by sodium-calcium exchange, inhibiting intracellular calcium release, and increases uptake of noradrenaline (norepinephrine) by the extraneuronal catecholamine transporter. Potassium channel activators cause vasodilatation of small and large arteries, but have little effect on the venous circulation. As glucose-stimulated insulin release is mediated by closure of pancreatic β-cell potassium channels, these agents would be expected to inhibit insulin response, but this does not occur with most members of the class.[40] The most extensively investigated agents are pinacidil, chromakalim and nicorandil.

Pinacidil has high oral absorption. Half-life is 1.6–2.9 hours. Plasma protein binding is 40%. Metabolism and elimination is by biotransformation in the liver via cytochrome P-450, followed by renal elimination.

Nicorandil has a nitrate moeity incorporated in the molecule. This significantly modifies the pharmacological vasodilator profile.[41] Thus, nicorandil increases smooth muscle cyclic GMP.[42,43] Reduction in systemic vascular resistance is associated with vasodilatation. Tachycardia is transient and cardiac output is not usually increased.

INDICATIONS AND CONTRAINDICATIONS

Adrenergic inhibitors

Ganglion blocking drugs

Because interference with transmission of the autonomic impulse at the ganglion level impairs adrenergic and parasympathetic impulse transmission, the clinical use of ganglion blockers is associated with severe side effects and unwanted parasympathetic inhibition. With the advent of newer agents, ganglion blockers have become mostly of academic interest.

The exception is trimetaphan, which is still used as an antihypertensive agent. Trimetaphan is delivered by slow intravenous infusion.[44] The starting dose is 0.5–2 mg/minute and the adequate dose is usually 0.5–6 mg/minute. Reduction of arterial pressure is immediate. Marked interindividual variability necessitates direct arterial BP monitoring. When the infusion is discontinued, return of arterial pressure to pre-infusion levels is prompt. Thus, when administered in severe hypertension, long-acting antihypertensive therapy must be initiated before discontinuing the infusion.

Volume constriction is associated with an augmented antihypertensive response and noradrenaline (norepinephrine) is associated with an enhanced pressor response. The phenomenon of denervation supersensitivity is extremely important in patients treated with sympatholytic agents.

Tachyphylaxis develops on prolonged use. Trimetaphan is rarely used in hypertensive crisis/emergencies because better agents are available. The drug is still used in hypertension with dissecting aortic aneurysm where trimetaphan reduces velocity of ventricular ejection and hence sheering force. Also, in controlling hypertension in acute aortic dissection, during surgery and in arteriography, trimetaphan may be more manageable than agents with more prolonged action. Under these circumstances, ganglion blockade will not be associated with the secondary reflexive stimulation of the heart that is found with other vasodilators.

There are several contraindications to trimetaphan including atheromatous vascular disease, because of reduced blood supply; pyloric stenosis, because of compromised gastric outflow via ganglionic blockade and, in pregnancy, because of the risk of paralytic or meconium ileus in the newborn. The duration of action of suxamethonium is prolonged by inhibition of pseudocholinesterase. The neuromuscular blocking action of trimetaphan enhances non-depolarizing muscle relaxants.

Rawolfia alkaloids

Reserpine and similar alkaloids are efficacious in reducing arterial pressure when used with a diuretic.[45,46] Reserpine is generally added to the treatment regimen if response to a thiazide (or thiazide-like) diuretic is inadequate. Reserpine is also useful in treating hypertensive emergencies.[47]

The maintenance dose of reserpine is up to 0.1 mg daily. Since reserpine has a long half-life, a loading dose is employed to obtain a reasonably rapid steady-state concentration.

Reserpine is contraindicated absolutely in depression and in those with a history of depression. The drug is also contraindicated in severe renal failure and is best avoided in peptic ulceration, ulcerative colitis or asthma. Reserpine may cause complications in the neonate if used in pregnancy. These include nasal obstruction (anosmia), bradycardia and hypothermia. Thus, reserpine is no longer a drug of choice in hypertensive emergencies in pregnancy. A reduced dose is recommended in the elderly.

Several drug interactions have been reported. There is enhanced peripheral vasodilatation and hypotension with alcohol. Enhanced falls in BP are also seen with glyceryl trinitrate, L-dopa, fenfluramine and phenothiazines. The pressor effects of phenylephrine and catecholamines are enhanced while the effect of direct acting amines, such as ephedrine, is diminished. There is excessive central nervous system excitation with monomine oxidase inhibitors. Reserpine lowers the convulsive threshold in epilepsy. The bradycardic effect of digoxin and the negative isotropic effects of anti-arrhythmic agents, such as disopyramide and quinidine, are enhanced. There is increased myocardial depression with halothane and increased prolactin/breast enlargement with the oral contraceptive steroids.

Adrenergic neurone-blocking agents

Guanethidine Because of prolonged action and because sympathetic inhibition is usually maximal at night, guanethidine needs to be administered only once daily. The starting dose of 10 mg is titrated to the required dose, usually 25–75 mg daily, although up to 200–300 mg daily may be needed. Antihypertensive effect can be hastened by initiation with a loading dose.

Because fluid retention and expanded intravascular and extracellular fluid volumes are prominent, a diuretic is indicated, with the caveat that patients should be monitored carefully for hypokalaemia and impaired renal excretory function. The phenomenon is due to fluid expansion, since impairment of drug absorption over time seems unlikely. However, the common adverse effect of diarrhoea may reduce absorption. Abrupt withdrawal is not associated with rebound hypertension because of the prolonged half-life.

The mechanism of action leads to postural hypotension particularly after exercise or circumstances favouring vasodilatation such as heat, alcohol or pyrexia. This is a particular risk in the elderly and when a diuretic is added.

When urgent reduction of BP is indicated, guanethidine can be given parenterally (intramuscular or intravenous). A slow intravenous infusion or intramuscular injection avoids the initial pressor response due to catecholamine release. The maximum effect after intramuscular use is seen in 1–2 hours.

Guanethidine is safe in pregnancy. Loss of BP control may be due to drug interactions; uptake into adrenergic nerve endings is reduced by concomitant tricyclic antidepressant therapy.

Bethanidine The initial dose 5–10 mg three times daily is titrated as necessary to a maximum dose of 200 mg daily. Bethanidine was widely used as third drug in combination with a thiazide and a β-blocker. The drug accumulates in renal failure where antihypertensive effect may be enhanced.

Debrisoquine The dose range is 20–400 mg daily administered by twice or thrice daily dosing regimens. Debrisoquine is used with β-blocker and diuretic to avoid fluid retention. Poor metabolizers respond to 10 mg twice daily which is, therefore, the usual starting dose unless the metabolic phenotype is known. The starting dose is 40 mg twice daily in extensive metabolizers.

Adrenergic neurone-blocking agents are contraindicated in phaeochromocytoma. Withdrawal of neurally released noradrenaline (norepinephrine) renders vasodilator-treated individuals extremely sensitive to circulating catecholamines. These drugs may exaggerate hypertension consequent on sudden release of catecholamines from the tumour.

Monoamine oxidase inhibitors

Monamine oxidase inhibitors may aggravate hypertension by inhibition of noradrenaline (norepinephrine) metabolism. Because monoamine oxidase is inhibited in the post-ganglionic nerve terminal, several weak pressor amines accumulate at this site. These substances are believed to act as false neurohumoral transmitters, tending to elevate BP.[48] Because of the potentially severe hypertensive crisis that may be associated with use of monoamine oxidase inhibitors, these drugs should be considered primarily of academic interest in the treatment of hypertension.

Veratrium alkaloids

Clinical use has been severely restricted by side effects.

Direct-acting smooth muscle relaxants

With the fall in total peripheral resistance and arterial pressure, reflex stimulation of the heart occurs so that tachycardia and palpitation results frequently, unless the cardiac reflex responses are offset by an adrenergic inhibitor, usually a β-blocker. These agents should not be administered to hypertensive patients with heart failure, myocardial infarction, angina or aortic dissection because the reflexive cardiac effects will aggravate the underlying cardiac condition.

Hydralazine

Hydralazine entered the therapeutic armamentarium shortly after the ganglion blocking agents and was one of the most effective drugs in the 1950s.[49] Usage declined rapidly in the 1960s with recognition of frequent lupus reactions and sympathetic nervous system activation. Hydralazine returned to regular usage in stepped-care regimens of the late 1960s, in combination with β-blocker and diuretic. The side effect profile is improved substantially by reduction of dose and combined use with a β-blocker. Hydralazine has largely been replaced by other peripheral acting drugs and is now not widely used, although the drug remains effective and safe in specialist hands.

Hydralazine is usually administered three or four times daily, preferably starting with an individual dose of 12.5–25 mg. A lower dose (10 mg) may be used if there are side effects. The dose is then increased as necessary to a maximum of 200–300 mg daily. Slow acetylators show greater lowering of BP;[22] the daily dose should not exceed 200 mg. High doses are more likely to be associated with development of anti-nuclear antibodies (ANA) and a lupus-like syndrome.[22] The acetylator phenotype can be determined readily by a simple urinary test of sulphonamide acetylation.[50] Periodic full blood count and ANA titres are recommended during chronic hydralazine therapy. Since hydralazine undergoes hepatic metabolism, dose adjustment is unnecessary in renal impairment. Hydralazine is rarely used alone, because increases in cardiac output lead to palpitation, headache and reduced BP reduction.

Pre-treatment with a β-blocker prevents sympathetic activation, reduces side effects, and potentiates the antihypertensive action.[51] Hydralazine is used with a β-blocker and diuretic to control moderate-to-severe hypertension. Where renal function is seriously impaired, a loop diuretic rather than a thiazide is needed to avoid oedema. A multicentre trial[52] evaluated hydralazine, labetalol, methyldopa, prazosin and placebo for value as a third drug when added to ongoing β-blocker and diuretic treatment. Overall, hydralazine was the most generally suitable third drug. No significant difference in antihypertensive effect was apparent between methyldopa, prazosin, labetalol and hydralazine, but hydralazine performed better than all other treatments for reported and observed side effects.

Hydralazine was the vasodilator used in several early major clinical outcome trials. Much of the early information demonstrated that antihypertensive therapy can diminish the morbidity and mortality involved hydralazine-treated patients.[45,46,53,54] A combination of reserpine, hydrochlorothiazide and hydralazine was used in the landmark Veterans Administration Co-operative Study Group Trials,[45,46] which demonstrated unequivocally the merits of antihypertensive therapy, not only in severe but also in moderate hypertension.

For urgent control of BP, hydralazine can be given parenterally. Onset of action is in 15 minutes,[3] but the dose and frequency of administration required for BP control is highly variable, the long duration of action makes dose titration difficult, and many patients do not respond adequately to any dose of hydralazine. Therefore, hydralazine is not an ideal drug for hypertensive emergencies. Sodium nitroprusside is more effective if continuous monitoring in an intensive therapy unit is available. Intramuscular hydralazine provides a simpler parenteral option. After a test dose of 10 mg, repeated doses can be given at 30-minute intervals in doubling doses up to an individual dose of 80 mg. Alternatively, hydralazine can be administered intravenously. BP control is usually achieved in 2–3 hours.

Although there have been no formal studies in pregnancy, and although the drug is teratogenic in some animals, hydralazine is widely used in pregnant women.[55] Hypertensive emergencies associated with pregnancy treated with hydralazine include pre-eclampsia and eclampsia.

The main contraindication is coronary artery disease, since increased cardiac output increases cardiac work and may provoke angina and myocardial ischaemia or infarction. However, if hypertension is severe, reduction in BP and cardiac work will more than compensate. In mitral valve disease, hydralazine may increase pulmonary artery pressure and induce congestive heart failure.

Endralazine lowers BP over 24 hours with once daily dosing.[56]

Minoxidil

Because of the severity of adverse effects, usage is limited to severe hypertension unresponsive to other treatments.[57] Minoxidil is usually administered twice daily with an initial dose of 2.5–5 mg. Once daily dosing is sometimes employed. The maximum daily dose is usually 50 mg, although doses up to 100 mg have been used.

Pre-treatment with a β-blocker limits sympathetic activation.[58] Sodium retention requires concomitant diuretic therapy in most. A loop diuretic is often necessary.

Minoxidil is excreted into breast milk and, therefore, is best avoided in breast-feeding mothers. Safety in pregnancy has not been established.

Diazoxide

Oral diazoxide can be used in resistant hypertension as a twice daily regimen, although the long half-life suggests that once daily treatment may be sufficient. A graded sustained fall in BP usually results. The initial dose is 50–100 mg twice daily, increasing as necessary to a total daily dose of 1 g.[59] The severity of side effects has rendered this usage largely obsolete.

Intravenous diazoxide is still occasionally used in the treatment of hypertensive emergencies. Diazoxide has been useful for the patient with hypertensive encephalopathy and severe, malignant or accelerated hypertension (without heart failure) in whom rapid and immediate reduction in arterial pressure is mandatory. BP is lowered rapidly and consistently but rarely below normal. The first dose is usually effective and the action persists for several hours. The maximal daily dose is 150 mg. Higher doses previously used were associated with unacceptable hypotension and exacerbation of ischaemic heart disease. For the same reason, rapid infusion is no longer recommended and the bolus should be administered over about 10 minutes.[60] Repeated doses can be administered every 5–15 minutes until target BP is achieved. After each dose, the patient should remain recumbent and should be closely monitored for 30 minutes. Diazoxide increases cardiac output and, therefore, maintains good tissue perfusion when BP is reduced. β-blockade increases the antihypertensive effect by antagonizing the reflex increase on cardiac output. Lower doses should be used in patients already receiving antihypertensive agents.

Diazoxide has been successful in severe hypertension in childhood. The usual effective dose is 5 mg/kg. Hypertensive crises induced by phaeochromocytoma or due to monoamine oxidase inhibitor therapy should not be treated with diazoxide since BP responds more specifically to α-blockers such as phentolamine. Safety in pregnancy has not been demonstrated conclusively.

Contraindications include subarachnoid haemorrhage, intracerebral haemorrhage and post-operative bleeding, functional hypoglycaemia, hypersensitivity to thiazides and dissecting aortic aneurysm where the increase in stroke volume and left-ventricular ejection rate reflexively induced by diazoxide augment stresses in the aortic wall. The antidiuretic properties of diazoxide may lead to significant fluid retention, which may precipitate congestive heart failure in patients with impaired cardiac reserve. Fluid retention responds to diuretics, but concomitant therapy may potentiate hyperglycaemia and hyperuricaemia.

Sodium nitroprusside

Sodium nitroprusside is used for the short-term treatment of severely hypertensive patients at high risk, to normalize BP before and during surgery for renal artery stenosis or phaeochromocytoma, in hypotensive anaesthesia and in dissecting aortic aneurysm. Sodium nitroprusside is useful in hypertensive emergencies because of rapid onset of action, titratability and rapid reversibility of excess BP reduction.

The absence of tachycardia in most patients means that sodium nitroprusside is free of the cardiac symptoms produced by some other vasodilators. The drug is administered dissolved in 5% dextrose in water as an intravenous infusion using an infusion pump or drip regulator. The infusion should be protected from light using aluminium foil.

The drip rate is titrated against BP. The average dose is 0.5–8.0 μg/kg/minute. The rate should be increased slowly to prevent or reduce compensatory reactions (sharp rises in catecholamines and renin, tachycardia and tachyphylaxis). The infusion should not be terminated abruptly to prevent excessive rebound in BP. The starting dose of 0.3–1.0 μg/kg/minute is increased gradually until the desired BP reduction is achieved, preferably while monitoring intra-arterial BP. To avoid excessive levels of cyanide and to lessen the possibility of precipitous BP reduction, the maximum recommended dose is 8 µg/kg/minute. If this is insufficient, another approach should be tried.

Prolonged infusions are undesirable because of the risk of thiocyanate intoxication, but if continuous therapy over several days is required, acid–base balance should be assessed by measurement of plasma bicarbonate, lactate and the lactate:pyruvate ratio. This is a more sensitive measure of intoxication than plasma concentration of the thiocyanate or cyanide under these conditions since toxicity is associated with the development of acidosis.

Sodium nitroprusside is contraindicated in severe liver impairment, Leber's optic atrophy or tobacco amblyopia. Precaution is needed in disturbed cerebral blood flow because of the risk of too rapid lowering of BP. Caution is also required in hypothyroidism because thiocyanate inhibits iodine uptake and binding by the thyroid. Care should be taken in renal failure because excretion of thiocyanate is decreased.

Potassium channel agonists

Pinacidil Greatest experience in hypertension is with this agent.[61] Pinacidil is usually administered as a sustained release preparation. In doses ranging from 12.5 to 37.5 mg twice daily, pinacidil has a useful BP lowering action. Dose-dependent oedema offsets the antihypertensive effect. This can be overcome by concomitant diuretic. Pinacidil is contraindicated in congestive heart failure and should be used with caution in coronary or cerebrovascular disease and tachyarrhythmias because of the tendency to tachycardia.

Since pinacidil undergoes hepatic metabolism, dose reduction is advised in severe hepatic dysfunction and in the elderly because renal clearance of the metabolite is reduced. Nevertheless, pinacidil has been used with success in renal hypertension.

Intravenous pinacidil can be used in emergencies. Because of tachycardia, pinacidil has no advantage over other drugs.

Nicorandil Intravenous use produces a fall in BP but oral treatment (20–40 mg daily) in normotensive subjects during exercise produces little effect on BP. The role in hypertension is therapeutically promising, but there are no adequate trial data.

Chromakalim This agent has been much less extensively investigated, but chromakalim lowers BP in both hypertensive and normotensive subjects following oral doses of 0.75–1.5 mg.[62,63] Whether chromakalim has advantages in adverse effect profile compared with pinacidil is unknown.

ADVERSE REACTIONS

Major complications are listed in Tables 10.2–10.5.

Adrenergic inhibitors

Ganglion blocking drugs
As a result of reduction in vasomotor tone, treated patients will pool blood in dependent capacitance vessels. This effect explains the phenomenon of

Table 10.2 Adverse reactions due to adrenergic inhibitors – ganglion blockers and rawolfia alkaloids

Drug	Common side effects	Other side effects
Ganglion blockers	Orthostatic hypotension Tachyphylaxis Reduced creatinine clearance	Paralytic ileus Urinary retention Asthma Respiratory arrest
Rawolfia alkaloids	Bradycardia Prolonged AV conduction Nasal stuffiness Depression	Peptic ulceration Diarrhoea Bronchospasm Increased appetite Fluid retention/weight gain Loss of libido/impotence Menstrual irregularities Amenorrhoea Galactorrhoea Ocular palsies Extrapyramidal symptoms

Table 10.3 Adverse reactions due to adrenergic inhibitors – adrenergic neurone-blocking agents, monoamine oxidase inhibitors and veratrium alkaloids

Drug	Common side effects	Other side effects
Adrenergic neurone-blockers	Orthostatic hypotension Muscle weakness Bradycardia Diarrhoea Retrograde ejaculation Fluid retention Dizziness Nasal stuffiness Lethargy	Nausea and vomiting Thrombocytopenia Loss of scalp hair Dry mouth Blurred vision Anorexia Epigastric discomfort Itch, rashes and urticaria
Monoamine oxidase inhibitors	Euphoria Insomnia Acute psychosis Severe hypertension with certain foods	Hepatocellular necrosis Blood dyscrasias
Veratrium alkaloids	Nausea and vomiting Excessive salivation Diaphoresis Blurred vision Mental confusion	

orthostatic hypotension that can be associated with syncope.[64] Because the orthostatic effect is so important, BP should be measured supine and erect. To enhance the antihypertensive effect in the supine posture, it is necessary to reduce intravascular (and extracellular) fluid volume and prevent the expansion of blood volume.[9,10] Prolonged therapy with trimetaphan for 48–72 hours is often associated with refractory responses (tachyphylaxis).[65] The most likely explanation is expansion of intravascular volume and better control of BP may be achieved by the introduction of a diuretic or more vigorous use of diuretics.[10,11]

Table 10.4 Adverse reactions due to direct acting vascular smooth muscle relaxants – hydralazine and minoxidil

Drugs	Common side effects	Other side effects
Hydralazine	Headache	Fluid retention/oedema
	Nasal stuffiness	Drug fever
	Tachycardia	Skin eruptions
	Palpitation	Blood dyscrasias
	Flushing	Purpura
	Sweating	
	Peripheral neuropathy	
	Lupus reaction	
Minoxidil	ECG changes	Nasal stuffiness
	Fluid retention/oedema	Nausea
	Hirsutism	Breast tenderness
	Flushing	Skin reactions
	Palpitation	
	Headache	

Table 10.5 Adverse reactions due to direct acting vascular smooth muscle relaxants – diazoxide, sodium nitroprusside and potassium channel agonists

Drug	Common side effects	Other side effects
Diazoxide	Hyperglycaemia	Chest pain
	Tachycardia	Extrapyrimidal reactions
	Palpitation	Skin rashes
	Fluid retention/oedema	Hypotension
	Hypertrichosis	Acute pancreatitis
	Headache	Fever
		Lymphadenopathy
		Gout
		Blood dyscrasias/purpura
		Nausea and vomiting
		Abdominal pain, ileus and diarrhoea
Sodium nitroprusside	Hypothyroidism	Restlessness
	Methaemoglobinaemia	Muscle twitching
	Nausea and vomiting	Cyanide intoxication
	Headache	
Potassium channel agonists	Headache	Hypertrichosis
	Dizziness	Nausea dyspepsia
	Palpitation	Rashes
	Tachycardia	Increased ANA titres
	Oedema	

Because cardiac output is reduced, there is at least proportionate reduction of renal blood flow, sometimes associated with reduced creatinine clearance.[66,67] Cerebral[65] and splanchnic[68] blood flow is also reduced.

Because parasympathetic inhibition also results from ganglionic blockade, tonic activation of the gastrointestinal and urinary tracts occurs with risk of paralytic ileus and acute urinary retention. Thus, abdominal pain with reduced bowel sounds, constipation, or reduced urinary output in a patient with aortic dissection may not reflect extension of the dissection into the mesenteric or renal arteries, but instead may be a side effect of treatment.

Other adverse drug reactions with trimetaphan include asthma attacks because of histamine release. Large doses may provoke muscle relaxation leading to cardiac arrest.

Rawolfia alkaloids

Parasympathetic activity remains unopposed, explaining many common side effects including bradycardia, prolonged atrio-ventricular conduction, increased gastric acid excretion with possible secondary peptic ulceration and frequency of bowel movements. These adverse effects may be counteracted by parasympathetic inhibitors.

Although arterial dilatation with increased blood flow has been considered greatest in the skin, other vascular beds are also involved. The frequent complaint of nasal mucosal congestion and stuffiness is ameliorated by nasally administered vasoconstrictors.[69,70] However, prolonged use may produce chemical rhinitis.

As a result of depletion of brain catecholamines and serotonin, there may be behavioural alterations and subtle or overt depression, sometimes leading to suicide.[71] Less severe central complications include drowsiness and nightmares.

Parkinsonism, dyskinesia and dystonia can result from dopamine depletion in the basal ganglia. Congestive heart failure may be precipitated or worsened.

Adrenergic neurone-blocking drugs

Because of coincidental inhibition of venous tone,[70] venous return to the heart is reduced by peripheral pooling of blood in dependent areas of the body with upright posture. As a result, orthostatic hypotension is prominent.[72]

Associated with the resulting fall in cardiac output, there is a proportionate reduction in organ blood flow. Severe hypotension may aggravate angina and lead to myocardial infarction, cerebrovascular insufficiency with syncope or even stroke. The renal and splanchnic territories may receive a smaller proportion of total cardiac output, but glomerular filtration rate and renal function appear to return to normal with time.[73] With reduced skeletal muscle blood flow and adrenergic innervation of skeletal muscle, weakness may result; this can be exacerbated by diuretic treatment.[74] Muscle weakness may be aggravated still further during and immediately after exercise.[75]

Some side effects (orthostatic hypotension, excessive hypotension, bradycardia, increased gastric excretion) result from unopposed parasympathetic activity and impaired adrenergic function. Similarly, diarrhoea, retrograde ejaculation and fluid retention may be explained by reduced adrenergic transmission. Many of these side effects may be counteracted by reducing dosage, or the addition of a parasympatholytic agent or a diuretic.

Because these agents act by entering the nerve terminal, any agent that prevents this will block the action. This is the means by which tricyclic antidepressants act,[76] and, therefore, these classes of drugs should not be prescribed concomitantly. Drugs that reduce efferent sympathetic output enhance postural hypotension and bradycardia. Examples include α-blockers, β-blockers and ganglion blockers. Cardiac glycosides may also enhance bradycardia.

Monoamine oxidase inhibitors

The major side effects are centrally mediated mental and emotional reactions including euphoria, insomnia and acute psychosis. More important is the severe hypertensive crisis following the ingestion of foods containing tyramine, such as aged cheeses, beer, sherry, Chianti and herring.[77]

Veratrium alkaloids

Because of the narrow therapeutic index, the effective control of arterial pressure is not infrequently associated with side effects. These can be reduced slightly by combined use with other antihypertensives.

Direct-acting vascular smooth muscle relaxants

Side effects common to these agents include headache and nasal stuffiness attributable to local vasodilatation, fluid retention and oedema. The latter effects can result in pseudotolerance.

Hydralazine

Peripheral neuropathy is dose-dependent and is rare at doses up to 200 mg daily.[78] This complication is more common in slow acetylators. Neuropathy is first manifest by paraesthesia, numbness and tingling of the extremities. Pyridoxine deficiency is the likely cause and correction can be achieved by administration of pyridoxine.[22]

The lupus reaction gives rise to malaise, myalgia and arthralgia/arthritis, and is associated with raised ANA titres.[79] Raised titres are often encountered in asymptomatic patients and are not a contraindication to continuation, although the lupus syndrome is. Hydralazine does not worsen idiopathic systemic lupus erythematosis.

There may be more severe signs of systemic illness such as weight loss, splenomegaly and effusions in serous cavities. Rashes may also occur. If not diagnosed promptly, the degree of temporary disability may be severe. Renal and cerebral involvement is rare. The hydralazine lupus reaction usually occurs after 6 months' therapy at doses over 400 mg daily and is almost always seen in slow acetylators. Patients with HLA DR4 phenotype are particularly susceptible.[80] The syndrome resolves when the drug is withdrawn, although months or years may be required for complete clearing.[22] After withdrawal of hydralazine, positive tests for ANA may persist for years.

Although the lupus reaction is reduced substantially at daily doses of 200 mg or less, there is still a significant incidence. In one study,[81] the incidence was 6.7% over 3 years. No cases were seen at 50 mg daily, 5.4% with 100 mg daily and 10.4% with 200 mg daily. The incidence was higher in women (11.6%) than in men (2.8%). In women taking 200 mg daily, the 3-year incidence was 19.4%. Thus, the true incidence of lupus syndrome is unacceptably high.

Concern about hydralazine lupus is frequently a deterrent to initiation of treatment and to adequately exploring the dose range in hypertension. To avoid an unacceptable incidence of hydralazine lupus, it appears that more effort than just dose containment may be necessary.[82] Determination of acetylator status, monitoring of ANA titres and even tissue typing may be required, but may represent unacceptably demanding prerequisites.

Decrease in white cell count is more common in blacks. Mild gastrointestinal side effects sometimes occur, but present no clinical problems at conventional doses. Hydralazine treatment is associated with a small reduction in total cholesterol.

Endralazine is not associated with the lupus syndrome.[83]

Minoxidil

Increase in cardiac work may account for ECG changes, which are often observed during the first few days of therapy. ECG changes include ST depression and T wave inversion,[84] but are not associated with cardiac enzyme elevation. However, reflex tachycardia may provoke angina in those with ischaemic heart disease. Pulmonary oedema may be the consequence of increased cardiac output. Flushing, palpitation and headache may occur if β-blocker is not taken concomitantly.

An uncommon cardiac adverse event is pericardial effusion, rarely associated with tamponade.[85] Deaths have been reported. Dependent oedema and ascites are extremely common. Fluid retention usually responds to diuretics, although high doses of loop diuretics may be necessary, particularly in renal failure where there is a predictable tendency to oedema.

A very common side effect of minoxidil is hirsutism, which is particularly bothersome in women. Hypertrichosis mainly affects the forehead and face and is most apparent in dark-haired individuals. There is no pharmacological treatment for excess hair growth, and the only remedy is removal of hair or discontinuation of the drug. After discontinuation, excessive hair growth reverses in a few months.

Diazoxide

Diazoxide shares the adverse effects of minoxidil. In addition, diazoxide causes impairment of glucose tolerance in the majority of patients.

Hyperglycaemia is due to inhibition of insulin secretion. The effect is probably mediated by action upon pancreatic islet cell potassium channels and can be reversed by sulfanylurea drugs.[59] Diabetic ketoacidosis and hyperosmolar, non-ketonic coma are infrequent, but can develop very rapidly. Conventional therapy with insulin and restoration of fluid and electrolyte balance is usually effective.

Hypotension occurs occasionally if thiazides are given concomitantly and usually responds to head-down tilt. The necessary, sympathomimetic agents, such as dopamine or noradrenaline (norepinephrine), may be used but the whole aim of treatment is to avoid excessive hypotension.

Increased hepatic enzymes, uraemia, reduced creatinine clearance, reversible nephrotic syndrome, decreased urine output, haematuria and albuminuria occur very occasionally. Thrombocytopenia with or without purpura may require discontinuation.

Drug interactions include bleeding with anticoagulants and hypotension with β-blockers. Diuretics potentiate hyperuricaemia by inhibition of tubular secretion of uric acid.

Sodium nitroprusside

Retrosternal discomfort, palpitation, dizziness and abdominal discomfort can occur if BP reduction is too rapid. Cyanide intoxication is rare unless the recommended dose is exceeded; metabolic acidosis may be followed by hypoxia and tetanic spasms.

Potassium channel agonists

When used as monotherapy, side effects of pinacidil are dose-related. ECG T wave changes have been reported in the initial phase of treatment.[61] Hypertrichosis is seen occasionally.[86]

CONCLUSIONS

Vasodilators are highly effective antihypertensive agents, which dominated the management of hypertension in the 1950s and 1960s. However, treatment with these agents is associated with an unacceptable level of adverse reactions. With the advent of newer and better tolerated antihypertensive agents, their use has declined dramatically. Many vasodilators can now be considered only of historical interest.

In developed countries, vasodilators have a limited clinical role. Some direct-acting vascular smooth muscle relaxants continue to have utility in the management of hypertensive emergencies (notably sodium nitroprusside) and in severe hypertension refractory to other antihypertensive agents (notably minoxidil). In developing countries, however, where the cost of newer agents may be prohibitive, vasodilators continue to be prescribed more widely. The safe and effective long-term use of those drugs requires careful attention to adverse reactions with concomitant administration of β-blockers and diuretics to avoid the consequences of reflex cardiac stimulation and salt and water retention.

References

1. Van Zwieten PA. Vasodilator drugs with direct action on smooth muscle. In: Van Zwieten PA, ed. *Handbook of hypertension, Vol 3*. Amsterdam: Elsevier; 1984:307–346.
2. Collier JG, Lorge RE, Robinson BF. Comparison of effects of tolmetozide (Rx 71107), diazoxide, hydralazine, prazosin, glyceryltrinitrate and sodium nitroprusside on forearm arteries and dorsal hand veins of man. *Br J Clin Pharmacol* 1978;5:35–44.
3. Ablad B. A study of the mechanism of the haemodynamic effects of hydralazine in man. *Acta Pharmacol Toxicol* 1963;20(Suppl 1):1–53.
4. Lin M-S, McNay JL, Shepherd AMM, et al. Increased plasma norepinephrine accompanies persistent tachycardia after hydralazine. *Hypertension* 1983;5:257–263.
5. Christensson B, Nordenvelt I, Westling H, et al. Haemodynamic effects of nitroglycerine in normal subjects during supine and sitting exercise. *Br Heart J* 1969;31:80–82.
6. O'Rourke M. Vasodilatation and arterial compliance. In: *Recent innovations in beta blockade: the role of vasodilatation*. RSM Round Table Series 1990;17:94–104.
7. Man in t'Veld AJ, Wenting GJ, Boomsma F, et al. Sympathetic and parasympathetic components of reflex cardiostimulation during vasodilator treatment of hypertension. *Br J Clin Pharmacol* 1980;9:547–551.
8. Koch-Weser J. Vasodilator drugs in the treatment of hypertension. *Arch Intern Med* 1974;133:1017–1027.
9. Dustan HP, Cumming GR, Corcoran AC, et al. A mechanism of chlorothiazide-enhanced effectiveness of antihypertensive ganglioplegic drugs. *Circulation* 1959;19:360–365.
10. Dustan HP, Tarazi RC, Bravo EL. Dependence of arterial pressure on intravascular volume in treated hypertensive patients. *N Engl J Med* 1972;286:861–866.
11. Weil JV, Chidsey CA. Plasma volume expansion resulting from interference with adrenergic function in normal man. *Circulation* 1968;37:54–61.
12. Patton WDM. Transmission and block in autonomic ganglia. *Pharmacol Rev* 1954;6:59–67.

13. Patton WDM, Zaimis EJ. The methonium compounds. *Pharmacol Rev* 1952;4:219–253.
14. Smirk FH. Methonium compounds in hypertension. *Lancet* 1950;2:477.
15. Veterans Administration Cooperative Study on Antihypertensive Agents. Double-blind controlled study of antihypertensive agents. II. Further report on the comparative effectiveness of reserpine, reserpine and hydralazine, and three ganglion blocking agents, chlorisondamine, mecylamine, and pentolinium tartrate. *Arch Intern Med* 1962;110:222–229.
16. Brest AN, Onesti G, Swartz C, et al. Mechanisms of antihypertensive drug therapy. *JAMA* 1970;211:480–484.
17. Pletschet A, Shore PA, Brodie BB. Serotonin release as a possible mechanism of reserpine action. *Science* 1955;122:374–375.
18. Moyer JH. Cardiovascular and renal hemodynamic response to reserpine (Serpasil) and clinical results of using this agent for treatment of hypertension. *Ann NY Acad Sci* 1954;59:82–94.
19. Emmelin N, Engstrom J. Supersensitivity of salivary glands following treatment with bretylium or guanethidine in dogs. *Br J Pharmacol Chemother* 1961;16:315–319.
20. McCubbin JW, Kaneto Y, Page IH. The peripheral cardiovascular actions of guanethidine in dogs. *J Pharmacol Exp Ther* 1961;181:346–354.
21. Richard DW. Paradoxical hypertension from tranylcypramine sulfate. Report of the Council on Drugs. *JAMA* 1963;186:854.
22. Koch-Weser J. Hydralazine. *N Eng J Med* 1976;295:320–323.
23. Rapaport RM, Draznin MB, Muirad F. Endothelial-dependent vasodilator and nitrovasodilator-induced relaxation may be mediated through cyclic GMP formation and cyclic GMP-dependent protein phosphosylation. *Trans Assoc Am Phys* 1983;96:19–30.
24. Krusyna H, Krusyna R, Smith RP, Wilcox DE. Red blood cells generate nitric oxide from directly acting nitrogenous vasodilators. *Toxicol Applied Pharmacol* 1987;91:429–438.
25. Spokas EG, Falco G, Quilley J, et al. Endothelial mechanisms in the vascular action of hydralazine. *Hypertension* 1983;5(Suppl 1):1107–1111.
26. Holmes DG, Bogers WA, Wideroe JE, et al. Endralazine, a new peripheral vasodilator: absence of effect of acetylators status on antihypertensive effect. *Lancet* 1983;1:670–671.
27. Reece PA, Cozamanis I, Zacest R. Influence of acetylators phenotype on the pharmacokinetics of a new vasodilator, antihypertensive endralazine. *Eur J Clin Pharmacol* 1982;23:523–527.
28. Bryan RK, Hoobler SW, Rosenzweig J, et al. Effect of minoxidil on blood pressure and haemodynamics in severe hypertension. *Am J Cardiol* 1977;39:796–801.
29. Andersson KE. Clinical pharmacology of potassium channel openers. *Pharmacol Toxicol* 1992;70:244–254.
30. Meisheri KD, Cipkus LA, Taylor CJ. Mechanism of action of minoxidil sulfate-induced vasodilatation: a role for increased K^+ permeability. *J Pharmacol Exp Ther* 1988;245:751–760.
31. Lowenthal DT, Affrime MB. Pharmacology and pharmacokinetics of minoxidil. *J Cardiovasc Pharmacol* 1980;2(Suppl 2):S93–S106.
32. Koch-Weser J. Diazoxide. *N Engl J Med* 1976;294:1271–1273.
33. Pohl JEF, Thurston H. Use of diazoxide in hypertension with renal failure. *BMJ* 1971;4:142–145.
34. Standen NB, Quayle JM, Davies NW, et al. Hyperpolarizing vasodilators activate ATP sensitive K^+ channels in arterial smooth muscle. *Science* 1989;245:177–180.
35. Cohn N, Burke P. Nitroprusside. *Ann Intern Med* 1979;91:752–757.
36. Palmer RF, Lasseter KD. Sodium nitroprusside. *N Engl J Med* 1975;293:294–297.
37. Schroder H, Noack E, Muller R. Evidence for a correlation between nitric oxide formation by cleavage of organic nitrates and activation of guanylate cyclase. *J Mol Cell Cardiol* 1985;17:931–934.
38. Verndier IR. Sodium nitroprusside: theory and practice. *Postgrad Med J* 1974;50:576–581.
39. Cook NS. The pharmacology of potassium channels and their therapeutic potential. *Trends Pharmacol Sci* 1988;9:21–28.
40. Richer C, Pratz J, Mulder P, et al. Cardiovascular and biological effects of K^+ channel openers: a class of drugs with vasorelaxant and cardioprotective properties. *Life Sci* 1990;47:1693–1705.
41. Frampton J, Buckley MM, Filton A. Nicorandil: a review of its pharmacology and therapeutic effects in angina pectoris. *Drugs* 1992;44:625–655.
42. Holzmann S. Cyclic GMP as possible mediator of coronary relaxation by nicorandil (SG - 75). *J Cardiovasc Pharmacol* 1983;5:364–370.
43. Kinoshita M, Sakai K. Pharmacology and therapeutic effects of nicorandil. *Cardiovasc Drug Ther* 1990;4:1075–1088.
44. Bhatia S, Frohlich ED. A hemodynamic comparison of agents useful in hypertensive emergencies. *Am Heart J* 1973;85:367–373.

45. Veterans Administration Co-operative Study Group on Antihypertensive Agents. Effects of treatment on morbidity in hypertension. I. Results in patients with diastolic blood pressures averaging 115 through 129 mmHg. *JAMA* 1967;202:116–122.

46. Veterans Administration Co-operative Study Group on Antihypertensive Agents. Effects of treatment on morbidity in hypertension. II. Results in patients with diastolic blood pressure averaging 90 through 114 mmHg. *JAMA* 1970;213:1143–1152.

47. Canary JJ, Schaaf M, Duffy BJ, et al. Effects of oral and intramuscular administration of reserpine in thyrotoxicosis. *N Engl J Med* 1957;257:435–442.

48. Onesti G, Novack P, Ramirez O, et al. Hemodynamic effects of pargyline in hypertensive patients. *Circulation* 1964;30:830–835.

49. Freis ED, Rose JC, Higgins TF, et al. The hemodynamic effects of hypotensive drugs in man: 41 - hydrazinophthalazine. *Circulation* 1953;8:197–204.

50. Schroder H. Simplified method for determining acetylators phenotype. *BMJ* 1972;3:506–507.

51. Zacest R, Gilmore E, Koch-Weser J. Treatment of essential hypertension with combined vasodilatation and beta adrenergic blockade. *N Engl J Med* 1972;286:617–622.

52. McAraevey D, Ramsey LE, Latham L, et al. "Third drug" trial: comparative study of antihypertensive agents added to treatment when blood pressure remains uncontrolled by beta-blocker plus thiazide diuretics. *BMJ* 1984;288:106–111.

53. Australian Therapeutic Trial in Mild Hypertension Management Committee. The Australian Therapeutic Trial in Mild Hypertension. *Lancet* 1980;i:1261–1267.

54. Hypertension Detection and Follow-Up Program Co-operative Group. Five year findings of the Hypertension Detection and Follow-Up Program. 1. Reduction in mortality of persons with high blood pressure, including mild hypertension. *JAMA* 1979;242:2562–2571.

55. Liedholm H, Melander A. Drug selection in the treatment of pregnancy hypertension. *Obstet Gynaecol* 1984;(Suppl 118):49–55.

56. McGourty JC, Silas JH, Pidgeon J. Comparison of once daily endralazine with placebo in the treatment of hypertension uncontrolled by a beta-blocker and diuretic. *Eur J Clin Pharmacol* 1985;29:401–403.

57. Swales JD, Bing RF, Heagerty AM, et al. Treatment of refractory hypertension. *Lancet* 1982;1:894–896.

58. Brunner HR, Jaeger P, Ferguson RK, et al. Need for beta blockade in hypertension reduced with long-term minoxidil. *BMJ* 1978;2:385–388.

59. Pohl JEF, Thurston H, Swales JD. Hypertension with renal impairment: influence of intensive therapy. *QJ Med* 1974;43:569–581.

60. Garrett BN, Kaplan NM. Efficacy of slow infusion of diazoxide in the treatment of severe hypertension without organ hyperperfusion. *Am Heart J* 1982;103:390–394.

61. Friedel HA, Brogden RN. Pinacidil. A review of its pharmacodynamic and pharmacokinetic properties and therapeutical potential in the treatment of hypertension. *Drugs* 1990;39:929–967.

62. Donnelly R, Elliott HL, Meredith PA, Reid JL. Clinical studies with a potassium channel activator chromakalin in normotensive and hypertensive subjects. *J Cardiovasc Pharmacol* 1990;16:790–795.

63. Singer DRJ, Markandu ND, Miller MA, et al. Potassium channel stimulation in normal subjects and in patients with essential hypertension: an acute study with chromakalim (BRL 34915). *J Hypertens* 1989;7(Suppl 6):S294–S295.

64. Freis ED, Rose JC, Partenope EA, et al. The hemodynamic effects of hypotensive drugs in man. II. Hexamethonium. *J Clin Invest* 1953;32:1285–1298.

65. Finnerty FA, Witkin L, Fazekas JF. Cerebral hemodynamics in acute hypotension. *J Clin Invest* 1954;33:933.

66. Ford RV, Moyer JH, Spurr CL. Hexamethonium in the chronic treatment of hypertension: its effects on renal hemodynamics and on the excretion of water and electrolytes. *J Clin Invest* 1953;32:1133–1139.

67. Ullmann TD, Menczel J. The effect of a ganglion blocking agent (hexamethonium) on renal function and on excretion of water and electrolytes in hypertension and in congestive heart failure. *Am Heart J* 1956;52:106–120.

68. Reynolds TB, Paton A, Freeman M, et al. The effect of hexamethonium bromide in splanchnic blood flow, oxygen consumption and glucose output in man. *J Clin Invest* 1953;32:793–800.

69. Frohlich ED. Inhibition of adrenergic function in the treatment of hypertension. *Arch Intern Med* 1974;133:1033–1048.

70. Gaffney FE, Bryant WM, Braunwald E. Effect of reserpine and guanethidine on venous reflexes. *Circ Res* 1962;11:889–894.

71. Freis ED. Mental depression in hypertensive patients treated for long periods with large doses of reserpine. *N Engl J Med* 1954;251:1006–1008.

72. Cohn JD, Liptak TE, Freis ED. Hemodynamic effect of guanethidine in man. *Circ Res* 1963;12:298–307.

73. Villareal H, Exaire JB, Rubio V, et al. Effects of guanethidine and bretylium tosylate on systemic and renal hemodynamics in essential hypertension. *Am J Cardiol* 1964;14:633–640.

74. Bowman WC, Notts MW. Actions of sympathomimetic amines and their antagonists on skeletal muscle. *Pharmacol Rev* 1969;21:27–72.

75. Khatri IM, Cohn HN. Mechanism of exercise hypotension after sympathetic blockade. *Am J Cardiol* 1970;25:329–338.

76. Mitchell JR, Cavenaugh JH, Arias L, et al. Guanethidine and related agents III. Antagonism by drugs which inhibit the norepinephrine pump in man. *J Clin Invest* 1970;49:1596–1604.

77. Goldberg LI. Monoamine oxidase inhibitors: adverse reactions and possible mechanisms. *JAMA* 1964;190:456–462.

78. Raskin NH, Fishman RA. Pyridoxine-deficiency neuropathy due to hydralazine. *N Engl J Med* 1965;273:1182–1185.

79. Perry HM, Tan EM, Karmody S, Sakamoto A. Relation of acetyl transferase activity to anti-nuclear antibodies and toxic symptoms in hypertensive patients treated with hydralazine. *J Lab Clin Med* 1970;76:114–125.

80. Batchelor JR, Welsh KI, Tinoco RM, et al. Hydralazine-induced systemic lupus erythematosus: influence of HLA DR and sex on susceptibility. *Lancet* 1980;1:1107–1109.

81. Cameron HA, Ramsay LE. The lupus syndrome induced by hydralazine: a common complication of low dose treatment. *BMJ* 1984;289:408–409.

82. Bing RF, Russell GI, Thurston H, Swales JD. Hydralazine in hypertension. Is there a safe dose? *BMJ* 1980;281:353–354.

83. Bogers WA, Meems L. Endralazine, a new peripheral vasodilator. Evaluation of safety and efficacy over a 3 year period. *Eur J Clin Pharmacol* 1983;24:301–305.

84. Hall D, Froer KL, Rudolph W. Serial electrocardiographic changes during long-term treatment of severe hypertension with minoxidil. *J Cardiovasc Pharmacol* 1980;2(Suppl 2): S200–S205.

85. Reichgott MJ. Minoxidil and pericardial effusion: an idiosyncratic reaction. *Clin Pharmacol Ther* 1981;30:64–70.

86. Goldberg MR. Clinical Pharmacology of pinacidil: a prototype for drugs that affect potassium channels. *J Cardiovasc Pharmacol* 1988;12(Suppl 2):S41–S47.

V

Beta-blocking agents

11 | β-adrenoceptor blocking drugs

Dennis Johnston

INTRODUCTION

In 1948 Ahlquist suggested the existence of two different adrenergic receptors; α and β, to explain the pharmacological effects of catecholamines on smooth and cardiac muscle.[1] The α-receptors, when stimulated, produced predominantly excitatory actions, e.g. vasoconstriction, except in the intestine where the effects were inhibitory. β-receptor stimulation generally produced inhibitory effects except for the heart where the action was excitatory. This theory did not achieve full acceptance, however, until the discovery of specific antagonists for the different receptors. The first β-adrenoceptor antagonist to be developed was dichloroisoprenaline (DCI) (Fig. 11.1).[2] DCI was effective in reducing catecholamine stimulation of the heart and relaxation of the guinea pig tracheal smooth muscle.[3] This compound was a partial agonist and was considered to be of little clinical value.

In the 1950s Sir James Black conceived the hypothesis that coronary heart disease would be improved if the work of the heart could be reduced by inhibition of the cardiac β-receptors.[4] This would result in a reduction in heart rate, myocardial contractility and myocardial oxygen demand. The first antagonist to be produced was pronethalol (Fig. 11.1), but development was abandoned because of the high incidence of thymic tumours in mice.[5] Eventually the work led to the synthesis of propranolol (Fig. 11.1), a non-selective β-adrenoceptor antagonist,[4] which, as predicted, proved effective in treating patients with ischaemic heart disease. It was a number of years later that the ability of adrenoceptor antagonists to lower blood pressure (BP) in hypertensive patients was finally confirmed.[6] Propranolol was followed by a number of other β-blockers with different pharmacology; β₁ selective agents, such as atenolol, metoprolol and bisoprolol, those with partial agonist activity, such as pindolol and oxprenolol, and those with additional α-antagonist and vasodilator properties, such as labetolol, carvedilol and nebivolol. Today β antagonists are used in the treatment of angina pectoris, hypertension, heart failure, myocardial infarction, arrhythmias, thyrotoxicosis, tremor, migraine and glaucoma, as well as

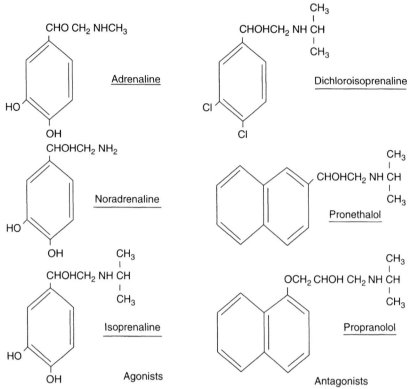

Fig. 11.1 Chemical structures of catecholamines, and the early beta adrenoceptor agonists and antagonists.

phaeochromocytoma, portal hypertension, obstructive cardiomyopathy and Fallot's tetralogy.[7]

CLASSIFICATION/CHEMISTRY

Classification

The early β-adrenoceptor antagonists, such as propranolol, were non-selective and had significant effects on the β_1- and β_2-receptors. Atenolol, metoprolol and bisoprolol introduced some years later, which were more selective for the β_1-receptors, particularly at low dose. β-blockers are now available with additional vasodilatory effects. Vasodilatation can be mediated by β_2-sympathomimetic activity (ISA), e.g. pindolol; added α-adrenergic blockade with labetolol and carvedilol; and, nitric oxide production with nebivolol.[7]

Non-selective agents

Non-selective β-adrenoceptor agents are as effective as β_1-selective drugs in reducing heart rate, myocardial contractility and conductivity, but tend to cause more smooth muscle contraction with an increased risk of bronchospasm in predisposed individuals. β_2-adrenergic blockade may have some advantages in migraine prophylaxis.[8]

Cardioselective agents

Cardioselective drugs are as effective in angina pectoris and hypertension as non-selective drugs. Selective drugs are preferred in patients with chronic obstructive lung disease[9] and insulin-dependent diabetes over non-selective agents. However, often it is better, if possible, to choose a drug from another class.[10] Cardioselectivity varies between different β-blockers, but is always greater at lower doses.[11]

Vasodilatory β-blockers

β-blockers with ISA (partial agonist activity; PAA) lower resting heart rate and cardiac output less than those without ISA. As with β-blockade, however, ISA may be non-selective or selective for the β_1- or β_2-receptors. The presence of β_1 ISA will result in a higher resting heart rate[12] when sympathetic tone is low, but major reductions in exercise heart rate when sympathetic activity is high.[13] It could be argued that β_1 ISA might be beneficial in patients with low cardiac output or in Afrocaribbeans in whom vasodilatation appears to increase the antihypertensive effect. To date, there is no clinical evidence that this is the case. In patients with ischaemic heart disease, particularly if they have angina at rest, it is better to avoid drugs with ISA. Labetalol, a drug with combined α- and β-blocking properties, appears to cause less bronchospasm and vasoconstriction than non-β_1-selective agents and has greater antihypertensive effects in Afrocaribbean populations. Labetalol has a rapid onset of action compared with standard β-blockers and is preferred in the emergency management of hypertensive crises.[14] This agent also continues to be one of the drugs of first choice in the management of hypertension of pregnancy.[15] Carvedilol is licensed for the treatment of heart failure,[16] but it remains unclear whether carvedilol has any advantages over β_1-selective β-blockers for this indication.

Antiarrhythmic β-blockers

All β-blockers are potentially antiarrhythmic, but propranolol has additional quinidine-like properties referred to as membrane stabilizing activity. This property has little clinical relevance except in overdose when it contributes to the much higher toxicity compared with β-blockers, which do not possess this property.[17] Sotalol is a unique β-blocker that has additional class III antiarrhythmic activity. As with propranolol this does not confer any clear benefit, but results in a higher incidence of serious rhythm disturbances when the drug is taken as an overdose.[17]

Chemistry

The β-adrenoceptor antagonists have similar structures to isoprenaline (Fig. 11.1). Three general structural features have been described[18,19] as necessary for β-adrenceptor antagonism: an ethanolamine or oxy-propanolamine side chain; an aromatic ring that can be benzenoid (atenolol), bicyclic aromatic (propranolol) or benzoheterocyclic (pindolol) and an amine component, which is a branched chain alkyl group (Fig. 11.2).

Intrinsic sympathomimetic activity

Full agonist activity is usually observed with compounds that retain the aromatic ring.[20] Loss of one or both hydroxyl groups of the catechol moiety in

Oxypropanolamines:

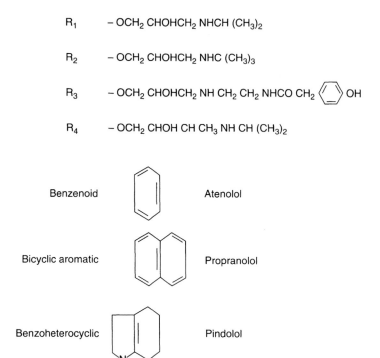

R_1 $- OCH_2 CHOHCH_2 NHCH (CH_3)_2$

R_2 $- OCH_2 CHOHCH_2 NHC (CH_3)_3$

R_3 $- OCH_2 CHOHCH_2 NH CH_2 CH_2 NHCO CH_2 \langle \bigcirc \rangle OH$

R_4 $- OCH_2 CHOH CH CH_3 NH CH (CH_3)_2$

Benzenoid   Atenolol

Bicyclic aromatic   Propranolol

Benzoheterocyclic   Pindolol

Fig. 11.2 Basic chemical structures of the beta adrenoceptor antagonists.

the aromatic ring results in partial agonism. Agonism is further reduced with large ortho-substitutions, as in the case of oxprenolol (o-$OCH_2 CHCH_2$). Partial agonism is also observed in the para position (e.g. practolol p-$NHCOCH_3$). ISA is lost altogether, as with atenolol and metoprolol, when a methylene group is inserted between the aromatic ring and these functions.[18,19]

The side chain is also important for agonist activity. Overall, ethanolamines have more ISA than have oxy-propanolamines and this property can be altered by changing the groups of the acyl portion of the acylaminoalkyl side chain.[18,19]

Cardioselectivity

Cardioselectivity for the β_1-receptor largely depends on substitution in the para position of the oxy-propanolamine type of compound with an amidic group (practolol, atenolol and acebutolol) or other moieties capable of participating in hydrogen-bond formation (metoprolol).[20]

Isomerism

All β-adrenoceptor antagonists contain an asymmetric carbon atom and so exist as pairs of optical isomers. In the oxy-propanolamine series, activity is usually related to the S enantiomer, which is 50–150 times more potent as an antagonist than the corresponding R enantiomer.[18] A number of the individual properties of β-adrenoceptor antagonists can be explained by the presence of different enantiomers. The (+) form of sotalol displays class III antiarrhythmic activity while the (−) form is a β-adrenoceptor antagonist.[21] Labetolol has two stereogenic centres and exists in stereoisomeric forms: RR, SS, RS and SR. The RR is predominantly the β-blocker and the SR the α-blocking component. The remaining isoforms SS and RS are almost completely devoid of significant biological activity.[22] The isomers of pindolol on the other hand express the same degree of ISA, although their potency values are different.[23]

MODE OF ACTION

β-adrenoceptors are present in the membranes of a number of different cells. $β_1$-adrenoceptors are generally close to the site of innervation and $β_2$-adrenoceptors are usually stimulated by circulating agonists.

Situated on the cardiac sarcolemma, the $β_1$-receptors are part of the adenylyl cyclase system (Fig. 11.3). This G protein system links the receptor to adenylyl cyclase when the G protein is in the stimulatory configuration (C_S). The G protein also exists in an inhibitory form (G_1), which increases following stimulation of the muscarinic receptors. When activated, adenylyl cyclase produces cyclic AMP from ATP (Fig. 11.3). This is the intracellular second messenger for $β_1$-stimulation and has important effects on calcium transport within the cell (Fig. 11.4). It promotes an opening of the calcium channels to produce a positive inotropic effect and increases the re-uptake of cytosolic calcium into the sacroplasmic reticulum resulting in an increased rate of relaxation or lusiotropic effect. In the sinus node the pacemaker current is increased, resulting in

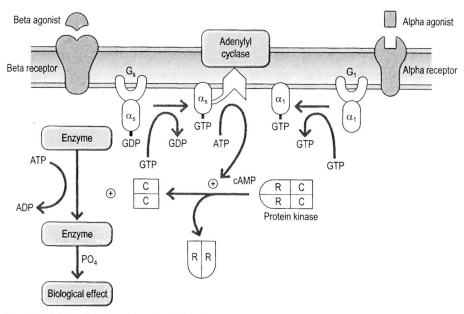

Fig. 11.3 Signal systems involved in the inotropic and chronic effects of adrenoceptor mediated responses.

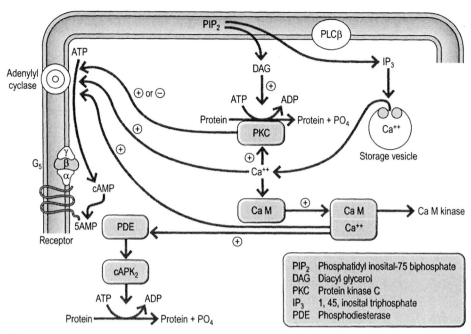

Fig. 11.4 Interactions between the second messangers, calcium and cyclic AMP.

an increased heart rate and accelerated conduction. Cardiac β_2-receptors also link to the G_S protein, but recent evidence suggests an additional link to the inhibitory protein G_i. It is possible that this inhibitory pathway could limit the adverse effects of catecholamines on the heart.[24,25]

Structure of β-adrenoceptors

The adrenoceptors constitute a family of closely related proteins that are structurally and functionally related to a wide variety of other neurotransmitters and hormones that are coupled to G proteins (Fig. 11.5).[26] These include receptors for biogenic amines, eicosanoids, peptide hormones and rhodopsin. The

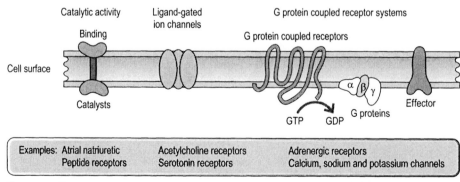

Fig. 11.5 Types of receptors for endogenous agonists involved in cardiovascular pharmacology.

different β-adrenoceptors share approximately 60% amino acid sequence identity within the membrane-spanning domains where the ligand-binding pocket for adrenaline and noradrenaline has been identified. For the β_2-receptor, the protonated amino group of the ligand appears to form a salt bridge within the acidic amino acid Asp^{113} in the third transmembrane-spanning domain. The Asp residue is conserved in all biogenic amine receptors. Other residues within the membrane domains have been identified as being involved with interactions with β-adrenoceptor antagonists. Asn^{312} in helix 7 appears to interact with the phenoxy oxygen found in many of the most potent β-adrenoceptor antagonists.[25]

Effects of β-adrenoceptor blockade

Following β-adrenoceptor stimulation, the greater and faster rise of cytosolic calcium and the increased metabolism of ATP by the myosin ATPase results in greater myocardial contractility. Increases in the rate of relaxation are linked to increased phosphorylation of phospholambin. In this form, phospholambin fails to inhibit the sarcoplasmic-endoplasmic reticulum calcium uptake pump. Increased cyclic AMP also increases the phosphorylation of troponin I, resulting in enhanced interaction between myosin heads and actin ends.[26]

β-adrenoceptor blockade will, therefore, cause the heart to beat more slowly by decreasing the force of contraction and the rate of relaxation as well as inhibiting the depolarizing currents in the sinoatrial node. These oxygen-conserving properties are clearly important in the treatment of angina pectoris, myocardial infarction and heart failure.[27]

RECEPTOR DOWN-REGULATION AND UP-REGULATION

The response of the β-adrenoceptor is decreased following prolonged β-adrenergic stimulation. This could be viewed as a self-protective mechanism to prevent excessive cyclic AMP production and increased third messenger calcium ions. The principal response to prolonged stimulation is to increase the activity of β_1-adrenergic receptor kinase (β_1ARK) as occurs in advanced heart failure. This enzyme phosphorylates the β_1-receptor, which becomes uncoupled from G_S in the presence of β-arrestin and internalizes. Prolonged stimulation of the receptor also results in lysosomal destruction and loss of receptor density. It remains unclear whether these changes occur in the β_2-receptor.[28]

Severe congestive heart failure provides the best clinical example of β-receptor down-regulation. During continued infusions of dobutamine, a β-agonist, progressive loss of therapeutic efficacy has been observed. This is sometimes referred to as tachyphylaxis. In heart failure the β_1-receptors are down-regulated by high circulating levels of catecholamines. In contrast, cardiac β_2-receptors appear to be unaffected, leading to the hypothesis that continued activity of the β_2-receptor may be beneficial in protecting myocardial cells from apoptosis.[25]

Up-regulation of the β-receptors[29] may provide an explanation of the clinical syndrome of 'β-blocker withdrawal', which results in sudden worsening of angina pectoris accompanied by an increase in heart rate and BP.[30] It is likely that an increase in β-receptor density, induced by prolonged blockade of the β-receptors, might trigger an increased response to physiological stimulation by circulating catecholamines.

PHARMACOKINETICS AND METABOLISM

β-adrenoceptor antagonists vary considerably in their lipid solubility. The highly lipid soluble drugs such as propranolol, oxprenolol and perbutolol are more likely to demonstrate first-pass metabolism, have greater variation in plasma concentrations, exhibit shorter half-lives and have a higher incidence of disturbed sleep than those of more water soluble agents, such as atenolol, sotalol or nadolol.[31]

Absorption

The majority of β-adrenoceptor antagonists are weak bases and undergo minimal gastric absorption. Most absorption takes place in the upper jejunum and is greatest with lipophilic compounds. For example, approximately 90% of the oral dose of propranolol is absorbed, with peak concentrations occurring within 2 hours of administration. For atenolol, intestinal absorption is usually less than 50% and peak plasma concentrations occur at about 4 hours.[32] Food decreases the absorption of atenolol and sotalol, and enhances that of propranolol and metoprolol. There are a number of sustained release formulations of lipid soluble compounds with delayed absorption and prolonged duration of effect.

Distribution

Lipophilic β-blockers distribute in the tissues more widely than hydrophilic agents and more readily enter the central nervous system. Propranolol, pindolol, labetalol and bisoprolol are highly protein bound, which will limit transfer across the blood–brain barrier even for drugs which are highly lipid soluble.[33,34]

Metabolism

At usual clinical doses, propranolol, labetalol and oxprenolol are metabolized when these compounds reach the liver via the splanchnic circulation (first-pass metabolism). The bioavailability of propranolol is reduced by about 30%. However, 4,hydroxy propranolol is as potent as the parent compound and, therefore, the therapeutic effect is not reduced. Acebutolol produces large amounts of diacetolol, a cardioselective metabolite with ISA, but with a longer half-life, mainly excreted by the kidneys. The plasma concentrations achieved after oral administration vary considerably, however, due to different rates of oxidative metabolism. Slow metabolizers tend to have higher concentrations of the parent compound compared with fast metabolizers. Inhibition of cytochrome P450 with enzyme inhibitors such as cimetidine will increase the plasma concentrations of metoprolol and propranolol and hence therapeutic effect.[35,36]

Excretion

Hydrophilic compounds, such as atenolol, sotalol and nadolol are excreted unchanged by the kidney, mostly by glomerular filtation. Half-lives are longer and reduced dosage will be required in the elderly and those with renal impairment.[37] Lipid soluble compounds are eliminated by the liver by metabolism and/or biliary excretion.[35]

PHARMACODYNAMICS

The principal effects of β-adrenoceptor antagonists relate to their inhibitory effects on the sinus node, the atrioventricular node and on myocardial contractility. These are, respectively, the negative chronotropic, dromotropic and inotropic effects. Slowing the heart and reducing the force of myocardial contraction, particularly following exercise, are useful in decreasing myocardial oxygen demand and producing symptomatic improvement in angina pectoris.[38] The inhibitory effect on the atrioventricular node is important in the treatment of atrial fibrillation and other supraventricular tachycardias.

Cardiac effects of β-adrenoceptor antagonists

β-adrenoceptor antagonists increase, decrease or have no important effect on stroke volume, although cardiac output is usually decreased. Decreases in the force of contraction also result in increases in heart size. As β-blockers are competitive antagonists, their effect depends critically on the level of sympathetic activity. A small decrease in heart rate and cardiac output is observed at rest, but during graduated exercise their effect progressively increases. There is little difference between selective and non-selective drugs following exercise, but compounds with ISA such as pindolol have less effect on cardiac output and heart rate.[39]

Following an intravenous bolus of a β-blocker, heart rate and cardiac output fall rapidly. Initially BP is not affected, but decreases occur some hours later. Two main actions of β-blockers have been proposed for the late fall in BP,[40] but neither fully explains the decrease.[41] The first hypothesis relates to inhibition of renin release and a fall in circulating renin has been linked by some investigators to a fall in BP.[42] The second explanation relates to resetting of the baroreceptor mechanism, which occurs secondary to reductions in heart rate and cardiac output.[43,44] An effect of β-blockade on the central control of BP has largely been discounted.[45,46] β-blockers have also been shown to prevent cardiac hypertrophy induced by exercise and reverse ventricular hypertrophy in hypertension,[47] although they seem to be less effective than most other antihypertensive agents.[48]

Effects of β-adrenoceptor antagonists on the peripheral and coronary arteries

Blood vessels supplying muscle beds have a rich supply of β_2-adrenoceptors. Non-selective agents, such as propranolol produce a small reduction in resting muscle blood flow.[49] Reductions in skin blood flow do not depend on β_1-selectivity and are probably due to a reflex response initiated by a fall in cardiac output.[50] The impact of β-blockade on the coronary circulation has been difficult to elucidate especially in patients with coronary artery disease. It has been suggested that β-blockers might cause coronary artery vasoconstriction due to unopposed α_1-agonist activity and a decrease in blood flow due to reduced cardiac output.[51] These effects have been described in experimental animal models, but in patients with coronary artery disease the longer diastolic filling time, due to reduced heart rate, leads to better myocardial perfusion during diastole and a reduction in ischaemic events.[52] The clear clinical benefit of monotherapy with β-blockers over other antianginal agents testifies to an improvement in overall cardiac function and improved coronary blood flow.[52]

Renal effects of β-adrenoceptor antagonists

β-adrenoceptor antagonists have a number of effects on renal function; some are due to a local action on the kidney while others occur secondary to changes in renal haemodynamics.[53] The effects on renal blood flow and glomerular filtration are variable and reductions are greater after acute β-blockade than following chronic therapy.[54] As previously mentioned, clinical doses of β-adrenoceptor antagonists reduce basal and stimulated renin release, an effect that may contribute to the antihypertensive activity.[55] Control of renin release is not only due to effects at the β_1-receptor, but sodium content of the tubular fluid, and renal perfusion pressures also have a role so that reductions in plasma renin are often modest following β-blockade.[55]

Neurological effects of β-adrenoceptor antagonists

β_1- and β_2-receptors are both present in the brain, particularly in the ascending reticular formation and hypothalamus, but only β_1-receptors are involved in cardiovascular control.[56] Non-selective lipophilic drugs, such as propranolol, produce EEG changes,[57] vivid dreams and insomnia, suggesting central effects for these types of β-adrenoceptor antagonists. Blockade of the β_2-receptor reduces tremor, and propranolol has been used with some success to reduce the tremor caused by anxiety and in the treatment of essential tremor.[58,59]

Metabolic effects of β-adrenoceptor antagonists

In general, β-adrenoceptor antagonists have little effect on blood glucose levels.[60] However, the hypoglycaemia response to insulin by non-selective agents can be prolonged, especially during fasting.[60] Insulin secretion is partially under the control of the β_2-receptors[61] and there is some clinical evidence that non-selective β-blockers are associated with 'hypoglycaemia unawareness'. More new cases of diabetes were also identified in hypertensive patients receiving an atenolol-based regimen than in those receiving a losartan-based regimen.[62]

Plasma triglycerides rise with selective and non-selective β-blockers and the LDL/HDL ratio tends to increase.[63] Drugs with ISA do not exhibit these effects and for celiprolol and pindolol favourable effects have been reported.[64,65]

β-blockers also increase serum potassium, an effect that is greatest with non-selective drugs.[66] Since hypokalaemia and excess adrenaline are associated with cardiac arrhythmias in patients with the acute coronary syndrome, the therapeutic benefit of β-blockers may, in part, be related to this metabolic effect.

Respiratory effects of β-adrenoceptor antagonists

Bronchial smooth muscle is innervated by the sympathetic nervous system and in humans, this exclusively involves the β$_2$-receptor.[67] In normal subjects β$_2$-blockade has very little effect on airways resistance. However, in asthmatic patients with sensitized, bronchial smooth muscle, β-blockers increase airways resistance.[68] Non-selective agents also tend to reverse the effects of bronchodilator drugs especially β$_2$-agonists.[69]

ADVERSE EFFECTS AND CONTRAINDICATIONS

A variety of minor adverse effects occur with propranolol, possibly due to high lipid solubility and central nervous system penetration (sedation, sleep disturbance and depression).[70,71] Rash, fever and allergic reactions are rare.[72] The major common adverse effects relate to β$_2$-adrenoceptor blockade. Mild asthma can become severe and patients with obstructive airways disease may experience increased breathlessness.[73,74] While β$_1$-selective drugs tend to have less effect on airways resistance than non-selective agents,[75] these drugs should be used cautiously, if at all, in patients with reversible airways obstruction.

β-adrenoceptor antagonists depress myocardial contractility and excitability. In patients with marked impairment of myocardial function, cardiac output is largely dependent on increased sympathetic activity. Removal of this activity can result in cardiac decompensation and severe congestive cardiac failure has been reported in some patients.[76] Almost 5% of patients on propranolol develop symptoms closely resembling those of Raynaud's phenomenon or complain that their claudication is worse.[77,78] This, in part, is due to unopposed α-stimulation resulting from β$_2$-blockade, but reduced cardiac output can contribute, particularly in patients with coronary artery disease. Sinus bradycardia is a normal response to β-adrenoceptor blockade. However, in patients with partial or complete atrioventricular blockade, this group of drugs can cause life-threatening bradyarrhythmias.[79] This is a particular problem in patients receiving other antiarrhythmic drugs (see drug interactions).

Catecholamines increase glycogenolysis and blood glucose levels. In addition, lipolysis is enhanced and free fatty acids are released from adipose tissue. β-blocking drugs (especially non-selective) antagonize these metabolic effects. Hypoglycaemic reactions have been reported during treatment with β-adrenoceptor antagonists in diabetic patients receiving insulin[80] and in healthy volunteers following exercise.[81] Of greater clinical importance is the effect in reducing the normal adrenergic responses to hypoglycaemia. β-adrenergic antagonists prolong the duration of the hypoglycaemia and make the clinical diagnosis of drug-induced hypoglycaemia more difficult.[82] Despite this, a large number of diabetic patients receive β-adrenoceptor antagonists without any major clinical effects. Renal function occasionally deteriorates during treatment with β-blockers, probably due to reduced renal blood flow,[83] and occasionally marked bradycardia results in orthostatic hypotension or syncope necessitating drug withdrawal or dose reduction.

Withdrawal reactions

Patients with coronary heart disease are at increased risk of developing sudden deterioration in their clinical condition following withdrawal of β-adrenoceptor antagonists.[84] Increased BP and prolonged chest pain can occur, especially in patients who have been receiving large doses of β-blockers for angina pectoris. The mechanism probably relates to up-regulation of the β-receptors and increased sensitivity to circulating catecholamines. Patients should be warned of the dangers of stopping these drugs suddenly and in those for whom withdrawal is necessary, gradual tapering of the dose is recommended.

Quality of life

In the first large quality-of-life study in hypertension, propranolol caused substantially more central nervous system effects than captopril.[85] Atenolol on the other hand compared favourably with enalapril, and acebutalol had no detrimental effect on measures of quality of life compared with placebo.[86] Overall, most β-blockers appear to have little negative impact on quality of life.

Contraindications

Absolute contraindications for the use of β-blockers are severe bradycardia, high degree atrioventricular blockade and severe left ventricular failure. Most patients with asthma should not receive a β-adrenoceptor antagonist and propranolol should be avoided in patients with depression or rest pain due to peripheral ischaemia. Relative contraindications are listed in Table 11.1.

CLINICAL INDICATIONS

β-adrenoceptor antagonists are most often used to treat cardiovascular disease. Beta blockers are drugs of first choice in the treatment of angina pectoris, hypertension, myocardial infarction and congestive cardiac failure. These drugs are also used to treat hypertrophic obstructive cardiomyopathy, Fallot's tetralogy and portal hypertension. β-blockade is used to reduce the symptoms

Table 11.1 Absolute and relative contra-indications for the use of beta adrenoceptor antagonists

	Absolute	Relative
Cardiac	Severe bradycardia Heart block	? Prinzmetal's angina Patient receiving drugs which depress SA or AV nodes – verapamil, diltiazem, digoxin, antiarrhythmic drugs.
Pulmonary	Severe asthma	Mild asthma or obstructive airways disease
Central nervous system	Severe depression	Visual hallucinations Vivid dreams Fatigue
Peripheral vascular	Severe peripheral vascular disease – gangrene, necrosis, rest pain	Cold extremities Raynaud's phenomenon Absent pulses
Diabetes	–	Avoid non-selective agents in patients prone to hypoglycaemia
Pregnancy	–	Avoid non-selective agents in favour of labetalol and atenolol

of sympathetic overactivity in hyperthyroidism, to block the effects of circulating catecholamines in phaeochromocytoma and to reduce intraocular pressure in glaucoma. Non-selective β-adrenoceptor antagonists are probably more effective than β_1-selective drugs in migraine prophylaxis, essential tremor and in acute alcohol and opioid withdrawal syndromes.

Angina pectoris

All drugs that antagonize the β_1-adrenoceptors are equally effective in the symptomatic treatment of angina pectoris.[38,87] Two properties may influence the choice of drug therapy: β_1-selectivity and intrinsic sympathomimetic or partial agonist activity. It is doubtful whether partial agonist activity confers a major advantage in the management of angina pectoris, but agents with this property may be less likely to cause reduced muscle blood flow in predisposed patients.[88] It has also been suggested that this property may protect against congestive heart failure, excessive bradycardia and depression of atrioventricular conduction. These potential benefits are counterbalanced by the consideration that intrinsic sympathomimetic activity is probably undesirable in angina that occurs at rest or after minimal exercise.[89]

Although β_1-selectivity offers some theoretical advantage by not blocking the cardiac β_2-receptors, no clinical superiority has been demonstrated. The incidence of adverse effects related to β_2-blockade (increased airways resistance, reduced peripheral circulation and prolonged hyperglycaemia) is, however, reduced. Similarly, although drugs with additional α-blocking properties have theoretical advantages over β-blockers without this property, they are no more efficacious in the treatment of angina pectoris.[38,87]

Evidence for the use of β-blockers in angina pectoris

β-blockers are the preferred agents in the treatment of angina pectoris for a number of reasons. First, for those patients with impaired left ventricular systolic function following a myocardial infarction, these drugs confer post-infarction protection and metoprolol, bisoprolol and carvedilol extend life expectancy in patients with chronic heart failure. Second, in patients thought to be at risk of developing unstable angina, the dihydropyridine calcium channel blockers are contraindicated because of the increased mortality associated with capsular nifedipine. Third, increased heart rate is an important risk factor for ischaemic heart disease and β-blockers are therefore preferred to the non-rate-limiting calcium channel antagonists, such as nifedipine.

A meta-analysis of 90 randomized or cross-over studies comparing β-blockers, calcium channel blockers and long-acting nitrates, demonstrated no difference in the rates of myocardial infarction and cardiac mortality between β-blockers and calcium channel blockers.[87] However, β-blockers were discontinued less often because of adverse effects.

The combination of a β-blocker with a calcium channel blocker provides greater anti-anginal efficacy than either drug given alone and appears to be safest when the combination involves a dihydropyridine. The combination with diltiazem or verapamil can be used, but more adverse events are likely to occur in patients with poor left ventricular function and impaired cardiac conduction.[38]

Acute coronary syndromes

No large-scale trials are available in unstable angina and non-Q wave infarction,[90,91] although β-blockers reduce early mortality after a myocardial infarction by 10–15%.[92] Prevention of malignant ventricular arrhythmias, re-infarction and possibly myocardial rupture appears to be the principal mechanism.[91] A meta-analysis of studies involving 4700 patients with unstable angina by Yusuf and colleagues in 1988, demonstrated a 13% reduction in the risk of myocardial infarction in patients receiving β-adrenoceptor antagonists.[93] The strong pathological and clinical link between angina pectoris and myocardial infarction has led to the general recommendation that these drugs should be used as first-line agents in all acute coronary syndromes.[25]

Myocardial infarction

Early myocardial infarction

Administration of intravenous metoprolol[94] or atenolol[95] within 4 hours of the onset of a myocardial infarction followed by oral therapy reduces the risk of ventricular fibrillation, decreases the severity of chest pain and limits infarct size. An analysis of 28 trials of β-blocker therapy in acute myocardial infarction demonstrated a reduction in deaths, re-infarction and cardiac arrest (Fig. 11.6). With continued oral administration early mortality is reduced. The addition of intravenous β-blockade to thrombolytic agents also seems to be beneficial.[96] Early outcome is improved and the incidence of intracranial haemorrhage is reduced, although atenolol therapy results in more hypotension, heart failure, recurrent ischaemia and the need for pacemaker insertion.[96]

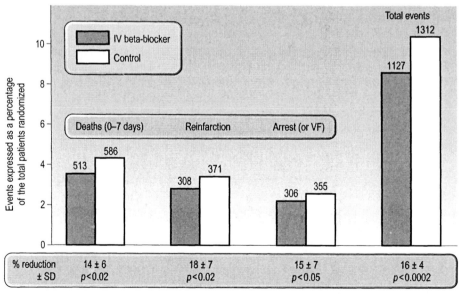

Fig. 11.6 Impact of intravenous β-adrenoceptor antagonist administration on early deaths, re-infarction rate and cardiac arrest following an acute myocardial infarction

Secondary prevention

In the period following a myocardial infarction β-blockade reduces mortality by 35% to 40%. Timolol, propranolol, metoprolol and atenolol are all effective, but drugs with intrinsic sympathomimetic effect, such as oxprenolol and pindolol, are relatively ineffective.[90–92,97]

Data from randomized clinical trials support the recommendation that β-blockers should be given to all patients with an acute myocardial infarction who do not have clear contraindications, such as pulmonary oedema, asthma, symptomatic hypotension, bradycardia or advanced atrioventricular block.[98] The greatest benefit, however, is observed in patients with the highest risk of death and, therefore, includes patients with these conditions.[98] If tolerated, β-blockers should be continued for at least 2–3 years and benefit up to 6 years has been described. Long-term β-blockade after an acute myocardial infarction reduces mortality by 23% (Fig. 11.7). Additional benefit has also been described when β-blockers are co-prescribed with ACE inhibitors following an acute myocardial infarction and treatment with calcium channel blockers and aspirin does not reduce the benefits of this treatment. Several mechanisms have been suggested to explain the dramatic effect of β-blockade in reducing the incidence of sudden death. These have included increasing the fibrillatory threshold,[99] attenuating the vagal withdrawal associated with stress and reducing the sympathetically driven adverse effects on heart rate, BP, shear stress, platelet function and thrombogenesis that promote atherosclerotic plaque rupture.[100,101]

Congestive heart failure

β-blockers are now recognized as an essential part of the treatment of congestive heart failure.[102] Important clinical aspects of the treatment are to start at a low dose with a gradual increase and to ensure that the patient is receiving optimal therapy with ACE inhibitors and diuretics. Three β-blockers are available for this indication: metoprolol,[103] carvedilol[16] and bisoprolol.[104] Bisoprolol and carvedilol reduce mortality (Table 11.2) and two recent meta-analyses

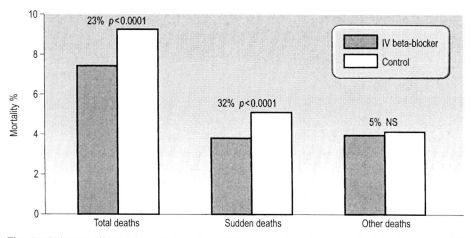

Fig. 11.7 Impact of beta-adrenoceptor antagonist therapy on long-term mortality following myocardial infarction.

Table 11.2 Effect of beta-adrenoceptor antagonist therapy on mortality in patients with congestive cardiac failure

Trial	Mean follow-up (months)	Number of deaths		Relative risk reduction	Lives saved per 1000
		Placebo	*β-blocker*		
MDC	15	19 (10.1%)	23 (11.9%)	n.s.	−18
CIBIS	21	67 (20.9%)	53 (16.6%)	20% n.s.	43
CIBIS II	15.6	228 (17.3%)	156 (11.8%)	32% ($p < 0.005$)	54
MERIT-HF	12	220 (11.0%)	143 (7.2%)	35% ($p = 0.006$)	39
COPERNICUS	10.4	209 (18.5%)	132 (11.4%)	35% ($p = 0.0014$)	66
ANZ	18	26 (12.5%)	20 (9.7%)	23% n.s.	28
US Trials	6.5	31 (7.8%)	22 (3.2%)	65% ($p = 0.0001$)	46

MDC = Metoprolol in Dilated Cardiomyopathy; CIBIS = Cardiac Insufficiency Bisoprolol Study; CIBIS II = Cardiac Insufficiency Bisoprolol Study II; MERIT-HF = Metoprolol Randomised Intervention Trial in Heart Failure; COPERNICUS = Carvedilol Prospective Randomised Cumulative Survival Trial; ANZ = Australia-New Zealand Heart Failure Trial; US Trials = US Carvedilol Heart Failure Trial Program; n.s. = not significant

assessing β-blockade in heart failure identified an overall relative risk reduction in mortality of over 30%. These analyses also suggested a greater effect of β-blockers in preventing non-sudden death than sudden death.[105,106]

A number of explanations have been advanced for the beneficial effects of β-blockers in heart failure. Reduction in heart rate, particularly when baseline resting heart rate is more than 80 beats/minute, will improve coronary blood flow and decrease myocardial oxygen demand.[105] High circulating levels of catecholamines increase the risk of cardiac arrhythmias and there is experimental evidence to show that they damage membranes and promote cellular destruction.[107] Reversal of these effects would clearly be beneficial in patients with heart failure. High levels of circulating catecholamines also result in down-regulation of the $β_1$-adrenoceptors. It has been suggested that β-adrenoceptor antagonists re-sensitize the down-regulated receptor system,[108] but such an explanation has not received widespread support because most investigators consider down-regulation to be beneficial overall in patients with heart failure.

Hypertension

A number of large outcome trials have used β-adrenoceptor antagonists as the principal group of antihypertensive agents. In the single-blind MRC trial of treatment of mild hypertension conducted in general practices in the UK, 17 354 subjects aged 35 to 64 years with diastolic BPs between 90 and 109 mmHg were studied.[109] Patients were randomized to active treatment (bendrofluazide 10 mg or propranolol up to 240 mg daily). Additional treatment with guanethidine or methyldopa was used as required to achieve the target diastolic BP of <90 mmHg. After 4.9 years average follow-up, systolic BP was reduced by 11 mmHg and diastolic BP by 6 mmHg in actively treated subjects compared with those on placebo. Those on active treatment had a 45% reduced risk of stroke compared with placebo and all cardiovascular disease events were reduced by 19% (Table 11.3). A number of deficiencies in the

Table 11.3 Impact of beta-adrenoceptor antagonist-based therapy on the incidence of stroke, coronary artery and total cardiovascular disease in pateints with essential hypetension

Trial	No.	Age (years)	Entry criteria	Follow-up (years)	Study design	Treatment	Outcomes % risk reduction (95% CI)		
							Stroke	Coronary heart disease	Total cardiovascular disease
MRC Trial 1985	17 354	35–64	Diastolic blood pressure (BP) 90–109 mmHg	4.9	Single-blind placebo controlled	Propranolol [bendrofluazide]	45 (25–60)	6 (–13–21)	19 (5–31)
Coope and Warrender 1986	884	60–79	Systolic BP >170 mmHg Diastolic BP >105 mmHg	4.4	Open No placebo	Atenolol	42 (4–65)	–3 (–63–37)	–
STOP-H 1991	1627	70–84	Systolic BP >180 mmHg Diastolic BP >90 mmHg or Diastolic BP 105–120 mmHg	2.1	Double-blind placebo controlled	β-blocker or [hydrochlorothiazide + amiloride]	47 (14–67)	13 (–65–51)	40 (15–57)
MRC Trial In Older People 1992	4396	65–74	Systolic BP >160 mmHg and Diastolic BP >115 mmHg	5.8	Single-blind placebo controlled	Atenolol or [hydrochlorothiazide + amiloride]	25 (3–42)	19 (–2–36)	17 (2–29)

study undermined the reliability of the data. Almost 20% were lost to follow-up and 43% of the diuretic group, 42% of the propranolol group and 47% of the placebo group at the end of the study were not taking the treatment to which they had been assigned at randomization. The doses of bendrofluazide used were substantially higher (10 mg) than those currently recommended (2.5 mg).

In a trial conducted by Coope and Warrender,[110] 884 subjects aged 60 to 79 years with systolic BPs of >170 mmHg or diastolic BPs of >105 mmHg (mean 196/99) were randomized to atenolol 100 mg or to an open control group. Two-thirds of subjects in the atenolol-treated group required the addition of a diuretic to achieve adequate BP control, which decreased by 18/11 mmHg. Active treatment resulted in a significant 42% decrease in stroke, a non-significant 22% reduction in cardiovascular death and no change in the number of coronary events (Table 11.3). Limitations of this trial included the relatively small sample size, major differences in the number of smokers in the two groups and a higher incidence of non-cardiovascular mortality in the treatment group (mainly lung cancer).

In the STOP-H trial, 1627 patients aged 70 to 84 years with systolic BPs between 180 and 230 mmHg and diastolic BPs at least 90 mmHg or diastolic BPs of 105–120 mmHg regardless of the systolic pressure, were randomized to active treatment or placebo.[111] The study was double-blind and active therapy was atenolol 50 mg, hydrochlorothiazide 25 mg with amiloride 2.5 mg, metoprolol 100 mg or pindolol 5 mg daily. Most patients completed the study on a combination of a β-blocker and a diuretic. The trial was terminated early at 25 months due to clear benefits in the active treatment group. Substantial and significant reductions in combined cardiovascular death (40%), stroke (47%) and vascular death (57%) were observed (Table 11.3). A smaller and non-significant reduction in myocardial infarction (13%) also occurred.

In a single-blind MRC trial of older adults, 4396 patients aged 65 to 74 years with systolic BPs of ≥160 mmHg and diastolic pressures of < 115 mmHg (mean 185/90 mmHg) were randomized to atenolol (50 mg), hydrochlorothiazide (25–50 mg) plus amiloride (2.5–5.0 mg) or placebo.[112] Over a mean of 5.8 years' follow-up, the active treatment group had a significant 25% reduction in stroke and a significant 17% reduction in total cardiovascular disease (Table 11.3). This study also had a high proportion of patients lost to follow-up or withdrawn from randomized treatment, so that by the end of the trial, 48% in the diuretic group, 63% in the β-blocker group and 53% in the placebo group were no longer on the original randomized treatment.

Overall, clinical outcome data from primary prevention trials support the efficacy of β-blocking in lowering BP and reducing the risk of stroke and total cardiovascular disease in middle-aged and older adults with hypertension. In an overview of 17 trials predominantly using β-blockers and diuretics, and involving 23 847 patients followed for 3–5 years, an average reduction of 5–6 mmHg diastolic BP was associated with a 16% reduction in coronary heart disease and a 38% reduction in total stroke.[113]

The efficacy of β-blockers, particularly atenolol, in the treatment of hypertension, however, has recently been questioned.[114] Four studies that compared atenolol with placebo or no treatment, and five clinical trials that compared atenolol with other antihypertensive drugs were identified for assessment. In the four studies comparing atenolol with placebo or no antihypertensive therapy and involving 6825 patients, there were no outcome differences in all-cause mortality, cardiovascular mortality and myocardial infarction. The risk of stroke was lower, however. When atenolol was compared with other antihypertensive drugs, hydrochlorothiazide, captopril, lacidipine, metoprolol or losartan, involving 17 671 patients, a higher mortality was observed in the atenolol-treated group for the same BP reduction. There was also a tendency for cardiovascular mortality and stroke to be more common in the atenolol-treated group.[114]

Most guidelines for the treatment of hypertension recommend diuretics and β-blockers as first-line therapies. Of these two major groups, diuretics have achieved more endpoint benefit[113] in meta-analyses and there remains a degree of doubt over atenolol as a first-line agent.[114] While primary prevention data are somewhat less than optimal for β-adrenoceptor antagonists, secondary cardiovascular protection is impressive and remains an important factor in recommending this group of drugs for hypertensive patients. These drugs are recommended as first-line therapy in angina pectoris, myocardial infarction, heart failure and to suppress a number of cardiac arrhythmias.

Cardiac arrhythmias

β-adrenoceptor antagonists are effective in the treatment of supraventricular and ventricular arrhythmias.[115,116] These drugs slow the ventricular response rates in atrial flutter and fibrillation by increasing the atrioventricular refractory period and reducing the frequency of ectopic beats related to excess catecholamine activity. They also suppress ventricular ectopic depolarizations in other clinical situations and their role in prevention of sudden cardiac death, in part, relates to their anti-arrhythmic activity.[117]

Other cardiac conditions

β-blocking drugs have been shown to increase stroke volume and improve diastolic function in patients with obstructive cardiomyopathy.[118] This beneficial effect probably relates to slowing of ventricular ejection and decreased outflow resistance. High-dose β-blockers are effective in relieving symptoms, such as dyspnoea, fatigue or angina in over 50% of patients with this condition. Other cardiac conditions that have been treated with β-adrenoceptor antagonists include mitral stenosis, mitral valve prolapse, Marfan's syndrome, Fallot's tetralogy and congenital QT prolongation.[117,119] In mitral stenosis, decreasing resting and exercise heart rates improves diastolic filling and exercise tolerance. In mitral valve prolapse β-blockers reduce the risk of arrhythmias and in Marfan's syndrome prevent aortic dilatation and dissection. In Fallot's tetralogy the beneficial effect is probably due to reduced right ventricular contractility and in the long QT syndrome, restoration of the imbalance between the right and left stellate ganglia.[26,117,119]

Glaucoma

Topical administration of β-adrenoceptor antagonists reduces intraocular pressure in patients with glaucoma. The mechanism appears to involve reduced production of aqueous humour by the ciliary body, which is activated by cyclic AMP.[120] Timolol is the drug of first choice, being a pure antagonist and devoid of local anaesthetic activity. Although the dose used is small, systemic effects have been reported in susceptible individuals.[121]

Hyperthyroidism

A number of features of hyperthyroidism resemble catecholamine over-activity: tachycardia, tremor and sweating. Reducing these effects by antagonizing the β-receptors and inhibiting the conversion of thyroxine to the more active form of thyroid hormone, tri-iodothyromine, contribute to the beneficial clinical response. Effects on this conversion vary from β-blocker to β-blocker, but propranolol appears to be particularly efficacious in a thyroid storm when tri-iodothyronine plays a major role.[122]

Neurological conditions

A number of studies have demonstrated that β-adrenoceptor antagonists reduce the frequency and intensity of migraine headache. The mechanism is unknown.[123] β-blockers have also been used in essential and other tremors, and to reduce the somatic features of anxiety and alcohol withdrawal.[58,124]

Portal hypertension

β-adrenoceptor antagonists reduce portal vein pressure in patients with hepatic cirrhosis. Propranolol and nadolol have been shown to reduce the risk of bleeding from oesophageal varices and to reduce the mortality rate associated with bleeding in patients with cirrhosis.[125]

DRUG INTERACTIONS

Important pharmacokinetic and pharmacodynamic interactions have been described between β-adrenoceptor antagonists and other drugs. Aluminium salts, cholestyramine and colestipol decrease the absorption of propranolol and atenolol. The impact of aluminium salts and other antacids is probably of little clinical significance[126,127] and the action of propranolol is not significantly affected by the exchange resins. Enzyme-inducing drugs rifampicin, pentobarbitone, phenobarbitone and tobacco smoking can reduce the plasma concentrations of β-blockers, which undergo hepatic metabolism: propranolol, alprenolol, bisoprolol, timolol and metoprolol.[128–132] An increase in the dose of β-blockers may be required to achieve the optimum therapeutic effect, particularly for drugs whose metabolites are inactive. Cimetidine increases the bioavailability of propranolol and metoprolol by reducing hepatic metabolism and decreasing liver blood flow[133–136] and hydralazine increases the area under the plasma concentration–time curve of propranolol, exprenolol and metoprolol by similar mechanisms.[137–139] β-adrenoceptor antagonists can also impair the clearance of lignocaine.[140]

Overall, pharmacodynamic interactions play a more important part in clinical practice. A number of drugs produce additive effects on cardiac contractility, conduction and BP. Serious cardiodepressant effects have been observed in patients receiving β-blockers with calcium channel blockers, nifedipine,[141,142] diltiazem[143,144] and verapamil.[145,146] β-blockers combine with other antihypertensive drugs, notably diuretics and vasodilators, to produce additive antihypertensive effects, which can result in severe hypotension in 'at-risk' patients. Conversely, the antihypertensive effects of β-blockers can be opposed by nonsteroidal anti-inflammatory agents: indometacin and piroxicam.[147,148]

OVERDOSAGE

Clinical features

Most patients who have taken a large dose of a β-blocker will demonstrate bradycardia and hypotension. With very large doses there will be coma, convulsions and profound hypotension. A variety of cardiac dysrhythmias and ECG abnormalities are described. The more serious of these can result in cardiorespiratory arrest. These include: heart block; intraventricular conduction defects; ST segment elevation; absent P waves; and ventricular fibrillation or asystole.[17,149,150]

Management

Gastric lavage and activated charcoal (50–100 g) may be considered if a large overdose has been taken within 1 hour of presentation, although evidence of efficacy for both is poor. Atropine (600–1200 µg) is commonly given to treat bradycardia and hypotension. If cardiogenic shock is unresponsive to atropine, glucagon is usually administered as a bolus of 50–150 µg/kg over 1 minute, although its reputation is mostly based on its widespread use rather than on results of comparative trials. Glucagon activates adenylyl cyclase to increase cyclic AMP production, which stimulates the β-receptors. A variety of other inotropes (e.g. isoprenaline, dopamine, dobutamine and phosphodiesterase inhibitors) have been used in resistant cases, and pacing is often required if the patient presents late. With the exception of propranolol overdose, convulsions are usually short-lived and rarely require treatment.[17,149,150]

Reference

1. Ahlquist RP. A study of the adrenotropic receptors. *Am J Physiol* 1948;153:586–600.
2. Slater IH, Powell CE. Blockade of adrenergic inhibitory receptor sites by 1-(3¹-4¹ dichloro-phenol)-2 isopropyl-aminoethanol hydrochloride. *Fed Proc* 1957;16:336.
3. Moran NC, Perkins ME. Adrenergic blockade of the mammalian heart by a dichloro analogue of isoproterenol. *J Pharmacol Exp Ther* 1958;124(3):223–237.
4. Black JW. Ahlquist and the development of beta-adrenoceptor antagonists. *Postgrad Med J* 1976;52(Suppl 4):11–13.
5. Black JW, Stephenson JS. Pharmacology of a new adrenergic beta-receptor-blocking compound (Nethalide). *Lancet* 1962;2:311–314.
6. Zacharias FJ, Cowen KJ. Controlled trial of propranolol in hypertension. *BMJ* 1970;1(694): 471–474.
7. Frishman WH. Alpha and beta adrenergic blocking drugs. In: Frishman WH, Sonnenblick EH, Sic D, eds. *Cardiovascular pharmacotherapies*. New York: McGaw-Hill; 2003:67–97.
8. Weerasuriya K, Patel L, Turner P. Beta-adrenoceptor blockade and migraine. *Cephalalgia* 1982;2(1):33–45.
9. Benson MK, Berrill WT, Cruickshank JM, Sterling GS. A comparison of four beta-adrenoceptor antagonists in patients with asthma. *Br J Clin Pharmacol* 1978;5(5):415–419.
10. Hampton JR. Choosing the right beta-blocker. A guide to selection. *Drugs* 1994;48(4): 549–568.

11. Cruickshank JM. The clinical importance of cardioselectivity and lipophilicity in beta blockers. *Am Heart J* 1980;100(2):160–178.

12. Kjekshus J. Heart rate reduction–a mechanism of benefit? *Eur Heart J* 1987;8(Suppl L):115–122.

13. Man In't Veld AJ, van den Meiracker AH. Effects of antihypertensive drugs on cardiovascular haemodynamics. In: Laragh JH, Brenner BM, eds. *Hypertension*. New York: Raven Press; 1990:2117–2130.

14. Lund-Johansen P. Pharmacology of combined alpha-beta-blockade. II. Haemodynamic effects of labetalol. *Drugs* 1984;28(Suppl 2):35–50.

15. Lamming GD, Broughton PF, Symonds EM. Comparison of the alpha and beta blocking drug, labetalol, and methyl dopa in the treatment of moderate and severe pregnancy-induced hypertension. *Clin Exp Hypertens* 1980;2(5):865–895.

16. Packer M, Bristow MR, Cohn JN, et al. The effect of carvedilol on morbidity and mortality in patients with chronic heart failure. U.S. Carvedilol Heart Failure Study Group. *N Engl J Med* 1996;334(21):1349–1355.

17. Johnston GD, Smith AMJ. Antihypertensive and anti-anginal drugs. In: Descotes J, ed. *Human Toxicology*. Amsterdam: Elsevier Science BV; 1996:395–409.

18. Main BG, Tucker H. Recent advances in beta-adrenergic blocking agents. In: Ellis GP, West GB, eds. *Prog Med Chem* 1985:(22)121–164.

19. Smith LH. Beta adrenergic blocking agents. *J Appl Chem Biotechnol* 1978;28:201–212.

20. Kaumann AJ, Blinks JR. beta-Adrenoceptor blocking agents as partial agonists in isolated heart muscle: dissociation of stimulation and blockade. *Naunyn Schmiedebergs Arch Pharmacol* 1980;311(3):237–248.

21. Johnston GD, Finch MB, McNeill JA, Shanks RG. A comparison of the cardiovascular effects of (+)-sotalol and (+/-)-sotalol following intravenous administration in normal volunteers. *Br J Clin Pharmacol* 1985;20(5):507–510.

22. Brittain RT, Drew GM, Levy GP. The alpha- and beta-adrenoceptor blocking potencies of labetalol and its individual stereoisomers in anaesthetized dogs and in isolated tissues. *Br J Pharmacol* 1982;77(1):105–114.

23. Walter M, Lemoine H, Kaumann AJ. Stimulant and blocking effects of optical isomers of pindolol on the sinoatrial node and trachea of guinea pig. Role of beta-adrenoceptor subtypes in the dissociation between blockade and stimulation. *Naunyn Schmiedebergs Arch Pharmacol* 1984;327(2):159–175.

24. Steinberg SF. The molecular basis for distinct beta-adrenergic receptor subtype actions in cardiomyocytes. *Circ Res* 1999;85(11):1101–1111.

25. Opie LH, Sonnenblick EH, Frishman WH, et al. Beta blocking agents. In: Opie LH, ed. *Drugs for the heart*. Philadelphia: WB Saunders; 1994:1–32.

26. Ross EM. G proteins and receptors in neuronal signaling. In: Hall ZW, ed. *An introduction to molecular neurobiology*, Massachusetts: Sinauer Associates; 1992:181–206.

27. Brodde OE. The functional importance of beta 1 and beta 2 adrenoceptors in the human heart. *Am J Cardiol* 1988;62(5):24C–29C.

28. Perkins JP, Hausdorff WP, Lefkowitz RJ. Mechanisms of ligand induced desensitization of beta adrenergic receptors. In: Perkins JP, ed. *The beta adrenergic receptors*. Clifton, New Jersey: The Humana Press; 1991:73–124.

29. Strader CD, Fong TM, Tota MR, et al. Structure and function of G protein-coupled receptors. *Annu Rev Biochem* 1994;63:101–132.

30. Wood AJ. Beta blocker withdrawal. *Drugs* 1983;25(Suppl 2):318–321.

31. Frishman WH, Alwarshetty M. Beta-adrenergic blockers in systemic hypertension: pharmacokinetic considerations related to the current guidelines. *Clin Pharmacokinet* 2002;41(7):505–516.

32. Fitzgerald JD, Ruffin R, Smedstad KG, et al. Studies on the pharmacokinetics and pharmacodynamics of atenolol in man. *Eur J Clin Pharmacol* 1978;13(2):81–89.

33. Neil-Dwyer G, Bartlett J, McAinsh J, Cruickshank JM. Beta-adrenoceptor blockers and the blood-brain barrier. *Br J Clin Pharmacol* 1981;11(6):549–553.

34. Gengo FM, Huntoon L, McHugh WB. Lipid-soluble and water-soluble beta-blockers. Comparison of the central nervous system depressant effect. *Arch Intern Med* 1987;147(1):39–43.

35. McDevitt DG. Comparison of pharmacokinetic properties of beta-adrenoceptor blocking drugs. *Eur Heart J* 1987;8(Suppl M):9–14.

36. Sotaniemi EA, Pelkonen RO, Arranto AJ, et al. Effect of liver function on beta blocker kinetics. *Drugs* 1983;25(Suppl 2):113–120.

37. Zech PY, Labeeuw M, Pozet N, et al. Response to atenolol in arterial hypertension in relation to renal function, pharmacokinetics and renin activity. *Postgrad Med J* 1977;53(Suppl 3):134–141.

38. Goldstein S. Beta-blockers in hypertensive and coronary heart disease. *Arch Intern Med* 1996;156(12):1267–1276.

39. Mani V, Schalekamp MA. Haemodynamic consequences of intrinsic sympathomimetic activity in relation to changes in plasma renin activity and noradrenaline during beta-blocker therapy for hypertension. *Postgrad Med J* 1983;59(Suppl 3):140–158.

40. Colfer HT, Cottier C, Sanchez R, Julius S. Role of cardiac factors in the initial hypotensive action by beta-adrenoreceptor blocking agents. *Hypertension* 1984;6(2 Pt 1):145–151.

41. Hollifield JW, Sherman K, Zwagg RV, Shand DG. Proposed mechanisms of propranolol's antihypertensive effect in essential hypertension. *N Engl J Med* 1976;295(2):68–73.

42. Amery A, Billiet L, Boel A, et al. Mechanism of hypotensive effect during betaadrenergic blockade in hypertensive patients. *Am Heart J* 1976;91(5):634–642.

43. Dunlop D, Shanks RG. Inhibition of the carotid sinus reflex by the chronic administration of propranolol. *Br J Pharmacol* 1969;36(1):132–143.

44. Scott EM. The effect of atenolol on the spontaneous and reflex activity of the sympathetic nerves in the cat: influence of cardiopulmonary receptors. *Br J Pharmacol* 1983;78(2):425–431.

45. Dahlof B, Andren L, Svensson A, Hansson L. Antihypertensive mechanism of beta-adrenoceptor antagonism – the role of beta 2-blockade. *J Hypertens Suppl* 1983;1(2):112–115.

46. Robb OJ, Petrie JC, Webster J, et al. ICI 118551 does not reduce BP in hypertensive patients responsive to atenolol and propranolol. *Br J Clin Pharmacol* 1985;19:541P–542P.

47. Gottdiener JS, Reda DJ, Massie BM, et al. Effect of single-drug therapy on reduction of left ventricular mass in mild to moderate hypertension: comparison of six antihypertensive agents. The Department of Veterans Affairs Cooperative Study Group on Antihypertensive Agents. *Circulation* 1997;95(8):2007–2014.

48. Dahlof B, Pennert K, Hansson L. Reversal of left ventricular hypertrophy in hypertensive patients. A metaanalysis of 109 treatment studies. *Am J Hypertens* 1992;5(2):95–110.

49. Hartling OJ, Noer I, Svendsen TL, et al. Selective and non-selective beta-adrenoreceptor blockade in the human forearm. *Clin Sci (Lond)* 1980;58(4):279–286.

50. McSorley PD, Warren DJ. Effects of propranolol and metoprolol on the peripheral circulation. *Br Med J* 1978;2(6152):1598–1600.

51. Yasue H, Touyama M, Shimamoto M, et al. Role of autonomic nervous system in the pathogenesis of Prinzmetal's variant form of angina. *Circulation* 1974;50(3):534–539.

52. Kaplinsky E. Management of angina pectoris modern concepts. *Drugs* 1987;59:37J.

53. van Baak MA, Struyker Boudier HA, Smits JF. Antihypertensive mechanisms of beta-adrenoceptor blockade: a review. *Clin Exp Hypertens A* 1985;7(1):1–72.

54. Buhler FR, Laragh JH, Baer L, et al. Propranolol inhibition of renin secretion. A specific approach to diagnosis and treatment of renin-dependent hypertensive diseases. *N Engl J Med* 1972;287(24):1209–1214.

55. de Leeuw PW, Birkenhager WH. Renal effects of beta blockade in essential hypertension. *Eur Heart J* 1983;4(Suppl D):13–17.

56. Philippu A, Stroehl U. beta-Adrenoreceptors of the posterior hypothalamus. *Clin Exp Hypertens* 1978;1(1):25–38.

57. Roubicek J. The effect of beta-adrenoceptor blocking drugs on EEG. *Br J Clin Pharmacol* 1976;3:661–665.

58. Arnold JMD, Johnston GD, Harron DWG, et al. The effect of ICI 118551 on isoprenaline-induced beta-adrenoceptor responses in man. *Br J Clin Pharmacol* 1983;15:133–134.

59. Shand DG. Drug therapy: propranolol. *N Engl J Med* 1975;293(6):280–285.

60. Smith U, Lager I. Beta blockade in diabetes. *N Engl J Med* 1978;299(26):1467–1468.

61. Harms HH, Gooren L, Spoelstra AJ, et al. Blockade of isoprenaline-induced changes in plasma free fatty acids, immunoreactive insulin levels and plasma renin activity in healthy human subjects, by propranolol, pindolol, practolol, atenolol, metoprolol and acebutolol. *Br J Clin Pharmacol* 1978;5(1):19–26.

62. Dahlof B, Devereux RB, Kjeldsen SE, et al. Cardiovascular morbidity and mortality in the Losartan Intervention For Endpoint reduction in hypertension study (LIFE): a randomised trial against atenolol. *Lancet* 2002;359(9311):995–1003.

63. Weidmann P, Gerber A, Mordasini R. Effects of antihypertensive therapy on serum lipoproteins. *Hypertension* 1983;5(5 Pt 2):III120–III131.

64. Johnston GD, Vyssoulis G, Feely J, et al. Effect of celiprolol and metoprolol on lipids, fibrinogen and airways function in hyperlipidaemic hypertensives: a randomised double-blind long-term parallel group trial. *J Hum Hypertens* 1995;9(2):123–129.

65. Frishman WH. Medical management of lipid disorders. In: Frishman WH, ed. *Focus on prevention of coronary artery disease.* New York: Futura Publishing Co.; 1992.

66. Struthers AD, Reid JL, Whitesmith R, Rodger JC. The effects of cardioselective and non-selective beta-adrenoceptor blockade on the hypokalaemic and cardiovascular responses to adrenomedullary hormones in man. *Clin Sci (Lond)* 1983;65(2):143–147.

67. Carstairs JR, Nimmo AJ, Barnes PJ. Autoradiographic visualization of beta-adrenoceptor subtypes in human lung. *Am Rev Respir Dis* 1985;132(3):541–547.
68. Tattersfield AE, Leaver DG, Pride NB. Effects of beta-adrenergic blockade and stimulation on normal human airways. *J Appl Physiol* 1973;35(5):613–619.
69. Johnsson G, Svedmyr N, Thiringer G. Effects of intravenous propranolol and metoprolol and their interaction with isoprenaline on pulmonary function, heart rate and blood pressure in asthmatics. *Eur J Clin Pharmacol* 1975;8(3–4):175–180.
70. Drayer DE. Lipophilicity, hydrophilicity, and the central nervous system side effects of beta blockers. *Pharmacotherapy* 1987;7(4):87–91.
71. Betts TA, Alford C. Beta-blockers and sleep: a controlled trial. *Eur J Clin Pharmacol* 1985;28 (Suppl:65–8):65–68.
72. Toogood JH. Beta blocker therapy and the risk of anaphylaxis. *Can Med Assoc J* 1989;136:929.
73. Committee on Safety of Medicines. Fatal bronchospasm associated with beta blockers. *Curr Problems* 1987;20:2–3.
74. Tattersfield AE. Respiratory function in the elderly and the effects of beta blockade. *Cardiovasc Drugs Ther* 1991;4(Suppl 6):1229–1232.
75. Ellis ME, Sahay JN, Chatterjee SS, et al. Cardioselectivity of atenolol in asthmatic patients. *Eur J Clin Pharmacol* 1981;21(3):173–176.
76. Barnett DB. Beta-blockers in heart failure: a therapeutic paradox. *Lancet* 1994;343 (8897):557–558.
77. Feleke E, Lyngstam O, Rastam L, Ryden L. Complaints of cold extremities among patients on antihypertensive treatment. *Acta Med Scand* 1983;213(5):381–385.
78. Lepantalo M. Beta blockade and intermittent claudication. *Acta Med Scand Suppl* 1985;700:1–48.
79. Cruickshank JM. Beta blockers, bradycardia and adverse effects. *Acta Ther* 1981;7:309.
80. Blohme G, Lager I, Lonnroth P, Smith U. Hypoglycemic symptoms in insulin-dependent diabetics. A prospective study of the influence of beta-blockade. *Diabete Metab* 1981;7(4):235–238.
81. Holm G, Herlitz J, Smith U. Severe hypoglycaemia during physical exercise and treatment with beta-blockers. *Br Med J (Clin Res Ed)* 1981;282(6273):1360.
82. Lager I, Attvall S, Blohme G, Smith U. Altered recognition of hypoglycaemic symptoms in type I diabetes during intensified control with continuous subcutaneous insulin infusion. *Diabet Med* 1986;3(4):322–325.
83. Wilkinson R. Beta-blockers and renal function. *Drugs* 1982;23(3):195–206.
84. Miller RR, Olson HG, Amsterdam EA, Mason DT. Propranolol-withdrawal rebound phenomenon. Exacerbation of coronary events after abrupt cessation of antianginal therapy. *N Engl J Med* 1975;293(9):416–418.
85. Croog SH, Levine S, Testa MA, et al. The effects of antihypertensive therapy on the quality of life. *N Engl J Med* 1986;314(26):1657–1664.
86. Grimm RH, Jr., Grandits GA, Cutler JA, et al. Relationships of quality-of-life measures to long-term lifestyle and drug treatment in the Treatment of Mild Hypertension Study. *Arch Intern Med* 1997;157(6):638–648.
87. Heidenreich PA, McDonald KM, Hastie T, et al. Meta-analysis of trials comparing beta-blockers, calcium antagonists, and nitrates for stable angina. *JAMA* 1999;281(20):1927–1936.
88. Fitzgerald JD. Do partial agonist beta-blockers have improved clinical utility? *Cardiovasc Drugs Ther* 1993;7(3):303–310.
89. Wilhelmsson C, Vedin A. Beta blockers in ischemic heart disease. *Am J Cardiol* 1983;20;52(2):108A–112A.
90. A randomized trial of propranolol in patients with acute myocardial infarction. I. Mortality results. *JAMA* 1982;247(12):1707–1714.
91. Olsson G, Wikstrand J, Warnold I, et al. Metoprolol-induced reduction in postinfarction mortality: pooled results from five double-blind randomized trials. *Eur Heart J* 1992;13(1):28–32.
92. Timolol-induced reduction in mortality and reinfarction in patients surviving acute myocardial infarction.*N Engl J Med* 1981;304(14):801–807.
93. Yusuf S, Wittes J, Friedman L. Overview of results of randomized clinical trials in heart disease. II. Unstable angina, heart failure, primary prevention with aspirin, and risk factor modification. *JAMA* 1988;260(15):2259–2263.
94. Metoprolol in acute myocardial infarction (MIAMI). A randomised placebo-controlled international trial. The MIAMI Trial Research Group. *Eur Heart J* 1985;6(3):199–226.
95. Randomised trial of intravenous atenolol among 16 027 cases of suspected acute myocardial infarction: ISIS-1. First International Study of Infarct Survival Collaborative Group. *Lancet* 1986;2(8498):57–66.
96. Roberts R, Rogers WJ, Mueller HS, et al. Immediate versus deferred beta-blockade following thrombolytic therapy in patients with acute myocardial infarction. Results

of the Thrombolysis in Myocardial Infarction (TIMI) II-B Study. *Circulation* 1991;83(2): 422–437.

97. Olsson G, Wikstrand J, Warnold I, et al. Metoprolol-induced reduction in postinfarction mortality: pooled results from five double-blind randomized trials. *Eur Heart J* 1992;13(1):28–32.

98. Held PH, Yusuf S. Effects of beta-blockers and calcium channel blockers in acute myocardial infarction. *Eur Heart J* 1993;14(Suppl F):18–25.

99. Khan MI, Hamilton JT, Manning GW. Protective effect of beta adrenoceptor blockade in experimental coronary occlusion in conscious dogs. *Am J Cardiol* 1972;30(8):832–837.

100. Kennedy HL. Beta blockade, ventricular arrhythmias, and sudden cardiac death. *Am J Cardiol* 1997;80(9B):29J–34J.

101. Parker GW, Michael LH, Hartley CJ, et al. Central beta-adrenergic mechanisms may modulate ischemic ventricular fibrillation in pigs. *Circ Res* 1990;66(2):259–270.

102. Bristow MR. Mechanism of action of beta-blocking agents in heart failure. *Am J Cardiol* 1997;80(11A):26L–40L.

103. Waagstein F, Bristow MR, Swedberg K, et al. Beneficial effects of metoprolol in idiopathic dilated cardiomyopathy. Metoprolol in Dilated Cardiomyopathy (MDC) Trial Study Group. *Lancet* 1993;342(8885):1441–1446.

104. A randomized trial of beta-blockade in heart failure. The Cardiac Insufficiency Bisoprolol Study (CIBIS). CIBIS Investigators and Committees. *Circulation* 1994;90(4):1765–1773.

105. Heidenreich PA, Lee TT, Massie BM. Effect of beta-blockade on mortality in patients with heart failure: a meta-analysis of randomized clinical trials. *J Am Coll Cardiol* 1997; 30(1):27–34.

106. Doughty RN, Rodgers A, Sharpe N, MacMahon S. Effects of beta-blocker therapy on mortality in patients with heart failure. A systematic overview of randomized controlled trials. *Eur Heart J* 1997;18(4):560–565.

107. Bristow MR. beta-Adrenergic receptor blockade in chronic heart failure. *Circulation* 2000; 101(5):558–569.

108. Koch WJ, Rockman HA. Exploring the role of the beta-adrenergic receptor kinase in cardiac disease using gene-targeted mice. *Trends Cardiovasc Med* 1999;9(3–4):77–81.

109. MRC trial of treatment of mild hypertension: principal results. Medical Research Council Working Party. *BMJ (Clin Res Ed)* 1985;291(6488):97–104.

110. Coope J, Warrender TS. Randomised trial of treatment of hypertension in elderly patients in primary care. *BMJ (Clin Res Ed)* 1986;293(6555):1145–1151.

111. Dahlof B, Lindholm LH, Hansson L, et al. Morbidity and mortality in the Swedish Trial in Old Patients with Hypertension (STOP-Hypertension). *Lancet* 1991;338(8778):1281–1285.

112. Medical Research Council trial of treatment of hypertension in older adults: principal results. MRC Working Party. *BMJ* 1992;304(6824):405–412.

113. Collins R, Peto R, MacMahon S, et al. Blood pressure, stroke, and coronary heart disease. Part 2, Short-term reductions in blood pressure: overview of randomised drug trials in their epidemiological context. *Lancet* 1990;335(8693):827–838.

114. Carlberg B, Samuelsson O, Lindholm LH. Atenolol in hypertension: is it a wise choice? *Lancet* 2004;364(9446):1684–1689.

115. Exner DV, Reiffel JA, Epstein AE, et al. Beta-blocker use and survival in patients with ventricular fibrillation or symptomatic ventricular tachycardia: the Antiarrhythmics Versus Implantable Defibrillators (AVID) trial. *J Am Coll Cardiol* 1999;34(2):325–333.

116. Gottlieb SS, McCarter RJ, Vogel RA. Effect of beta-blockade on mortality among high-risk and low-risk patients after myocardial infarction. *N Engl J Med* 1998;%20;339(8):489–497.

117. Marcus FI, Opie LH. Antiarrhythmic agents. In: Opie LH, ed. *Drugs for the Heart.* Philadelphia: WB Saunders; 1994:207–246.

118. Wigle ED, Rakowski H, Kimball BP, Williams WG. Hypertrophic cardiomyopathy. Clinical spectrum and treatment. *Circulation* 1995;92(7):1680–1692.

119. Moss AJ, Zareba W, Hall WJ, et al. Effectiveness and limitations of beta-blocker therapy in congenital long-QT syndrome. *Circulation* 2000;101(6):616–623.

120. Potter DE. Adrenergic pharmacology of aqueous humor dynamics. *Pharmacol Rev* 1981;33 (3):133–153.

121. Alward WL. Medical management of glaucoma. *N Engl J Med* 1998;339(18):1298–1307.

122. Geffner DL, Hershman JM. Beta-adrenergic blockade for the treatment of hyperthyroidism. *Am J Med* 1992;93(1):61–68.

123. Tfelt-Hansen P. Efficacy of beta-blockers in migraine. A critical review. *Cephalalgia* 1986; 6(Suppl 5):15–24.

124. Brantigan CO, Brantigan TA, Joseph N. Effect of beta blockade and beta stimulation on stage fright. *Am J Med* 1982;72(1):88–94.

125. Pagliaro L, D'Amico G, Sorensen TI, et al. Prevention of first bleeding in cirrhosis. A meta-analysis of randomized trials of nonsurgical treatment. *Ann Intern Med* 1992; 117(1):59–70.

126. Dobbs JH, Skoutakis VA, Acchardio SR, et al. Effects of aluminium hydroxide on the absorption of propranolol. *Curr Ther Res* 1977;21:887.

127. Hibbard DM, Peters JR, Hunninghake DB. Effects of cholestyramine and colestipol on the plasma concentrations of propranolol. *Br J Clin Pharmacol* 1984;18(3):337–342.

128. Alvan G, Piafsky K, Lind M, von Bahr C. Effect of pentobarbital on the disposition of alprenolol. *Clin Pharmacol Ther* 1977;22(3):316–321.

129. Sotaniemi EA, Anttila M, Pelkonen RO, et al. Plasma clearance of propranolol and sotalol and hepatic drug-metabolizing enzyme activity. *Clin Pharmacol Ther* 1979;26(2):153–161.

130. Fox K, Deanfield J, Krikler S, et al. The interaction of cigarette smoking and beta-adrenoceptor blockade. *Br J Clin Pharmacol* 1984;17(Suppl 1):92S–93S.

131. Herman RJ, Nakamura K, Wilkinson GR, Wood AJ. Induction of propranolol metabolism by rifampicin. *Br J Clin Pharmacol* 1983;16(5):565–569.

132. Bennett PN, John VA, Whitmarsh VB. Effect of rifampicin on metoprolol and antipyrine kinetics. *Br J Clin Pharmacol* 1982;13(3):387–391.

133. Reimann IW, Klotz U, Frolich JC. Effects of cimetidine and ranitidine on steady-state propranolol kinetics and dynamics. *Clin Pharmacol Ther* 1982;32(6):749–757.

134. Kirch W, Ramsch K, Janisch HD, Ohnhaus EE. The influence of two histamine H2-receptor antagonists, cimetidine and ranitidine, on the plasma levels and clinical effect of nifedipine and metoprolol. *Arch Toxicol* 1984;7(Suppl):256–259.

135. Kirch W, Rose I, Klingmann I, et al. Interaction of bisoprolol with cimetidine and rifampicin. *Eur J Clin Pharmacol* 1986;31(1):59–62.

136. Spahn H, Kirch W, Mutschler E. The interaction of cimetidine with metoprolol, atenolol, propranolol, pindolol and penbutolol. *Br J Clin Pharmacol* 1983;15(4):500–501.

137. Hawksworth GM, Dart AM, Chiang K, et al. Effect of oxprenolol on the pharmacokinetics and pharmacodynamics of hydralazine. *Drugs* 1983;25(Suppl 2):136–140.

138. McLean AJ, Skews H, Bobik A, Dudley FJ. Interaction between oral propranolol and hydralazine. *Clin Pharmacol Ther* 1982;27(6):726–732.

139. Jack DB, Kendall MJ, Dean S, et al. The effect of hydralazine on the pharmacokinetics of three different beta adrenoceptor antagonists: metoprolol, nadolol, and acebutolol. *Biopharm Drug Dispos* 1982;3(1):47–54.

140. Wyse DG, Kellen J, Tam Y, Rademaker AW. Increased efficacy and toxicity of lidocaine in patients on beta-blockers. *Int J Cardiol* 1988;21(1):59–70.

141. Opie LH, White DA. Adverse interaction between nifedipine and beta-blockade. *BMJ* 1980;281(6253):1462.

142. Vetrovec GW, Parker VE. Nifedipine, beta-blocker interaction:effect on left ventricular function. *Clin Res* 1984;32:833A.

143. Rocha P, Baron B, Delestrain A, et al. Hemodynamic effects of intravenous diltiazem in patients treated chronically with propranolol. *Am Heart J* 1986;111(1):62–68.

144. O'Hara MJ, Khurmi NS, Bowles MJ, Raftery EB. Diltiazem and propranolol combination for the treatment of chronic stable angina pectoris. *Clin Cardiol* 1987;10(2):115–123.

145. McAllister RG, Todd GD, Slack JD, et al. Haemodynamic and pharmacokinetic aspects of the interaction between propranolol and verapamil. *Clin Res* 1981;29:755A.

146. Misra M, Thakur R, Bhandari K. Sinus arrest caused by atenolol-verapamil combination. *Clin Cardiol* 1987;10(6):365–367.

147. Watkins J, Abbott EC, Hensby CN, et al. Attenuation of hypotensive effect of propranolol and thiazide diuretics by indomethacin. *BMJ* 1980;281(6242):702–705.

148. Wong DG, Spence JD, Lamki L, et al. Effect of non-steroidal anti-inflammatory drugs on control of hypertension by beta-blockers and diuretics. *Lancet* 1986;1(8488):997–1001.

149. Love JN, Howell JM, Litovitz TL, Klein-Schwartz W. Acute beta blocker overdose: factors associated with the development of cardiovascular morbidity. *J Toxicol Clin Toxicol* 2000; 38(3):275–281.

150. Kerns W, Kline J, Ford MD. Beta-blocker and calcium channel blocker toxicity. *Emerg Med Clin North Am* 1994;12(2):365–390.

VI

Drugs acting on the renin–angiotensin system

12 | Angiotensin converting enzyme inhibitors

M. Gary Nicholls, Georg Petroianu and S. George Carruthers

INTRODUCTION

The angiotensin converting enzyme ACE inhibitors, developed in the 1970s and thereafter, have been used in the treatment of hypertension, cardiac failure, various forms of renal disease, and post-myocardial infarction. Widespread utilization has awakened interest in and understanding of two hormonal systems which underpin the actions of these drugs, the renin–angiotensin system (RAS) and the kallikrein–kinin system. In fact, whilst the ACE inhibitors are neither selective nor complete blockers of the RAS, development of ACE inhibitors along with the subsequent synthesis of specific angiotensin II type-1 and type-2 receptor blockers (see Chapter 13), has spawned an extensive literature which attests to the widespread, complex and important actions of the RAS in health and disease. Likewise, the advent of ACE inhibitors along with the development of bradykinin-receptor blocking agents, has encouraged research into and understanding of the kallikrein–kinin system. In this chapter, we discuss the ACE inhibitors and use of these drugs in the treatment of hypertension. A description of the RAS and the kallikrein–kinin system is given as the basis for understanding most of the known actions and side effects of these drugs. We will concentrate mostly, though not exclusively, on recently published information.

The renin–angiotensin system (RAS)

A historical review of the RAS was provided in 1993, 95 years after the discovery of renin.[1] An account of its phylogeny and comparative physiology is given by Henderson and Deacon.[2] The enzyme renin cleaves the biologically inactive decapeptide angiotensin I from its α2-globulin substrate and this, through removal of two carboxy-terminal amino-acids by ACE, forms the biologically active octapeptide, angiotensin II (Ang II). Until recent decades, the view was of a uniquely 'circulatory' RAS wherein renin, synthesized and stored within the juxta-glomerular (JG) cells of the kidney was released into the circulation under the influence of input from the afferent renal arteriolar baroreceptor, the macula densa (sensing tubular chloride concentration), and sympathetic innervation of the JG apparatus, to act on its substrate, secreted by the liver, producing angiotensin I which, as it passed through the pulmonary circuit, was converted by ACE to Ang II. This, the final end-product of the system, was released into the arterial limb of the circulation where Ang II induced arteriolar constriction, an immediate and incremental ('slow-pressor') elevation in arterial blood pressure (BP), stimulation of aldosterone from the adrenal glomerulosa and antidiuretic hormone from the pituitary, numerous and complex actions within the kidney, augmentation of thirst, activation of the sympathetic nervous system, inhibition of the parasympathetic nervous system, and stimulation of cardiac contractility. The biological effects of Ang II were seen broadly to be maintaining homeostasis through prevention of sodium and fluid loss, hypotension or excessive vasodilatation when body sodium and volume status were under threat. Whereas this early perspective is still valid in broad terms, it is now clear that the RAS is considerably more complex (Fig. 12.1).

Regulation of renin production in, and release from, the JG apparatus is subject to numerous input signals beyond the three noted above. These include the cardiac natriuretic peptides, adrenomedullin, prostaglandins, endothelin-I, Ang II itself, and antidiuretic hormone. Changes in JG or macula densa intracellular calcium, cyclic AMP, nitric oxide and possibly cyclic GMP and adenosine, are central to the renin-modulating action of many of these stimuli.[3,4] Most of the 'classical' biological actions of Ang II occur via stimulation of AT-1 receptors but some are through activation of AT-2 receptors which are thought, in some cases, to oppose the responses via AT-1 receptor stimulation.[5,6] The ACE inhibitors, by limiting Ang II formation via ACE, result in reduced stimulation of both of these receptors. By contrast, the angiotensin receptor blockers

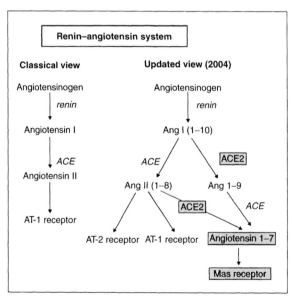

Fig. 12.1 An updated view of the renin–angiotensin system. In the classical view, angiotensin II mediates all known effects via the AT-1 receptor. The updated view on the right shows ACE2 degrading angiotensin I to angiotensin 1–9 and angiotensin II to the vasodilator, angiotensin 1–7. Angiotensin II also mediates effects via the G-protein coupled AT-2 receptor, and angiotensin 1–7 acts via its Mas receptor. From Burrell et al.[48] with permission.

(ARBs) selectively block AT-1 receptors, thereby enhancing renin release and Ang II formation and heightening stimulation of AT-2 receptors. Clearly therefore, if actions of Ang II via the AT-2 receptor are of importance, there is every reason to hypothesize that these two groups of drugs, the ACE inhibitors and the ARBs, both designed to inhibit actions of the RAS, might be associated with quite different outcomes in the treatment of cardiovascular and renal disorders.[7] Another reason that these two drug groups might have disparate therapeutic outcomes is that Ang II can be produced by non-ACE pathways, for example by chymases in vascular and cardiac tissues.[8,9] Accordingly, the effects of Ang II production via non-ACE pathways will be unaltered by administration of ACE inhibitors whereas ARBs, provided the drugs have access to the relevant AT-1 receptors, will block the biological effects of Ang II via that receptor whatever the source of the octapeptide.

Whereas the traditional view was of renin and renin-substrate being produced uniquely in the kidney and liver respectively, and Ang II, the end-product hormone being transported in the circulation with a brief half-life to targets in a few specific organs, it is now clear that many tissues and organs are able to produce, or take up from the circulation, components of the RAS and locally produce Ang II, which acts in a paracrine and possibly an intracrine manner. There are, for example, RASs in the heart,[10,11] vasculature,[12] brain,[13] pancreas,[14,15] eye,[16,17] adrenal,[18] testis[19] and adipose tissue[20] as well as in the kidney. The importance of these local systems in humans is gradually being unravelled. Should these indeed be pivotal to disease progression in, for example essential hypertension or diabetic organopathy, the ability of the individual ACE inhibitors (and ARBs) to achieve access to ACE (and AT-1 receptors) in these tissues and organs will be central to individual protective potential.[21]

Apart from the 'classical' biological effects of Ang II described above, it has become evident that the octapeptide has numerous additional actions which have the potential to contribute to cardiovascular disease. For example, Ang II has been shown experimentally to be a growth factor for vascular, cardiac and renal cells with potential to induce cellular proliferation, hypertrophy, apoptosis and differentiation,[22] to be a proinflammatory molecule, to have pro-fibrotic activity, and to be capable of inducing a procoagulant/prothrombotic state and stimulating erythropoietin, inflammatory cytokines and adhesion molecules.[23,24] Ang II may also play a role in angiogenesis under certain circumstances.[25,26] There is speculation, therefore, that the RAS, through these diverse actions, might be involved in the development and progression of atherosclerotic disease, in contributing to instability of atherosclerotic plaques, and in the development or spread of neoplasms.[27–32] Such experimental data have been brought into sharp focus by clinical and epidemiological studies suggesting that ACE inhibitors might have anti-atherosclerotic, anti-fibrotic, anti-thrombotic, anti-arrhythmic and anti-neoplastic effects – as discussed below.

The cellular and cardiovascular toxic effects of Ang II, first documented in the 1940s,[33] seem likely to be mediated, at least in part, via oxidative stress directly or via Ang II-induced endothelin-1 production.[34,35] Whether these effects result from a direct toxic action of the peptide and/or endothelin-1, or from Ang II-induced hypertension, however, can be difficult to determine.[36]

A number of the biological actions of Ang II are modified in a coordinated and coherent manner according to the prevailing state of sodium and water balance. Thus, sodium-loading enhances the pressor potency of infused Ang II whereas aldosterone-stimulating action is inhibited. The result is an enhanced ability of the kidney to excrete excess sodium, thus returning sodium and fluid balance to 'normal'. The opposite occurs with sodium deprivation wherein the pressor action of Ang II is diminished whilst its aldosterone-stimulation potency is enhanced. Under circumstances where body fluid status and circulating volume are under threat, the RAS is protective through the marshalling and enhancing of sodium-retaining mechanisms at a low renal arterial perfusion pressure. In this regard, the RAS is counterbalanced by other systems, most notably the natriuretic peptides, adrenomedullin and the kallikrein–kinin system, which are protective against excessive vasoconstriction and sodium and fluid overload. The last of these systems is discussed later.

The cardiac natriuretic peptides, atrial and B-type or brain natriuretic peptide (ANP and BNP), are released from the heart in response to increased stretch of the cardiac chambers, as seen inter alia with sodium and fluid loading, heart failure and cardiac tachyarrhythmias. ANP and BNP act on the JG apparatus to inhibit renin release and, under some circumstances, on the adrenal glomerulosa to restrain aldosterone secretion. Some of the most striking biological effects of ANP and BNP (vasodilatation, natriuresis, and inhibition of aldosterone secretion, for example) are the opposite of those elicited by Ang II. The two systems move in opposite directions in healthy volunteers during perturbations in body fluid status. This regular, reciprocal relationship between the RAS and the cardiac natriuretic peptides, which serves to maintain body sodium and fluid homeostasis, is lost in some pathological states, most obviously in heart failure.[37] The positive association between the two systems in cardiac failure may result, in part, from the stimulatory action of Ang II on secretion of the cardiac natriuretic peptides.[38]

The reciprocal relationship between the two contrary systems provided the rationale for the development of drugs which both blocked ACE and sustained the actions of the natriuretic peptides through inhibiting their breakdown by neutral endopeptidase (NEP) 24.11. Such combined NEP/ACE or vasopeptidase inhibitors, by reducing plasma Ang II levels and increasing ANP and BNP concentrations should, in theory, have an antihypertensive action greater than that of ACE or NEP inhibition alone. This prediction turned out to be true but so did the prediction that bradykinin levels would rise beyond those observed with either inhibitor alone, resulting in an excessive incidence of angio-oedema.[39] (see Chapter 14).

The third member of the natriuretic peptide family, C-type natriuretic peptide (CNP), is secreted prominently within the vascular endothelium and in selected areas of the brain. Like ANP and BNP, CNP interacts, at least experimentally, with the RAS.[40,41] Clearly, therefore, ACE inhibition has the potential to alter the production and/or actions of the natriuretic peptides within tissues (especially blood vessels) and organs (including the heart) as well as the circulation, and these effects may contribute to the various haemodynamic/ cardiovascular responses to ACE inhibitors in patients with hypertension.

Adrenomedullin, a 52-amino acid peptide, is produced in many tissues including heart and blood vessels where it functions largely as a paracrine hormone. Circulating adrenomedullin, derived mostly from endothelial cells, is in the low picomolar range. Adrenomedullin has unique interactions with the

RAS.[42] This peptide is a potent stimulus to renin release through a direct action on the JG apparatus[43] and perhaps, when infused intravenously, via activation of the sympathetic nervous system and a fall in renal perfusion pressure. Yet adrenomedullin selectively inhibits some actions of Ang II while enhancing others. Thus, adrenomedullin inhibits the aldosterone-stimulating and pressor actions of Ang II, but the positive inotropic effect of Ang II is enhanced.[42,44] Adrenomedullin also inhibits Ang II-induced generation of reactive oxygen species in vascular smooth muscle cells.[45] These unique interactions between adrenomedullin and the RAS are likely to be physiologically and pathophysiologically important, and therapeutic implications are possible.[42]

In addition to these hormone systems which interact with and counterbalance the RAS, there is now described an additional limb within an expanded RAS which may also serve to modulate the biological actions of Ang II. This concept is based on the discovery in 2000 of a second angiotensin converting enzyme, ACE2[46] which cleaves a single amino acid residue from Ang II to form angiotensin 1–7 (Fig. 12.1), a peptide found in low picomolar concentrations in plasma.[47] Through stimulation of nitric oxide and prostaglandin 1_2 formation, angiotensin 1–7 has vasodilator, natriuretic, diuretic, anti-growth and anti-proliferative actions and hence may have a protective effect within the cardiovascular system.[48] ACE2 also catalyses the cleavage of angiotensin I to angiotensin 1–9 which is biologically inactive but can be converted by ACE to angiotensin 1–7[48] (Fig. 12.1). Unlike ACE, the distribution of which is widespread, ACE2 is expressed predominantly in the heart, kidneys and testis and is not affected by ACE inhibitor drugs. Whereas importance in humans remains to be elucidated,[49] reduced ACE2 protein expression occurs in the kidney of diabetic rats[50] and targeted disruption of ACE2 in mice results in a severe cardiac contractility defect and elevated levels of Ang II in plasma, heart and kidneys.[51] On the other hand, cardiac overexpression of ACE2 in mice is associated with cardiac arrhythmias.[52] Even though ACE2 is not blocked by ACE inhibitors, it is possible that changes in angiotensin 1–7 levels in the circulation or in tissues of vital organs account for some of the biological effects of the ACE inhibitors since ACE (which is inhibited by the ACE inhibitors) contributes both to the formation of the heptapeptide (via angiotensin 1–9) and to its enzymatic breakdown.[53,54] Ang II is metabolized by a number of enzymes into peptides other than angiotensin 1–7, including angiotensin III (angiotensin 2–8) and angiotensin IV (angiotensin 3–8), both of which are biologically active but considerably less so than Ang II.

Clearly, the RAS is more complex than was suspected even a decade ago.[55] Accordingly, the numerous biological effects of ACE inhibitors are not as readily explained as had been thought in the years immediately following the introduction of this class of drugs into clinical medicine.

The RAS in hypertension

There is considerable controversy regarding activity of the RAS, and circulating levels of various components, in patients with essential hypertension.[56] An overview is that there is no bimodal pattern of plasma renin or Ang II levels separating essential hypertensives from normotensives – rather, there is a continuum: renin and Ang II levels may be slightly higher in young subjects with or prone to develop essential hypertension than in normotensives, but the age-related fall in both indices is greater in essential hypertensives; responsiveness of renin and Ang II levels to stimulation (by sodium-depletion, orthostasis etc.) is inhibited in essential hypertensives; there is a weak inverse association between renin levels and BP in population surveys which include both essential hypertensives and normotensives, and among essential hypertensives; and evidence for elevated levels of plasma angiotensinogen (renin-substrate) or prorenin, and for abnormalities in ACE or Ang II receptor genotypes in essential hypertension is far from robust.[56]

Activity of the RAS may not be the same in all racial groups. In Britain and the USA, blacks have consistently been found to have plasma renin levels lower than in whites, although the possibility that the intra-renal RAS is activated in blacks has been raised.[57] Whether these aforementioned perturbations in activity of the 'circulatory' RAS according to age (with the development and evolution of essential hypertension) and race translate into differences in the blood pressure response to ACE inhibitor drugs, has been a focus of debate over the years and is discussed below.

Also in dispute is whether or not the degree of activation of the RAS in essential hypertension provides an index of cardiovascular risk and prognosis. There are many reasons why heightened activity of the system, resulting in elevated plasma and tissue levels of Ang II would, for any given level of BP, predispose to cardiac, vascular, atherosclerotic or renal disease. The outcome of the Losartan Intervention for Endpoint Reduction (LIFE) trial in patients with essential hypertension and left ventricular hypertrophy (LVH) in which antihypertensive treatment based on an ARB was associated with a superior outcome (for the composite primary endpoint of cardiovascular death, myocardial infarction and stroke) compared with a beta-blocker-based regimen,[58] has been taken by some as confirmatory evidence that 'Ang II (exerts) detrimental effects beyond the mechanical damage of high BP'.[59] But the sum total of data from epidemiological studies and drug trials has failed to clarify this issue to everyone's satisfaction.

Involvement of the RAS in the pathogenesis of various secondary forms of hypertension varies considerably. At one end of the spectrum, the system is central to development and maintenance of hypertension associated with, for example, renin or angiotensinogen-secreting tumours, scleroderma renal crisis and renal artery stenosis due to unilateral renal arterial narrowing with a normal circulation to the contralateral kidney. At the other extreme are states where activity of the circulatory RAS is suppressed and probably plays little role in the pathophysiology – as in mineralocorticoid hypertension, Gordon's syndrome (familial hyperkalaemia and hypertension) and primary renin deficiency. Between these extremes are disorders such as phaeochromocytoma, coarctation of the aorta and connective tissue diseases, in which involvement of the RAS in the hypertension is less clear-cut but a supportive or contributory role appears likely.

The kallikrein–kinin system

This system has similarities with the RAS. Activators (kallikreins) hydrolyze substrates (kininogens) to release vasoactive peptides (kinins), most notably bradykinin and its intermediate kallidin which, via B1 and especially B2 receptors and thence the release of prostacyclin, nitric oxide and endothelial-derived hyperpolarizing factor, contribute to the regulation of vascular tone and permeability, sodium homeostasis, inflammation and nociception.[60,61]

Bradykinin also has, at least experimentally, antihypertrophic and antiproliferative effects on cardiomyocytes and fibroblasts,[62] and antithrombotic actions. Bradykinin has a brief plasma half-life (<30 seconds) due to degradation by kininases including ACE, NEP and aminopeptidase P. It is generally assumed that bradykinin is synthesized largely within tissues, and indeed concentrations in tissues are higher than in plasma.[61]

Studies from the 1960s revealed that the bioactivity of bradykinin disappeared during passage through the pulmonary circulation, and the suggestion from Ng and Vane[63] was that the same pulmonary enzyme (ACE or kininase-11) might catalyze conversion of angiotensin I to Ang II and inactivation of bradykinin. This indeed turned out to be so. ACE has a higher affinity for bradykinin than for angiotensin I.[60] ACE/kininase-II is not the only degradative pathway for bradykinin, there being other specific and non-specific peptidases. ACE inhibition need not necessarily result in elevated plasma (or tissue) bradykinin levels. Swiss researchers, however, reported a twofold rise in venous bradykinin levels in healthy volunteers within eight hours of a single oral dose of the ACE inhibitor, quinapril.[64] Furthermore, inhibition of ACE potentiates the vasodilator action of exogenous bradykinin in human forearm and coronary circulations[65,66] and the release of tissue plasminogen activator in the coronary circulation of patients with hypertension.[67]

The pivotal position of ACE in the functioning of the RAS and the kallikrein–kinin system is now well known. However functional linkages and interactions between the two systems are complex (Fig. 12.2) and remain ill-understood.

In summary, plasma kallikrein can activate prorenin to renin; the endothelial enzyme prolylcarboxypeptidase activates prekallikrein and inactivates Ang II; there is cross-talk between bradykinin and angiotensin 1–7 actions; the AT-1

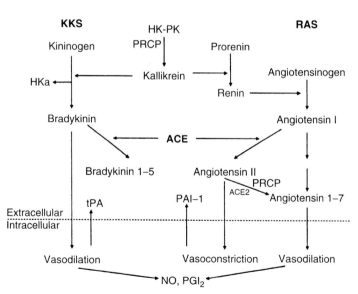

Fig. 12.2 Interactions of the plasma kallikrein–kinin system (KKS) with the renin–angiotensin system (RAS). HK, high molecular weight kininogen; PK, prekallikrein; PRCP, prolylcarboxypeptidase; Hka, plasma kallikrein-cleaved, high molecular weight kininogen free of bradykinin; ACE2, angiotensin converting enzyme 2; tPA, tissue plasminogen activator; PAI-1, plasminogen activator inhibitor 1; PGI2, prostaglandin I2 or prostacyclin. From Schmaier et al.[69] with permission.

Ang II receptor forms heterodimers with the AT-2 and bradykinin B2 receptors; and the B2 receptor interacts with ACE.[62,68,69] Nevertheless, overall the two systems appear to counterbalance one another with regard to control of BP, regulation of sodium and fluid balance, growth of cardiovascular tissues, thrombosis, fibrinolysis and angiogenesis.[69] Accordingly, the ACE inhibitors should, in theory, favour an alteration in homeostasis towards lower BP, loss of body sodium, reduced growth of cardiovascular tissues, an impaired thrombotic and increased fibrinolytic tendency, and an anti-neoplastic effect.

The kallikrein–kinin system in hypertension

Genetic engineering studies in experimental animals point to the potential for bradykinin to modulate BP[70] but the situation in humans is less clear. Studies in the 1970s reported reduced kallikrein levels in the urine of patients with essential hypertension and in hypertensive rodents.[71] Subsequent research in the 1980s suggested that compared with normotensive controls, essential hypertensives had low plasma levels of kininogen and a kininogen-potentiating factor. The modulating effects of the kallikrein–kinin system with changes in dietary sodium intake seen in normotensive volunteers, are reportedly blunted in essential hypertensives and have been considered likely to contribute to the development or maintenance of hypertension in some patients.[72]

If indeed the kallikrein–kinin system is suppressed in some patients with essential hypertension, could this explain in part not only the elevation in BP but also the cardiovascular damage attending hypertension? Possibly so, since mice deficient in tissue kallikrein develop cardiovascular abnormalities even when BP is unaltered.[73] The question is also germane to the cardioprotective and metabolic effects of ACE inhibitor treatment in human hypertension where increased tissue and/or circulating bradykinin levels may play a protective role.

CLASSIFICATION/CHEMISTRY

The story of the development of the first oral non-peptide ACE inhibitor (captopril) at Squibb – an early example of rational drug design – is well known. The terminal residue in naturally occurring inhibitors (peptides from snake venom) of ACE is proline, so this was chosen as part of the inhibitor. Benzyl-succinate had been shown to be a good competitive inhibitor of carboxypeptidase (an ACE-related enzyme), so succinate and proline were combined to yield succinylproline, which, while having the right molecular size, was still a weak inhibitor. By replacing the carboxyl group in the succinate moiety with a thiol group, attachment to the zinc ion in ACE was enhanced, resulting in the potent oral ACE inhibitor, captopril, which was approved by the Federal Drug Administration (FDA) in 1981.[74–77]

While captopril can be viewed as a di-peptide substrate analogue, the subsequently synthesized enalapril (FDA approved in 1985) and all other ACE inhibitors are tri-peptide substrate analogues.[78,79] These molecules have the same basic structure. Proline or an equivalent cyclic structure (indole, indane, pyrrole, isoquinoline, thiazepin, benzazepine, diazepine or thiazolidine) is attached to a second amino acid (alanine, lysine) and linked to a phenyl moiety; the exception is perindopril which lacks the phenyl ring. A functional residue that allows the drug to adhere to the zinc component of the active site of ACE, is attached. Functional groups can be sulfhydryl, phosphonyl or carboxyl, thus allowing a classification of ACE inhibitors based on chemical structure (Table 12.1).[79,80]

The clinical relevance of a particular functional group (and of a functional group-based classification) is unclear. Initially sulfhydryl ACE inhibitors were considered less desirable due to sulfonamide-like side effects such as neutropenia, rash and proteinuria.[81,82] The relatively high incidence of such adverse drug reactions in early studies with captopril was due mainly to its administration at dosages now recognized to be in excess of those necessary for drug action.[83] This perception has changed and sulfhydryl ACE inhibitors are often now looked upon more favourably. For example, in a direct comparison between captopril (sulfhydryl group) and enalapril (carboxyl group), patients receiving captopril had a significantly better quality of life[84] at the doses tested. The sulfhydryl ACE inhibitors have been claimed to have particular benefits such as attenuating nitrate tolerance and scavenging free radicals.[82,85–88] However, the situation is complex since, for example, two non-sulfhydryl ACE inhibitors (imidaprilat and enalaprilat) were reported, like captopril, to be capable of scavenging hydroxyl radicals.[89]

Molecular weight (MW)

Captopril, a di-peptide substrate analogue, is the smallest molecule among ACE inhibitors with a MW of 217. The tri-peptide substrate analogue ACE inhibitors have MWs between that of perindopril (340) and moexipril (535).

Fat solubility

The logarithm of the (organic/aqueous) partition coefficient (Log P) varies according to the conditions under which it is measured and the choice of partitioning solvent. Therefore comparing values from different sources is difficult if not impossible. The values listed below are for orientation purposes only. Log P=1 indicates 10:1 organic/aqueous, Log P=0 indicates 1:1 organic/aqueous, while a Log P=−1 indicates 1:10 organic/aqueous.

For the prodrugs (prils), the values range from extremely fat soluble (zofenopril 3.5, fosinopril 2.7; trandolapril 2.1; quinapril 1.8; benazepril 1.7; ramipril 1.6) through both fat and water soluble (perindopril 1.3; captopril and moexipril 1; enalapril 0.7; spirapril 0.6; delapril 0.2) to water soluble (lisinopril −1.8).[79,90,91]

Metabolic activation (pril→prilat) drastically changes Log P. Zofenopril Log P changes from 3.5 (pril) to 0.2 (prilat), fosinopril from 2.7 (pril) to −0.5 (prilat), enalapril from 0.7 (pril) to −3 (prilat), while ramipril changes from 1.6 (pril) to −2 (prilat).[90]

Essentially these numbers indicate that the pril form is approximately 3 orders of magnitude more fat soluble than the prilat. The clinical relevance of fat solubility is not clearly established. Conceptually high fat solubility prodrugs have a superior tissue penetration allowing for inhibition of tissue ACEs. Whether or not this actually translates into different outcomes in the treatment of hypertension with the various ACE inhibitors, is not known.

Table 12.1 Categorization of the ACE inhibitors based on chemical structure

Sulfhydryl ACE inhibitor

ACE inhibitor	Cyclical structure	MW	LogP	Bio-availability (%) of prilat after p.o. administration of pril	Protein binding (%)	V_d in L BW = 70 kg	Half-life $t_{1/2}$ (h)	Clearance (C) mL/min RC = Renal clearance TBC = Total body clearance	Elimination	CNS penetration
Alacepril (Cetapril®)	Proline	407		60–70	60		Captopril 2 Deacetyl-Alacepril 5		R	yes
Captopril (Capoten®)	Proline	217	Pril 1	70 ↓↓ Decreased by food	20–40	40–60 L	2	RC 187 RC 310–370	R	yes
Zofenopril (Zoprace®)	Proline	449	Pril 3.5 Prilat 0.2	65–80	Pril > 80 Prilat>90	Prilat 110 L	Prilat 5,5	Prilat TBC 800; RC 220	H + R	yes

Phosphonyl ACE inhibitor

ACE inhibitor	Cyclical structure	MW	LogP	Bio-availability (%) of prilat after p.o. administration of pril	Protein binding (%)	V_d in L BW = 70 kg	Half-life $t_{1/2}$ (h)	Clearance (C) mL/min RC = Renal clearance TBC = Total body clearance	Elimination	CNS penetration
Fosinopril (Monopril®)	Proline	453	Pril 2.7 Prilat 0.5	25–35	Pril > 90 Prilat >90	Prilat 10 L	Prilat 2; 12	Prilat TBC 40 RC 17	H + R	(?) no

Carboxyl ACE inhibitor

ACE inhibitor	Cyclical structure	MW	LogP	Bio-availability (%) of prilat after p.o. administration of pril	Protein binding (%)	V_d in L BW = 70 kg	Half-life $t_{1/2}$ (h)	Clearance (C) mL/min RC = Renal clearance TBC = Total body clearance	Elimination	CNS penetration
Bonazepril (Lotensin®)	Benzazepine	424	Pril 1.7	30–40	Pril 96 Prilat 94	Prilat 9 L	Pril 0.6 Prilat 3–10; 22	Prilat TBC 30; RC 15–25	R+H	no
Cilazapril (Vascace®)	Diazepine	389		57–77	Pril < 50 Prilat 24–90	Pril 25 L Prilat 31–46 L	Pril 1–2 Prilat 9;45	Prilat TBC 240 Prilat TBC 205–230 RC 180–200	R	no
Delapril (Adecut®)	Indane	424	Pril 0.2 Prilat	57	Pril > 90		Pril 0.3 Prilat 1.2; 9 5-OH-prilat 1.4		R + H	?
Enalapril (Vasotec®)	Proline	348	Pril 0.7 Prilat-3	40–60	Pril 50 Prilat 50	Prilat 12	Pril 2 Prilat 11;35	Prilat TBC 120–164	R	no
Imidapril (Tanatril®)	Proline	450		20 ↓↓ Decreased by food	Pril 85 Prilat 53		Pril 2 Prilat 8;24		R + H	no
Lisinopril (Zestril®)	Proline	405	Pril–1.8 Pril 1	25	< 10 Pril 70 Prilat 50	120 L Prilat 180 L	10; 40	RC 50–110	R	no
Moexipril (Univasc®)	Isoquinoline	535		15; ↓↓ Decreased by food			Prilat 10	Pril TBC 430 Prilat TBC 230	R + H	no
Pentopril	Indole			60–70		Pril 60 L Prilat 40 L	Pril 0.7 Prilat 2.2	Pril RC 210 Prilat RC 250–400	R + H	?

Continued

Table 12.1 Categorization of the ACE inhibitors based on chemical structure—Cont'd

ACE inhibitor	Cyclical structure	MW	LogP	Bio-availability (%) of prilat after p.o. administration of pril	Carboxyl ACE inhibitor		Half-life t$_{1/2}$ (h)	Clearance (C) mL/min RC = Renal clearance TBC = Total body clearance	Elimination	CNS penetration
					Protein binding (%)	V$_d$ in L BW = 70 kg				
Perindopril (Aceon®)	Indole	340	Pril 1.3	20–25	Pril 30–60; Prilat < 10	Pril 300 L	Pril 1; Prilat 8;40	Pril TBC 220–360; RC 25; Prilat RC 110	R + H	yes
Quinapril (Accupril®)	Isoquinoline	396	Pril 1.8	40	Pril 97; Prilat 35–97	Pril at 50 L	Pril 1–2; Prilat 2; 24	Pril TBC 1.850; Prilat TBC 220	R	no
Ramipril (Altace®)	Pyrrole	388	Pril 1.6; Prilat-2	40–60	Pril 70; Prilat 50	Pril 90 L; Prilat 500 L	Pril 13–17; 100	Pril RC 10–15; Prilat RC 100–50	R + H	yes
Spirapril (Renormax®)	Proline	521	Pril 0.6	40–50		Pril 28–60 L; Prilat 43 L	Pril 1.4; Prilat 1.5; 35	Pril TBC 900; RC 180; Prilat TBC 320; RC 50	H + R	yes
Temocapril (Acecol®)	Thiazepin	513		65			Prilat 7–9	Pril RC 50; Prilat RC 24	H + R	?
Trandolapril (Mavik®)	Indole	430	Pril 2.1	70	Pril 80; Prilat 65–95	Pril 20–30 L	Pril 2–4; Prilat 16; 20+	Pril TBC 870; Prilat TBC 120; RC 20–60	H + R	yes

R=renal, H=hepatic. R+H=renal (predominant)+hepatic. H+R=hepatic (predominant)+renal.
References – see under individually named drugs in the Pharmacokinetics/Metabolism section.

MECHANISMS OF ACTION

Blockade of the RAS

Antihypertensive action

The favoured explanation for the antihypertensive action of ACE inhibitors has been inhibition of Ang II formation. The consequences are dependent upon the level of activity of the RAS. When the system is activated, as can occur in malignant or accelerated hypertension, with diuretic administration or with dietary sodium restriction, the fall in BP may be profound and precipitous after the first dose of an ACE inhibitor especially one with a rapid onset of action such as captopril. On the other hand, inhibition of the RAS in, for example, primary hyperaldosteronism or an essential hypertensive taking a diet high in sodium content, is associated with little if any initial decline in BP. The fall in BP with ACE inhibitors in the short term relates inversely to the prevailing degree of activation of the RAS[92,93] (Fig. 12.3).

The observation that baseline plasma renin levels correlate less clearly with the longer-term antihypertensive action of these drugs could be interpreted to indicate the importance of other mechanisms, especially enhanced activity of the kallikrein–kinin system. It might also reflect the finding that whereas some actions of Ang II are of rapid onset (and offset when blocked), other actions

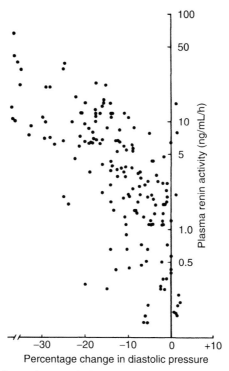

Fig. 12.3 Percentage change in seated diastolic arterial pressure 90 minutes after a single oral dose of captopril 25 mg in 166 patients with a variety of forms of hypertension (r=0.71). From Cody et al.[92] with permission.

have a more sluggish time of onset profile (and offset when blocked). For example, as mentioned earlier, Ang II has a slow pressor action wherein a constant infusion of the peptide, via a number of mechanisms,[94,95] has an incremental effect on BP. Accordingly, reduced Ang II formation through ACE inhibition will lower BP with a temporal profile reflecting reversal of these various, complex actions of the octapeptide. Another issue of relevance here is that Ang II formation via ACE may not be blocked completely through 24 hours by ACE inhibitors given once daily and in usual doses.[96] The absence of a robust statistical association between baseline plasma renin levels and the magnitude of the fall in BP with ACE inhibitor monotherapy should not be taken alone, as firm evidence against the primacy of Ang II withdrawal in the antihypertensive action of ACE inhibitors.

Plasma aldosterone levels fall with the introduction of an ACE inhibitor but return to, or close to, baseline values after weeks or months of continued administration.[97] Whatever the reasons for this 'breakthrough' (increased secretion due to a rise in plasma potassium and perhaps decreased clearance of aldosterone resulting from a decline in hepatic blood flow), aldosterone 'breakthrough' provides part of the rationale for the use of aldosterone receptor blockers in combination with an ACE inhibitor in patients with resistant hypertension. Careful plasma potassium and renal function is needed when this drug combination is used.

Electrolyte balance is altered variably with the introduction of ACE inhibitor therapy, but the tendency is for a small negative cumulative balance of sodium and a positive balance of potassium.[98] The pressor action of any residual Ang II under these circumstances will be reduced, thereby contributing to the antihypertensive effect of ACE inhibition.

Cardiovascular protection

Regarding the cardiovascular protective effects of ACE inhibitors in patients with essential hypertension, the fall in BP alone may be sufficient explanation.[99–102] Some commentators consider that the ACE inhibitors (and ARBs) offer substantially greater cardiovascular protection for any given level of achieved BP than other antihypertensive drug groups,[31,59,103] and this can be explained by withdrawal of the cardiovascular growth-promoting, pro-fibrotic, prothrombotic and toxic actions of Ang II.[104] As discussed later, antihypertensive drugs designed to specifically interfere with the RAS, the ACE inhibitors and ARBs, are arguably the most effective of all drug groups in reversing LVH. The explanation is thought to reside in withdrawal of the myocardial hypertrophic and pro-fibrotic actions of Ang II through the AT-1 receptor and the effect of ACE inhibitors in reducing central (aortic) systolic BP to a greater extent than is suggested by brachial artery recordings.[105]

It is likely that ACE inhibitors reduce the occurrence of cardiac arrhythmias, particularly atrial fibrillation in hypertensive patients.[106] ACE inhibitor therapy reduces not only left ventricular mass, but also QT and QTc dispersion, indicators of ventricular arrhythmias and sudden death, in patients with essential hypertension and LVH.[107] A reduction in the incidence of atrial fibrillation might be explained by reversal of LVH, since left ventricular mass relates closely to left atrial volume[108,109] which, in turn, is a major determinant of the development of atrial fibrillation.[108,110] Withdrawal of the tendency for Ang II to encourage myocardial fibrosis[104] and to alter activity of the autonomic system in favour of the sympathetic, over the parasympathetic limb, might also contribute to any antiarrhythmic effect of ACE inhibitors, as might slight increments in plasma levels of potassium and magnesium.

Renal protection

There are many mechanisms by which Ang II might contribute to progression of nephropathy in hypertensive patients, especially in those with diabetes mellitus (Fig. 12.4).[111,112] These data, along with the observations that the intra-renal RAS appears to be activated in the diabetic kidney,[113] that experimentally-increased expression of ACE exacerbates renal complications in the diabetic mouse,[114] and that blockade of the RAS with either ARBs or ACE inhibitors in humans is especially nephroprotective, provides powerful evidence to support a pivotal role for a reduction in Ang II levels in the renoprotective effect of ACE inhibitors in diabetes. This does not rule out a contribution from increased bradykinin levels, as is discussed below.

Metabolic effects

ACE inhibitors improve insulin sensitivity and prevent the development of glucose intolerance and type 2 diabetes in essential hypertensives. Whereas most data come from studies comparing ACE inhibitor-based treatment with therapy based on diuretics or beta-adrenergic blockers, other studies show a lesser incidence of new onset diabetes with blockers of the RAS than with placebo control[115,116] (see below).

What are the underlying mechanisms? First, in animals at least, there exists a pancreatic RAS.[14,15] Ang II produced by this local system or from elsewhere, is capable of reducing the microcirculation of the islets and delaying glucose-induced insulin release whereas ACE inhibitors preferentially increase islet blood flow.[117] Zucker diabetic fatty rats exhibit increased expression of components of the RAS within pancreatic islets correlating with islet fibrosis,

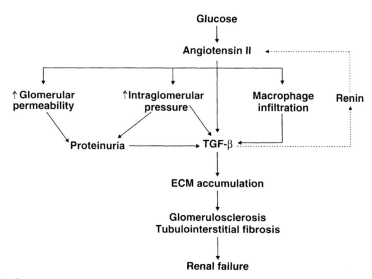

Fig. 12.4 Possible mechanisms by which angiotensin II contributes to the development of diabetic nephropathy. ECM, extracellular matrix; TGF-β, transforming growth factor-beta. From Gilbert et al.[111] with permission.

apoptosis and oxidative stress, and ACE inhibitors (or ARBs) in these animals attenuate the distorted architecure.[118] Second, there is speculation, largely from experiments in animals, that adipose tissue RAS may play a role in the development of the metabolic syndrome and type 2 diabetes and that ACE inhibitors might be beneficial, in part, by limiting local Ang II production.[20,119] Third, withdrawal or diminution of Ang II's action to inhibit skeletal muscle glucose transport through ACE inhibition (or ARB administration), should enhance glucose transport into cells.[120]

Enhanced activity of the kallikrien–kinin system

Antihypertensive action

The possibility that a delay in the breakdown of bradykinin contributes to the antihypertensive action of ACE inhibitors has been entertained, initially from animal and in-vitro evidence.[121,122] Accumulation of comparable data in humans was hindered by difficulties in measuring accurately bradykinin in plasma and tissue samples, and the unavailability, until recently, of selective antagonists of the peptide which could be administered safely. Despite conflicting earlier reports,[60] Pellacani et al. developed a sensitive radioimmuno-assay for measuring bradykinin and showed that venous concentrations of the peptide increased twofold in healthy volunteers within 8 hours of a single oral dose (20 mg) of the ACE inhibitor, quinapril.[64]

Blockade of the bradykinin B2 receptor was shown to inhibit the ACE inhibitor-induced increase in flow-dependent dilatation in the radial artery of healthy volunteers,[123] pointing to a central role of endogenous bradykinin in the short-term vasodilatating action of ACE inhibitors. Gainer et al. reported that a bradykinin receptor antagonist decreased by 53% the fall in BP in response to a single 25 mg dose of captopril in essential hypertensive patients (and nor-motensives) studied on a sodium-restricted diet.[124] Whereas these data are consistent with an important role for the kinins in the acute BP response to an ACE inhibitor, aspects of the study have been criticized,[125,126] and the results provide no information regarding the place of kinins in the long-term antihypertensive action of ACE inhibitors. In healthy volunteers, a bradykinin antagonist attenuated the BP response to acute ACE inhibition,[127] again suggesting that the early response in BP to these drugs depends, at least in part, on the kinin system.

The interaction of ACE inhibitors and the kinins and their contribution to the antihypertensive effects of these drugs, is far from simple. As explained by Tom et al.,[62] there is evidence for bradykinin-potentiating effects of ACE inhibitors that are independent of bradykinin hydrolysis. For example, ACE-bradykinin B2 receptor 'cross-talk' might result in receptor up-regulation and/or more efficient activation of signal transduction pathways; there may be direct activation of bradykinin receptors by ACE inhibitors; and angiotensin 1–7 levels, which increase during ACE inhibition, are thought to reduce BP via a bradykinin-dependent manner and to act as an endogenous ACE inhibitor. Decreased catabolism of bradykinin may contribute to the fall in BP during ACE inhibition also by opposing the actions of the potent vasoconstrictor, endothelin-1.[128] Whatever the contribution of these various mechanisms, it does appear that, at least in the shortterm, delayed breakdown of bradykinin contributes to the antihypertensive action of the ACE inhibitors. But the relative contribution of increased circulating and tissue bradykinin levels versus decreased circulating and tissue Ang II levels is not clear and may vary according to the baseline state of activity of the kallikrein–kinin system and the RAS.

Cardiovascular protection

Supportive evidence for a role for kinins in the cardiovascular protection afforded by ACE inhibitors in essential hypertension has accumulated over the past decade. Almost all of this evidence comes from experiments in vitro or from animal studies,[121,122,129] and extrapolation to circumstances in humans needs to be cautious. Particular note is made of the beneficial cardiac and vascular effects of an ACE inhibitor given in doses insufficient to lower BP in various experimental animal models, and that these effects were abolished by selective blockade of bradykinin B2 receptors.[130] Some of the positive findings from these studies could not be reproduced by other workers, however.[131]

Renal protection

The observation by Tschope et al.[132] that the antiproteinuric action of ACE inhibition in experimental diabetic nephropathy is explained, in part, by the action of kinins is of interest in that other evidence, collected under experimental circumstances in animal models and summarized by Takahashi et al.,[133] points toward low levels of bradykinin contributing to progression of diabetic nephropathy. Indeed, diabetic nephropathy is exacerbated in mice lacking the bradykinin B2 receptor.[134]

Metabolic effects

Literature supporting a role for bradykinin in the increased insulin sensitivity associated with ACE inhibition is persuasive. Whereas most evidence, again, comes from experiments in animals or in vitro, reports from studies in humans are considerable in number and, in general, congruent with animal data. For example, Frossard et al. showed that the ACE inhibitor enalapril or bradykinin, but not the ARB losartan, when injected locally into the interstitial space fluid in skeletal muscle of healthy volunteers, augmented the transcapillary transport of glucose.[135]

It is evident that increased bradykinin levels with ACE inhibition have the potential to improve insulin sensitivity through a number of mechanisms.[136] Here again the situation is far from simple since kininogen-deficient rats and bradykinin B2 receptor knockout mice have little disturbance in the handling of glucose. Further, the kinins are thought to contribute to the development of streptozotocin-induced diabetes in mice.[136] Nevertheless the balance of evidence is that increased activity of the kallikrein–kinin system contributes importantly to the protective effect of ACE inhibition against glucose intolerance and type 2 diabetes in humans. However, recent evidence that ARBs also reduce the tendency to new-onset diabetes in hypertension[58] argues against a pivotal contribution of activation of the kallikrein–kinin system.

PHARMACOKINETICS/METABOLISM

Pharmacokinetics

Bioavailability

Values (of a prilat after oral administration of a pril) range from low (<20%) for moexipril to high (70%) for zofenopril and trandolapril. Although the differences in bioavailability are marked, this is of limited clinical significance. Co-ingestion of food decreases more the rate than the extent of absorption; captopril, imidapril and moexipril are the most affected by food so spacing between food intake and drug administration is sometimes advised.[88]

Protein binding (PB)

Values range from <10% (lisinopril) to >90% (benazepril, delapril, fosinopril, quinapril, spirapril, trandolapril, zofenopril). Essentially, lisinopril does not bind to plasma proteins other than ACE.[137] The differences in PB are marked and this is of some clinical significance in the context of patients undergoing dialysis.[80]

While numerous factors influence the PB of a substance, Harrold suggests that fat solubility (Log P) shows the best correlation.[79] Since activation (pril→prilat) changes Log P it is reasonable to assume that PB will also be affected. As a general rule the less fat soluble active metabolites (prilats) will have a lower PB than that of the precursor drug.

The PB of ramipril is about 70% as opposed to that of ramiprilat which is approximately 50%.[138] For imidapril/imidaprilat the values are 85 and 53% respectively. The less fat soluble perindopril has a PB of <30 while perindoprilat essentially does not bind to proteins other than ACE.[139] For the very fat soluble prils, the difference in PB subsequent to activation is not relevant: benazepril and benazeprilat have almost identical PB values (96 and 94%, respectively).[140] The same applies to quinapril/quinaprilat, zofenopril/zofenoprilat[141] and fosinopril/fosinoprilat.[142]

Volume of distribution (V_d)

While numerous factors influence the volume of distribution of a substance, PB and fat solubility are major determinants with opposite effects on V_d. Since activation (pril→prilat) changes both Log P and PB it is reasonable to assume that V_d will also be affected i.e. each form will have a different V_d. The differences in V_d are marked and this is of some clinical relevance in patients undergoing dialysis.

T_{max}

Captopril has the shortest time required to reach maximal plasma concentrations (C_{max}) after oral administration ($\approx$ 1 hour). While the subsequently developed non-sulfhydryl prils have comparable t_{max} values, this is irrelevant since the prodrugs are inactive. The corresponding t_{max} values for the prilats are generally longer: trandolapril, enalapril, perindopril and lisinopril have tmax values $\approx$ 6 hours.[143]

The newer ACE inhibitors (quinapril, cilazapril, fosinopril, benazepril, delapril, pentopril, spirapril, zofenopril) have t_{max} values for the prilat (time needed to reach the maximal concentration C_{max} of prilat after oral administration of the pril) in the 1–2 hour range. Clinically this is not especially relevant since hypertension requiring emergency treatment is better controlled with other medications.

Half-life ($t_{1/2}$)

The half-life of pril prodrugs is generally short (< 2 hours), reflecting both rapid metabolic conversion to the active prilat and some degree of elimination. The only exception is trandolapril.

The plasma concentration of the active substance (prilat) over time after intravenous administration is triphasic. The initial distribution phase is short ($t_{1/2}$ <1 hour), followed by a second phase most commonly referred to as the apparent or accumulation phase which reflects total body clearance, and a third protracted (terminal) phase which reflects the binding/dissociation kinetics of the prilat–ACE complex before elimination. When ACE inhibitors are given orally (almost always the case) the initial prilat distribution phase is masked by the slow conversion of pril to prilat.

There is a poor correlation between accumulation $t_{1/2}$ and clinical duration of action of ACE inhibitors. The conventional view is that drugs with short accumulation half-lives (captopril) need to be administered twice daily at least; all other ACE inhibitors can be administered once/day[88] although, with the inception of trandolapril, duration of action is dose-dependent. Thus at low doses, multiple daily doses are appropriate for most agents.

Although most ACE inhibitors are recommended for once-daily administration, few have trough-to-peak effect ratios in excess of 50%.[144] For some of the newer drugs, data are not available. Again, trough-to-peak ratios are dose-dependent, with those for trandolapril least affected by dose.

Metabolism

Activation

The vast majority of ACE inhibitors are inactive prodrugs identifiable by the suffix –pril and require metabolic activation to the active form –prilat. Activation occurs during intestinal absorption and hepatic first pass through ester hydrolysis. As a rule of thumb, the prils are weak ACE inhibitors but have acceptable bioavailability as opposed to prilats which are potent inhibitors with poor bioavailability. The exceptions are captopril and lisinopril which do not require intestinal or hepatic activation. Enalaprilat is available for parenteral use. Delapril is converted to two active metabolites[145] while alacepril and moveltipril are converted to captopril.

Degradation and elimination

Most ACE inhibitors, as the active prilats and some minor metabolites, are cleared by the kidney via glomerular filtration with or without tubular secretion. The often quoted presence of drug in the faeces is due mostly to incomplete absorption and should not be interpreted as proof of biliary/hepatic elimination. Predominantly renal elimination (>90%) occurs with alacepril, captopril, cilazapril, enalapril, lisinopril and quinapril, while some additional hepatic elimination (15–40%) is described for benazepril, delapril, imidapril, moexipril, pentopril, perindopril and ramipril. Therefore drug dosage for the vast majority of ACE inhibitors must be modified according to renal function.

For fosinopril, temocapril, trandolapril, spirapril and zofenopril total body clearance of the respective prilats greatly exceeds renal clearance and therefore the issue of dose adjustment in impaired renal function is less important. For some of these drugs it has been proposed that decreases in renal clearance are compensated for by increases in hepatic clearance, so that total clearance is maintained.[146,147] The effect of hepatic dysfunction is difficult to estimate but under most circumstances it appears to be of minor relevance. If in doubt the advice is to use a drug, such as lisinopril, which does not require hepatic activation or metabolism.

Alacepril[148] (renal): This drug is metabolized to deacetyl-alacepril (active) which then liberates phenyl-alanine to form captopril (active). Alacepril and captopril are eliminated in the urine unchanged and as captopril and alacepril disulfide dimers and as cysteine conjugates.

Benazepril[149,150] (renal and hepatic): Elimination is in the urine and bile as the prilat and pril (20%) and the corresponding glucuronides.

Captopril[151–153] (renal): Approximately 50% of captopril is eliminated in the urine unchanged, the remainder as captopril disulfide dimers and as cysteine conjugate. Non-renal excretion is of no relevance.

Cilazapril[154–158] (renal): This drug is eliminated in the urine as the prilat.

Delapril[159–161] (renal and hepatic): Elimination is in the urine (60%) as prilat, 5-OH-prilat and pril.

Enalapril[161–164] (renal): Enalapril is eliminated in the urine as prilat and pril.

Fosinipril[165–168] (renal and hepatic): Elimination is in the urine (40%) and bile (60%) as prilat (75%) and the corresponding glucuronide (20%). Since fosinoprilat is not biotransformed after intravenous administration, fosinopril, not fosinoprilat, appears to be the precursor for the glucuronide metabolites. A dose adjustment in altered renal function is not necessary for fosinopril (total body clearance for the prilat is greater than twice the renal clearance).

Imidapril[169] (renal and hepatic): Elimination is via the urine and bile.

Lisinopril[170,171] (renal): Not metabolized; eliminated in the urine.

Moexipril[172,173] (renal and hepatic): Elimination is in the urine as prilat (40%) and pril (26%) and other metabolites resulting from cyclization via dehydration (diketopiperazines). About 20% is eliminated via the bile.

Pentopril[174–176] (renal and hepatic): Elimination is in the urine (1/3 as pril and 2/3 as prilat) and bile.

Perindopril[177–180] (renal and hepatic): Elimination is in the urine as prilat and pril (<10%), the corresponding glucuronides and other metabolites resulting from cyclization via dehydration (diketopiperazines). Some elimination is via the bile.

Quinapril[181–183] (renal): Elimination is in the urine as prilat and pril and the corresponding glucuronides and other metabolites (6%) resulting from cyclization via dehydration (diketopiperazines).

Ramipril[184,185] (renal and hepatic): Elimination is in urine (2/3) and bile (1/3) as prilat and pril, the corresponding glucuronides and other metabolites resulting from cyclization via dehydration (diketopiperazines). Dosage adjustment is needed in renal insufficiency.

Spirapril[186] (hepatic and renal): Spirapril is eliminated mainly in the bile (>50%) and the urine as prilat (prilat total body clearance is much greater than renal clearance). Dosage adjustment is probably not needed in moderate renal insufficiency.

Temocapril[187,188] (hepatic and renal): Elimination is in urine and bile. Decreases in renal clearance are compensated for by increases in hepatic clearance, so that total clearance is maintained in patients with renal impairment. Dosage adjustment is probably not needed in moderate renal insufficiency.

Trandolapril[189,190] (hepatic and renal): Eliminated in the urine (1/3) and bile (2/3) as prilat and pril and the corresponding glucuronides (prilat total body clearance is more than twice the renal clearance). Dosage adjustment is probably not needed in moderate renal insufficiency.

Zofenopril[191–194] (hepatic and renal): Elimination is in urine (2/3) and bile (1/3) as prilat (prilat total body clearance is greater than three times renal clearance). Dosage adjustment is probably not needed in moderate renal insufficiency.

It should be remembered that when elimination is impaired, peak ACE inhibition is little affected but clearance is prolonged. Thus in severe renal impairment, the pharmacological action of a single dose of trandolapril may persist for one week.[195]

PHARMACODYNAMICS

Haemodynamics

ACE inhibitor/BP dose–response information, as with most antihypertensive drug groups, is difficult to obtain. Distinct dose–response relationships have, however, been developed for a number of ACE inhibitors by plotting the BP response to infused angiotensin I against the plasma level of the ACE inhibitor or the active metabolite.[196]

The fall in BP with ACE inhibitors relates to a decrease in total peripheral resistance, with blood flow increasing to the kidneys and being maintained elsewhere,[197] except possibly to the liver.[198] A tendency for coronary blood flow to fall is matched by a decline in myocardial oxygen requirement,[199] hence precipitation or exacerbation of angina pectoris is unusual. At low doses, ACE inhibitors induce preferential dilatation of arterioles and at higher doses also increase the diameter of larger arteries.[200] The vasodilator effect is associated with little or no change in cardiac output or heart rate, the latter perhaps reflecting reduced activity of the sympathetic nervous system with or without augmentation of parasympathetic activity. Orthostatic hypotension is not common since important cardiac reflexes remain intact.[201] Venous capacitance is increased, at least in the short-term.[202]

Although by no means all studies are congruent, the following are generalizations regarding the response in BP to ACE inhibitors in patients with essential hypertension. First, if younger patients have a greater fall in BP with ACE inhibitors than older patients, as might be predicted from their higher pre-treatment levels of circulating Ang II, the differences are small.[203,204] In this regard and although experience is limited, a recent report[205] confirms earlier studies suggesting that ACE inhibitors are both effective and safe in children with hypertension. Second, blacks have a lesser BP response to ACE inhibitors than whites,[206–208] due presumably to relative suppression of the circulatory RAS, but also to reduced vascular reactivity to bradykinin.[209] Recent observations have, however, cast doubt on the often-accepted adage that the BP response of black patients to thiazide-like diuretics is greater than that to ACE inhibitors.[210] Third, the proportional fall in systolic BP is greater than that for diastolic pressure from brachial artery recordings,[211] and these underestimate the fall in peak central aortic pressure with ACE inhibitors,[212] perhaps reflecting improved vessel wall structure.[213] Fourth, the fall in BP with ACE inhibitors is rather similar to that with other groups of antihypertensive agents[214] although potency is modulated considerably by the level of dietary sodium intake compared with, in particular, calcium channel antagonists. Accordingly, both the rapidity and magnitude of fall in BP is greater with calcium channel blockers in, for example, hypertensive diabetics receiving a liberal sodium diet.[215] Fifth, the fall in BP in hypertensives with type 2 diabetes is greatest in those with preserved renal function, good glycaemic control and least suppression of the circulatory RAS and aldosterone.[215]

Renal haemodynamics and renal function

Renal vasodilatation with an increase in renal blood flow and little or no change in glomerular filtration rate is the typical response to ACE inhibition in essential hypertension.[216] In the short term urinary sodium is unaltered or increased and urinary potassium is reduced giving, respectively, a small decrease in cumulative sodium balance and a small positive balance in potassium.[98]

ADVERSE EFFECTS/CONTRAINDICATIONS

Adverse effects

Some adverse effects reported with high-dose captopril therapy, including disturbances of taste, leucopenia and tongue ulceration, have largely disappeared with current dosing schedules. Numerous other reported side effects, including Guillain-Barré syndrome, lymphadenopathy, exacerbation of Huntingdon's disease, and proteinuria are not now considered as side effects of ACE inhibitors.

Cough

This unexpected side effect of disputed incidence,[217] more common in females, non-smokers,[218] Chinese[219] and blacks and perhaps in diabetics,[220] is presumed to result from a bradykinin-induced[221] imbalance of thromboxane and prostacyclin[222] rather than perturbations in the RAS.[223] Typically dry and irritating, sometimes worse at night, occasionally associated with voice change and a sore throat,[224] the cough may come on weeks or months after initiation of ACE inhibitor therapy, can disappear spontaneously despite continued treatment,[225] sometimes persists for weeks after cessation of treatment[226] and may not occur in re-challenge.[227] Evidence that some ACE inhibitors are less associated with this side effect than are others is fragile.

Angio-oedema

Angio-oedema with ACE inhibitors is related to increased bradykinin levels.[228,229] This adverse effect affects the tongue, lips, throat, face and abdominal viscera and can develop immediately or after years of ACE inhibitor treatment. Approximately 0.7% of hypertensives exposed to these drugs will develop the side effect.[230] Angio-oedema afflicts blacks more commonly than whites,[231] is liable to recur with continued exposure to the offending drug,[232] and can be life-threatening. Avoidance of all ACE inhibitors is recommended for afflicted patients in whom an ARB might be considered as substitution therapy – but with caution since recurrence of angio-oedema has been reported under these circumstances.[233,234]

Anaphylaxis during haemodialysis or low-density lipoprotein apharesis

Reports from a number of centres in the early 1990s indicated that anaphylactoid reactions could occur during haemodialyses using AN69 membranes,[235] or during apheresis,[236] in patients taking ACE inhibitors. Increased bradykinin generation appears central to the problem although the phenomenon has been reported also in a patient receiving an ARB.[237] This adverse event with ACE inhibitors is now well recognised. Accordingly, few case reports have appeared over recent years.[238]

Fluid loss, renal failure, hyperkalaemia

Soon after the introduction of ACE inhibitors it became apparent that these drugs could contribute to severe dehydration and renal failure, sometimes with hyperkalaemia. These problems are most likely to occur in elderly patients who develop incidental fever, diarrhoea or vomiting.[239,240] Those taking a NSAID or a diuretic, particularly spironolactone or eplerenone in addition to an ACE inhibitor, are especially prone to such problems.[239–241] Renal failure under these circumstances is usually reversible.

First-dose hypotension

This complication, more common in heart failure than hypertension, is most likely in patients with gross activation of the RAS as in malignant hypertension, renovascular hypertension, the hypertensive-hyponatraemic syndrome, scleroderma renal crisis and patients already taking diuretics. Warning signals are severe grades or secondary forms of hypertension, baseline postural hypotension, hyponatraemia and high plasma levels of renin.[92,93,242,243] In susceptible patients, it is wise to begin cautiously with a small dose of ACE inhibitor and at a time when the patient is able to remain supine or sitting until after the expected nadir of BP, depending on characteristics of the individual ACE inhibitor chosen.

Contraindications

Pregnancy

Whilst the ACE inhibitors have been used successfully in pregnant women under exceptional circumstances[244,245] and without apparent harm during the first trimester, adverse effects from their use during the second and third trimesters include intrauterine growth retardation, renal tract defects and functional renal impairment, skull hypoplasia and oligohydramnios. The European Society of Hypertension[246] and the British Hypertension Society guidelines[247] are clear that ACE inhibitors are contraindicated during pregnancy and the JNC 7 report goes further in advising that they should be avoided by women who are likely to become pregnant.[248] The FDA rates use of the ACE inhibitors in the first trimester under Category C (animal studies show adverse effects and there are no adequate and well-controlled studies in pregnant women) and thereafter in pregnancy under Category D (adequate well-controlled or observational studies in pregnant women have demonstrated a risk to the fetus).

Renovascular hypertension

ACE inhibitors can induce renal failure, usually reversible, in patients with hypertension due to bilateral renal artery stenosis or narrowing of the artery to a single kidney, so should generally be avoided under these circumstances. The situation is less clear for patients with hypertension due to stenosis of the renal artery to one kidney, the arterial supply to the contralateral kidney being unimpeded (see below).

Areas of uncertainty

Testicular function

The male reproductive system has several sites of intrinsic renin–angiotensin activity with possible,[249] though of uncertain involvement in reproductive function and the development of prostatic hypertrophy.[19] Whereas some ACE inhibitors such as enalapril have little or no access to testicular ACE because of a blood–testis barrier,[250] it is not clear whether this is so for all ACE inhibitors. Nor is it clear what might be the consequences on reproductive function should an ACE inhibitor gain access to testicular ACE.

Quality of life, cognitive function, dementia

There have been reports, summarized by Fletcher and Dollery,[251] that ACE inhibitors, compared with other antihypertensive drug groups, have a favourable effect on quality of life and cognition. These issues remain in dispute.[252]

Hypertension is linked with the subsequent development of dementia, and antihypertensive drug treatment is protective.[253] Whether ACE inhibitors offer protection beyond that of alternative drug groups for a similar achieved level of BP, is unclear.[254] Within the group of ACE inhibitors, Ohrui et al. provided evidence that those drugs capable of penetration into the brain (captopril or perindopril) slowed the rate of cognitive decline in hypertensive patients with mild-to-moderate Alzheimer's disease compared to those (enalapril or imidapril) without brain-penetrating capacity or a calcium channel blocker (nifedipine or nilvadipine).[255]

DRUG INTERACTIONS

Drug–drug interactions can be classified as pharmacokinetic or pharmacodynamic, the former being further subdivided into four categories involving drug absorption, distribution, metabolism and elimination. Pharmacodynamic interactions address pharmacological, therapeutic and toxic effects, both predictable and unpredictable, of concurrently administered drugs from the same or different medication classes.

Ensuring that drugs have little likelihood of kinetic or dynamic interaction is a necessary part of early phase drug development. This is especially important for medicines that are to be used widely in primary care for chronic conditions like hypertension. Ultimately the drug needs to be accepted as a useful medication that can be used extensively and safely by average practitioners and patients without the need for detailed lists of contraindications or potentially interacting medications that should be avoided. In general, ACE inhibitors fall into this category.

Knowledge of the patient, and his or her diseases and drug combinations, enables the informed prescriber to forecast with reasonable accuracy the potential for interactions, especially when one of the numerous drug–drug interaction texts, charts or software programs is consulted a priori. However, the actual extent of interaction in the individual patient is much more difficult to predict and demands careful follow-up, especially when serious and potentially lethal adverse effects are anticipated.

Whereas individual ACE inhibitors used as monotherapy are remarkably free of serious adverse effects and are generally well tolerated across a wide range of doses, pharmacodynamic interactions with ACE inhibitors are more likely to be problematic. Hypotension can occur in the presence of other BP-lowering drug classes, especially in the setting of sodium or volume depletion or a patient's inability to mount an adequate physiological response (as with autonomic blockade). Hyperkalaemia and reduced creatinine clearance may be worsened by ACE inhibitors against a background of impaired renal function or medications that reduce glomerular filtration or impair potassium homeostasis. Given the widespread and growing use of ACE inhibitors in patients with hypertension, it is hardly surprising that older age, renal dysfunction, heart disease, diabetes, arthritis and polypharmacy feature commonly in reports of interactions with ACE inhibitors.

When prescribing an ACE inhibitor de novo the importance of considering the patient's age, clinical state and concurrent treatments cannot be over-stated. Likewise, when adding drugs likely to lower blood pressure (other anti-hypertensives), impair renal perfusion (NSAIDs), increase potassium load (K^+ preparations) or reduce potassium elimination (aldosterone antagonists, non-selective beta-blockers) in a patient already on an ACE inhibitor, caution must be exercised. If these simple considerations are respected, the likelihood of serious interactions with ACE inhibitors can be largely avoided.

Epidemiology of ACE inhibitor interactions

The use of ACE inhibitors with other potassium-sparing drugs is a matter of concern. Bjerrum et al. studied potential drug interactions in Swedish patients receiving multiple medications.[256] Drugs accounting for the highest number of potential interactions were diuretics, NSAIDs, ACE inhibitors, digoxin, oral antidiabetic agents, calcium channel blockers, anticoagulants and beta-blockers. A population-based, case-control study investigated the risk associated with receiving a potassium-sparing medication while being treated with an ACE inhibitor in persons aged 66 years or older in the Ontario Pharmacare programme.[257] During a 7-year period, patients treated with ACE inhibitors admitted with a diagnosis of hyperkalaemia were about 20 times more likely to have been treated with a potassium-sparing diuretic in the previous week. With current knowledge of drug–drug interactions, many of these episodes could have been avoided. The risk of hyperkalaemia is especially high in patients with severe grades of heart failure receiving both an ACE inhibitor and spironolactone as observed following publication of the Randomised Aldactone Evaluation Study (RALES).[258,259]

Interactions with food and antacids

The relative bioavailability of captopril is 0.66 and 0.48 after administration with antacid and after food, respectively. Food, but not antacid, delayed the BP-lowering effect of captopril.[260] Apart from captopril, food interactions with ACE inhibitors are not considered important.

Interactions with other antihypertensive and cardiovascular drugs

We will focus mainly on pharmacokinetic and toxic interactions and will not address here the many studies in which ACE inhibitors were used with other antihypertensive drugs to lower BP as the primary therapeutic objective.

Diuretics

In renally impaired subjects, fosinopril and hydrochlorothiazide (HCTZ) can be coadministered without undue increases in fosinoprilat concentrations or clinically significant pharmacodynamic effects.[261] Interactions of the ACE inhibitor imidapril with other medications used in hypertension and heart failure were investigated.[262] There was no pharmacokinetic interaction with HCTZ and haemodynamic effects were additive.

Aldosterone antagonists

The combination of an ACE inhibitor and spironolactone or eplerenone may have considerable cardiac and renal protective potential, but the combination enhances the risk of hyperkalaemia. The new, more selective aldosterone antagonist eplerenone is devoid of some side effects of spironolactone but it is likely that metabolic interactions with ACE inhibitors will not differ from those with spironolactone.

Beta-blockers

The combination of an ACE inhibitor and a beta-blocker has limited anti-hypertensive efficacy, although a potential greater than the additive effects on BP lowering with propranolol and cilazapril were reported by Belz et al.[263] Neither the combination of cilazapril and propranolol,[264] nor imidapril with bisoprolol[262] was accompanied by pharmacokinetic interactions.

Calcium channel antagonists

The combination of imidapril and nilvadipine was not accompanied by pharmacokinetic interactions and BP-lowering effects were additive.[262]

Neither verapamil nor amlodipine added to trandolapril significantly improved the antiproteinuric effect of the ACE inhibitor in patients with non-diabetic nephropathies.[265] In hypertensive patients with acute renal function impairment secondary to ACE inhibitor treatment, the addition of verapamil appeared to restore serum creatinine towards baseline values.[266]

Angiotensin receptor blockers (ARBs)

While the combination of an ACE inhibitor and ARB may enable complete blockade of the RAS, high doses given to rats produced a syndrome that resulted in death.[267] Such dire consequences are not seen in humans.

BP was measured by telemetry in spontaneously hypertensive rats and the acute response to losartan, captopril, or their combination was studied.[268] The effect of the combination of low doses of the two drugs was more than additive. In higher doses the response was less than additive, but a greater decrease in systolic BP was achieved with the combination than with captopril, the response to which was in turn greater than that with losartan. The interaction between ACE inhibitors and ARBs depends on the dose used, but the combination has greater BP-lowering effects than either drug alone.[269]

The effects of adding an ARB to an ACE inhibitor on augmentation pressure, a measure of arterial stiffness, and pulse pressure amplification were studied in patients with poorly controlled essential hypertension.[270] The beneficial haemodynamic response, which was sustained over several weeks,[271] suggests that this combined treatment may have more beneficial effects than the simple reduction in BP.

When enalapril and losartan were coadministered to patients with IgA nephropathy, proteinuria decreased by a greater extent than with either drug alone. An additional reduction in proteinuria was observed when doses of each constituent were doubled.[272] Reductions in diastolic and mean ambulatory BP were significantly correlated with the decrease in proteinuria, as well as with creatinine clearance. Combination therapy has an additive, dose-dependent antiproteinuric effect that is likely induced in part by the drug-related reduction in systemic BP and by altered intraglomerular haemodynamics because efferent arteriolar regulation is hampered more completely by the coadministration of ACE inhibitors and ARBs.

Nitrates

Among hypertensive subjects use of ACE inhibitors is associated with a reduced risk of headache caused by nitrates.[273] Whether this depends on the type of ACE inhibitor (sulfhydryl or not) is unclear.

Aspirin (ASA)

Several studies have suggested that ASA attenuates the beneficial effects of ACE inhibitors in hypertension, congestive heart failure or coronary artery disease and have questioned the safety of using ASA concomitantly with these agents. Others have concluded that there is no detrimental effect.

In rats rendered hypertensive by administration of methylprednisolone, concurrent ASA treatment (100 and 25 mg/kg/day p.o.) with lisinopril did not hinder the BP-lowering effect of the ACE inhibitor.[274] However ASA 100 mg/kg/day increased the mortality rate and produced cardiac necrosis and renal damage. Clearly, ASA attenuates the beneficial effects of ACE inhibitors on survival in hypertensive rats and this effect is more pronounced at higher doses of ASA. The relevance of these observations to humans can be debated, given the ASA dosage used in rats.

A systematic review has examined all mortality studies of treatment with ACE inhibitors and aspirin in patients with coronary artery disease.[275] Studies were included if these provided data on mortality of patients who received both drugs, either drug and no drug. The pooled synergy index S indicated slight antagonism between ACE inhibitors and aspirin (S = 0.91; 95% CI 0.80–1.03). The investigators concluded that there seems to be an antagonistic interaction between ACE inhibitors and aspirin.

The significance of this interaction in heart failure has received considerable attention but is complex and beyond the focus of this review.

Lithium

The use of lithium in the elderly as acute and maintenance therapy in bipolar disorder and augmentation therapy for major depression is well documented.[276] The association between hospital admission for lithium toxicity and the use of diuretics, ACE inhibitors and NSAIDs was studied in the elderly using a Canadian data base.[277] After adjustment for potential confounders, a dramatically increased risk of lithium toxicity was seen within a month of initiating treatment with a loop diuretic (RR=5.5, 95% CI=1.9–16.1) or an ACE inhibitor (RR=7.6, 95% CI=2.6–22.0). Neither thiazide diuretics nor NSAIDs were independently associated with an increased risk of hospitalization for lithium toxicity.

Miscellaneous

Tizanidine
Patients treated chronically with ACE inhibitors may have a limited ability to respond to hypotension when the sympathetic response is simultaneously blocked. A 10-year-old boy chronically treated with lisinopril for hypertension developed hypotension following the addition of tizanidine, an alpha-2 agonist, for the treatment of spasticity.[278]

Cyclooxygenase-2 (COX 2) inhibitors
An inducible isoform of COX-2, insulin-like growth factor (IGF) II, and the IGF-I receptor are up-regulated in colon carcinoma and might have crucial roles in tumour growth and invasion. The effects of COX-2 inhibition, ACE inhibitor and ARB treatment on IGF-IR expression and tumour growth were studied in vivo in mice.[279] The study results suggested that combination therapy with COX-2 and ACE inhibitors might be a promising strategy for the chemoprevention of colon cancer. However, a higher rate of cardiovascular disease in a study examining rofecoxib's impact on colon cancer prevention led to voluntary withdrawal and has cast a cloud over the entire COX-2 class.[280,281]

Antipsychotic drugs
A review of pharmacokinetic and pharmacodynamic interactions between antipsychotics and antihypertensives was undertaken by searching the English-language literature for human and animal studies, reviews, and case reports.[282] Hypotension and postural syncope were reported in a patient given therapeutic dosages of chlorpromazine and captopril, and in two patients when clozapine was added to enalapril therapy. No antipsychotic–antihypertensive combination is absolutely contraindicated, but no combination should be considered to be completely without risk. The authors recommend careful patient monitoring for attenuated or enhanced activity of either agent whenever antipsychotics and antihypertensives are given concurrently, but ACE inhibitors appear fairly innocuous.

Aprotinin
Aprotinin is a protease inhibitor that has effects on many homeostatic functions including coagulation, platelet function and inflammation.[283] Since patients with cardiovascular diseases are treated frequently with ACE inhibitors and also often need cardiopulmonary bypass surgery and receive aprotinin, there are potential interactions. However, the available information indicates that the advantages of its application outweigh its potential disadvantages.

N-acetylcysteine (NAC)
It has been observed that the hypotensive effect of ACE inhibitors is, at least partially, mediated by nitric oxide (NO). Sulfhydryl group donors, such as

NAC, may enhance the antihypertensive effect of some drugs through a NO mechanism.[284] The potential effect of NAC on the ACE inhibitor antihypertensive action was studied in hypertensive patients who were smokers. The addition of NAC to the ACE inhibitor potentiated the latter's antihypertensive effect.[282]

CLINICAL USE INCLUDING OUTCOME DATA

Whereas ACE inhibitors are used in essential hypertension primarily as antihypertensive agents, ACE inhibitors have effects beyond the lowering of BP, which has seen these drugs accepted as drugs of first choice in special situations. Furthermore, reported effects on the heart, blood vessels, renal function and metabolic indices have led many clinicians to consider ACE inhibitors to be actually, or potentially, more protective than other drug groups against the cardiovascular complications of hypertension, with the possible exception of the ARBs. This postulate is controversial.

The relative acceptability to patients of the various antihypertensive drugs, and hence persistence with therapy, is an important practical issue. In this regard, the ACE inhibitors fare well, better than diuretics though less well than ARBs, according to a European study which reported in 2002.[285]

Essential hypertension: outcome data

ACE inhibitor-based treatment protects against the major complications of hypertension. Cumulative results from five trials, analysed by the Blood Pressure Lowering Treatment Trialists' Collaboration, indicate that ACE inhibitor-based treatment versus placebo, given over a period of 2.3–4.7 years with a mean difference in BP of 5.4/2.3 mmHg, reduced significantly the relative risk of stroke (RR 0.72, 95% CI 0.64–0.81), coronary heart disease (RR 0.80, 0.73–0.88), heart failure (RR 0.82, 0.69–0.98), cardiovascular death (RR 0.80, 0.71–0.89) and total mortality (RR 0.88, 0.81–0.96).[99] For one study included in this analysis, HOPE, patients were at high risk of cardiovascular disease but the mean baseline BP was only 139/79 mmHg and only 47% of patients were diagnosed as hypertensive.[286] The incidence of cardiovascular endpoints was not statistically different between those with, or without hypertension.[286]

Further analysis by the Trialists' Collaboration reported no significant difference in total major cardiovascular events, cardiovascular death or total mortality in a meta-analysis of studies using antihypertensive regimens based on ACE inhibitors, calcium antagonists, or beta-blockers or diuretics.[284] There are three caveats here. First, ACE inhibitor-based treatment reduced BP less overall than diuretic/beta-blocker-based, or calcium blocker-based treatment (1.9/0.2 and 0.6/0.9 mmHg, respectively). One interpretation is that the protective effects of the ACE inhibitors would likely have been superior had identical levels of BP been achieved. Second, specific cardiovascular outcomes were said to be altered differently according to the drug-based regimen. In particular, ACE inhibitors were said to be more effective than calcium blockers in preventing heart failure. While this may be so, uncertainties regarding the diagnosis of heart failure in most studies, particularly ALLHAT,[287,288] leave an air of uncertainty on this point. The 'trend' for calcium antagonist-based treatment to show a lesser risk of stroke than with ACE inhibitors is also difficult to interpret given the difference in achieved levels of BP between the two regimens.

The third caveat is particularly contentious. It relates to the question of what constitutes best clinical advice in the absence of evidence derived from formal, interventional studies.[289] The mean age of patients in the trials included in the above meta-analysis was 65 years, and the duration of drug treatment was 2–8.4 years. How far should practising clinicians extrapolate these findings to young and middle-aged hypertensives for whom many decades of drug therapy will be required? On the one hand it might be argued that thiazide-like diuretics should be drugs of first choice in view of low cost and the evidence of similar cardiovascular protection to ACE inhibitors in the meta-analysis.[99] An alternative view is that ACE inhibitors should be first choice on the basis that their beneficial effects on the heart, blood vessels and kidneys, together with neutral or salutary metabolic effects (especially regarding glucose tolerance), will protect the cardiovascular system over 30–60 years for a given level of achieved BP better than diuretics with an inferior metabolic profile, stimulatory actions on the RAS and sympathetic system and, arguably, less obvious benefits on cardiac and vascular structure and function. Commentators of the latter persuasion would not accept the premise that perturbations in metabolic indices (glucose, lipids and potassium levels) during chlorthalidone versus lisinopril therapy in ALLHAT which 'did not translate into more cardiovascular events or into higher all-cause mortality'[208] can be accepted as innocuous for younger hypertensives requiring antihypertensive drug treatment over decades.

Guidelines for the use of ACE inhibitors

There are special indications for the use of ACE inhibitors with broad agreement across recent major guidelines[246–248] (Table 12.2). Likewise the cautions and contraindications shown in Table 12.2 are generally accepted. The situation in renovascular hypertension is contentious (see below).

Regarding initial choice of antihypertensive therapy where there is no compelling indication for one drug group over another, ACE inhibitors are seen as a suitable option in the 2003 European[246] and JNC 7 guidelines, although the latter suggest 'thiazide-type diuretics for most (patients)'.[248]

Table 12.2 Indications, cautions and contraindications for ACE inhibitors

Compelling indications	Possible indications	Caution	Compelling contraindications
Heart failure	Chronic renal disease*	Renal impairment*	Pregnancy
Left ventricular dysfunction, post-myocardial infarction or established coronary heart disease	Type 2 diabetic nephropathy	Peripheral vascular disease†	Renovascular disease‡
Type 1 diabetic nephropathy	Proteinuric renal disease		
Secondary stroke prevention**			

*ACE inhibitors may be beneficial in chronic renal failure but should only be used with caution, close supervision and specialist advice when there is established and significant renal impairment.
†Caution because of association between peripheral vascular disease and renovascular disease.
‡ACE inhibitors sometimes used under specialist supervision.
**In combination with thiazide or thiazide-like diuretic.

The British Hypertension Society recommends, in its AB/CD algorithm, use of an ACE inhibitor (ARB) or beta-blocker as first-line drug therapy for essential hypertensives who are white and younger than 55 years, based on the premise that such patients have relatively high plasma levels of renin and show a superior BP response to drugs which block the RAS compared with those who are older and/or black.[246] Where a drug combination is required to achieve goal BP, then one of the CD drugs (calcium channel blocker or thiazide-like diuretic) should be added to the ACE inhibitor (ARB) (or beta-blocker). This suggestion for combination ACE inhibitor therapy is consistent with that from the recent European guidelines.[246] An ACE inhibitor/beta-blocker combination has long been suggested to have limited antihypertensive efficacy.[290] For resistant essential hypertension, Brown et al.[291] propose the triple combination of an ACE inhibitor (or ARB), a calcium channel blocker and a diuretic. Thereafter and if normotension is not achieved, addition of spironolactone (or eplerenone), an alpha-receptor blocker or another diuretic, is advised (Fig. 12.5).

The combination of an ACE inhibitor and spironolactone or eplerenone, considered by some to have particular cardiac and renoprotective potential,[292–294] requires careful patient follow-up in order to avoid hyperkalaemia and azotaemia. The possibility that a combined approach to blockade of the RAS using both an ACE inhibitor and an ARB might afford superior cardiovascular protection, is an intriguing, but largely untested possibility.[295,296]

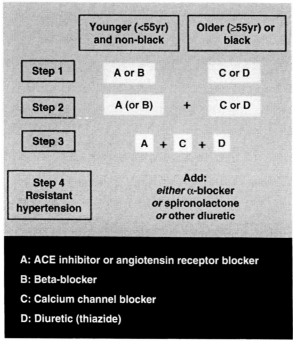

Fig. 12.5 Modified Cambridge AB/CD Rule. Initial monotherapy (step 1) is selected according to age and ethnic group, as surrogates for plasma renin. In step 2, one drug from each of the AB and CD categories combined. Because of the diabetogenic potential of the older classes in older patients, B is shown in parenthesis in step 2 and is dropped altogether from step 3 (triple therapy). Recommendations for step 4 (quadruple therapy) are more anecdotal and may require secondary referral. Non-thiazide diuretic therapy is most appropriate in patients with normal renal function and suppression of plasma renin despite receiving the A+C+D combination. From Brown et al.[291] with permission.

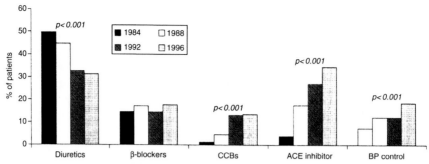

Fig. 12.6 Time trends in the use of different classes of first-line antihypertensive drugs by female patients in the Brisighella Heart Study from 1984 to 1996. The pattern of use was similar for male patients. CCBs, calcium channel blockers; ACE inhibitor, ACE inhibitors; BP, blood pressure. From Borghi et al.[301] with permission.

Reported effects of ACE inhibitors which might be taken to favour these drugs as first choice antihypertensive agents, particularly in younger age groups where long-term therapy is needed and where features of the 'metabolic syndrome' are evident, may have had an impact on clinician prescribing habits. Notwithstanding cost-benefit analyses[297,298] and recommendations of many guidelines and government promotion to the effect that unless there are compelling reasons to choose otherwise a thiazide-like diuretic should be drug of first choice,[299] the ACE inhibitors have been increasingly chosen as first-line therapy in many[300,301] (Fig. 12.6), though not all countries.[302]

Special effects of ACE inhibitors

Cardiac effects

Left ventricular hypertrophy (LVH) and cardiac fibrosis LVH is an important adverse prognostic sign in essential hypertension, and a reduction in left ventricular mass with antihypertensive drug therapy is associated with a markedly reduced risk of subsequent cardiovascular disease.[303] The balance of evidence is that drugs interfering specifically with the RAS, the ACE inhibitors and ARBs, are at least as, or more effective in reversing LVH than are calcium channel blockers and diuretics, and clearly more effective compared with beta-blockers.[58,304–306]

ACE inhibition in essential hypertensives has been shown on myocardial biopsies to induce regression of cardiac fibrosis, and to improve left ventricular diastolic function whereas other antihypertensive agents (not including an ARB or aldosterone receptor antagonist) had no, or lesser effects.[307,308] Since Ang II can, experimentally, stimulate cardiac fibrosis whilst inhibiting collagenase activity,[104] and an ARB (but not a beta-blocker) reduced myocardial collagen content in patients with essential hypertension,[309] it is difficult not to conclude that inhibition of Ang II formation is central to the ability of ACE inhibitors to reverse myocardial fibrosis.

Arrhythmias

The possibility that ACE inhibitors reduce the occurrence of atrial fibrillation in essential hypertensives has been raised.[106] An alternative explanation of the results from the study by L'Allier[106] is that ACE inhibitors had little or no effect on the development of atrial fibrillation, but the comparator agents, calcium channel antagonists, were pro-arrhythmic, perhaps through activation of the sympathetic nervous system. Nevertheless, the ACE inhibitors (and ARBs) are, in theory, likely to be effective in preventing cardiac arrhythmias as has been demonstrated in many experimental and clinical situations.[310–313] Prevention of atrial fibrillation is certainly possible in essential hypertensives since the ACE inhibitors are particularly effective in reducing left ventricular mass, one determinant of left atrial volume that, in turn, contributes importantly to the risk of developing atrial fibrillation.[108] In this regard, Dernellis et al. demonstrated that an ACE inhibitor normalized left atrial function in parallel with regression of LVH in hypertensive patients.[314] Further support for this anti-arrhythmic potential comes from the report by Anne et al. that treatment with ACE inhibitors (or ARBs or diuretics) was associated with a lesser incidence of atrial fibrillation over a median follow-up period of 2.2 years after radiofrequency ablation in 196 patients with atrial flutter, though only a minority were known to have hypertension.[315] Tsai et al. reported an association between gene polymorphisms of the RAS and atrial fibrillation and listed mechanisms linking Ang II with arrhythmogenesis,[316] thus providing a rationale for formally investigating the place of ACE inhibitors (and ARBs) in treating or preventing atrial fibrillation.

Effects on blood vessels and atherosclerosis

Many reasons have been cited as to why ACE inhibitors might retard the development of atherosclerosis in humans, and studies in animals show that these agents are capable of inducing regression of experimentally-induced atherosclerosis.[317] However, firm evidence that the favourable actions of ACE inhibitors on vessel walls, endothelial function, thrombotic/fibrinolytic tendency, rheology, inflammation and metabolic indices translate in humans into retardation of the atherosclerotic process, is lacking. The possibility that an ACE inhibitor–statin combination will prove especially protective against atherogenesis is an intriguing possibility.[318]

Effects on the kidneys

A protective effect of ACE inhibitors on renal function, cardiovascular and retinal complications and on survival, has been amply demonstrated for patients with diabetic nephropathy.[319] Accordingly, ACE inhibitors are recommended (for example by the American Diabetes Association) as first-line agents in diabetic type1 or type 2 patients with hypertension. It has been claimed that the ACE inhibitors are more effective than other antihypertensive agents in slowing the deterioration of renal function in patients with non-diabetic renal disease[320] although interpretation of available data is fraught with difficulty since levels of achieved BP in key comparative studies favoured the ACE inhibitors.

Metabolic effects

The effect of ACE inhibitors on metabolic indices, in particular glucose homeostasis (Fig. 12.7), has been discussed earlier.

Since thiazide-like diuretics and beta-blockers can impair glucose tolerance and provoke diabetes, and such effects may have adverse cardiovascular

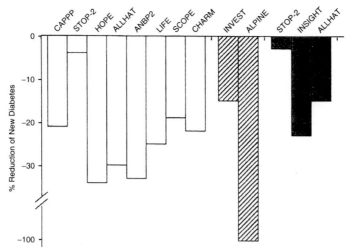

Fig. 12.7 Percentage reduction in new diabetes mellitus in randomized clinical trials with treatment groups using predominantly an ACE inhibitor or ARB (open bars), calcium channel blocker plus ACE inhibitor or ARB (striped bars), or calcium channel blocker alone (solid bars). The comparator groups contained predominantly thiazide diuretics and/or beta-blockers or, in the case of the HOPE trial, placebo. CAPPP, Captopril Prevention Project; STOP-2, Swedish Trial in Old Patients with Hypertension-2; HOPE, Heart Outcomes Prevention Evaluation; ALLHAT, Antihypertensive and Lipid-Lowering treatment to Prevent Heart Attack Trial; ANBP2, Second Australian National Blood Pressure Study; LIFE, Losartan Intervention For Endpoint reduction; SCOPE, Study on Cognition and Prognosis in the Elderly; CHARM, Candesartan in Heart Failure Assessment and Reduction in Mortality and Morbidity; INVEST, International Verapamil-Trandolapril Study; ALPINE, Antihypertensive Treatment and Lipid Profile in a North of Sweden Efficacy Evaluation; INSIGHT, Intervention as a Goal in Hypertension Treatment. From Pepine et al.[116] with permission.

effects in hypertensive patients over the long term,[321,322] a case can be made to prefer ACE inhibitors for patients predisposed to diabetes, especially where long-term treatment seems likely.

Antineoplasic effects

There are a number of mechanisms by which ACE inhibitors might, in theory, be antineoplasic and experimental studies have demonstrated a tumour-inhibitory effect of these drugs. Whereas a retrospective cohort study in Scotland raised the possibility that long-term treatment of hypertension with ACE inhibitors protects against some cancers,[323] no association between ACE inhibition and cancer was found in relatively short-term follow-up of a Swedish population of hypertensives.[324]

ACE inhibitors in special circumstances

Hypertension in adults with diabetes

The American Diabetes Association recommendation in 2003 that the established practice of choosing an ACE inhibitor as the first-line agent for patients with either mild or severe hypertension and type 1 or type 2 diabetes[325] appears reasonable. The evidence supporting this recommendation relates more convincingly to the renal than the cardiovascular protection afforded by the ACE inhibitors.[326] It is possible that in the future, albuminuria may become one target of a cardiovascular (as well as renal) protection strategy beyond or additional to BP reduction, and blockers of the RAS would be central to this strategy.[327] Certainly, ACE inhibitor therapy, compared with a non-dihydropyridine calcium channel blocker, prevented the development of microalbuminuria in type 2 diabetics with hypertension[328] – a key treatment goal for renoprotection.

Apart from renal and cardiovascular protection, the ACE inhibitors also slow the progression of retinopathy, at least in normotensive type 1 diabetics.[329] Whether this protective action is superior to that of other antihypertensive agents, including ARBs,[330] and whether ACE inhibitors are similarly, or more protective in diabetics who are hypertensive, is unclear.

Combination therapy of an ACE inhibitor, usually with a calcium channel antagonist and/or a diuretic, is often needed to achieve BP control in hypertensive diabetics. The combination of an ACE inhibitor and an ARB has shown promise regarding control of BP and reducing proteinuria in hypertensive type 1[331] or type 2 diabetics.[332]

Hypertension and non-diabetic renal disease

A meta-analysis of 11 studies suggested that antihypertensive regimens which included an ACE inhibitor were more effective than other regimens in slowing progression of non-diabetic renal disease.[320] As pointed out in the 2003 European Guidelines, however, it is unclear whether this advantage was due to ACE inhibition or the lower achieved level of BP.[246] The possibility that an ACE inhibitor-ARB combination provides superior renal protection for patients with non-diabetic renal disease than either alone has been raised by encouraging results from preliminary studies.[333–335]

Hypertension and end-stage renal disease

Cardiovascular disease mortality is 10–30 times higher in patients with end-stage renal failure than in the general population,[336] and hypertension, one contributor to this problem, is present in the vast majority of cases.[337] Whereas there was hesitation initially amongst clinicians to use ACE inhibitors for such patients, recent evidence is that these drugs can control the BP[338] whilst also improving large vessel function,[339] inducing regression of LVH[340] and improving blood rheology.[341] Whether ACE inhibitors improve outcome in such patients remains to be tested formally but a retrospective, non-randomized study in patients on haemodialysis showed that there was a mortality risk reduction of 52% for those receiving an ACE inhibitor compared with those not receiving an ACE inhibitor.[342] Whilst a careful watch for hyperkalaemia is needed,[343] and the haematocrit may fall,[341] there is increasing enthusiasm for ACE inhibitors (or ARBs) in end-stage renal failure for control of BP, to slow the decline in residual renal function, and perhaps to reduce cardiovascular morbidity and mortality.[344] The possibility that ACE inhibitors also have a beneficial effect on post-renal transplant graft function, has been raised.[345] Dual blockade of the RAS with an ACE inhibitor and ARB shows promise regarding a reduction in proteinuria and control of BP in patients with chronic renal disease.[346]

Renovascular hypertension

The ACE inhibitors must be used with extreme caution in patients with hypertension resulting from bilateral renal artery stenosis or stenosis of the artery feeding a solitary kidney in order to avoid a major decline in glomerular filtration rate.[347] For the more common circumstance of hypertension due to unilateral renal artery stenosis when medical, rather than interventional treatment is indicated, the place of ACE inhibitors is disputed.[348,349] There is logic behind blockade of the RAS since it is involved in the pathophysiology to an extent that varies with the stage of the disorder.[350] Certainly, activation of the RAS contributes to the proteinuria (sometimes in the nephrotic range) that accompanies stenosis or occlusion of a renal artery, since ACE inhibitors correct the abnormality.[351,352] Concern revolves around the observation that the glomerular filtration rate may fall substantially in the stenotic kidney with ACE inhibition, and that this is not reflected accurately by plasma creatinine levels.[353] Nevertheless, BP is usually difficult to control without an ACE inhibitor or ARB. Furthermore, drug regimens which included an ACE inhibitor reportedly achieved a BP lower than with alternative regimens,[353,354] and were associated with a superior survival outcome.[355] Whilst the aforementioned studies were either small or non-randomized and cannot be seen as definitive, they do support use of ACE inhibitors, usually in combination with other hypertensives, provided careful monitoring of renal function is carried out.[356] It is reassuring that the decline in glomerular filtration rate which may occur in the ischaemic kidney during ACE inhibition usually recovers upon withdrawal of therapy even when the drug has been administered for sustained periods.[356, 357]

One approach to the patient with hypertension due to atherosclerotic unilateral renal artery stenosis, is to assess the effect of an ACE inhibitor on both BP and differential glomerular filtration rate using a nuclear medicine scan. Where BP control is inadequate or severe impairment of glomerular function occurs in the stenosed kidney, an alternative approach (angioplasty, stent or surgery) can be considered.[358]

Concern has been expressed that the introduction of ACE inhibitor therapy might, presumably through a sudden fall in BP, provoke thrombosis within a stenotic renal artery.[359] Whether such concern is warranted is not known, but retrospective studies suggest that the natural history is for 9–16% of renal arteries affected by atherosclerotic stenosis to progress to total occlusion over a 2–3 year period.[360] Furthermore, renal artery thrombosis has been reported upon withdrawal, as well as introduction, of ACE inhibitors.[361] Overall, it is difficult to be convinced that renal artery thrombosis is a specific complication of ACE inhibition. Nevertheless, avoidance of a sudden and vigorous decline in BP with the first dose seems a prudent precaution.

A special situation is the *hypertensive–hyponatraemic syndrome* associated with renal artery stenosis or occlusion.[353] In this not-so-rare disorder,[362] there is extreme activation of the RAS with volume depletion[363] and often hypokalaemia.[362,363] In order to avoid a precipitous decline in BP, volume repletion should be considered before an ACE inhibitor is administered, the first dose of which should be small. Careful monitoring of both BP and renal function is needed.

The hypertension of *segmental renal infarction*, which is often transient, is renin-dependent.[364,365] Accordingly, treatment with an ACE inhibitor (or ARB) is logical and has been successful in control of BP and correction of hypokalaemia and hyponatraemia.[364,365]

Scleroderma renal crisis

This complication of diffuse scleroderma is best treated with ACE inhibitors which improve survival and sometimes allow discontinuation of dialysis.[366,367]

Prophylactic ACE inhibition has been proposed for patients considered to be at high risk of developing scleroderma renal crisis.[368] Not only do the ACE inhibitors frequently stabilize or improve renal function, but they also increase myocardial perfusion and improve systolic and diastolic left ventricular function.[369,370] Claims that ACE inhibitors also have salutory effects on the skin and the digital circulation in patients with scleroderma require confirmation.

Secondary polycythaemia

A low dose of enalapril induced a fall in haematocrit, proteinuria and BP in Bolivians with altitude polycythaemia.[371] The effects are reminiscent of those seen with ACE inhibitors in patients with other forms of secondary polycythaemia,[372] most notably following renal transplantation.[373]

CONCLUSIONS

The ACE inhibitors have been a major advance in the treatment of hypertension. ACE inhibitors are drugs of choice for some secondary forms of hypertension, and their use alone and in combination in the treatment of essential hypertension is established. Debate continues as to the place of ACE inhibitors versus thiazide-like diuretics as initial therapy for essential hypertensives, especially where long-term administration is contemplated and in patients considered prone to diabetes mellitus. Compared with many older antihypertensive agents, the side-effect profile of ACE inhibitors has been excellent. The high-profile position of ACE inhibitors in the therapeutics of hypertension looks secure, at least for the near future.

References

1. Robertson JIS. Renin and angiotensin: a historical review. In: Robertson JIS, Nicholls MG, eds. *The renin-angiotensin system.* London: Mosby; 1993:1.1–1.18.
2. Henderson IW, Deacon CF. Physiology and comparative physiology of the renin-angiotensin system. In: Robertson JIS, Nicholls MG, eds. *The renin-angiotensin system.* London: Mosby; 1993:2.1–2.28.
3. Persson PB. Renin: origin, secretion and synthesis. *J Physiol* 2003;552:667–671.
4. Schnermann J. The juxtaglomerular apparatus: from anatomical peculiarity to physiological relevance. *J Am Soc Nephrol* 2003;14:1681–1694.
5. Dinh DT, Frauman AG, Johnston CI, et al. Angiotensin receptors: distribution, signalling and function. *Clin Sci (Lond)* 2001;100:481–492.
6. Johren O, Dendorfer A, Dominiak P. Cardiovascular and renal function of angiotensin II type-2 receptors. *Cardiovasc Res* 2004;62:460–467.
7. Levy BI. Can angiotensin II type 2 receptors have deleterious effects in cardiovascular disease? Implications for therapeutic blockade of the renin-angiotensin system. *Circulation* 2004;109:8–13.
8. McDonald JE, Padmanabhan N, Petrie MC, et al. Vasoconstrictor effect of the angiotensin-converting enzyme-resistant, chymase-specific substrate [Pro^{11} (D)-Ala^{12}] angiotensin I in human dorsal hand veins. *Circulation* 2001;104:1805–1808.
9. Petrie MC, Padmanabhan N, McDonald JE, et al. Angiotensin converting enzyme (ACE) and non-ACE dependent angiotensin II generation in resistance arteries from patients with heart failure and coronary heart disease. *J Am Coll Cardiol* 2001;37:1056–1061.
10. Schuijt MP, Danser AHJ. Cardiac angiotensin II: an intracrine hormone? *Am J Hypertens* 2002;15:1109–1116.
11. De Mello W. Effect of extracellular and intracellular angiotensins on heart cell function; on the cardiac renin-angiotensin system. *Regul Pept* 2003;114:87–90.
12. Hilgers KF, Veelken R, Muller DN, et al. Renin uptake by the endothelium mediates vascular angiotensin formation. *Hypertension* 2001;38:243–248.
13. McKinley MJ, Albiston AL, Allen AM, et al. The brain renin-angiotensin system: location and physiological roles. *Int J Biochem Cell Biol* 2003;35:901–918.

14. Leung PS, Chappell MC. A local pancreatic renin-angiotensin system: endocrine and exocrine roles. *Int J Biochem Cell Biol* 2003;35:838–846.

15. Lau T, Carlsson PO, Leung PS. Evidence for a local angiotensin-generating system and dose-dependent inhibition of glucose-stimulated insulin release by angiotensin II in isolated pancreatic islets. *Diabetologia* 2004;47:240–248.

16. Wagner J, Danser AHJ, Derkx FHM, et al. Demonstration of renin mRNA, angiotensinogen mRNA, and angiotensin converting enzyme mRNA expression in the human eye: evidence for an intraocular renin-angiotensin system. *Br J Ophthalmol* 1996;80:159–163.

17. Cullinane AB, Leung PS, Ortego J, et al. Renin-angiotensin system expression and secretory function in cultured human ciliary body non-pigmented epithelium. *Br J Ophthalmol* 2002;86:676–683.

18. Mulrow PJ. The adrenal cortical renin-angiotensin system. In: Robertson JIS, Nicholls MG, eds. *The renin-angiotensin system*, London: Mosby; 1993:44.1–44.9.

19. Leung PS, Sernia C. The renin-angiotensin system and male reproduction: new functions for old hormones. *J Mol Endocrinol* 2003;30:263–270.

20. Engeli S, Schling P, Gorzelniak K, et al. The adipose-tissue renin-angiotensin-aldosterone system: role in the metabolic syndrome? *Int J Biochem Cell Biol* 2003;35:807–825.

21. Dzau VJ, Bernstein K, Celermajer D, et al. The relevance of tissue angiotensin-converting enzyme: manifestations in mechanistic and endpoint data. *Am J Cardiol* 2001;88(Supplement 1):1–20.

22. Wolf G, Wenzel UO. Angiotensin II and cell cycle regulation. *Hypertension* 2004;43:693–698.

23. Brasier AR, Recinos A, Eledrisi MS. Vascular inflammation and the renin-angiotensin system. *Arterioscler Thromb Vasc Biol* 2002;22:1257–1266.

24. Taubman MB, Angiotensin II. a vasoactive hormone with ever-increasing biological roles. *Circ Res* 2003;92:9–11.

25. Egami K, Murohara T, Shimada T, et al. Role of host angiotensin II type 1 receptor in tumor angiogenesis and growth. *J Clin Invest* 2003;112:67–75.

26. Ichiki T. Role of renin angiotensin system in angiogenesis: it is still elusive. *Arterioscler Thromb Vasc Biol* 2004;24:622–624.

27. Landmesser U, Drexler H. Oxidative stress, the renin-angiotensin system, and atherosclerosis. *Eur Heart J* 2003;5(Supplement A):A3–A7.

28. Schieffer B. Interaction of interleukin-6 and angiotensin II in atherosclerosis: culprit for inflammation? *Eur Heart J* 2003;5(Supplement A):A25–A30.

29. Cipollone F, Fazia M, Iezzi A, et al. Blockade of the angiotensin II type 1 receptor stabilizes atherosclerotic plaques in humans by inhibiting prostaglandin E2-dependent matrix metalloproteinase activity. *Circulation* 2004;109:1482–1488.

30. Candido R, Allen TJ, Lassila M, et al. Irbesartan but not amlodipine suppresses diabetes-associated atherosclerosis. *Circulation* 2004;109:1536–1542.

31. Muscella A, Greco S, Elia MG, et al. Angiotensin II stimulation of Na^+/K^+ ATPase activity and cell growth by calcium-independent pathway in MCF-7 breast cancer cells. *J Endocrinol* 2002;173:315–323.

32. Kikkawa F, Mizuno M, Shibata K, et al. Activation of invasiveness of cervical carcinoma cells by angiotensin II. *Am J Obstet Gynecol* 2004;190:1258–1263.

33. Gavras I, Gavras H. Angtiotensin II – possible adverse effects on arteries, heart, brain, and kidney: experimental, clinical, and epidemiological evidence. In: Robertson JIS, Nicholls MG, eds. *The renin-angiotensin system*, London: Mosby; 1993:40.1–40.11.

34. Luft FC, Mervaala E, Muller DN, et al. Hypertension-induced end-organ damage. A new transgenic approach to an old problem. *Hypertension* 1999;33:212–218.

35. Xia Y, Karmazyn M. Obligatory role for endogenous endothelin in mediating the hypertrophic effects of phenylephrine and angiotensin II in neonatal rat ventricular myocytes: evidence for two distinct mechanisms for endothelin regulation. *J Pharmacol Exp Ther* 2004;310:43–51.

36. Mori T, Cowley AW. Role of pressure in angiotensin II-induced renal injury. Chronic servo-control of renal perfusion pressure in rats. *Hypertension* 2004;43:752–759.

37. Richards AM, Tonolo G, Tree M, et al. Atrial natriuretic peptides and renin release. *Am J Med* 1988;84(Supplement 3A):112–118.

38. Suo M, Hautala N, Foldes G, et al. Posttranscriptional control of BNP gene expression in angiotensin II-induced hypertension. *Hypertension* 2002;39:803–808.

39. Worthley MI, Corti R, Worthley SG. Vasopeptidase inhibitors: will they have a role in clinical practice? *Br J Clin Pharmacol* 2003;57:27–36.

40. Davidson NC, Barr CS, Struthers AD. C-type natriuretic peptide: an endogenous inhibitor of vascular angiotensin-converting enzyme activity. *Circulation* 1996;93:1155–1159.

41. Kohno M, Horio T, Yokokawa K, et al. C-type natriuretic peptide inhibits thrombin- and angiotensin II-stimulated endothelin release via cyclic guanosine 3′,5′-monophosphate. *Hypertension* 1992;19:320–325.

42. Charles CJ, Lainchbury JG, Nicholls MG, et al. Adrenomedullin and the renin-angiotensin-aldosterone system. *Regul Pept* 2003;112:41–49.
43. Jensen BL, Kramer BK, Kurtz A. Adrenomedullin stimulates renin release and renin mRNA in mouse juxtaglomerular granular cells. *Hypertension* 1997;29:1148–1155.
44. Luodonpaa M, Leskinen H, Ilves M, et al. Adrenomedullin modulates hemodynamic and cardiac effects of angiotensin II in conscious rats. *Am J Physiol* 2004;286:R1085–R1092.
45. Yoshimoto T, Fukai N, Sato R, et al. Antioxidant effect of adrenomedullin on angiotensin II-induced reactive oxygen species generation in vascular smooth muscle cells. *Endocrinology* 2004;145:3331–3337.
46. Donoghue M, Hsieh F, Baronas E, et al. A novel angiotensin-converting enzyme-related carboxypeptidase (ACE2) converts angiotensin I to angiotensin 1–9. *Circ Res* 2000;87:e1–e9.
47. Nussberger J, Brunner DB, Nyfeler JA, et al. Measurement of immunoreactive angiotensin-(1–7) heptapeptide in human blood. *Clin Chem* 2001;47:726–729.
48. Burrell LM, Johnston CI, Tikellis C, et al. ACE2, a new regulator of the renin-angiotensin system. *Trends Endocrinol Metab* 2004;15:166–169.
49. Yagil Y, Yagil C. Hypothesis: ACE2 modulates blood pressure in the mammalian organism. *Hypertension* 2003;41:871–873.
50. Tikellis C, Johnston CI, Forbes JM, et al. Characterization of renal angiotensin-converting enzyme 2 in diabetic nephropathy. *Hypertension* 2003;41:392–397.
51. Crackower MA, Sarao R, Oudit GY, et al. Angiotensin-converting enzyme 2 is an essential regulator of heart function. *Nature* 2002;417:822–828.
52. Donoghue M, Wakimoto H, Maguire CT, et al. Heart block, ventricular tachycardia, and sudden death in ACE2 transgenic mice with downregulated connexins. *J Mol Cell Cardiol* 2003;35:1043–1053.
53. Zisman LS, Meixell GE, Bristow MR, et al. Angiotensin-(1–7) formation in the intact human heart: in vivo dependence on angiotensin II as substrate. *Circulation* 2003;108:1679–1681.
54. Carey RM. Angiotensin type-1 receptor blockade increases ACE 2 expression in the heart. *Hypertension* 2004;43:943–944.
55. Carey RM, Siragy HM. Newly recognized components of the renin-angiotensin system: potential roles in cardiovascular and renal regulation. *Endocr Rev* 2003;24:261–271.
56. Nicholls MG, Robertson JIS. The renin system and hypertension. In: Birkenhager WH, Robertson JIS, Zanchetti A, eds. *Handbook of Hypertension*. Amsterdam: Elsevier; 2004:262–297.
57. Price DA, Fisher NDL. The renin-angiotensin system in blacks: active, passive, or what? *Curr Hypertens Rep* 2003;5:225–230.
58. Dahlöf B, Devereux RB, Kjeldsen SE, et al. Cardiovascular morbidity and mortality in the Losartan Intervention For Endpoint reduction in hypertension study (LIFE): a randomised trial against atenolol. *Lancet* 2002;359:995–1003.
59. Brunner HR, Gavras H. Angiotensin blockade for hypertension: a promise fulfilled. *Lancet* 2002;359:990–992.
60. Adam A, Blais CJr, Marceau F. The contribution of angiotensin-converting enzyme (ACE) to the metabolism of kinins (bradykinin and des-Arg^9-bradykinin) and effect of ACE inhibitors on their in *vitro* and in *vivo* metabolism. In: Juste PD, Plante GE, eds. *ACE Inhibitors*. Switzerland: Verlag; 2001:129–144.
61. Campbell DJ. The kallikrein-kinin system in humans. *Clin Exp Pharmacol Physiol* 2001;28:1060–1065.
62. Tom B, Dendorfer A, Danser AHJ. Bradykinin, angiotensin-(1–7), and ACE inhibitors: how do they interact? *Int J Biochem Cell Biol* 2003;35:792–801.
63. Ng KKF, Vane JR. Fate of angiotensin I in the circulation. *Nature* 1968;218:144–150.
64. Pellacani A, Brunner HR, Nussberger J. Plasma kinins increase after angiotensin-converting enzyme inhibition in human subjects. *Clin Sci (Lond)* 1994;87:567–574.
65. Benjamin N, Cockcroft JR, Collier JG, et al. Local inhibition of converting enzyme and vascular response angiotensin and bradykinin in the human forearm. *J Physiol* 1989;412:543–555.
66. Kuga T, Mohri M, Egashira K, et al. Bradykinin-induced vasodilation of human coronary arteries in vivo: role of nitric oxide and angiotensin-converting enzyme. *J Am Coll Cardiol* 1997;30:108–112.
67. Matsumoto T, Mina K, Horie H, et al. Angiotensin-converting enzyme inhibition but not angiotensin II type 1 receptor antagonism augments coronary release of tissue plasminogen activator in hypertensive patients. *J Am Coll Cardiol* 2003;41:1373–1379.
68. Campbell DJ. The renin-angiotensin and the kallikrein-kinin systems. *Int J Biochem Cell Biol* 2003;35:784–791.
69. Schmaier AH. The kallikrein-kinin and the renin-angiotensin systems have a multilayered interaction. *Am J Physiol* 2003;285:R1–R13.
70. Alfie ME, Yang XP, Hess F, et al. Salt-sensitive hypertension in bradykinin B2 receptor knockout mice. *Biochem Biophys Res Commun* 1996;224:625–630.
71. Sharma JN. Does the kinin system mediate in cardiovascular abnormalities? An overview. *J Clin Pharmacol* 2003;43:1187–1195.

72. Murphey LJ, Eccles WK, Williams GH, et al. Loss of sodium modulation of plasma kinins in human hypertension. *J Pharmacol Exp Ther* 2004;308:1046–1052.
73. Meneton P, Bloch-Faure M, Hagege AA, et al. Cardiovascular abnormalities with normal blood pressure in tissue kallikrein-deficient mice. *Proc Natl Acad Sci USA* 2001;98:2634–2639.
74. Cushman DW, Ondetti MA. Design of angiotensin converting enzyme inhibitors. *Nat Med* 1999;5:1110–1113.
75. Cushman DW, Ondetti MA. History of the design of captopril and related inhibitors of angiotensin converting enzyme. *Hypertension* 1991;17:589–592.
76. Vane JR. The history of inhibitors of angiotensin converting enzyme. *J Physiol Pharmacol* 1999;50:489–498.
77. Smith CG, Vane JR. The discovery of captopril. *FASEB J* 2003;17:788–789.
78. Jackson EK. Renin and angiotensin. In: Hardman JG, Limbird LE, eds. *The pharmacological basis of therapeutics*, New York: McGraw-Hill; 2002:809–841.
79. Harrold MW. Angiotensin converting enzyme inhibitors/angiotensin antagonists/calcium blockers. In: Lemke TL, Williams DA, eds. *Foye's principles of medicinal chemistry*. Baltimore: Willliams and Wilkins; 2002:533–561.
80. White CM. Pharmacologic, pharmacokinetic, and therapeutic differences among ACE inhibitors. *Pharmacotherapy* 1998;18:588–599.
81. Kayanakis JG, Doat P, Grenet B, et al. Side effects induced by captopril. *Arch Mal Coeur Vaiss* 1983;76:1065–1071.
82. Brown NJ, Vaughan DE. Angiotensin-converting enzyme inhibitors. *Circulation* 1998;97:1411–1420.
83. DiBianco R. Adverse reactions with angiotensin converting enzyme (ACE) inhibitors. *Med Toxicol* 1986;1:122–141.
84. Testa MA, Anderson RB, Nackley JF, et al. Quality of life and antihypertensive therapy in men. A comparison of captopril with enalapril. The Quality-of-Life Hypertension Study Group. *N Engl J Med* 1993;328:907–913.
85. Pizzulli L, Hagendorff A, Zirbes M, et al. Influence of captopril on nitroglycerin-mediated vasodilation and development of nitrate tolerance in arterial and venous circulation. *Am Heart J* 1996;131:342–349.
86. Kleinman HK, Lourdes PM. The good side of side effects: captopril blocks vessel and tumor growth. *J Clin Invest* 1996;98:599.
87. Noda Y, Mori A, Packer L. Free radical scavenging properties of alacepril metabolites and lisinopril. *Res Commun Mol Pathol Pharmacol* 1997;96:125–136.
88. Fischler MP, Follath F. Comparative evaluation of ACE inhibitors: which differences are relevant? *Schweiz Med Wochenschr* 1999;129:1053–1060.
89. Obata T, Yamanaka Y. Effect of OH scavenging by non-SH-containing angiotensin converting enzyme inhibitor imidaprilat using microdialysis. *J Physiol Paris* 1998;92:1–4.
90. Subissi A, Evangelista S, Giachetti A. Preclinical profile of Zofenopril. *Cardiovascular Drug Reviews* 1999;17:115–133.
91. Cawello W, Boekens H, Waitzinger J, et al. Moexipril shows a long duration of action related to an extended pharmacokinetic half-life and prolonged ACE inhibition. *Int J Clin Pharmacol Ther* 2002;40:9–17.
92. Cody RJ, Laragh JH, Case DB, et al. Converting enzyme inhibition to identify and treat renin-mediated or sodium-volume related forms of increased peripheral resistance in hypertension and in congestive heart failure. *J Hypertens* 1983;1(Supplement 1):77–84.
93. Hodsman GP, Isles CG, Murray GD, et al. Factors related to first dose hypotensive effect of captopril: prediction and treatment. *Br Med J* 1983;286:832–834.
94. Lever AF. The fast and the slowly developing pressor effect of angiotensin II. In: Robertson JIS, Nicholls MG, eds. *The renin-angiotensin system*. London: Mosby; 1993:28.1–28.9.
95. Reckelhoff JF, Romero JC. Role of oxidative stress in angiotensin-induced hypertension. *Am J Physiol* 2003;284:R893–R912.
96. Juillerat L, Nussberger J, Ménard J, et al. Determinants of angiotensin II generation during converting enzyme inhibition. *Hypertension* 1990;16:564–572.
97. Sato A, Saruta T. Aldosterone breakthrough during angiotensin-converting enzyme inhibitor therapy. *Am J Hypertens* 2003;16:781–788.
98. Atlas SA, Case DB, Yu ZY, et al. Hormonal and metabolic effects of angiotensin converting enzyme inhibitors. *Am J Med* 1984;77:13–17.
99. Blood Pressure Lowering Treatment Trialists' Collaboration. Effects of different blood-pressure-lowering regimens on major cardiovascular events: results of prospectively-designed overviews of randomised trials. *Lancet.* 2003;362:1527–1535.
100. Psaty BM, Lumley T, Furberg CD, et al. Health outcomes associated with various antihypertensive therapies used as first-line agents: a network meta-analysis. *JAMA* 2003;289:2534–2544.

101. Williams B. VALUE and supremacy of blood pressure control for cardiovascular protection. *J Hypertens* 2004;22:1435–1437.

102. Staessen JA, Birkenhager WH. VALUE: to the heart of the matter. *J Hypertens* 2004;22:1431–1434.

103. Sleight P, Yusuf S. New evidence on the importance of the renin-angiotensin system in the treatment of higher-risk patients with hypertension. *J Hypertens* 2003;21: 1599–1608.

104. Brilla CG, Zhou G, Matsubara L, et al. Collagen metabolism in cultured adult rat cardiac fibroblasts: response to angiotensin II and aldosterone. *J Mol Cell Cardiol* 1994;26: 809–820.

105. de Luca N, Asmar RG, London GM, et al. Selective reduction of cardiac mass and central blood pressure on low-dose combination perindopril/indapamide in hypertensive subjects. *J Hypertens* 2004;22:1623–1630.

106. L'Allier PL, Ducharme A, Keller P-F, et al. Angiotensin-converting enzyme inhibition in hypertensive patients is associated with a reduction in the occurrence of atrial fibrillation. *J Am Coll Cardiol* 2004;44:159–164.

107. Gonzalez-Juanatey JR, Garcia-Acuna JM, Pose A, et al. Reduction of QT and QTc dispersion during long-term treatment of systemic hypertension with enalapril. *Am J Cardiol* 1998;81:170–174.

108. Verdecchia P, Reboldi GP, Gattobigio R, et al. Atrial fibrillation in hypertension: predictors and outcome. *Hypertension* 2003;41:218–223.

109. Cioffi G, Mureddu GF, Stefenelli C, et al. Relationship between left ventricular geometry and left atrial size and function in patients with systemic hypertension. *J Hypertens* 2004;22:1589–1596.

110. Jennings GLR. The left atrium in hypertension: next to the chamber of power. *J Hypertens* 2004;22:1473–1474.

111. Gilbert RE, Krum H, Wilkinson-Berka J, et al. The renin-angiotensin system and the long-term complications of diabetes: pathophysiological and therapeutic considerations. *Diabet Med* 2003;20:607–621.

112. Vidotti DB, Casarini DE, Cristovam PC, et al. High glucose concentration stimulates intracellular renin activity and angiotensin II generation in rat mesangial cells. *Am J Physiol* 2004;286:F1039–F1045.

113. Carey RM, Siragy HM. The intrarenal renin-angiotensin system and diabetic nephropathy. *Trends Endocrinol Metab* 2003;14:274–281.

114. Huang W, Gallois Y, Bouby N, et al. Genetically increased angiotensin I-converting enzyme level and renal complications in the diabetic mouse. *Proc Natl Acad Sci USA* 2001;98:13330–13334.

115. Opie LH, Schall R. Old antihypertensives and new diabetes. *J Hypertens* 2004;22:1453–1458.

116. Pepine CJ, Cooper-DeHoff RM. Cardiovascular therapies and risk for development of diabetes. *J Am Coll Cardiol* 2004;44:509–512.

117. Carlsson P-O, Berne C, Jansson L. Angiotensin II and the endocrine pancreas: effects on islet blood flow and insulin secretion in rats. *Diabetologia* 1998;41:127–133.

118. Tikellis C, Wookey PJ, Candido R, et al. Improved islet morphology after blockade of the renin-angiotensin system in the ZDF rat. *Diabetes* 2004;53:989–997.

119. Sharma AM. Is there a rationale for angiotensin blockade in the management of obesity hypertension? *Hypertension* 2004;44:12–19.

120. Henriksen EJ, Jacob S. Modulation of metabolic control by angiotensin converting enzyme (ACE) inhibition. *J Cell Physiol* 2003;196:171–179.

121. Linz W, Wiemer G, Gohlke P, et al. Contribution of kinins to the cardiovascular actions of angiotensin-converting enzyme inhibitors. *Pharmacol Rev* 1995;47:25–49.

122. Bonner G. The role of kinins in the antihypertensive and cardioprotective effects of ACE inhibitors. *Drugs* 1997;54(Supplement 5):23–30.

123. Hornig B, Kohler C, Drexler H. Role of bradykinin in mediating vascular effects of angiotensin-converting enzyme inhibitors in humans. *Circulation* 1997;95:1115–1118.

124. Gainer JV, Morrow JD, Loveland A, et al. Effect of bradykinin-receptor blockade on the response to angiotensin-converting-enzyme inhibitor in normotensive and hypertensive subjects. *N Engl J Med* 1998;339:1285–1292.

125. Azizi N. Bradykinin and inhibition of angiotensin-converting enzyme in hypertension. *N Engl J Med* 1998;340:967.

126. Agarwal R. Bradykinin and inhibition of angiotensin-converting enzyme in hypertension. *N Engl J Med* 1998;340:967–968.

127. Squire IB, O'Kane KPJ, Anderson N, et al. Bradykinin B2 receptor antagonism attenuates blood pressure response to acute angiotensin-converting enzyme inhibition in normal men. *Hypertension* 2000;36:132–136.

128. Elmarakby AA, Morsing P, Pollock DM. Enalapril attenuates endothelin-1-induced hypertension via increased kinin survival. *Am J Physiol* 2003;284:H1899–H1903.

129. Meneton P, Bloch-Faure M, Hagege AA, et al. Cardiovascular abnormalities with normal blood pressure in tissue kallikrein-deficient mice. *Proc Natl Acad Sci USA* 2001;98:2634–2639.

130. Linz W, Wiemer G, Scholkens BA. Contribution of bradykinin to the cardiovascular effects of ramipril. *J Cardiovasc Pharmacol* 1993;22(Supplement 9):S1–S8.

131. Scicli AG. Increases in cardiac kinins as a new mechanism to protect the heart. *Hypertension* 1994;23:419–421.

132. Tschope C, Seidl U, Reinecke A, et al. Kinins are involved in the antiproteinuric effect of angiotensin-converting enzyme inhibition in experimental diabetic nephropathy. *Int Immunopharmacol* 2003;3:335–344.

133. Takahashi N, Hagaen JR, Kim H-S. Computer simulations of blood pressure regulation by the renin-angiotensin system. *Endocrinology* 2003;144:2184–2190.

134. Kakoki M, Takahashi N, Jennette JC, et al. Diabetic nephropathy is markedly enhanced in mice lacking the bradykinin B2 receptor. *Proc Natl Acad Sci USA* 2004;101:13302–13305.

135. Frossard M, Joukhadar Ch, Steffen G, et al. Paracrine effects of angiotensin-converting-enzyme-and angiotensin-II-receptor-inhibition on transcapillary glucose transport in humans. *Life Sci* 2000;66:2728–2732.

136. Damas J, Garbacki N, Lefebvre PJ. The kallikrein-kinin system, angiotensin converting enzyme inhibitors and insulin sensitivity. *Diabetes Metab Res Rev* 2004;20:288–297.

137. Goa KL, Haria M, Wilde MI. Lisinopril. A review of its pharmacology and use in the management of the complications of diabetes mellitus. *Drugs* 1997;53:1081–1105.

138. Meisel S, Shamiss A, Rosenthal T. Clinical pharmacokinetics of ramipril. *Clin Pharmacokinet* 1994;26:7–15.

139. Devissaguet JP, Ammoury N, Devissaguet M, et al. Pharmacokinetics of perindopril and its metabolites in healthy volunteers. *Fundam Clin Pharmacol* 1990;4:175–189.

140. Kaiser G, Ackermann R, Gschwind HP, et al. The influence of hepatic cirrhosis on the pharmacokinetics of benazepril hydrochloride. *Biopharm Drug Dispos* 1990;11:753–764.

141. Borghi C, Ambrosioni E. Zofenopril: A review of the evidence of its benefits in hypertension and acute myocardial infarction. *Clin Drug Invest* 2000;20:371–384.

142. Ford NF, Lasseter KC, Van Harken DR, et al. Single-dose and steady-state pharmacokinetics of fosinopril and fosinoprilat in patients with hepatic impairment. *J Clin Pharmacol* 1995;35:145–150.

143. Ulm EH, Vassil TC. Total serum angiotensin converting enzyme activity in rats and dogs after enalapril maleate (MK-421). *Life Sci* 1982;30:1225–1230.

144. Song JC, White CM. Clinical pharmacokinetics and selective pharmacodynamics of new angiotensin converting enzyme inhibitors: an update. *Clin Pharmacokinet* 2002;41:207–224.

145. Razzetti R, Acerbi D. Pharmacokinetic and pharmacologic properties of delapril, a lipophilic nonsulfhydryl angiotensin-converting enzyme inhibitor. *Am J Cardiol* 1995;75:7F–12F.

146. Hui KK, Duchin KL, Kripalani KJ, et al. Pharmacokinetics of fosinopril in patients with various degrees of renal function. *Clin Pharmacol Ther* 1991;49:457–467.

147. Arakawa M, Sasaki M, Ohmori M, et al. Pharmacokinetics and pharmacodynamics of temocapril during repeated dosing in elderly hypertensive patients. *Eur J Clin Pharmacol* 2001;56:775–779.

148. Onoyama K, Hirakata H, Tsuruda H, et al. Pharmacokinetics of a new angiotensin I converting enzyme inhibitor (alacepril) after oral dosing in fasting or fed states. *Clin Pharmacol Ther* 1985;38:462–468.

149. Kaiser G, Ackermann R, Dieterle W, et al. Pharmacokinetics and pharmacodynamics of the ace inhibitor benazepril hydrochloride in the elderly. *Eur J Clin Pharmacol* 1990;38: 379–385.

150. Macdonald NJ, Elliott HL, Hughes DM, et al. A comparison in young and elderly subjects of the pharmacokinetics and pharmacodynamics of single and multiple doses of benazepril. *Br J Clin Pharmacol* 1993;36:201–204.

151. Duchin KL, McKinstry DN, Cohen AI, et al. Pharmacokinetics of captopril in healthy subjects and in patients with cardiovascular diseases. *Clin Pharmacokinet* 1988;14:241–259.

152. Creasey WA, Funke PT, McKinstry DN, et al. Pharmacokinetics of captopril in elderly healthy male volunteers. *J Clin Pharmacol* 1986;26:264–268.

153. Richer C, Giroux B, Plouin PF, et al. Captopril: pharmacokinetics, antihypertensive and biological effects in hypertensive patients. *Br J Clin Pharmacol* 1984;17:243–250.

154. Anderson PJ, Critchley JA, Tomlinson B. A comparison of the pharmacokinetics and pharmacodynamics of cilazapril between Chinese and Caucasian healthy, normotensive volunteers. *Eur J Clin Pharmacol* 1996;50:57–62.

155. Massarella J, DeFeo T, Lin A, et al. The pharmacokinetics and dose proportionality of cilazapril. *Br J Clin Pharmacol* 1989;27:199S–204S.

156. Williams PE, Brown AN, Rajaguru S, et al. The pharmacokinetics and bioavailability of cilazapril in normal man. *Br J Clin Pharmacol* 1989;27(Supplement 2):181S–188S.

157. Meredith PA, Elliott HL, Reid JL, et al. The pharmacokinetics and angiotensin converting enzyme inhibition dynamics of cilazapril in essential hypertension. *Br J Clin Pharmacol* 1989;27:263S–266S.

158. Fillastre JP, Moulin B, Godin M, et al. Pharmacokinetics of cilazapril in patients with renal failure. *Br J Clin Pharmacol* 1989;27(Supplement 2):275S–282S.

159. Shionoiri H, Yasuda G, Ikeda A, et al. Pharmacokinetics and depressor effect of delapril in patients with essential hypertension. *Clin Pharmacol Ther* 1987;41:74–79.

160. Saruta T, Nishikawa K. Characteristics of a new angiotensin converting enzyme inhibitor: delapril. *Am J Hypertens* 1991;4:23S–28S.

161. Onoyama K, Nanishi F, Okuda S, et al. Pharmacokinetics of a new angiotensin I converting enzyme inhibitor (delapril) in patients with deteriorated kidney function and in normal control subjects. *Clin Pharmacol Ther* 1988;43:242–249.

162. MacFadyen RJ, Meredith PA, Elliott HL. Enalapril clinical pharmacokinetics and pharmacokinetic-pharmacodynamic relationships. *An overview. Clin Pharmacokinet* 1993;25:274–282.

163. Hockings N, Ajayi AA, Reid JL. Age and the pharmacokinetics of angiotensin converting enzyme inhibitors enalapril and enalaprilat. *Br J Clin Pharmacol* 1986;21:341–348.

164. Lees KR, Reid JL. Age and the pharmacokinetics and pharmacodynamics of chronic enalapril treatment. *Clin Pharmacol Ther* 1987;41:597–602.

165. Hui KK, Duchin KL, Kripalani KJ, et al. Pharmacokinetics of fosinopril in patients with various degrees of renal function. *Clin Pharmacol Ther* 1991;49:457–467.

166. Singhvi SM, Duchin KL, Morrison RA, et al. Disposition of fosinopril sodium in healthy subjects. *Br J Clin Pharmacol* 1988;25:9–15.

167. Kostis JB, Garland WT, Delaney C, et al. Fosinopril: pharmacokinetics and pharmacodynamics in congestive heart failure. *Clin Pharmacol Ther* 1995;58:660–665.

168. Ford NF, Lasseter KC, Van Harken DR, et al. Single-dose and steady-state pharmacokinetics of fosinopril and fosinoprilat in patients with hepatic impairment. *J Clin Pharmacol* 1995;35:145–150.

169. Harder S, Thurmahh PA, Ungethum W. Single dose and steady state pharmacokinetics and pharmacodynamics of the ACE-inhibitor imidapril in hypertensive patients. *J Clin Pharmacol* 1998;45:377–380.

170. Gautam PC, Vargas E, Lye M. Pharmacokinetics of lisinopril (MK521) in healthy young and elderly subjects and in elderly patients with cardiac failure. *J Pharm Pharmacol* 1987;39:929–931.

171. Beermann B. Pharmacokinetics of lisinopril. *Am J Med* 1988;85:25–30.

172. Cawello W, Boekens H, Waitzinger J, et al. Moexipril shows a long duration of action related to an extended pharmacokinetic half life and prolonged ACE inhibition. *Int J Clin Pharmacol Ther* 2002;40:9–17.

173. Brogden RN, Wiseman LR. Moexipril. A review of its use in the management of essential hypertension. *Drugs* 1998;55:845–860.

174. Rakhit A, Hurley ME, Tipnis V, et al. Pharmacokinetics and pharmacodynamics of pentopril, a new angiotensin-converting-enzyme inhibitor in humans. *J Clin Pharmacol* 1986;26:156–164.

175. Rakhit A, Kochak GM, Tipnis V, et al. Pharmacokinetics of pentopril in the elderly. *Br J Clin Pharmacol* 1987;24:351–357.

176. Rakhit A, Radensky P, Szerlip HM, et al. Effect of renal impairment on disposition of pentopril and its active metabolite. *Clin Pharmacol Ther* 1988;44:39–48.

177. Louis WJ, Workman BS, Conway EL, et al. Single-dose and steady-state pharmacokinetics and pharmacodynamics of perindopril in hypertensive subjects. *J Cardiovasc Pharmacol* 1992;20:505–511.

178. Macfadyen RJ, Lees KR, Reid JL. Perindopril. *A review of its pharmacokinetics and clinical pharmacology. Drugs* 1990;39:49–63.

179. Lees KR. Clinical pharmacology of perindopril. *J Human Hypertens* 1990;4:7–11.

180. Lees KR, Green ST, Reid JL. Influence of age on the pharmacokinetics and pharmacodynamics of perindopril. *Clin Pharmacol Ther* 1988;44:418–425.

181. Olson SC, Horvath AM, Michniewicz BM, et al. The clinical pharmacokinetics of quinapril. *Angiology* 1989;40:351–359.

182. Kaplan HR, Taylor DG, Olson SC, et al. Quinapril–a preclinical review of the pharmacology, pharmacokinetics, and toxicology. *Angiology* 1989;40:335–350.

183. Blumer JL, Daniels SR, Dreyer WJ, et al. Pharmacokinetics of quinapril in children: assessment during substitution for chronic angiotensin-converting enzyme inhibitor treatment. *J Clin Pharmacol* 2003;43:128–132.

184. Meisel S, Shamiss A, Rosenthal T. Clinical pharmacokinetics of ramipril. *Clin Pharmacokinet* 1994;26:7–15.

185. van Griensven JM, Schoemaker RC, Cohen AF, et al. Pharmacokinetics, pharmacodynamics and bioavailability of the ACE inhibitor ramipril. *Eur J Clin Pharmacol* 1995;47:513–518.

186. Krahenbuhl S, Grass P, Surve A, et al. Pharmacokinetics and haemodynamic effects of a single oral dose of the novel ACE inhibitor spirapril in patients with chronic liver disease. *Eur J Clin Pharmacol* 1993;56:247–253.

187. Puchler K, Sierakowski B, Roots I. Single dose and steady state pharmacokinetics of temocapril and temocaprilat in young and elderly hypertensive patients. *Br J Clin Pharmacol* 1998;46:363–367.

188. Arakawa M, Sasaki M, Ohmori M, et al. Pharmacokinetics and pharmacodynamics of temocapril during repeated dosing in elderly hypertensive patients. *Eur J Clin Pharmacol* 2001;56:775–779.

189. Lenfant B, Mouren M, Bryce T, et al. Trandolapril: pharmacokinetics of single oral doses in healthy male volunteers. *J Cardiovasc Pharmacol* 1994;23:S38–S43.

190. Arner P, Wade A, Engfeldt P, et al. Pharmacokinetics and pharmacodynamics of trandolapril after repeated administration of 2 mg to young and elderly patients with mild-to-moderate hypertension. *J Cardiovasc Pharmacol* 1994;23(Supplement 4):S44–S49.

191. Borghi C. Zofenopril: A review of the evidence of its benefits in hypertension and acute myocardial infarction. *Clin Drug Invest* 2000;20:371–384.

192. Subissi A, Evangelista S, Giachetti A. Preclinical profile of zofenopril: an angiotensin converting enzyme inhibitor with peculiar cardioprotective properties. *Cardiovasc Drug Rev* 1999;17:115–133.

193. DeForrest JM, Waldron TL, Krapcho J, et al. Preclinical pharmacology of zofenopril, an inhibitor of angiotensin I converting enzyme. *J Cardiovasc Pharmacol* 1989;13:887–894.

194. Singhvi SM, Foley JE, Willard DA, et al. Disposition of zofenopril calcium in healthy subjects. *J Pharm Sci* 1990;79:970–973.

195. Bevan EG, McInnes GT, Aldigier JC, et al. Effect of renal function in the pharmacokinetics and pharmacodynamics of tranolapril. *Br J Clin Pharmacol* 1993;38:128–135.

196. Brunner HR, Nussberger J, Waeber B. Dose-response relationships of ACE inhibitors and angiotensin II blockers. *Eur Heart J* 1994;15(Supplement D):123–128.

197. Ventura HO, Frohlich ED, Messerli FH, et al. Immediate regional blood flow distribution following angiotensin converting enzyme inhibition in patients with essential hypertension. *Am J Med* 1984;76(Supplement 5B):58–61.

198. Crossley IR, Bihari D, Gimson AES, et al. Effects of converting enzyme inhibitor on hepatic blood flow in man. *Am J Med* 1984;76(Supplement 5B):62–65.

199. Daly P, Rouleau J-L, Cousineau D, et al. Acute effects of captopril on the coronary circulation of patients with hypertension and angina. *Am J Med* 1984;76(Supplement 5B):111–115.

200. Safar ME, Boudier HA JS, Van Bortel LM AB, et al. Arterial structure and function and blockade of the renin-angiotensin system in hypertension. In: D'Orleans-Juste P, Plante GE, eds. *ACE Inhibitors.* Switzerland: Birkhauser Verlag; 2001:105–114.

201. Veerman DP, Douma CE, Jacobs MC, et al. Effects of acute and chronic angiotensin converting enzyme inhibition by spirapril on cardiovascular regulation in essential hypertensive patients. Assessment by spectral analysis and haemodynamic measurements. *Br J Clin Pharmacol* 1996;41:49–56.

202. Duprez D, Clement DL. Vasodilator effects of enalapril in patients with arterial hypertension. *Acta Cardiol* 1986;41:359–364.

203. Breckenridge A. Age-related effects of angiotensin converting enzyme inhibitors. *J Cardiovasc Pharmacol* 1988;12(Supplement 8):S100–S104.

204. Ball SG. Age-related effects of converting enzyme inhibitors: a commentary. *J Cardiovasc Pharmacol* 1988;12(Supplement 8):S105–S108.

205. Soffer B, Zhang Z, Miller K, et al. A double-blind, placebo-controlled, dose-response study of the effectiveness and safety of lisinopril for children with hypertension. *Am J Hypertens* 2003;16:795–800.

206. Cohn JN, Julius S, Neutel J, et al. Clinical experience with perindopril in African-American hypertensive patients: a large United States community trial. *Am J Hypertens* 2004;17:134–138.

207. Mokwe E, Ohmit SE, Nasser SA, et al. Determinants of blood pressure response to quinapril in black and white hypertensive patients: the Quinapril Titration Interval Management Evaluation trial. *Hypertension* 2004;43:1202–1207.

208. The ALLHAT officers and coordinators for the ALLHAT collaborative research group. Major outcomes in high-risk hypertensive patients randomized to angiotensin-converting enzyme inhibitor or calcium channel blocker vs diuretic: The Antihypertensive and Lipid-Lowering Treatment to Prevent Heart Attack Trial (ALLHAT). *JAMA* 2002;288:2981–2997.

209. Gainer JV, Stein CM, Neal T, et al. Interactive effect of ethnicity and ACE insertion/deletion polymorphism on vascular reactivity. *Hypertension* 2001;37:46–51.

210. Falconnet C, Bochud M, Bovet P, et al. Gender difference in the response to an angiotensin-converting enzyme inhibitor and a diuretic in hypertensive patients of African descent. *J Hypertens* 2004;22:1213–1220.

211. Asmar RG, Pannier BM, Santoni JP, et al. Angiotensin converting enzyme inhibition decreases systolic blood pressure more than diastolic pressure as shown by ambulatory blood pressure monitoring. *J Hypertens* 1988;6(Supplement 3):S79–S81.

212. Morgan T, Lauri J, Bertram D, et al. Effect of different antihypertensive drug classes on central aortic pressure. *Am J Hypertens* 2004;17:118–123.

213. London GM, Asmar RG, O'Rourke MF, et al. Mechanism(s) of selective systolic blood pressure reduction after a low-dose combination of perindopril/indapamide in hypertensive subjects: comparison with atenolol. *J Am Coll Cardiol* 2004;43:92–99.

214. Hansson L, Dahlöf B, Himmelmann A, et al. Angiotensin-converting enzyme inhibitors the treatment of essential hypertension. In: Robertson JIS, Nicholls MG, eds. *The renin-angiotensin system*. London: Mosby; 1993:91.1–91.24.

215. Chan JCN, Nicholls MG, Cheung C-K, et al. Factors determining the blood pressure response to enalapril and nifedipine in hypertension associated with NIDDM. *Diabetes Care* 1995;18:1001–1006.

216. de Zeeuw D, Navis GJ, Donker AJM, et al. The angiotensin converting enzyme inhibitor enalapril and its effects on renal function. *J Hypertens* 1983;1(Supplement 1):93–97.

217. Yeo WW, Ramsay LE. Persistent dry cough with enalapril: incidence depends on methods used. *J Hum Hypertens* 1990;4:517–520.

218. Os I, Bratland B, Dahlof B, et al. Female preponderance for lisinopril-induced cough in hypertension. *Am J Hypertens* 1994;7:1012–1015.

219. Woo KS, Norris RM, Nicholls G. Racial difference in incidence of cough with angiotensin-converting enzyme inhibitors (a tale of two cities). *Am J Cardiol* 1995;75:967–968.

220. Malini PL, Strocchi E, Fiumi N, et al. ACE inhibitor-induced cough in hypertensive type 2 diabetic patients. *Diabetes Care* 1999;22:1586–1587.

221. Fox AJ, Lalloo UG, Belvisi MG, et al. Bradykinin-evoked sensitization of airway sensory nerves: a mechanism for ACE- inhibitor cough. *Nat Med* 1996;2:814–817.

222. Mailini PL, Strocchi E, Zanardi M, et al. Thromboxane antagonism and cough induced by angiotensin-converting-enzyme inhibitor. *Lancet* 1997;350:15–18.

223. Lacourciere Y, Brunner H, Irwin R, et al. Effects of modulators of the renin-angiotensin-aldosterone system on cough. *J Hypertens* 1994;12:1387–1393.

224. Yeo WW, Foster G, Ramsay LE. Prevalence of persistent cough during long-term enalapril treatment: controlled study versus nifedipine. *Q J Med* 1991;81:763–770.

225. Reisin L, Schneeweiss A. Spontaneous disappearance of cough induced by angiotensin-converting enzyme inhibitors (captopril or enalapril). *Am J Cardiol* 1992;70:398–399.

226. Lip GYH, Zarifis J, Beevers M, et al. Duration of cough following cessation of ACE inhibitor therapy. *Am J Hypertens* 1995;8:98.

227. Charlon V, Dollow S, Fidel J, et al. Reproducibility of angiotensin converting enzyme inhibitor induced cough: a double-blind randomized study. *Br J Clin Pharmacol* 1995;39:125–129.

228. Nussberger J, Cugno M, Amstutz C, et al. Plasma bradykinin in angio-oedema. *Lancet* 1998;351:1693–1697.

229. Molinaro G, Cugno M, Perez M, et al. Angiotensin- converting enzyme inhibitor-associated angioedema is characterized by a slower degradation of des- arginine^9-bradykinin. *J Pharmacol Exp Ther* 2002;303:232–237.

230. Coats AJS. Omapatrilat–the story of Overture and Octave. *Int J Cardiol* 2002;86:1–4.

231. Brown NJ, Ray WA, Snowden M, et al. Black Americans have an increased rate of angiotensin converting enzyme inhibitor-associated angioedema. *Clin Pharmacol Ther* 1996;60:8–13.

232. Brown NJ, Snowden M, Griffin MR. Recurrent angiotensin- converting enzyme inhibitor-associated angioedema. *JAMA* 1997;278:232–233.

233. Howes LG, Tran D. Can angiotensin receptor antagonists be used safely in patients with previous ACE inhibitor-induced angioedema? *Drug Saf* 2002;25:73–76.

234. Cicardi M, Zingale LC, Bergamaschini L, et al. Angioedema associated with angiotensin-converting enzyme inhibitor use: outcome after switching to a different treatment. *Arch Intern Med* 2004;164:910–913.

235. Verresen L, Waer M, Vanrenterghem Y, et al. Angiotensin- converting-enzyme inhibitors and anaphylactoid reactions to high- flux membrane dialysis. *Lancet* 1990;336:1360–1362.

236. Davidson DC, Peart I, Turner S, et al. Prevention with icatibant of anaphylactoid reactions to ACE inhibitor during LDL apheresis. *Lancet* 1994;343:1575.

237. John B, Anijeet HKI, Ahmad R. Anaphylactic reaction during haemodialysis on AN69 membrane in a patient receiving angiotensin II receptor antagonist. *Nephrol Dial Transplant* 2001;16:1955–1956.

238. Kammerl MC, Schaefer RM, Schweda F, et al. Extracorporal therapy with AN69 membranes in combination with ACE inhibition causing severe anaphylactoid reactions: still a current problem? *Clin Nephrol* 2000;53:486–488.

239. Wynckel A, Ebikili B, Melin J-P, et al. Long-term follow-up of acute renal failure caused by angiotensin converting enzyme inhibitors. *Am J Hypertens* 1998;11:1080–1086.

240. Stirling C, Houston J, Robertson S, et al. Diarrhoea, vomiting and ACE inhibitors:-an important cause of acute renal failure. *J Hum Hypertens* 2003;17:419–423.

241. Palmer BF. Managing hyperkalemia caused by inhibitors of the renin-angiotensin-aldosterone system. *N Engl J Med* 2004;351:585–592.

242. Webster J. Angiotensin converting enzyme inhibitors in the clinic: first-dose hypotension. *J Hypertens Suppl* 1987;5(Supplement 3):S27–S30.

243. Postma CT, Dennesen PJW, de Boo T, et al. First dose hypotension after captopril; can it be predicted? A study of 240 patients. *J Hum Hypertens* 1992;6:205–209.

244. Easterling TR, Carr DB, Davis C, et al. Low-dose, short- acting, angiotensin-converting enzyme inhibitors as rescue therapy in pregnancy. *Obstet Gynecol* 2000;96:956–961.

245. Tomlinson AJ, Campbell J, Walker JJ, et al. Malignant primary hypertension in pregnancy treated with lisinopril. *Ann Pharmacother* 2000;34:180–182.

246. Guidelines Committee. European Society of Hypertension – European Society of Cardiology guidelines for the management of arterial hypertension. *J Hypertens* 2003;21:1011–1053.

247. Williams B, Poulter NR, Brown MJ, et al. British Hypertension Society guidelines for hypertension management 2004 (BHS-IV): summary. *BMJ* 2004;328:634–640.

248. Chobanian AV, Bakris GL, Black HR, et al. Seventh report of the Joint National Committee on Prevention, Detection, Evaluation, and Treatment of High Blood Pressure. The JNC 7 report. . *JAMA* 2003;289:2560–2572.

249. Krege JH, John SWM, Langenbach LL, et al. Male-female differences in fertility and blood pressure in ACE-deficient mice. *Nature* 1995;375:146–148.

250. Johnston CI. Angiotensin-converting enzyme inhibitors. In: Robertson JIS, Nicholls MG, eds. *The renin-angiotensin system*, London: Mosby; 1993:87.1–87.15.

251. Fletcher AE, Dollery CT. Side effects associated with inhibitors of angiotensin-converting enzyme. In: Robertson JIS, Nicholls MG, eds. *The renin-angiotensin system*. London: Mosby; 1993:99.1–99.15.

252. Herrick AL, Waller PC, Berkin KE, et al. Comparison of enalapril and atenolol in mild to moderate hypertension. *Am J Med* 1989;86:421–427.

253. Rigaud A-S, Hanon O, Seux M-L, et al. Hypertension and dementia. *Curr Hypertens Rep* 2001;3:454–457.

254. Spence JD. Preventing dementia by treating hypertension and preventing stroke. *Hypertension* 2004;44:20–21.

255. Ohrui T, Tomita N, Sato-Nakagawa T, et al. Effects of brain-penetrating ACE inhibitors on Alzheimer disease progression. *Neurology* 2004;63:1324–1325.

256. Bjerrum L, Andersen M, Petersen G, et al. Exposure to potential drug interactions in primary health care. *Scand J Prim Health Care* 2003;21:153–158.

257. Juurlink DN, Mamdani M, Kopp A, et al. Drug-drug interactions among elderly patients hospitalized for drug toxicity. *JAMA* 2003;289:1652–1658.

258. Pitt B, Zannad F, Remme WJ, et al. The effect of spironolactone on morbidity and mortality in patients with severe heart failure. Randomized Aldactone Evaluation Study Investigators. *N Engl J Med.* 1999;341:709–717.

259. Juurlink DN, Mamdani MM, Lee DS, et al. Rates of hyperkalemia after publication of the Randomized Aldactone Evaluation Study. *N Engl J Med* 2004;351:543–551.

260. Mantyla R, Mannisto PT, Vuorela A, et al. Impairment of captopril bioavailability by concomitant food and antacid intake. *Int J Clin Pharmacol Ther Toxicol* 1984;22:626–629.

261. O'Grady P, Yee KF, Lins R, et al. Fosinopril/hydrochlorothiazide: single dose and steady-state pharmacokinetics and pharmacodynamics. *Br J Clin Pharmacol* 1999;48:375–381.

262. Breithaupt-Grogler K, Ungethum W, Meurer-Witt B, et al. Pharmacokinetic and dynamic interactions of the angiotensin-converting enzyme inhibitor imidapril with hydrochlorothiazide, bisoprolol and nilvadipine. *Eur J Clin Pharmacol* 2001;57:275–284.

263. Belz GG, Essig J, Erb K, et al. Pharmacokinetic and pharmacodynamic interactions between the ACE inhibitor cilazapril and beta-adrenoceptor antagonist propranolol in healthy subjects and in hypertensive patients. *Br J Clin Pharmacol* 1989;27(Suppl 2):317S–322S.

264. Erb KA, Essig J, Breithaupt K, et al. Clinical pharmacodynamic studies with cilazapril and a combination of cilazapril and propranolol. *Drugs* 1991;41(Suppl 1):11–17.

265. Boero R, Rollino C, Massara C, et al. The verapamil versus amlodipine in nondiabetic nephropathies treated with trandolapril (VVANNTT) study. *Am J Kidney Dis* 2003;42:67–75.

266. Macias-Nunez JF, Fernandez R, Calvo C, et al. Verapamil reverts acute renal functional impairment induced by angiotensin II converting enzyme inhibitors. *Ren Fail* 2003;25:727–737.

267. Griffiths CD, Morgan TO, Delbridge LM. Effects of combined administration of ACE inhibitor and angiotensin II receptor antagonist are prevented by a high NaCl intake. *J Hypertens* 2001;19:2087–2095.

268. Morgan T, Griffiths C, Delbridge L. Interaction of ACE inhibitors and AT(1)-receptor blockers on maximum blood pressure response in spontaneous hypertensive rats. *J Renin Angiotensin Aldosterone Syst* 2002;3:16–18.

269. Morgan T, Griffiths C, Delbridge L. Low doses of angiotensin converting enzyme inhibitors and angiotensin type 1 blockers have a synergistic effect but high doses are less than additive. *Am J Hypertens* 2002;15:1003–1005.

270. Mahmud A, Feely J. Favourable effects on arterial wave reflection and pulse pressure amplification of adding angiotensin II receptor blockade in resistant hypertension. *J Human Hypertens* 2000;14:541–546.

271. Mahmud A, Feely J. Reduction in arterial stiffness with angiotensin II antagonist is comparable with and additive to ACE inhibition. *Am J Hypertens* 2002;15:321–325.

272. Russo D, Minutolo R, Pisani A, et al. Coadministration of losartan and enalapril exerts additive antiproteinuric effect in IgA nephropathy. *Am J Kidney Dis* 2001;38:18–25.

273. Onder G, Pahor M, Gambassi M, et al. Association between ACE inhibitors use and headache caused by nitrates among hypertensive patients: results from the Italian group of pharmacoepidemiology in the elderly (GIFA). *Cephalalgia* 2003;23:901–906.

274. Dubey K, Balani DK, Pillai KK. Potential adverse interaction between aspirin and lisinopril in hypertensive rats. *Hum Exp Toxicol* 2003;22:143–147.

275. Takkouche B, Etminan M, Caamano F, et al. Interaction between aspirin and ACE inhibitors: resolving discrepancies using a meta-analysis. *Drug Saf* 2002;25:373–378.

276. Sproule BA, Hardy BG, Shulman KI. Differential pharmacokinetics of lithium in elderly patients. *Drugs Aging* 2000;16:165–177.

277. Juurlink DN, Mamdani MM, Kopp A, et al. Drug-induced lithium toxicity in the elderly: a population-based study. *J Am Geriatr Soc* 2004;52:794–798.

278. Johnson TR, Tobias JD. Hypotension following the initiation of tizanidine in a patient treated with an angiotensin converting enzyme inhibitor for chronic hypertension. *J Child Neurol* 2000;15:818–819.

279. Yasumaru M, Tsuji S, Tsujii M, et al. Inhibition of angiotensin II activity enhanced the antitumor effect of cyclooxygenase-2 inhibitors via insulin-like growth factor I receptor pathway. *Cancer Res* 2003;63:6726–6734.

280. Warner TD, Mitchell JA. Cyclooxygenases: new forms, new inhibitors, and lessons from the clinic. *FASEB J* 2004;18:790–804.

281. Fitzgerald GA. Coxibs and cardiovascular disease. *N Engl J Med* 2004;351:1709–1711.

282. Markowitz JS, Wells BG, Carson WH. Interactions between antipsychotic and antihypertensive drugs. *Ann Pharmacother* 1995;29:603–609.

283. Waxler B, Rabito SF. Aprotinin: a serine protease inhibitor with therapeutic actions: its interaction with ACE inhibitors. *Curr Pharm Des* 2003;9:777–787.

284. Barrios V, Calderon A, Navarro-Cid J, et al. N-acetylcysteine potentiates the antihypertensive effect of ACE inhibitors in hypertensive patients. *Blood Press* 2002;11:235–239.

285. Hasford J, Mimran A, Simons WR. A population-based European cohort study of persistence in newly diagnosed hypertensive patients. *J Hum Hypertens* 2002;16:569–575.

286. The Heart Outcomes Prevention Evaluation Study Investigators. Effects of an angiotensin-converting-enzyme inhibitor, ramipril, on cardiovascular events in high-risk patients. *N Engl J Med* 2000;342:145–153.

287. McInnes GT. Size isn't everything -ALLHAT in perspective. *J Hypertens* 2003;21:459–461.

288. Weber MA. The ALLHAT report: a case of information and misinformation. *J Clin Hypertens (Greenwich)* 2003;5:9–13.

289. Burgers JS, van Everdingen JJ. Beyond the evidence in clinical guidelines. *Lancet* 2004;364:392–393.

290. Wing LMH, Chalmers JP, West MJ, et al. Treatment of hypertension with enalapril and hydrochlorothiazide or enalapril and atenolol: contrasts in hypotensive interactions. *J Hypertens Suppl* 1987;5(Supplement 5):S603–S606.

291. Brown MJ, Cruickshank JK, Dominiczak JK, et al. Better blood pressure control: how to combine drugs. *J Hum Hypertens* 2003;17:81–86.

292. Pitt B, Reichek N, Willenbrock R, et al. Effects of eplerenone, enalapril, and eplerenone/enalapril in patients with essential hypertension and left ventricular hypertrophy: the 4E-left ventricular hypertrophy study. *Circulation* 2003;108:1831–1838.

293. Black HR. Evolving role of aldosterone blockers alone and in combination with angiotensin-converting enzyme inhibitors or angiotensin II receptor blockers in hypertension management: a review of mechanistic and clinical data. *Am Heart J* 2004;147:564–572.

294. Hollenberg NK. Aldosterone in the development and progression of renal injury. *Kidney Int* 2004;66:1–9.

295. Forclaz A, Maillard M, Nussberger J, et al. Angiotensin II receptor blockade: is there truly a benefit of adding an ACE inhibitor? *Hypertension* 2003;41:31–36.

296. Azizi M, Menard J. Combined blockade of the renin-angiotensin system with angiotensin-converting enzyme inhibitors and angiotensin II type 1 receptor antagonists. *Circulation* 2004;109:2492–2499.

297. Johannesson M. The cost-effectiveness of the switch towards more expensive antihypertensive drugs. *Health Policy* 1994;28:1–13.

298. Fretheim A, Aaserud M, Oxman AD. The potential savings of using thiazides as the first choice antihypertensive drug: cost-minimisation analysis. *BMC Health Serv Res* 2003;3:18–25.

299. Spurgeon D. NIH promotes use of lower cost drugs for hypertension. *BMJ* 2004;328:539.

300. Siegel D, Lopez J, Meier J, et al. Changes in the phamacologic treatment of hypertension in the Department of Veterans Affairs 1997–1999: decreased use of calcium antagonists and increased use of beta-blockers and thiazide diuretics. *Am J Hypertens* 2001;14:957–962.

301. Borghi C, Dormi A, D'Addato S, et al. Trends in blood pressure control and antihypertensive treatment in clinical practice: the Brisighella Heart Study. *J Hypertens* 2004;22:1707–1716.

302. Dias da Costa JS, Fuchs SC, Olinto MTA, et al. Cost-effectiveness of hypertension treatment: a population-based study. *Sao Paulo Med J* 2002;120:100–104.

303. Verdecchia P, Angeli F, Borgioni C, et al. Changes in cardiovascular risk by reduction of left ventricular mass in hypertension: a meta-analysis. *Am J Hypertens* 2003;16:895–899.

304. Dahlöf B, Pennert K, Hansson L. Reversal of left ventricular hypertrophy in hypertensive patients. A metaanalysis of 109 treatment studies. *Am J Hypertens* 1992;5:95–110.

305. Klingbeil AU, Schneider M, Martus P, et al. A meta-analysis of the effects of treatment on left ventricular mass in essential hypertension. *Am J Med* 2003;115:41–46.

306. Zhang R, Crump J, Reisin E. Regression of left ventricular hypertrophy is a key goal of hypertension management. *Curr Hypertens Rep* 2003;5:301–308.

307. Brilla CG, Funck RC, Rupp H. Lisinopril-mediated regression of myocardial fibrosis in patients with hypertensive heart disease. *Circulation* 2000;102:1388–1393.

308. Brilla CG, Rupp H, Maisch B. Effects of ACE inhibition versus non-ACE inhibitor antihypertensive treatment on myocardial fibrosis in patients with arterial hypertension. Retrospective analysis of 120 patients with left ventricular endomyocardial biopsies. *Herz* 2003;28:744–753.

309. Ciulla MM, Paliotti R, Esposito A, et al. Different effects of antihypertensive therapies based on losartan or atenolol on ultrasound and biochemical markers of myocardial fibrosis: results of a randomized trial. *Circulation* 2004;110:552–557.

310. Madrid AH, Bueno MG, Rebollo JMG, et al. Use of irbesartan to maintain sinus rhythm in patients with long-lasting persistent atrial fibrillation: a prospective and randomized study. *Circulation* 2002;106:331–336.

311. Al-Khatib SM. Angiotensin-converting enzyme inhibitors: a new therapy for atrial fibrillation? *Am Heart J* 2004;147:751–752.

312. Finkielstein D, Schweitzer P. Role of angiotensin-converting enzyme inhibitors in the prevention of atrial fibrillation. *Am J Cardiol* 2004;93:734–736.

313. Freestone B, Beevers DG, Lip GYH. The renin-angiotensin-aldosterone system in atrial fibrillation: a new therapeutic target? *J Hum Hypertens* 2004;18:461–465.

314. Dernellis JM, Vyssoulis GP, Zacharoulis AA, et al. Effects of antihypertensive therapy on left atrial function. *J Hum Hypertens* 1996;10:789–794.

315. Anne W, Willems R, Van der Merwe N, et al. Atrial fibrillation after radiofrequency ablation of atrial flutter: preventive effect of angiotensin converting enzyme inhibitors, angiotensin II receptor blockers, and diuretics. *Heart* 2004;90:1025–1030.

316. Tsai CT, Lai LP, Lin JL, et al. Renin-angiotensin system gene polymorphisms and atrial fibrillation. *Circulation* 2004;109:1640–1646.

317. Halkin A, Keren G. Potential indications for angiotensin-converting enzyme inhibitors in atherosclerotic vascular disease. *Am J Med* 2002;112:126–134.

318. Koh KK, Son JW, Ahn JY, et al. Simvastatin combined with ramipril treatment in hypercholesterolemic patients. *Hypertension* 2004;44:180–185.

319. Strippoli GFM, Craig M, Deeks JJ, et al. Effects of angiotensin converting enzyme inhibitors and angiotensin II receptor antagonists on mortality and renal outcomes in diabetic nephropathy: systematic review. *BMJ* 2004;329:828.

320. Jafar TH, Schmid CH, Landa M, et al. Angiotensin-converting enzyme inhibitors and progression of nondiabetic renal disease. *Ann Intern Med* 2001;135:73–87.

321. Dunder K, Lind L, Zethelius B, et al. Increase in blood glucose concentration during antihypertensive treatment as a predictor of myocardial infarction: population based cohort study. *BMJ* 2003;326:681–686.

322. Verdecchia P, Reboldi G, Angeli F, et al. Adverse prognostic significance of new diabetes in treated hypertensive subjects. *Hypertension* 2004;43:963–969.

323. Lever AF, Hole DJ, Gillis CR, et al. Do inhibitors of angiotensin-I-converting enzyme protect against risk of cancer? *Lancet* 1998;352:179–184.

324. Lindholm LH, Anderson H, Ekbom T, et al. Relation between drug treatment and cancer in hypertensives in the Swedish Trial in Old Patients with Hypertension 2: a 5-year, prospective, randomised, controlled trial. *Lancet* 2001;358:539–544.

325. American Diabetes Association. Treatment of hypertension in adults with diabetes. *Diabetes Care* 2003;26(Supplement 1):S80–S82.

326. Marshall SM. Inhibition of the renin-angiotensin system: added value in reducing cardiovascular and renal risk? *Diabet Med* 2004;21:1–3.

327. de Zeeuw D, Remuzzi G, Parving H-H, et al. Albuminuria, a therapeutic target for cardiovascular protection in type 2 diabetic patients with nephropathy. *Circulation* 2004;110:921–927.

328. Ruggenenti P, Fassi A, Ilieva AP, et al. Preventing microalbuminuria in type 2 diabetes. *N Engl J Med* 2004;351:1941–1951.

329. Chaturvedi N, Sjolie A-K, Stephenson JM, et al. Effect of lisinopril on progression of retinopathy in normotensive people with type 1 diabetes. *Lancet* 1998;351:28–31.

330. Sjolie AK, Chaturvedi N. The retinal renin-angiotensin system: implications for therapy in diabetic retinopathy. *J Hum Hypertens* 2002;16:S42–S46.

331. Jacobsen P, Andersen S, Rossing K, et al. Dual blockade of the renin-angiotensin system versus maximal recommended dose of ACE inhibition in diabetic nephropathy. *Kidney Int* 2003;63:1874–1880.

332. Mogensen CE, Neldam S, Tikkanen I, et al. Randomised controlled trial of dual blockade of renin-angiotensin system in patients with hypertension, microalbuminuria, and non-insulin dependent diabetes: the candesartan and lisinopril microalbuminuria (CALM) study. *BMJ* 2000;321:1440–1444.

333. Laverman GD, Navis G, Henning RH, et al. Dual renin-angiotensin system blockade at optimal doses for proteinuria. *Kidney Int* 2002;62:1020–1025.

334. Campbell R, Sangalli F, Perticucci E, et al. Effects of combined ACE inhibitor and angiotensin II antagonist treatment in human chronic nephropathies. *Kidney Int* 2003;63:1094–1103.

335. Nakao N, Yoshimura A, Morita H, et al. Combination treatment of angiotensin-II receptor blocker and angiotensin-converting-enzyme inhibitor in non-diabetic renal disease (COOPERATE): a randomised controlled trial. *Lancet* 2003;361:117–124.

336. Sarnak MJ, Levey AS, Schoolwerth AC, et al. Kidney disease as a risk factor for development of cardiovascular disease. *Circulation* 2003;108:2154–2169.

337. Agarwal R, Nissenson AR, Batlle D, et al. Prevalence, treatment, and control of hypertension in chronic hemodialysis patients in the United States. *Am J Med* 2003;115:291–297.

338. Agarwal R, Lewis R, Davis JL, et al. Lisinopril therapy for hemodialysis hypertension: hemodynamic and endocrine responses. *Am J Kidney Dis* 2001;38:1245–1250.

339. Safar ME, London GM, Plante GE. Arterial stiffness and kidney function. *Hypertension* 2004;43:163–168.

340. Cannella G, Paoletti E, Delfino R, et al. Prolonged therapy with ACE inhibitors induces a regression of left ventricular hypertrophy of dialyzed uremic patients independently from hypotensive effects. *Am J Kidney Dis* 1997;30:659–664.

341. Shand BI, Bailey RR, Lynn KL, et al. Effect of enalapril on erythrocytosis in hypertensive patients with renal disease. *Clin Exp Hypertens* 1995;17:689–700.

342. Efrati S, Zaidenstein R, Dishy V, et al. ACE inhibitors and survival of hemodialysis patients. *Am J Kidney Dis* 2002;40:1023–1029.

343. Knoll GA, Sahgal A, Nair RC, et al. Renin-angiotensin system blockade and the risk of hyperkalemia in chronic hemodialysis patients. *Am J Med* 2002;112:110–114.

344. Thomas MC, Cooper ME. Blockade of the renin-angiotensin system: better late than never. *Am J Kidney Dis* 2004;43:1113–1115.

345. Lorenz M, Billensteiner E, Bodingbauer M, et al. The effect of ACE inhibitor and angiotensin II blocker therapy on early posttransplant kidney graft function. *Am J Kidney Dis* 2004;43:1065–1070.

346. Kincaid-Smith P, Fairley KF, Packham D. Dual blockade of the renin-angiotensin system compared with a 50% increase in the dose of angiotensin-converting enzyme inhibitor: effects on proteinuria and blood pressure. *Nephrol Dial Transplant* 2004;19:2272–2274.

347. Hricik DE, Browning PJ, Kopelman R, et al. Captopril-induced functional renal insufficiency in patients with bilateral renal-artery stenoses or renal-artery stenosis in a solitary kidney. *N Engl J Med* 1983;308:373–376.

348. Menard J, Michel JP, Plouin P-F. A cautious view of the value of angiotensin-converting enzyme inhibition in renovascular disease. In: Robertson JIS, Nicholls MG, eds. *The renin-angiotensin system*. London: Mosby; 1993:89.1–89.9.

349. Hollenberg NK. A buoyant view of the value of angiotensin-converting enzyme inhibition in renovascular disease. In: Robertson JIS, Nicholls MG, eds. *The renin-angiotensin system*. Mosby: London; 1993:90.1–90.8.

350. Robertson JIS. Renin and the pathophysiology of renovascular hypertension. In: Robertson JIS, Nicholls MG, eds. *The renin-angiotensin system*. London: Mosby; 1993:55.1–55.34.

351. Ie EH-Y, Karschner JK, Shapiro AP. Reversible nephrotic syndrome due to high renin state in renovascular hypertension. *Neth J Med* 1995;46:136–141.

352. Rossignol P, Chatellier G, Azizi M, et al. Proteinuria in renal artery occlusion is related to active renin concentration and contralateral kidney size. *J Hypertens* 2002;20:139–144.

353. Robertson JIS. Angiotensin-converting enzyme inhibitors in clinical renovascular hypertension. In: Robertson JIS, Nicholls MG, eds. *The renin-angiotensin system*. London: Mosby; 1993:88.1–88.13.

354. Tullis MJ, Caps MT, Zierler RE, et al. Blood pressure, antihypertensive medication, and atherosclerotic renal artery stenosis. *Am J Kidney Dis* 1999;33:675–681.

355. Losito A, Gaburri M, Errico R, et al. Survival of patients with renovascular disease and ACE inhibition. *Clin Nephrol* 1999;52:339–343.

356. van de Ven PJG, Beutler JJ, Kaatee R, et al. Angiotensin converting enzyme inhibitor-induced renal dysfunction in atherosclerotic renovascular disease. *Kidney Int* 1998;53:986–993.

357. Salahudeen AK, Pingle A. Reversibility of captopril- induced renal insufficiency after prolonged use in an unusual case of renovascular hypertension. *J Hum Hypertens* 1988;2:57–59.

358. Spence JD. Treatment options for renovascular hypertension. *Expert Opin Pharmacother* 2002;3:411–416.

359. Hannedouche T, Godin M, Fries D, et al. Acute renal thrombosis induced by angiotensin-converting enzyme inhibitors in patients with renovascular hypertension. *Nephron* 1991;57:230–231.

360. Novick AC. Atherosclerotic ischemic nephropathy. *Urol Clin North Am* 1994;21:195–200.

361. Svarstad E, Hultstrom D, Jensen D, et al. Renal artery thrombosis with acute renal failure after withdrawal of angiotensin converting enzyme inhibitor: a case report. *Nephrol Dial Transplant* 2002;17:687–689.

362. Agarwal M, Lynn KL, Richards AM, et al. Hyponatremic-hypertensive syndrome with renal ischemia: an underrecognized disorder. *Hypertension* 1999;33:1020–1024.

363. McAreavey D, Brown JJ, Cumming AMM, et al. Inverse relation of exchangeable sodium and blood pressure in hypertensive patients with renal artery stenosis. *J Hypertens* 1983;1:297–302.

364. Elkik F, Corvol P, Idatte J-M, et al. Renal segmental infarction: a cause of reversible malignant hypertension. *J Hypertens* 1984;2:149–156.

365. Fay MF, Nicholls MG, Richards AM. A man with severe, transient hypertension due to acute renal infarction. *J Hum Hypertens* 1999;13:343–344.

366. Steen VD, Costantino JP, Shapiro AP, et al. Outcome of renal crisis in systemic sclerosis: relation to availability of angiotensin converting enzyme (ACE) inhibitors. *Ann Intern Med* 1990;113:352–357.

367. Steen VD. Scleroderma renal crisis. *Rheum Dis Clin North Am* 2003;29:315–333.

368. Walker JG, Ahern MJ, Smith MD, et al. Scleroderma renal crisis: poor outcome despite aggressive antihypertensive treatment. *Intern Med J* 2003;33:216–220.

369. Kahan A, Devaux JY, Amor B, et al. The effect of captopril on thallium 201 myocardial perfusion in systemic sclerosis. *Clin Pharmacol Ther* 1990;47:483–489.

370. Kazzam E, Caidahl K, Hallgren R, et al. Non-invasive evaluation of long-term cardiac effects of captopril in systemic sclerosis. *Intern Med* 1991;230:203–212.

371. Plata R, Cornejo A, Arratia C, et al. Angiotensin- converting-enzyme inhibition therapy in altitude polycythaemia: a prospective randomised trial. *Lancet* 2002;359:663–666.

372. Fakhouri F, Grunfeld J-P, Hermine O, et al. Angiotensin- converting enzyme inhibitors for secondary erythrocytosis. *Ann Intern Med* 2004;140:492–493.

373. Vlahakos DV, Marathias KP, Agroyannis B, et al. Posttransplant erythrocytosis. *Kidney Int* 2003;63:1187–1194.

13 | Angiotensin receptor blockers

Marc de Gasparo and Gordon T. McInnes

INTRODUCTION

After the discovery of angiotensin converting enzyme (ACE), blockade of this enzyme became a successful approach to effective lowering of blood pressure (BP) in hypertension. Moreover, this class of drug improves morbidity and mortality by blocking angiotensin II (Ang II) formation in diseases with left ventricular dysfunction. Over the years, the results of large interventional trials have consistently shown cardiac risk reduction with ACE inhibitors. However, ACE is a relatively non-specific enzyme, which also catalyses the breakdown of many proteins, such as bradykinin, substance P, encephalin and LHRH. Blockade of ACE results in accumulation of bradykinin, which facilitates vasodilation; however, it may also be responsible for the irritating dry cough occurring in about 15% of ACE-inhibitor-treated patients and for rare life-threatening angio-oedema. In addition, a so-called escape phenomenon was reported after ACE inhibition; although BP remains decreased, Ang II and aldosterone returned to the pretreatment baseline. This could be due to a reactive rise of plasma renin activity and/or the stimulation of alternative pathways for Ang II production. It was, therefore, postulated that Ang II receptor antagonism would provide a more complete and selective blockade of the Ang II effect and would prevent the interaction of Ang II with its specific receptor on the target tissue, independently of the Ang II pathways of synthesis.

ANGIOTENSIN II

Ang II, an octapeptide, is the final effective product of the renin–angiotensin (RA) cascade, which regulates arterial pressure and fluid and electrolyte balance. This peptide acts on blood vessels producing vasoconstriction, on the kidney regulating sodium and fluid retention, but also contracting efferent arterioles preferentially compared with afferent arterioles,[1,2] on the adrenals, nerve terminals and the sympathetic system-stimulating catecholamines release.

Moreover, Ang II affects aldosterone and vasopressin activities, regulating salt excretion and circulating volume.[3,4]

Through these various mechanisms, Ang II increases vascular resistance and regulates fluid volume in order to maintain arterial pressure in circumstances associated with extracellular volume depletion.[5] Overactivity or dysregulation of the system causes hypertension.

The RA system (RAS), and, therefore, Ang II production, is stimulated by a decrease in plasma volume, plasma sodium concentration and renal perfusion pressure. Diuretics are potent stimuli of the RAS, whereas β-blockers and central sympatholytic drugs decrease activity. Hypotension, dehydration, high plasma potassium and low-sodium diet also stimulate the RAS.

Ang II is more than a hormone causing vasoconstriction and regulating fluid and electrolyte balance. Ang II stimulates various genes leading to hypertrophy of the cardiomyocytes and of the vascular smooth muscle cells. It affects extracellular matrix formation in regulating collagen and fibronectin synthesis.[6] Ang II also has mitogenic properties.[7] Ang II, through activation of cytokines, such as TGF-β, promotes mesangial cell proliferation and extracellular matrix deposition.[8] Glomerular hypertension and Ang II have also been shown to increase the rate of glomerular podocyte loss.[9] In ageing and several disease states, these local actions of Ang II are likely to contribute importantly to glomerulosclerosis and progressive decline of glomerular filtration rate (GFR).

Although Ang II has been viewed as a blood-borne, systemically active hormone producing an immediate effect, it is also formed in many tissues, such as brain, kidney, heart and blood vessels, where it functions locally as a paracrine and autocrine substance, having late, but sustained consequences. Indeed, the whole RAS machinery exists to produce Ang II locally in the tissue and/or interstitial compartment. The cardiac interstitial fluid concentration of Ang I and II are over 100-fold that of plasma, and even 1000-fold higher in the renal interstitium. Some Ang II is formed in cardiac and renal tissue through the action of proteolytic enzymes other than ACE, such as chymase and enthepsin, on the decapeptide AI.[10,11]

Ang II has direct effects on endothelial and vascular smooth muscle cells and locally formed Ang II plays an essential role in inflammatory reactions and the development of atherosclerosis. Elevated tissue levels of Ang II are demonstrated in hypertension, congestive heart failure (CHF), myocardial infarction (MI), atherosclerosis, kidney diseases and diabetes.

The multiple actions of Ang II are mediated through two specific cell-surface receptors, AT1 and AT2, which have been cloned and characterized.[12] Ang II does not distinguish between the two receptors. The AT1 receptor mediates virtually all the well-known physiological effects of Ang II.[13,14] The clinical relevance of the AT2 receptors is less clear.[15]

AT1 receptors have been demonstrated in many tissues, including vascular smooth muscle, adrenal zona glomerulosa, mesangial and tubular epithelial cells of the kidney, myocardium, neuronal tissue, and the choroid plexus.[16] Receptor density and magnitude of response to Ang II are not always related. For example, vascular smooth muscle cells have a density of AT1 receptors much lower than that in cells of the adrenal glomerulosa, yet have a more rapid and dramatic response to Ang II.[17] The multiple actions of Ang II are listed in Table 13.1.

Table 13.1 Actions of angiotensin ii

Tissue	Action
Vasculature	Vasoconstriction
	Smooth muscle hypertrophy
Adrenal cortex	Synthesis and secretion of aldosterone
Adrenal medulla	Release of epinephrine
Kidney	Vasoconstriction of efferent (and afferent) arterioles
	Inhibition of renin release
	Sodium reabsorption
	Mesangial growth and matrix deposition
Heart	Myocardial hypertrophy and collagen synthesis
Brain	Stimulation of thirst and vasopression
	Increased central sympathetic outflow
Peripheral sympathetic nerve terminals	Presynaptic augmentation of norepinephrine release

AT1 RECEPTOR

The AT1 receptor belongs to the G-protein coupled receptor (GPCR) super family. The signalling mechanisms are highly complex. In addition to the five classic pathways for GPCR, namely adenylate cyclase, phospholipase C, A_2, D and calcium channels, the AT1 receptor binds various cytosolic kinases (e.g. Src, JAK-STAT, Tyk2, Fak, Pyk2) and activates members of the MAP kinase family, which play important roles in Ang II-stimulated cell proliferation, hypertrophy and migration. Notably, the NADPH oxidase responsible for superoxide formation is also under control of the AT1 receptor. Moreover, Ang II, through AT1 receptor binding, can transactivate growth factor tyrosine kinase receptors such as EGF and PDFG. Blockade of the AT1 receptor, therefore, appears a potential target to control the overactivity of the RAS.

The discovery, isolation and synthesis of Ang II were followed by a series of investigations into the structure–activity relationship of analogues with the hope of finding an antagonist. Saralasin was the first peptide antagonist synthesized. Sarcosine replaced aspartic acid, the first amino acid of Ang II, whereas alanine substituted for the last (eighth) phenylalanine. Due to its peptidic nature, saralasin is not orally active and had a short half-life. In addition, saralasin is a partial agonist, having a pressor effect in low-renin hypertensive patients.[18] For these reasons, saralasin was essentially used only for diagnostic purposes.[19]

It was only in 1982 that the first non-peptidic molecule with uncomplicated chemical structure and having Ang II antagonistic properties was discovered and patented by Furakawa of Takeda Chemical industries in Osaka, Japan. This 1-benzyl-imidazole-5 acetic-acid derivative bound significantly to Ang II receptor, but had only weak antihypertensive effect.[20] Using this new information, the chemists in DuPont and in Smith-Kline-Beecham started molecular modelling overlapping the Takeda molecule and Ang II. The 2 chlorobenzyl substitute of the Takeda lead was spatially equivalent to the Tyr[4] of Ang II, whereas the aliphatic butyl group pointed towards the Ile.[5] This approach was successful, leading to losartan in 1989[21] and later to eprosartan in 1991.[22]

Change in the imidazole ring of losartan gave rise to various AT1 receptor antagonists containing the two biphenyl rings and an acidic (tetrazole or carboxylic acid) function.

CLASSIFICATION/CHEMISTRY

The available AT1 receptor blockers differ somewhat in binding affinity and pharmacokinetics (see Pharmacokinetics/metabolism below).

Losartan

Compared with the Takeda lead, it was observed that the acidic group at the ortho position was essential. The length of the alkyl chain on the position of the imidazole was also critical. This chain should be short. Finally, linkage between the two phenyl groups added to the receptor affinity. Extensive molecular modelling resulted in losartan, characterized by an imidazole group, a biphenyl ring and a tetrazole acidic function. Losartan was the first non-peptide orally active AT1 receptor blocker to be commercially available.[23,24]

Losartan is described chemically as 2-butyl-4-chloro-1- [p-(o-1H-tetrazole-5-ylphenyl)-benzyl] imidazole-5-methanol monopotassium salt. Maximum pharmacological action requires the oxidation of the 5-hydroxymethyl group on the imidazole ring to form EXP3174, the carboxylic metabolite of losartan.[25] EXP3174 is essentially responsible for the whole activity of losartan. This metabolite has two-fold greater affinity for the AT1 receptor and is 15 to 30 times more potent than losartan.[26]

Valsartan

Valsartan is unique since the heterocyclic imidazole ring of losartan is replaced by a non-planar, acetylated amino acid[27,28] Valsartan, N-(1-oxypentyl)-[[2^1-(1H-tetrazol-5-yl) [1, 1^1-biphenyl]-4-yl] methyl]-2-valine[29] is, like EXP3174, a diacid. Unlike losartan, valsartan does not require metabolic oxidation to achieve maximum pharmacological effect.[29]

Irbesartan

The imidazole ring of losartan is replaced by imidazolinone where a carbonyl is substituted for the hydroxymethyl group.[27] Irbesartan is described chemically as 2-butyl-(1H-tetrazol-5-yl) [1, 1^1-biphenyl]-4-yl[methyl]-1, 3-diazospiro [4,4] nor-1-en. This agent possesses a high affinity and specificity for AT1 receptors. Irbesartan does not require biotransformation to achieve efficacy.[30]

Candesartan

Candesartan is also derived from losartan where the imidazole moiety is replaced by an ethoxy-benzimidazole carboxylic acid ring.[31] This prodrug is rapidly metabolized to a highly potent AT1 receptor antagonist with a C7 carboxyl group positioned in a fashion similar to the imidazole carboxyl moiety of EXP3174.[32]

Eprosartan

This angiotensin receptor blocker (ARB) differs from others in the class. It is derived from the Furakawa lead, but does not contain the biphenyl-tetrazole ring of losartan. Eprosartan is described chemically as (E)-α-[[2-butyl-1(1-carboxyphenyl) methyl]-1H-imidazol-5-yl] methylene-2-thiophenepropionic acid.[33,34]

Telmisartan

In telmisartan, 4^1-[(1, 4^1-dimethyl-2^1-propyl [2, 6^1-bi-1H-benzimidazol]-1^1-yl) methyl]-[1, 1^1-biphenyl]-2-carboxylic acid, the imidazole moiety of losartan is replaced by a benzimidazole. The molecule contains the biphenyl ring, but tetrazole is replaced by a carboxylic acid group.[35,36]

Olmesartan

This is the most recently introduced ARB. The substitution at the 4-carboxy-imidazole of EXP 3176 has been modified as follows: chlorine (position 5) is replaced by 1-hydroxy-1-methyl-ethyl and the n-butyl side chain (position 2) is replaced by an n-propyl chain. Olmesartan minoximil is described chemically as 2,3 hydroxy-2-butenyl-4-(1-hydroxy-1-methylethyl)-2-propyl-1-[P-O-1H-tetrazol-5-ylphenyl)benzyl] imidazole-5-carboxylate, cyclic 2,3 carbonate.

The chemical structures of the available ARB are illustrated in Figure 13.1.

MECHANISM OF ACTION

Binding

The AT1 receptor antagonists bind specifically to the Ang II receptor. There is no blockade of bradykinin, as with the ACE inhibitors, and no interference with other receptors such as adrenergic, muscarinic, dopaminergic and calcium channels. ARBs bind selectively to the AT1 receptor. None of the available ARB has a significant affinity for the AT2 receptor. Binding to the AT1 receptor occurs in a competitive manner following the law of mass action. The binding is saturable and reversible. In contrast to saralasin, the non-peptidic antagonists have no agonistic properties.

The affinity of the ARBs is variable depending on the tissue source, the radioactive ligand, and the assay conditions.[22,36,37] In two different assays, the relative affinity of candesartan and losartan varied between 13 000- and 170-fold. Therefore, a precise comparison requires that all the ARBs be tested simultaneously. From the published data, the rank-order of potency approximates to candesartan > EXP3174 (the active metabolite of losartan) > eprosartan = valsartan = irbesartan > telmisartan > olmesartan > losartan.

Stimulation of isolated aortic rings with Ang II allows another distinction between available ARBs. After pretreatment with the antagonist, there is a shift to the right of the Ang II dose–response curve. In some cases, there is also a decrease in the maximal contraction. This observation suggests a difference between the ARBs in the receptor-binding mechanism. Cells expressing endogenous AT1 receptor, such as vascular smooth muscle cells or cell lines

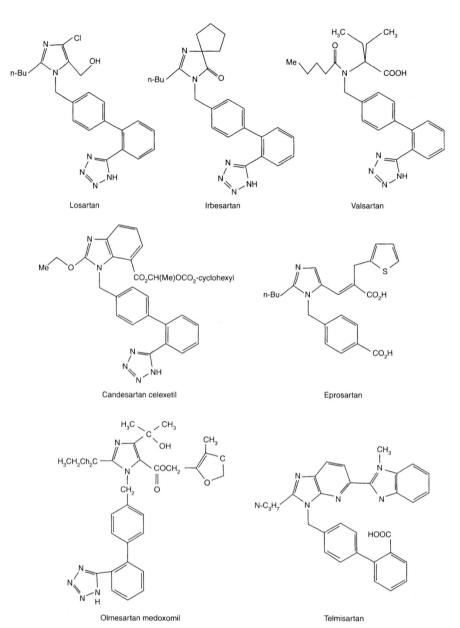

Fig. 13.1 Chemical structure of available angiotensin receptor blockers.

transfected with the gene coding for the AT1 receptor have been used to evaluate the binding characteristics and the biochemical response, such as IP3 formation. In these studies, the antagonist is administered ahead of Ang II. Losartan tested at increasing concentrations produces a parallel rightward shift of the dose–response curve without change in maximal binding.

Losartan is the prototype competitive surmountable antagonist. Eprosartan is also a member of this class. In contrast, other antagonists are also able to reduce the maximal response to Ang II leading to a non-parallel displacement of the response curve. The extent of the maximal response depression is variable. This is almost complete for candesartan[37] and telmisartan (competitive insurmountable antagonism), but only partial for valsartan, irbesartan, olmesartan and EXP3174, which are, therefore, competitive mixed surmountable/insurmountable antagonists.[30,38] The different behaviour is only observed when there is a pre-incubation and does not occur when the antagonist is co-incubated directly with Ang II. In this experimental condition, all the ARBs produce rightward shifts without decreased maximal response.

Insurmountable antagonists either bind in an irreversible way and the receptor number available for binding is permanently reduced or, alternatively, they dissociate very slowly[37] and the number of receptors available for further binding is reduced. Indeed, in AT1 transfected CHO cells at 57°C, the surmountable antagonist losartan dissociates very rapidly (5 minutes), whereas the dissociation half-life was, 7, 17, 30 and 120 minutes for irbesartan, valsartan, EXP3174 and candesartan, respectively. Access to the receptor binding site is, therefore, limited by occupancy. It was proposed by Vauquelin and colleagues[39] that all the ARBs bind to a fast-dissociating site on the receptor. However, the insurmountable antagonists convert the fast-dissociating complex into a tight-binding form. The mixed-type antagonists bind to both a high affinity, slow-dissociating state and a low-affinity high dissociating state in various ratios: 73/27, 55/45, 42/58 for EXP3174, valsartan and irbesartan, respectively. Depending on the dissociation rate, there is a progressive restoration of the functional response to Ang II.

Slowly-dissociating antagonists may have clinical benefit because of long-lasting blockade of the receptor. The elimination half-life probably also plays an important role in controlling the duration of action.[40] However, whereas plasma levels of candesartan cannot be detected 24 hours after oral administration in the rat, the hypertensive response to intravenous Ang II is still blocked by 75%.[41] Similarly, there is anticlockwise hysteresis in healthy volunteers when relating plasma levels of candesartan to the inhibition of the pressor response to Ang II. There is a sustained effect of candesartan when concentration is failing.[42] Accumulation of the antagonists in fat cells and binding to plasma protein may also be involved in the duration of action of the various ARBs.

ARBs inhibit Ang II-induced contraction of isolated aortic rings, catecholamine release from adrenal medulla and neural endings, and arginine vasopressin (AVP), aldosterone and endothelin release. In vivo, the ARBs not only affect haemodynamics, but also act directly on the heart, kidney and nervous system. ARBs reduce peripheral resistance, and decrease BP in the pithed rat following Ang I injection, as well as in spontaneously hypertensive or two-kidney, one-clip renal hypertensive rats. In the latter model, there is marked activation of the RAS and the effect of the ARB is more marked than in the spontaneous hypertensive rat (SHR). Volume expansion or bilateral nephrectomy attenuates or even abolishes the effect of the ARB,[43] underlining the importance of the RAS in the beneficial effect of AT1 receptor blockade.

Owing to blockade of peripheral sympathetic sites, there is no major change in heart rate despite the decreased vascular resistance. In addition, the ARBs have antifibrotic and antiproliferative effects and attenuate left ventricular hypertrophy. These drugs also improve coronary reserve.

Blockade of the AT1 receptor affects kidney-regulated circulating volume and this acts together with decreased vascular resistance on BP control. ARBs produce renal vasodilation with a small increase in GFR. There is a modest natriuresis following blockade of proximal convoluted tubular receptors. The effect increases after volume depletion, which stimulates the RAS. The natriuretic effect is also partly due to a decrease in aldosterone synthesis and release, affecting distal tubule sodium reabsorption.[44]

The ARBs decrease the peripheral sympathetic activity essentially by blocking the pre-synaptic AT1 receptor. When injected directly into the cerebral ventricles, ARBs decrease sympathetic nervous outflow at the paraventricular nucleus level, involved in the pathway leading to AVP release.[45] As well as decreasing AVP, ARBs alter drinking behaviours.[46]

Following blockade of the AT1 receptor at the juxtaglomerular level, there is inhibition of the regulatory negative feedback mechanism of Ang II leading to an increase in renin release, and Ang I and II production. High circulating levels of Ang II following blockade of the AT1 receptor may stimulate the unblocked AT2 receptor, which appears to counterbalance the effect of the AT1 receptor in a Yin-Yang manner. Although a number of preclinical studies support this hypothesis,[47–49] relevance has not yet been established in the clinic.

The haemodynamic and neurohumoral effects of ARBs are summarized in Table 13.2.

Haemodynamic effects

ARBs reduce peripheral resistance and systemic arterial pressure in hypertensive animals.[50] The effect is more marked and more consistent in models dependent on RAS activation.[51,52] Volume expansion or bilateral nephrectomy attenuates or abolishes the antihypertensive effect.[43] In euvolaemic normotensive animals and humans, ARBs have little effect. In the majority of hypertensive individuals, these agents reduce significantly peripheral resistance and BP.[53,54]

Lowering of peripheral resistance is mainly due to direct binding to and antagonism of vascular Ang II receptors and hence reversal of the vasoconstrictor action of Ang II.[43] Augmentation of this effect may arise from blockade of Ang II receptors on sympathetic nerve terminals and consequent attenuation of sympathetically mediated vasoconstriction[55]. ARBs also enhance nitric oxide-mediated vascular endothelial actions[56]. In normotensives, ARB-induced decline in arterial compliance and BP correlate with pretreatment plasma renin activity[57].

Table 13.2 Haemodynamic and neurohumoral effects of angiotensin receptor blockers

Arterial vasodilatation
Decrease in peripheral resistance
Reduction in aldosterone
Increase in renin
Increase in angiotensin II
Inhibition of peripheral sympathetic activity
Decrease in glomerular filtration rate (in volume depleted states)
Increase in glomerular filtration of fraction (in volume depleted states)

Cardiac effects

Despite the decline in peripheral resistance, heart rate is little affected in euvo-laemic hypertensive animals and humans during ARB treatment. This may be due to antagonism of Ang II receptors at peripheral sympathetic sites as well as centrally mediated actions.[58]

Plasma Ang II levels tend to increase during therapy with ARBs as a result of AT1 receptor-mediated disinhibition of renin release by cells of the renal juxtaglomerular apparatus.[59] Thus, administration of a selective AT1 antagonist would not only attenuate the cardiac-growth-promoting effects mediated by the AT1 receptor, but also may enhance the antiproliferative effect mediated by the unblocked AT2 receptor subtype.[60]

ARBs prevent Ang II-mediated cardiac growth and remodelling.[61] These effects may be important in the prevention or treatment of hypertensive cardiomyopathies. In experimental models of coronary ischaemia, losartan has beneficial effects on survival and on myocardial growth and remodelling.[62] ARBs may also benefit the heart by decreasing collagen deposition and cardiac fibrosis, by blocking Ang II effects directly or aldosterone effects indirectly, and may prevent the development of atrial fibrillation by attenuation of structural remodelling of the atrial myocardium.[63] ARBs improve coronary reserve in hypertensive animals concomitant with a reduction in cardiac mass.[64,65]

Renal effects

Through binding to AT1 receptor sites, ARBs inhibit the intrarenal actions of Ang II. In healthy persons on a low-salt diet, orally administered ARB produces a prompt dose-related increase in renal plasma flow and a slightly delayed, but more prolonged, increase in plasma renin activity.[66] In patients with essential hypertension, ARBs generally have no discernible effect on GFR as assessed by creatinine clearance.[67] Renal blood flow is usually unaffected by ARBs in euvolaemic animals or people.[68]

The overall effect of Ang II blockade on renal haemodynamics depends on the nature and degree of local and systemic counteracting responses. In healthy men on a very-low salt diet, renal blood flow increases with ARB administration to an extent that equals or exceeds that following ACE inhibitor infusion.[69] However, compensatory activation of the sympathetic nervous system in response to a pronounced fall in systemic BP may result in net renal vasoconstriction and a decline in renal function.[70] In the clinical setting of salt or volume depletion, ARBs may also produce a decline in GFR, perhaps by interference with glomerular blood flow autoregulation.[71]

In experimental models of unilateral renal artery stenosis, ARBs consistently produce a decline in GFR in the affected kidney. Effects on glomerular filtration and renal blood flow in the contralateral kidney are variable. In patients with renal impairment and renovascular occlusive disease, increases in serum creatinine follow ARB treatment.[71]

ARBs produce a modest natriuretic action through blockade of proximal tubular AT1 receptor sites that mediate sodium reabsorption.[71] The effect is most evident in the volume-depleted state, in which renin activation and the influence of the RAS are greatest.[71,72] An additional natriuretic action results from inhibition of aldosterone synthesis and release by the adrenal zona glomerulosa cells.[44,73] Reduced aldosterone-mediated distal tubular sodium reabsorption may contribute to the diuretic effect of ARBs.

Because Ang II has the potential for growth promoting effects at the mesangial tissue level, it has been speculated that Ang II receptor blockade may exert additional effects on glomerular filtration at the basement-membrane filtration barrier.[74] In hypertensive patients with proteinuric renal disorders, administration of losartan is associated with a decrease in urine protein, an increase in effective renal blood flow and stable GFR.[75] The degree and time course of the anti-proteinuric response to ARBs vary considerably and appear to differ from that of the antihypertensive effect. The peak of the ARB-anti-proteinuric dose–response relationship is yet to be defined.

Losartan has a unique property of exerting a modest uricosuric effect.[76] The effect is dose-dependent and has been documented in normotensive and hypertensive individuals with and without renal impairment. It is independent of the activity of the RAS and is not affected by changes in salt intake. Infusion of the active metabolite of losartan, EXP3174, has no effect on uric acid exertion, indicating that the effect is specific to the parent molecule.[76] The mechanism is unknown, but may be related to renal tubular anion load competing with urate at tubular transport sites.

Nervous system effects

Ang II antagonism inhibits peripheral sympathetic activity via blockade of pre-synaptic AT1 receptors that normally amplify release of neurotransmitters.[77] When administered intracerebrally to experimental animals, ARBs also inhibit centrally mediated sympathetic nervous outflow at the level of the paraventricular nucleus.[45] Drinking behaviour and release of AVP are also suppressed following central administration of these agents.[46]

Behaviour, affect, cognition and other effects

In experimental animals, ARBs improve cognitive function and anxiety associated deficits.[78] In humans, compared with amlodipine, losartan-treated patients had higher scores for the Psychological Well-Being Index after 12 weeks of double-blind therapy, despite similar blood pressure lowering.[79]

Blockade of the brain AT1 receptors in animals reduces the sympathoadrenal and hormonal responses to stress and prevents stress-induced gastric injury.[80] It has been suggested that there may be a role for ARBs in the treatment of stress-related disorders and in the preservation of cognition.[80]

In the Study on Cognition and Prognosis in the Elderly (SCOPE) in 4500 elderly hypertensive patients,[81] cognitive function was equally preserved on candesartan and placebo. In elderly hypertensive patients, 16 weeks of treatment with valsartan (unlike enalapril) improved some of the components of cognitive function, particularly episodic memory.[82]

The findings of one group have suggested beneficial effects of ARBs on sexual function. In hypertensive men[83] and in postmenopausal, sexually active hypertensive women,[84] valsartan improved sexual function, at least in some respects, compared with β-blockers.

PHARMACOKINETICS/METABOLISM

The ARBs differ in oral bioavailability, rate of absorption, tissue distribution, metabolism and rate of elimination. Several of these agents act as prodrugs with conversion to more biologically active metabolites (Table 13.3).

Losartan

Losartan is not a prodrug. The potassium salt is well absorbed orally with systemic bioavailability of 33%.[85–87] After oral absorption, peak plasma concentration (C_{max}) is reached after 1 hour. Food slows absorption and delays C_{max} without affecting significantly the area under the curve (AUC).[88] Terminal half-life ($T_{1/2}$) is 1.5–2.5 hours.[26] Losartan undergoes substantial first-pass metabolism to form an active compound, EXP3174,[89] which represents 14% of the ingested dose. The 5-hydroxy methyl group of the imidazole ring is biooxidized to its carboxylic acid through a CYP 450 2C9 and 3A4-dependent mechanism.[89] The formation of EXP3174 involves an intermediate aldehyde.

After oral administration, EXP3174 peaks at 2–4 hours and the $T_{1/2}$ is 6–9 hours.[26] The volume of distribution and plasma clearance are low, 12 L and 2.8 L/hour, respectively. EXP3174 is excreted in bile (58%) and in urine (30–35%).[88]

In plasma, losartan and its metabolites are highly protein bound (98.7–99.8%) in a non-surmountable manner. These compounds penetrate the blood–brain barrier poorly.

A lower starting dose is recommended in patients with hepatic dysfunction. Less than one-third of the absorbed drug and its metabolites are cleared by renal filtration.[88] Dose adjustment is not necessary in patients with renal impairment including those requiring dialysis, unless they are volume depleted or have occlusive vascular disease.[90] Neither losartan nor EXP3174 can be removed by dialysis.

Valsartan

The activity of valsartan is independent of hepatic metabolism.[91] Bioavailability is low (25%)[92] and is further reduced by 46% when administered with food. C_{max} of valsartan administered in the fasting state occurs at 2 hours, but is delayed with food[93] suggesting that the rate of absorption is slowed. However, the AUC between 6 and 24 hours is similar in the fed and fasted state. The $T_{1/2}$ varies between 6 and 9 hours. Valsartan is highly bound to serum protein (95%), primarily albumin.[94]

Volume of distribution is 17 L and plasma clearance is low (2 L/hour). Seventy per cent of the drug is excreted unchanged in bile[92] and 30% in the kidney. An inactive metabolite (valeryl-4-hydroxy valsartan) is found in small amounts (10%) and excreted in faeces.

Valsartan does not accumulate following repeated administration. However, patients with hepatic or biliary tract impairment have an increase in AUC, indicating a slowed plasma clearance rate.[95] The pharmacokinetics of valsartan do not appear to be affected appreciably by renal impairment.

Table 13.3 Pharmacokinetics and metabolism of angiotensin receptor blockers

Parameter	Product					
	Candesartan	Eprosartan	Irbesartan	Losartan	Valsartan	Olmesartan
Prodrug	Yes	No	No	No	No	Yes
Active metabolite	Yes	No	No	Yes	No	Yes
Metabolism by CYP_{450}	Low	No	Yes	Yes	Yes	No
Effect of food	No	25% reduction	No	Minimal	48% reduction	No
Affinity AT_1 (IC50) mol/L	0.6	1.5–9.2	1.3	1.4–200	1.9–8.2	37*
						7.7
Selectivity AT_1/AT_2	>10 000*		>10 000	3000 >30 000*	>30 000	>100 000
t_{max} (hours)	3–4	1.5	2	3–4	2	2
Half-life (hours)	3.5–4	5–8	11–15	2 6–9*	6–9	11–15
Bioavailability %	42	13	60–80	33	23	25–30
Protein-binding (%)	99.5	98–99	90	99 100*	94–97	94.4–99.3
Elimination (%)	Urine 30 Faeces 70	Urine 10 Faeces 90	Urine 20 Faeces 80	Urine 40 Faeces 60	Urine 30 Faeces 70	Urine 10–16 Faeces 78–85

*Metabolite

Irbesartan

Irbesartan does not require biotransformation for pharmacological action.[96] Bioavailability (60–80%)[97] is the greatest amongst available ARBs. In elderly, C_{max} and AUC are increased by 20–50%. There is no interference with food.[97] C_{max} after oral administration occurs after 1.5–2 hours and the $T_{1/2}$ is prolonged, 11–15 hours.

Volume of distribution is large, 53–93 L, indicating that the drug has access to the intracellular compartment. Plasma clearance is 10 L/hour, amongst the highest in the class. Although initially reported to have low protein binding, irbesartan is 99.5% protein bound, similar to other ARBs.

Irbesartan is eliminated mainly in bile (75%),[98] but only 1% is unchanged. The drug is glucuronidated and oxidized via CYP450 2C9. Drug accumulation does not appear to occur in hepatic or renal insufficiency.[96] Dose adjustment is not necessary in these conditions or in the elderly.

Candesartan

Because of poor oral absorption, candesartan is administered as a cilexetil ester prodrug, which is rapidly hydralized to the active compound in the gastrointestinal tract. Food does not interfere with absorption.[99]

The bioavailability of the prodrug is 42%, but only 15% for candesartan. In the elderly, AUC increases by 30–50%.[100] C_{max} is observed after 3–4 hours and the $T_{1/2}$ is 8–11 hours. AUC increases linearly with dosage between 2 and 16 mg.

Candesartan is excreted unchanged in bile (70%) and the kidney (30%).[101] Volume of distribution is 9.1 L, indicating low tissue penetration. Plasma clearance is very low (1.4 L/hour).

The pharmacokinetic profile of candesartan is not altered in patients with mild-to-moderate hepatic dysfunction.[102] In patients with renal impairment, AUC, C_{max} and $T_{1/2}$ are significantly greater than in healthy subjects. Thus, lower doses may be advisable in severe renal dysfunction. The drug is not dialysable.[102]

Eprosartan

The bioavailability of eprosartan is low (13–15%),[103] but increases slightly with age.[104] C_{max} is reached after 1–3 hours and $T_{1/2}$ is 4.5–9 hours. Food delays and reduces absorption by 25%, without clinical significance.[104] Plasma concentration increases in a slightly less than proportional manner over the 100–800 mg dose range. The volume of distribution is 13 L and plasma clearance 7.8 L/hour. Eprosartan is eliminated largely in bile (90%), primarily as the unchanged compound. A glucuronide metabolite is formed by a CYP450-independent mechanism[105] and excreted in urine.

Eprosartan is highly protein bound (98%) in plasma.[105] Both renal and hepatic impairment delay the elimination of eprosartan.

Telmisartan

The bioavailability of telmisartan is high (40–60%) and is dose-dependent. Pharmacokinetics are not linear over the dose range 20–160 mg, with greater than proportional increases in C_{max} and AUC with increasing dose. Peak plasma concentration occurs between 0.5 and 1 hour. Interference with food is negligible (6% and 20% for 40 and 160 mg doses, respectively). The $T_{1/2}$ is extremely long at 20–24 hours.[36]

The distribution volume (500 L) is the greatest amongst the available ARBs. Telmisartan is the most lipophylic ARB with excellent tissue penetration and access to the intracellular compartment. The plasma clearance is also high (60 L/hour). Telmisartan is excreted essentially in bile (98%). Glucuronidation is minimal and independent of CYP450.

Telmisartan is highly protein bound (>99.5%) in plasma. Due to the biliary route of elimination, telmisartan should be used with caution in patients with hepatic insufficiency.

Olmesartan

Due to poor absorption, olmesartan is administered as an inactive ester pro-drug, which is hydrolysed in the gastrointestinal tract.[106] The absolute bioavailability of the prodrug is 28% and is unaffected by food. The C_{max} is reached after 1–3 hours and the $T_{1/2}$ is 10–15 hours.[107]

Following the rapid and complete conversion of olmesartan medoxomil to olmesartan, there is virtually no further metabolism. Volume of distribution is approximately 17 L. Olmesartan is excreted mainly in bile (60%). Pharmacokinetics are linear up to a dose of 320 mg.

PHARMACODYNAMICS

The ARBs occupy space among the seven transmembrane helices of the receptor protein. Interaction with amino acid residues in these regions of the receptor molecule prevents the binding of Ang II to the receptor.[108] All currently available ARBs have been shown to attenuate the circulatory, renal, endocrine, and neurohumoral actions normally mediated by Ang II. Unlike the earlier non-selective peptide antagonist, saralasin, these agents are devoid of partial agonist activity. The ARBs cause a two-fold to three-fold rise in plasma renin activity and a consequent rise in Ang II concentration.[109]

The ARBs were characterized in healthy volunteers infused with Ang II or after sodium depletion with a low sodium diet and pretreatment with a diuretic to stimulate the endogenous RAS. The degree of AT1 receptor blockade was also directly measured using the capacity of the plasma of the treated volunteer to inhibit Ang II binding in isolated vascular smooth muscle cells. This approach was also used to measure plasma concentration of the active drug.

Whereas plasma renin activity and Ang II increase proportionally to the extent of receptor blockade, this is a less sensitive marker. The reduction in plasma aldosterone levels is inconsistent, confirming that other pathways, such as ACTH and plasma potassium levels modulate aldosterone secretion.

The fall of BP in hypertensive patients allows the comparison of various ARBs, which differ in their AT1 receptor affinity, and specific pharmacokinetic and pharmacodynamic properties. Losartan at a dose of 100 mg inhibits the pressor effect of Ang II by 25% after 24 hours. With valsartan, the Ang II pressor response is still abolished by 30%, 24 hours after an 80 mg dose. For most patients, the onset of antihypertensive effect is at about 2 hours, with the maximum reduction of BP at about 6 hours.[91,93] The Ang II pressure effect is still inhibited by 40 and 60%, 24 hours after irbesartan 150 mg and 300 mg, respectively. Candesartan cilexetil 8 mg inhibits the Ang II pressure effect by 50% at 24 hours. Eprosartan 300 mg inhibits the Ang II pressure effect by about 30% at 24 hours. However, telmisartan 80 mg gives only approximately 40% Ang II inhibition at 24 hours. At doses greater than 40 mg, olmesartan gives more than 90% inhibition of the Ang II pressure effect at 24 hours.

Comparative studies of different ARBs in either normal volunteers or in hypertensive patients are sometimes difficult to reconcile. Compared with placebo, a single dose of irbesartan (150 mg) caused a greater and more sustained blockade of the AT1 receptor than that of a single dose of losartan (50 mg) or valsartan (80 mg) in healthy volunteers challenged with Ang II. In contrast, changes in 24-hour AUC of plasma active renin and Ang II indicate that losartan 50 mg, valsartan 80 mg and candesartan 8 mg are equivalent, whereas valsartan 160 mg and candesartan 16 mg are not different. Valsartan, telmisartan, losartan and candesartan dose-dependently inhibit the Ang II-induced increase in diastolic BP. The rightward shift of the dose–response was statistically not different for candesartan, irbesartan, losartan and valsartan (mean 18.75 mg + 1.25) whereas it was significantly lower for telmisartan (8 mg). The results were different using the Schild regression technique. The calculated 24-hour Ki, i.e. the dose required to induce a two-fold shift in the dose–response corresponding to 50% receptor blockade was 1, 123, 54 and 93 mg for candesartan, irbesartan, telmisartan and valsartan, respectively.

Direct comparison of drugs within the class gives very variable results. A meta-analysis[110] of the first 43 randomized placebo-controlled clinical trials with losartan, valsartan, irbesartan and candesartan suggested equivalent antihypertensive efficacy. This analysis, however, was performed on trials having very different designs, treatment durations, comparators and patient populations. Dissimilar results were obtained in different comparative trials using valsartan, losartan or irbesartan.[111] In a cross-over study, the calculated equipotent antihypertensive doses were 80.5 mg for losartan, 115.5 mg for valsartan, 216.6 mg for irbesartan and 13.5 mg for candesartan. Recently, reviewing comparative studies of different ARBs, Maillard and Burnier[112] wrote: 'Yet one must take into account that all studies have been sponsored by the pharmaceutical industry and came generally to the same conclusion i.e. the new compound is better than the older one.'

Independent, multicentre, randomized, double-blind studies, with sufficient subjects and across a large dose range are required. Except for irbesartan evaluated between 1 and 900 mg, the dose–response relationship was defined in too small cohorts of patients and over too narrow dose-ranges, neglecting the lower and upper extremes of dose–response. This failure has led to recommending clearly inadequate starting and maintenance doses for losartan[113] and perhaps valsartan.[114]

The calculated trough:peak ratio and 24-hour ambulatory blood pressure monitoring were used to estimate the duration of action of the various ARBs. All the ARBs available have a trough:peak ratio greater than 50% and, therefore, are appropriate for once-a-day administration: losartan 50–100 mg: 50–75%; valsartan 80–160 mg: 66%; candesartan 8–16 mg: >80%; irbesartan 150–300 mg:

58–74%; eprosartan 400–800 mg: 67–85%; telmisartan 100–200 mg: >50%. The duration of action is dose-dependent.

Ambulatory blood pressure monitoring suggests that losartan 50 mg should be administered twice a day, as the BP during the last 6 hours of the 240-hour cycle does not differ from placebo. Using the smoothness index to assess the homogeneity of blood pressure reduction may be superior to the required trough:peak ratio. This index better identifies the occurrence of a balanced 24-hour blood pressure reduction with treatment.

Comparative trials against other antihypertensive drugs have been performed. ARBs, ACE inhibitors or β-blockers are equally efficient in lowering BP in various pathological environments. Calcium channel blockers (CCBs) and ARBs have similar efficacy, but amlodipine may perhaps induce a greater fall in BP.[114] Such differences may depend on the dosage employed.

Overall, ARBs have a gradual onset of action and a smooth antihypertensive effect. There is no first-dose hypotension. The maximal effects of the ARBs occur between 2 and 5 weeks, depending on the drug and the dose. Sodium and volume depletion activating the RAS should be corrected to avoid excessive BP fall.

Losartan, unlike its metabolite EXP3174, has a unique uricosuric property in healthy volunteers and in hypertensive patients. The effect is independent of AT1 receptor blockade and is caused by inhibition of the urate/anion exchanger in the brush border of the renal proximal tubule. This property may be of importance in patients receiving ciclosporin, which induces uricaemia. In contrast, this effect may favour the formation of urate stones in predisposed patients with nephrolithiasis, low urinary flow and academia. This complication has not been reported.

In addition to blockade of the AT1 receptor, irbesartan inhibits platelet aggregation in vitro and reduces TXA/PGH2 receptor binding. Valsartan also produces sustained inhibition of platelet aggregation and major platelet receptors.[115] The antiplatelet properties of valsartan do not appear to be dose- or time-dependent and are more marked in patients with diabetes and mild-to-moderate hypertension.

Telmisartan interests at physiological concentrations with a ligand-binding domain of the PPAR γ-receptor. This agent acts as a partial agonist, stabilizing the receptor in an active conformation in rats fed a high-fat, high-carbohydrate diet, as well as in isolated adipocytes. This effect occurs in the absence of the AT1 receptor.[116] Irbesartan may have a similar property in vitro.

Recent evidence suggests that the RAS may have a direct role in the pathogenesis of diabetes.[117] Angiotensin-mediated increases in oxidative stress, inflammation and free fatty acid concentrations potentially contribute to β-cell dysfunction in diabetes. In addition, activation of the RAS appears to potentiate the action of other pathogenic pathways, including glucotoxicity, lipotoxicity and advanced glycation. In experimental models of type 2 diabetes, angiotensin receptor blockade results in improvement of islet structure and function. In the ICARUS substudy of LIFE,[118] losartan treatment was associated with improved insulin sensitivity.

In the prospective Val-MARC trial,[119] valsartan reduced high-sensitivity C-reactive protein (hsCRP) levels in a manner independent of the degree of blood pressure reduction. These data raise the hypothesis that ARBs may have anti-inflammatory effects in addition to blood pressure lowering effects.

Olmesartan

Olmesartan has minimal or no inhibitory activity on human cytochrome P450. Co-administration of olmesartan with digoxin or warfarin did not result in clinically significant steady-state pharmacokinetic interactions.[107]

CLINICAL USE INCLUDING OUTCOME DATA

Blockade of the AT1 receptor inhibits direct and indirect effects of Ang II and catecholamines. This results in decreased vascular resistance and improvement of the hydroelectrolytic balance with reduction of circulating volume. As a consequence ARBs effectively lower BP. Heart rate remains unchanged because of blockade of the adrenergic system. Improvement of vascular smooth muscle cell hypertrophy and extracellular matrix formation is also observed (Table 13.4).

Numerous clinical studies have demonstrated the beneficial effect of ARBs on BP in mild-to-moderate or severe hypertension, irrespective of age or gender. The responder rate, defined as diastolic BP of <90 mmHg or fall in diastolic BP of >10 mmHg, varies between 50 and 65%. Approximately 50–60% of hypertensive individuals have a clinically significant response to ARBs.[54,136] This is comparable to monotherapy with diuretics, β-blockers, ACE inhibitors and CCBs.[137,138] The usual doses of ARBs are shown in Table 13.5. The antihypertensive efficacy of ARBs depends at least partially on the activity of the RAS.[57] Approximately 80% of patients demonstrate a significant blood pressure-lowering response when an ARB is combined with a thiazide diuretic.[139] The antihypertensive response is attenuated following volume expansion.[140] The full therapeutic profile of the ARBs has yet to be fully elucidated. The effects of age, race and concomitant medical conditions on the antihypertensive efficacy of these agents await further clarification.

Several studies have compared the relative efficacy of ARBs. In general, the observed differences have been modest.[141,142] The incidence of adverse effects in patients receiving either candesartan or irbesartan was similar to that experienced by patients receiving losartan.

Table 13.4 Antihypertensive mechanisms of angiotensin receptor blockers

---

Vascular actions
Direct blockade of Ang II–mediated vasoconstriction
Reversal of vascular hypertrophy
Augmentation of nitric oxide-mediated endothelial function

Renal actions
Augmentation of renal blood flow
Direct and indirect enhancement of proximal tubular natriuresis
Inhibition of aldosterone release and distal tubular reabsorption

Central and central nervous system actions
Attenuation of sympathetic activation
Inhibition of Ang II-mediated central sympathetic outflow
Inhibition of Ang II-mediated thirst and vasopressin release

Table 13.5 Angiotensin receptor blocker doses in hypertension

Drug	Starting daily dose	Maximum daily dose
Losartan	50 mg	100 mg
Valsartan	80 mg	320 mg
Irbesartan	150 mg	300 mg
Candesartan	4 mg	32 mg
Eprosartan	200 mg	600 mg
Telmisartan	40 mg	80 mg
Olmesartan	20 mg	80 mg

The highly insurmountable receptor antagonists may have a greater amplitude and duration of action.[143,144] However, a meta-analysis of 43 controlled trials involving the use of losartan, valsartan, irbesartan and candesartan concluded that within the ARB class, there is similar antihypertensive efficacy and a flat dose–response.[110] All the agents studied showed substantial augmentation of antihypertensive effect with the addition of thiazide diuretics.

The effects of ARBs in patients with left ventricular hypertrophy have also been studied. In a 10-month study of 89 hypertensive patients, losartan given as monotherapy or in association with hydrochlorothiazide produced not only a significant reduction in BP, but also a decrease in left ventricular mass studied by echocardiography.[145] Similarly, valsartan[146] and irbesartan[147] are superior to atenolol in reducing echocardiographic left ventricular mass in hypertensive patients with left ventricular hypertrophy. Valsartan is also superior to amlodipine in reducing left ventricular mass in left ventricular hypertrophy, independent of BP.[121] In hypertensive patients with left ventricular hypertrophy, losartan decreases myocardial collagen content, whereas atenolol does not.[148] Treatment based on atenolol or irbesartan improves diastolic function in patients with hypertensive left ventricular hypertrophy to the same degree, but through different mechanisms.[149]

Four large trials (LIFE with losartan,[150] SCOPE with candesartan,[81] VALUE with valsartan[114] and MOSES with eprosartan[151]) have reported on the long-term efficacy of ARBs in hypertensive patients. A further trial, evaluating telmisartan, ramipril, and their combination, and comparing telmisartan and placebo in ACE-inhibitor-intolerant subjects, in high-risk patients (ONTARGET/TRANSCEND) is underway and should report in 2008.[152]

Losartan Intervention For Endpoint (LIFE) Reduction in Hypertension

The LIFE trial[150] was a direct comparison of losartan with the β-blocker atenolol in hypertensive patients with ECG evidence of left ventricular hypertrophy. LIFE randomized 9139 patients aged 55–80 years. Forced titration was employed to achieve a target BP of <140/<90 mmHg. The primary endpoint was a composite of cardiovascular mortality, MI or stroke. BP fall after a mean follow-up of 4.8 years was identical in both groups (30.2/12.6 mmHg and 29.1/12.8 mmHg) in the losartan and atenolol groups, respectively. Mean doses were losartan 82 mg and atenolol 79 mg. Concomitant hydrochlorothiazide was used in about 70% of each group. The adjusted risk reduction (RR) was 13% in favour of losartan. There was no significant difference for MI, but RR reduction for stroke was 24.9%. RR reduction for the composite endpoint was 24.5% in the diabetic sub-population of 1195 subjects.[153] In this diabetic sub-group, RR reduction was 17.1% for fatal and non-fatal MI and 39% for cardiovascular mortality. Sudden arrhythmic cardiac death was also reduced in diabetic patients treated with losartan,[154] suggesting that blockade of the AT1 receptor offers protection better than atenolol against repolarization abnormalities. Greater regression of left ventricular hypertrophy[155] and reduced incidence of atrial fibrillation[156] may be the mechanisms for the beneficial effects.

Compared with patients randomized to atenolol, the losartan group exhibited a reduced incidence of new cases of diabetes,[157] suggesting that losartan acts beyond BP. This observation has been confirmed with irbesartan, candesartan and valsartan, and appears to be a class effect, perhaps mediated by improved insulin sensitivity.[118] Losartan was also superior to atenolol in 1326 patients with isolated systolic hypertension.[158]

In the whole LIFE population, the beneficial effect of losartan was mainly due to a reduction of stroke. Compared with conventional therapy, the number needed to treat for 5 years to prevent one stroke was 54 for the average participant, declining to 25, 24 and nine for patients with cardiovascular disease, isolated systolic hypertension and atrial fibrillation, respectively.[159] In LIFE, the clinical benefit of losartan was achieved at a cost well within accepted thresholds for cost-effectiveness.[160]

Although the results of LIFE are convincing, there are several imponderables. Losartan reduced left ventricular mass more in women (−33 g) than in men (−23 g) despite similar BP falls in both genders. More than 50% of losartan-treated patients received doses less than 100 mg, doses which do not block the RAS for 24 hours. Moreover, the comparator, atenolol, may not have been the best choice of first-line antihypertensive in an elderly population (mean age 67 years).

Study on Cognition and Prognosis in the Elderly (SCOPE)

SCOPE[81] was a randomized double-blind trial in 4964 patients aged 70–89 years with systolic BP of 160–179 mmHg and/or diastolic BP of 90–99 mmHg. The objective was to assess the effect of candesartan 8–16 mg compared with placebo on cardiovascular events and cognitive function. In fact, most of the placebo group received other antihypertensive agents. BP fell by 21.7/10.8 mmHg in the candesartan group and by 18.5/9.2 mmHg in the control group (a mean between group difference of 3.2/1.6 mmHg). Although the reduced risk of a first major cardiovascular event (11%) after 4 years' treatment with candesartan was not significant, there was a significant (28%) reduction in fatal stroke.

In patients who did not receive add-on antihypertensive therapy after randomization,[161] BP fell by 21.8/11.0 mmHg in the candesartan group and by 17.2/8.4 mmHg in the placebo group. There were significant RR reductions with candesartan in major cardiovascular events (32%; $p = 0.013$), cardiovascular mortality (29%; $p = 0.045$) and fatal mortality (27%; $p = 0.018$). These findings may best reflect the original intention of the placebo-controlled trial.

In elderly patients with isolated systolic hypertension, antihypertensive therapy based on candesartan resulted in a significant (42%) relative risk reduction in stroke in comparison with other antihypertensive treatments, despite little difference in BP.[162] The results of ACCESS (Acute Candesartan Cilexetil Therapy in Stroke Survivors) trial in 500 patients also suggest that a beneficial effect of candesartan may be unrelated to antihypertensive efficacy since there was no difference in BP between the study arms.[163]

The results of SCOPE did not show any improvement of cognitive function after candesartan. When the population was divided on the basis of baseline cognitive function, however, those with lower cognitive performance exhibited greater improvement after candesartan.[164]

Valsartan Antihypertensive Long-term Use Evaluation (VALUE)

VALUE is currently the largest double-blind, randomized, prospective comparative trial with ARBs in hypertension to have reported.[114] VALUE compared valsartan- and amlodipine-based therapy in 15 254 patients at high cardiovascular risk. The target was to achieve BP less than 140/90 mmHg. The median daily doses were valsartan 151.7 mg and amlodipine 8.5 mg. Blood pressure reduction after 1 month was 4.0/2.1 mmHg lower on amlodipine than in the valsartan group, and the difference in favour of amlodipine averaged about 3/2 mmHg throughout the trial. The target BP was achieved in 56% of patients randomized to valsartan and in 62% of those given amlodipine. Despite a greater decrease in BP in the amlodipine group, the primary composite cardiac morbidity and mortality outcome did not differ between the groups. However, the incidence of MI was less in the amlodipine-based group. The results of VALUE indicate that the rate of achieving adequate blood pressure control is of paramount importance in hypertensive patients at high cardiovascular risk.

A technique for serial median matching applied at 6 months, when treatment adjustments intended to achieve control were complete, created 5006 valsartan:amlodipine patient pairs, matched exactly for systolic BP, age, gender, and the presence or absence of previous coronary heart disease, stroke or diabetes. Subsequent combined cardiovascular events, MI, stroke and mortality were almost identical in the two cohorts, but admissions to hospital for heart failure were significantly lower in the valsartan group.[165] Despite lower absolute event rates in patients maintained on monotherapy, a sub-population with similar BP control in the two groups, the relative risk of heart failure and new onset diabetes favoured valsartan.[166]

Morbidity and Mortality after Stroke, Eprosartan compared with Nitrendipine for Secondary Prevention (MOSES)

The MOSES trial addressed secondary stroke prevention.[151] In those patients at high risk of stroke, good BP control was achieved in both groups. The combined primary endpoint (total mortality and all cardiovascular and cerebrovascular events including recurrent events) was significantly lower in the eprosartan group (21%; 95% confidence interval 4, 34%, $p = 0.014$) and recurrent stroke was reduced by 25% (95% confidence interval 3, 42%, $p = 0.03$).

An ARB-MI paradox has been proposed,[167,168] suggesting that ARB therapy may increase the risk of MI. This hypothesis is controversial and is difficult to substantiate in the face of blood pressure differences between treatment regimens.[169,170] It depends on assumptions concerning blood pressure-independent benefits of ACE inhibitor-based therapy and lack of benefits with CCBs and β-blockers. Discussion will continue until further comparative information becomes available.

A meta-analysis[171] of large outcome trials in hypertension involving 29 375 subjects indicates that ARBs reduce the primary endpoint and stroke compared with active controls. Compared with other antihypertensive drugs, ARB treatment was associated with no change in all-cause mortality. MI was increased but a decrease in new-onset diabetes at least partially offsets the increased risk of MI.

Several recent clinical trials have suggested that ARBs may protect against the development of de novo diabetes in 'at risk' patients.[117,172] The beneficial effect appears to outweigh both the metabolic effects of agents used in the control arms of these studies and the control of blood pressure achieved. In patients after acute MI, ARBs appear to be as effective as ACE inhibitors in reducing the incidence of new MI.[173]

Cardiac diseases

ARBs have also been shown to have benefits in heart failure. The ELITE (Evaluation of Losartan in the Elderly) study was designed to determine whether the ARB, losartan, offered advantages over the ACE inhibitor, captopril, in older patients with heart failure.[174] In this randomized, double-blind study of 722 patients with heart failure and ejection fraction <40%, losartan was titrated to 50 mg once daily and captopril to 50 mg three times daily for 48 weeks. The losartan treatment group had a 46% lower risk of death, 64% reduction in sudden death, and 26% reduction in hospitalization rate compared with the captopril-treated group. Improvement in symptoms was similar in both groups, as was the rate of hospitalization for progressive heart failure. Fewer losartan patients discontinued therapy because of adverse experiences (12.2% vs. 20.8%).

To confirm these findings, ELITE II was conducted on 3152 patients with similar characteristics and in a protocol similar to ELITE. All-cause mortality was slightly but not significantly higher for losartan (11.7%) compared with captopril (10.4%).[113] Losartan was again somewhat better tolerated than captopril.

In Val-HeFT (Valsartan Heart failure Trial), valsartan 160 mg twice daily was compared with placebo in patients with heart failure treated with digitalis, diuretics and ACE inhibitor in the majority, and β-blockers in some.[175,176] The combined endpoint of worsening heart failure, resuscitated cardiac arrest, or mortality occurred 13% less frequently in the valsartan group, primarily because of a decrease in heart failure hospitalizations. Significant improvements in heart failure symptoms, ejection fraction, quality of life indices were observed. The beneficial effect of valsartan in patients who were not on background ACE inhibitor therapy was marked.

The CHARM (Candesartan in Heart failure Assessment of Reduction in Mortality and morbidity) trial compared candesartan titrated to 32 mg once daily with placebo in three distinct populations: patients with left ventricular ejection fraction <40% who were not receiving ACE inhibitors (CHARM – alternative trial, 2028 patients); patients with left ventricular ejection fraction <40% who were receiving ACE inhibitors (CHARM – added trial, 2548 patients):

and patients with left ventricular ejection fraction >40% (CHARM – preserved trial, 3023 patients). Overall, when all three studies were analysed together, candesartan was generally well tolerated and significantly reduced cardiovascular deaths and hospital admissions for heart failure.[177–180]

OPTIMAAL (OPtimal Trial in Myocardial Infarction with the Angiotensin II Antagonist Losartan) compared losartan, target dose 50 mg daily, with captopril 50 mg three times daily in 4577 patients with acute MI.[181] After an average follow-up of 2.7 years, mortality was 17% in the losartan group and 16% in the captopril group ($p = 0.7$). In VALIANT, a study of 14 703 patients with MI complicated by left ventricular systolic dysfunction, heart failure or both, valsartan was equivalent to captopril for the composite endpoint of fatal and non-fatal cardiovascular events.[182]

Taken together, these trials indicate that ARBs confer benefits similar to those of ACE inhibitors in patients with coronary heart disease and heart failure. The combination of an ARB with an ACE inhibitor may convey additional benefits, especially in preventing hospitalization for heart failure.

Treatment with ARBs reduced the incidence of atrial fibrillation in the CHARM programme[183] and the effectiveness of ARBs in prevention of atrial fibrillation has been confirmed in a meta-analysis.[184] New-onset atrial fibrillation and associated stroke were reduced significantly by losartan, compared with atenolol-based antihypertensive treatment with similar BP reduction in LIFE.[154] Losartan was also more effective than atenolol-based therapy in reducing the risk of the primary composite endpoint of cardiovascular morbidity and mortality as well as stroke and cardiovascular death in hypertensive patients with ECG left ventricular hypertrophy and atrial fibrillation.[185] Losartan compared with atenolol reduced the risk of stroke, new-onset diabetes and new-onset atrial fibrillation in lower-risk as well as higher-risk patients in LIFE.[186] In a prospective, randomized study, use of an ARB facilitated maintenance of sinus rhythm in patients with long-lasting persistent atrial fibrillation.[187] It has been suggested that the benefit in prevention of atrial fibrillation may be limited to patients with left ventricular dysfunction or hypertrophy.[184] However, the role of ARBs requires further study.

Renal disease

Several randomized clinical trials have demonstrated the renal protective effects of ARBs in proteinuric diabetes. The Reduction of Endpoints in NIDDM with the Angiotensin II Antagonist Losartan (RENAAL) study and the Irbesartan Diabetic Nephropathy Trial (IDNT) were comparisons of the long-term effects of ARB therapy with conventional antihypertensive therapy on the composite primary endpoint of doubling of serum creatinine, occurrence of end-stage renal disease, or death.[188,189] Both the ARB-treated groups showed a significant reduction of the composite risk of 16–20%. The RR reductions in the ARB groups were also significant for the renal specific outcomes of doubling of serum creatinine (33% in IDNT and 25% in RENAAL) and end-stage renal disease (28% in IDNT and 25% in RENAAL).

The presence of microalbuminuria may reflect a generalized defect in vascular permeability leading to artherogenesis. Therapy with ARBs is associated with a reduction in microalbuminura and a slowing of progression to microalbuminuria.[190–192] In non-diabetic renal disease and proteinuria, therapy with

ARBs significantly reduces protein excretion in a dose-dependent manner.[193–195] The beneficial effect of losartan on the reduction of risk for hospitalization for new atrial fibrillation has been demonstrated in patients with high renal (RENAAL) as well as high cardiovascular risk (LIFE).[196]

The greatest anti-proteinuric efficacy of ARBs is often observed at the highest tested dosage, which is frequently the upper end of the blood pressure dosing range.[197,198] However, the optimal renoprotective doses have yet to be clearly established and are the subject of ongoing investigation.[197] The ROAD-MAP Study with olmesartan[199]addresses the question of whether an ARB can prevent or delay the onset of microalbuminuria in type 2 diabetes and whether this translates into protection against cardiovascular and renal disease.

The clinical effects of ARBs are summarized in Table 13.6.

A recent meta-analysis[200] suggests that in patients with diabetes, additional renoprotective actions of ARBs, beyond blood pressure lowering, remain unproven, and that there is uncertainty about the greater renoprotection afforded in non-diabetic renal disease. A renoprotective effect over and above the effect of blood pressure lowering cannot be excluded reliably, but better designed randomized trials with sufficient power to detect realistic reductions in clinically relevant endpoints are needed.

Combination therapy

Combination of an ARB with a diuretic increases the efficacy of AT1 receptor blockade as a non-responder is converted into a responder by stimulation of the RAS. BP becomes more sensitive to volume depletion induced by the diuretic. Only about 25% of hypertensive patients have high plasma renin–angiotensin with increased responsiveness to RAS blockade. Moreover, ARBs attenuate the metabolic side effects of diuretics, e.g. hypokalaemia, hyperglycaemia, hyperuricaemia (losartan) and hypercholesterolaemia.

Combining an ACE inhibitor and an ARB may produce more complete blockade of the RAS. During ACE inhibition, Ang II may be produced by

Table 13.6 Clinical effects of angiotensin receptor blockers: results from randomized clinical trials

---

Uncomplicated hypertension
Decreased blood pressure

Hypertension with left ventricular hypertrophy
Decreased mortality
Decreased incidence of new onset diabetes

Chronic heart failure
Decreased hospitalization
Decreased cardiovascular mortality

Acute myocardial infarction with or without left ventricular dysfunction
Reduced cardiovascular mortality

Proteinuric kidney disease
Decreased proteinuria

Hypertension with type 2 diabetes and proteinuria
Preservation of renal function

---

alternative pathways, independent of ACE and from a variety of peptide substrates. Therefore, generation of Ang II can proceed in an unbridled way irrespective of ACE inhibitor treatment. These pathways may be upregulated during chronic ACE blockade, explaining the escape phenomenon. With ARBs, the receptor on the target tissue is blocked independently of the pathway of Ang II synthesis. The beneficial effect of bradykinin following ACE inhibition is also preserved in combination with an ARB.

There is little information on the efficacy of the combination of an ACE inhibitor and ARB and the trials published are difficult to generalize as only small patient populations have been studied for short periods. Valsartan added to benazapril reduced the average awake ambulatory BP by a further 6.5/4.5 mmHg compared with benazapril alone.[201] Addition of candesartan to an ACE inhibitor produced an incremental reduction of BP of 15.3/10.0 mmHg.[202]

Other findings suggest a less than additive effect with ACE inhibitors and ARBs in combination. In patients in whom BP was not controlled by full dose ARB monotherapy, a diuretic, a calcium channel blocker or an ACE inhibitor provided significant additional antihypertensive effect.[203] The antihypertensive effect of the ARB-diuretic and ARB-CCB was superior to that of the ARB-ACE inhibitor combination.

ACE inhibitors and ARBs slow the progression of renal impairment in diabetic and non-diabetic kidney disease.[204] Both classes of antihypertensive agent inhibit the vasoconstrictive effects of Ang II at the efferent arteriole. In addition, ARBs and ACE inhibitors exert non-haemodynamic actions. Increases in bradykinin and other small peptides may contribute to the renoprotective effect of ACE inhibitors. In contrast, the renal production of Ang II is not completely blocked by ACE inhibition and the ARBs are selective for AT1 receptors; AT2 receptors that are unblocked mediate production of nitric oxide and attenuation of cell proliferation in the kidney.[205,206] Thus, ARBs and ACE inhibitors have overlapping and complementary mechanisms of action.

The combination of ACE inhibitor and ARB is associated with a greater antiproteinuric effect than that with either agent alone.[207,208] In COOPERATE,[209] 263 patients with non-diabetic proteinuric renal disease were randomized to receive losartan 100 mg daily, trandolapril 3 mg daily or the combination at the same doses. During a 3-year follow-up, the combination group achieved a highly significant 50% relative risk reduction for the combined endpoint of doubling of serum creatinine or end-stage renal disease. Many patients in COOPERATE had Ig A nephropathy. Whether the findings can be extrapolated to the treatment of other forms of renal disease remains to be determined. In the 12 month Candesartan and Lisinopril Microalbuminuria (CALM) II trial of patients with type 1 and type 2 diabetes, no significant differences in systolic BP or the albumin:creatinine ratio were seen when combination therapy of ACE inhibitor and ARB were compared with higher doses of the ACE inhibitor.[210]

In may be speculated that blockade of the RAS with an ACE inhibitor or an ARB should be sufficient to reduce BP effectively if the dose is optimized. The positive results with the combination of ACE inhibitor and ARB may be linked to dosage of the ACE inhibitor or ARB as monotherapy sub-optimal for complete blockade of the RAS. The Ongoing Telmisartan Alone and in Combination with Ramipril Global Endpoint Trial (ONTARGET) will provide definitive answers to many questions regarding the combination of an ACE inhibitor with an ARB.[152]

In patients with BP uncontrolled on an ARB, the addition of eplerenone at 8 weeks significantly lowers both systolic and diastolic BP. Combination of an ARB with an aldosterone receptor antagonist could improve the cardiovascular outcome in hypertensive patients. Although myocardial hypertrophy is related to increased haemodynamic workload as a consequence of hypertension, the resulting myocardial fibrosis is exaggerated by endocrine changes involving activation of the RAS, particularly aldosterone. Local production of aldosterone has been demonstrated in the heart and the vasculature. During chronic treatment with an ARB, aldosterone may not be completely suppressed; an escape phenomenon and local production of aldosterone lead to collagen deposits in the heart. Through more complete blockade of the RAS, the combination of an ARB with an aldosterone receptor antagonist should prevent the development of cardiac fibrosis and lessen the consequences of left ventricular hypertrophy.

CONCLUSIONS

The ARBs are effective antihypertensive agents in a broad range of patients and appear to have an incidence of adverse effects lower than those with other currently available drugs. National and international guidelines for the management of hypertension[211–213] recognize that hypertension often exists with other serious conditions for which, based on clinical trial data, there are 'compelling' indications for the use of ARBs. These include CHF, chronic kidney disease and diabetes mellitus. Promising results from a number of clinical trials suggest that ARBs may confer important benefits for patients with other serious conditions, such as chronic coronary artery disease, left ventricular hypertrophy, acute coronary syndromes and non-diabetic kidney disease, as well as primary and secondary prevention of cerebrovascular events.[140]

References

1. Edwards R. Segmental effects of norepinephrine and angiotensin II on isolated renal microvessels. *Am J Physiol* 1983;244:F526–F535.
2. Hura C, Kunau R. Angiotensin II – stimulated prostaglandin production by canine renal afferent arterioles. *Am J Physiol* 1983;254:F734–F745.
3. Ganong W. Neuropeptides in cardiovascular control. *J Hypertens* 1984;2(Suppl 3):15–22.
4. Zimmerman B, Sybertz E, Wong P. Interactions between sympathetic and renin-angiotensin system. *J Hypertens* 1984;2:581–588.
5. Sancho J, Re R, Burton J. The role of the renin-angiotensin-aldosterone system in cardiovascular homeostasis in normal human subjects. *Circulation* 1976;53:400–412.
6. Kjato H, Suzuki H, Tajima S, et al. Angiotensin II stimulates collagen synthesis in cultured vascular smooth muscle cells. *J Hypertens* 1991;9:17–22.
7. Zachary I, Woll P, Rozengurt E. A role for neuropeptides in the control of cell proliferation. *Dev Biol* 1987;124:295–311.
8. Wolf G, Ziyadeh FN. The role of angiotensin II in diabetic nephropathy: emphasis on non-hemodynamic mechanisms. *Am J Kidney Dis* 1997;29:153–163.
9. Durvasula R, Peterman A, Hiromura K, et al. Activation of a local tissue angiotensin system in podocytes by mechanical strain. *Kidney Int* 2004;65:30–39.
10. Nishyama A, Seth DB, Navar LG. Renal interstitial fluid angiotensin I and angiotensin II concentration during local angiotensin converting enzyme inhibition. *J Am Soc Nephrol* 2002;13:2207–2212.
11. Urata H, Kimoshita A, Misono K, et al. Identification of a highly specific chymase as a major angiotensin II-forming enzyme in the human heart. *J Biol Chem* 1990;265:22348–22357.
12. Sandberg K. Structural analysis and regulation of angiotensin receptors. *Trends Endocrinol Metab* 1994;5:28–35.

13. Catt K. Angiotensin II receptors. In: Robertson J, Nicholson J, eds. *The Renin-Angiotensin System*. London: Gower Medical; 1993:12.1–12.14.
14. Quinn S, Williams G. Regulation of aldosterone secretion. In: James VT, ed. *The Adrenal Gland*, New York: Raven Press; 1992:159–189.
15. Dzau V, Horiuchi M. Differential expression of angiotensin receptor subtypes in the myocardium: a hypothesis. *Eur Heart J* 1996;17:978–980.
16. Griedling K, Lasegue B, Alexander R. Angiotensin receptors and their therapeutic implications. *Annu Rev Pharmacol Toxicol* 1996;36:281–306.
17. Goodfriend TL. Angiotensin receptors: history and mysteries. *Am J Hypertens* 2000;13:442–449.
18. Keeton TK, Campbell WS. The pharmacologic alteration of renin release. *Pharmacol Rev* 1980;32:81–227.
19. Streeten D, Anderson G, Freiberg J, Dalakos T. Use of an angiotensin II antagonist (saralasin) in the recognition of angiotensinogenic hypertension. *N Engl J Med* 1975;292:657–662.
20. Wong PC, Chiu AT, Price WA, et al. Nonpeptide ARBs. I. Pharmacologica characterization of 2-n-butyl-4-chloro-1 (2-chlorobenzyl) imidazole-5-acetic acid, sodium salt (S-8307). *J Pharmacol Exp Ther* 1988;247:1–7.
21. Chiu AT, Duncia JV, McCall DE, et al. Nonpeptide ARBS. III. Structure function studies. *J Pharmacol Exp Ther* 1988;250:867–874.
22. Edwards RM, Aiyar N, Ohlstein EH, et al. Pharmacological characterization of the nonpeptide ARB, SK and F108566. *J Pharmacol Exp Ther* 1992;260:175–181.
23. Beevers D. Losartan: the first angiotensin receptor antagonist in clinical use. *J Hum Hypertens* 1995;9(Suppl 5):S1–S3.
24. Wexler RR, Greenlee WJ, Irvin JD, et al. Nonpeptide ARBs: the next generation in antihypertensive therapy. *J Med Chem* 1996;39:625–656.
25. Wong PC, Price WA, Chiu AT, et al. Nonpeptide angiotensin antagonists. IX. Pharmacology of EXP 3174: an active metabolite of DuP 753, an orally active antihypertensive agent. *J Pharmacol Exp Ther* 1990;255:211–217.
26. Burnier M, Waeber B, Brunner H. Clinical pharmacology of the ARB losartan in healthy subjects. *J Hypertension* 1995;13(Suppl 1):S23–S28.
27. Bernhart CA, Perreaut PM, Ferrari BP, et al. A new series of imidazolines: highly specific and potent nonpeptide AT1 ARB. *J Med Chem* 1993;36:3371–3380.
28. Buhlmeyer P, Furet P, Criscione L, et al. Valsartan, a potent, orally active angiotensin II antagonist developed from the structurally new amino acid series. *Bioorg Med Chem Lett* 1994;4:29–34.
29. Criscione L, de Gaspero M, Buhlmeyer P, et al. Pharmacologic profile of CGP-48933, a novel, nonpeptide antagonist of AT1 angiotensin II receptor subtype. *Br J Pharmacol* 1993;110:761–771.
30. Cazaubon C, Gougat J, Bouscet F, et al. Pharmacologic characterization of SR 47436: a new nonpeptide AT1 subtype ARB. *J Pharmacol Exp Ther* 1993;265:826–834.
31. Kubo K, Kohara Y, Inamya E, et al. Nonpeptide ARBs. Synthesis and biological activity of benzimidazolecarboxylic acids. *J Med Chem* 1993;36:2182–2195.
32. Kubo K, Kohara Y, Yoshimura Y, et al. Nonpeptide ARBs. Synthesis and biologic activity of potential prodrugs of benzimidazole-7-carboxylic acids. *J Med Chem* 1993;36:2343–2349.
33. Keenen RM, Weinstock J, Finkelstein JA, et al. Potent nonpeptide ARBs. 1-(carboxybenzyl) imidazole-5-acrylic acids. *J Med Chem* 1993;36:1880–1892.
34. Samamen JM, Peishoff CE, Keenen RM, Weinstock J. Refinement of a molecular model of angiotensin II employed in the discovery of potent nonpeptide antagonists. *Bioorg Med Chem Lett* 1993;3:909–914.
35. Ries UJ, Mihm G, Narr B, et al. 6-substituted benzimidazoles as new nonpeptide ARBs: synthesis, biological activity, and structure activity relationships. *J Med Chem* 1993;36:4040–4051.
36. Wienen W, Hauel N, Van Mecl JC, et al. Pharmacologic characterization of the novel nonpeptide ARB, BIBR277. *Br J Pharmacol* 1993;110:245–252.
37. Nishikawa K, Naka T, Chatani F, Yoshimura Y. Candesartan cilexetil: a review of its preclinical pharmacology. *J Hum Hypertension* 1997;11(Suppl 2):S9–S17.
38. Johnston CI, Risvanis J. Preclinical pharmacology of ARBs. *Am J Hypertens* 1997;10(Part 2):306s–310s.
39. Vauquelin G, Fierens FLP, Verheijen I, Vanderheyden PML. Distinctions between non-peptide angiotensin II AT_1 receptor antagonists. *JRAAS* 2001;2:S24–S31.
40. Sever P. Candesartan cilexetil: a new, long-acting, effective angiotensin II type 1 receptor blocker. *J Hum Hypertens* 1997;11(Suppl 2):S91–S95.
41. Morsing P, Adler G, Brandt-Eliasson U, et al. Mechanistic differences of various AT_1-receptor blockers in isolated vessels of different origin. *Hypertension* 1999;33:1406–1413.

42. Delacr(taz E, Nussberger J, Biollaz J, et al. Characterisation of the angiotensin II receptor antagonist TCV-116 in healthy volunteers. *Hypertension* 1995;25l:14–21.
43. Messerli FH, Weber MA, Brunner HR. Angiotensin II receptor inhibition. A new therapeutic principle. *Arch Intern Med* 1996;156:1957–1965.
44. Balta T, Bankal AJ, Eng S, Catt KJ. Angiotensin II receptor subtypes and biological responses in the adrenal cortex and medulla. *Mol Pharmacol* 1991;40:401–406.
45. Stadler T, Veltmar A, Qadri F, Unger T. Angiotensin II evokes noradrenaline release from the paraventricular nucleus in conscious rats. *Brain Res* 1992;569:117–122.
46. Blair-West JR, Carey K, Denton DA, et al. Evidence that brain angiotensin II is involved in both thirst and sodium appetite in baboons. *Am J Physiol* 1998;275R1639–R1639–R1646.
47. Booz EW, Baker KM. Role of type 1 and type 2 angiotensin receptors in angiotensin II induced cardiomyocyte hypertrophy. *Hypertension* 1996;28:635–640.
48. Haywood GA, Gullestand L, Katsuya T, et al. AT_1 and AT_2 angiotensin receptor gene expression in human heart failure. *Circulation* 1997;95:1201–1206.
49. Rogg H, de Gaspero M, Graedel E, et al. Angiotensin II-receptor subtypes in human atria and evidence for alterations in patients with cardiac dysfunction. *Eur Heart J* 1996;17:1112–1120.
50. Cody RJ, Haas GJ, Binkley PF, Brown DM. Hemodynamic and vascular characteristics of DuP 753: a specific angiotensin II antagonist in the spontaneous hypertensive rat (SHR). *J Am Coll Cardiol* 1991;17(Suppl A):202A.
51. Lacour C, Canals F, Galindo G, et al. Efficacy of SR 47436 (BMS - 186295), a nonpeptide angiotensin AT_1 receptor antagonist in hypertensive rat models. *Eur J Pharmacol* 1994;264:307–316.
52. Timmermans PB, Duncia JV, Carini DJ, et al. Discovery of losartan, the first ARB. *J Hum Hypertens* 1995;9(Suppl 5):S3–S18.
53. Brunner HR, Delacretaz E, Nussberger J, et al. Angiotensin II antagonists DuP 753 and TCV 116. *J Hypertens* 1994;12(Suppl 9):S29–S34.
54. Gradman AH, Arcuri KE, Goldberg AI, et al. A randomized, placebo-controlled, double-blind, parallel study of various doses of losartan potassium compared with enalapril maleate in patients with essential hypertension. *Hypertension* 1995;25:1345–1350.
55. Wong PC, Hart SD, Timmermans PB. Effect of angiotensin II antagonism on canine renal sympathetic nerve function. *Hypertension* 1991;17(Part 2):1127–1134.
56. Schiffrin E. Vascular changes in hypertension response to drug treatment: effects of angiotensin receptor blockers. *Can J Cardiol* 2002;18(Suppl A):15A–18A.
57. Resnick L, Cantanzaro D, Sealey J, Laragh J. Acute vascular effects of the angiotensin II receptor antagonist olmesartan in normal subjects: relation to the renin aldosterone system. *Am J Hypertens* 2004;17:203–208.
58. Reid IA. Interactions between ANGII, sympathetic nervous system, and baroreceptor reflexes in regulation of blood pressure. *Am J Physiol* 1992;262:E763–E778.
59. Goldberg M, Tanaka W, Burchowsky A, et al. Effects of losartan on blood pressure, plasma renin activity and angiotensin II in volunteers. *Hypertension* 1993;21:704–713.
60. Dzau VJ, Sasamura H, Hein J. Heterogeneity of angiotensin synthetic pathways and receptor subtypes: physiological and pharmacological implications. *Curr Opin Hypertens* 1993;1:3–9.
61. Bunkenberg B, Van Amelsvoort T, Roog H, Wood JM. Receptor-mediated effects of angiotensin II on growth of vascular smooth muscle cells from spontaneous hypertensive rats. *Hypertension* 1992;20:746–754.
62. Smits JF, Van Krimpen C, Schoemaker RG, et al. Angiotensin II receptor blockade after myocardial infarction in rats: effects on hemodynamics, myocardial DNA synthesis, and interstitial collagen content. *J Cardiovasc Pharmacol* 1992;20:772–778.
63. Kumagai K, Nakashima H, Urata H, et al. Effects of angiotensin II type 1 receptor antagonist on electrical and structural remodeling in atrial fibrillation. *J Am Coll Cardiol* 2003;41:2197–2204.
64. Dahlöf B. Effect of angiotensin II blockade on cardiac hypertrophy and remodelling: a review. *J Hum Hypertens* 1995;9(Suppl 5):S37–S44.
65. Kaneko R, Susic D, Nunez E, Frohlich E. Losartan reduces cardiac mass and improves coronary flow reserve in the spontaneously hypertensive rat. *J Hypertens* 1996;14:645–654.
66. Lansang M, Osei S, Price D, et al. Renal hemodynamic and hormonal responses to the angiotensin II antagonist candesartan. *Hypertension* 2000;36:834–838.
67. Burnier M, Brunner HR. Angiotensin II receptor antagonists. *Lancet* 2000;355:637–645.
68. Bauer JH, Reams GP. The angiotensin II type I receptor antagonists. A new class of antihypertensive drugs. *Arch Intern Med* 1995;155:1361–1368.
69. Price DA, D'Oliveira JM, Fisher ND, Hollenberg NK. Renal hemodynamic response to an angiotensin antagonist, eprosartan, in healthy men. *Hypertension* 1997;30:240–246.

70. Takishita S, Muratani H, Sesoko S. Short-term effects of angiotensin II blockade on renal blood flow and sympathetic activity in awake rats. *Hypertension* 1994;24:445–450.
71. Burnier M, Roch-Ramel F, Brunner HR. Renal effects of angiotensin II receptor blockade in normotensive subjects. *Kidney Int* 1996;49:1787–1790.
72. Fenoy FJ, Milicic I, Smith RD, et al. Effects of DuP 753 on renal function of normotensive and spontaneously hypertensive rats. *Am J Hypertens* 1991;4(Part 2):321s–326s.
73. Goldberg MR, Bradstreet TE, McWilliams EJ, et al. Biochemical effects of losartan, a nonpeptide ARB, on the renin-angiotensin-aldosterone system in hypertensive patients. Hypertension 995; 25 :37–46.
74. Burnier M, Brunner H. ARBs and the kidney. *Curr Opin Hypertens* 1995;1:92–100.
75. Gansevoort RT, de Zeeuw D, Shahinfar S, et al. Effects of the angiotensin II antagonist losartan in hypertensive patients with renal disease. *J Hypertens* 1994;12(Suppl): s37–s42.
76. Nakashima M, Uematsu T, Kosuge K, Kanamaru M. Pilot study of the uricosuric effect of DuP-753, a new ARB in healthy subjects. *Eur J Clin Pharmacol* 1992;42:333–335.
77. Moan A, Hoieggen A, Nordby G, et al. Effects of losartan on insulin sensitivity in severe hypertension:connections through sympathetic nervous activity? *J Hum Hypertens* 1995;9 (Suppl 5):S45–S50.
78. Braszko J. The contribution of AT_1 and AT_2 angiotensin receptors to its cognitive effects. *Acta Neurobiol Exp* 1996;56:49–54.
79. Dahlöf B, Lindholm L, Carney S, et al. Main results of the losartan versus amlodipine (LOA) study on drug tolerability and psychological well-being. *J Hypertens* 1997;15:1327–1335.
80. Armando I, Seltzer A, Bregonzio C, Saavedra J. Stress and angiotensin II: novel therapeutic opportunities. *Curr Drug Target Neurol Disord* 2003;2:413–419.
81. Lithell H, Hansson L, Skoog I, et al for the SCOPE Study Group. The Study of Cognition and Prognosis in the Elderly (SCOPE): principal results of randomised double-blind intervention trial. *J Hypertens* 2003;21:875–886.
82. Fogari R, Mugellini A, Zoppi I, et al. Effects of valsartan compared with enalapril on blood pressure and cognitive function in elderly patients with essential hypertension. *Eur J Clin Pharmacol* 2004;59:863–868.
83. Fogari R, Zoppi A, Poletti L, et al. Sexual activity in hypertensive men treated with valsartan or carvedilol: a crossover study. *Am J Hypertens* 2001;14:27–31.
84. Fogari R, Preti P, Zoppi A, et al. Effect of valsartan and atenolol on sexual behavior in hypertensive postmenopausal women. *Am J Hypertens* 2004;17:77–81.
85. Munafo A, Christen Y, Nussberger J, et al. Drug concentration response relationships in normal volunteers after oral administration of losartan, an angiotensin antagonist. *Clin Pharmacol Ther* 1992;51:513–521.
86. Ohtawa M, Takayama F, Saitoh K, et al. Pharmacokinetics and biochemical efficacy after single and multiple oral administration of losartan, on orally active nonpeptide angiotensin receptor antagonist, in humans. *Br J Pharmacol* 1993;35:290–297.
87. Weber MA. Clinical experience with the angiotensin receptor antagonist losartan: a preliminary report. *Am J Hypertens* 1992;5:S247–S251.
88. Lo M, Goldberg M, McCrea J, et al. Pharmacokinetics of losartan, an ARB, and its active metabolite EXP3174 in humans. *Clin Pharmacol Ther* 1995;58:641–649.
89. Stearns R, Chakravarty P, Chen R, Chiu S. Biotransformation of losartan to its active carboxylic acid metabolite in human liver microsomes. Role of cytochrome P450C and 3A subfamily members. *Drug Metab Dispos* 1995;23:207–215.
90. Sica D, Lo M, Shaw W, et al. The pharmacokinetics of losartan in renal insufficiency. *J Hypertens* 1995;13(Suppl 1):S49–S52.
91. Muller P, Flesch G, de Gasparo M, et al. Pharmacokinetics and pharmacodynamic effects of the angiotensin II antagonist valsartan at steady state in healthy, normotensive subjects. *Eur J Clin Pharmacol* 1997;52:441–449.
92. Flesch G, Muller P, Lloyd P. Absolute bioavailability and pharmacokinetics of valsartan, on angiotensin II antagonist, in man. *Eur J Clin Pharmacol* 1997;52:115–120.
93. Markham A, Goa K. Valsartan. A review of its pharmacology and therapeutic use in essential hypertension. *Drugs* 1997;54:299–311.
94. Colussi D, Parisot C, Rossolino M, et al. Protein binding in plasma of valsartan, a new ARB. *J Clin Pharmacol* 1997;37:214–221.
95. Brookman L, Rolan P, Benjamin I, et al. Pharmacokinetics of valsartan in patients with liver disease. *Clin Pharmacol Ther* 1997;62:272–278.
96. Ruilope L. Human pharmacokinetic/pharmacodynamic profile of irbesartan: a new potent ARB. *J Hypertens* 1997;15(Suppl 7):S15–S20.
97. Marino M, Langenbacher K, Ford N, Uderman H. Pharmacokinetics of irbesartan in healthy subjects. *J Clin Pharmacol* 1998;38:246–255.

98. Brunner H. The new ARB, irbesartan, pharmacokinetic and pharmacodynamic considerations. *Am J Hypertens* 1997;10(Part 2):S311–S317.

99. Riddell JG. Bioavailability of candesartan is unaffected by food in healthy volunteers administered candesartan cilexetil. *J Hum Hypertens* 1997;11(Suppl 2):S29–S30.

100. Hubner R, Hogemann A, Sunzel M, Riddell J. Pharmacokinetics of candesartan after single and repeated doses of candesartan cilexetil in young and elderly healthy volunteers. *J Hum Hypertens* 1997;11(Suppl 2):S19–S25.

101. van Lier JJ, van Heiningen PNM, Sunzel M. Absorption, metabolism and excretion of 14C-candesartan and 14C-candesartan cilexetil in healthy volunteers. *J Hum Hypertens* 1997; 11(Suppl 2):S27–S28.

102. de Zeeuw D, Remuzzi G, Kirch W. Pharmacokinetics of candesartan cilexetil in patients with renal and hepatic impairment. *J Hum Hypertens* 1997;11(Suppl 2):S37–S42.

103. Cox PJ, Bush BD, Gorycki PD, et al. The metabolic fate of eprosartan in healthy subjects. *Exp Toxicol Pathol* 1996;48(Suppl II):75–82.

104. Martin D, Chapelsky MC, Ilson B, et al. Pharmacokinetics and protein binding of eprosartan in healthy volunteers and in patients with varying degrees of renal impairment. *J Clin Pharmacol* 1998;38:129–137.

105. McClellan KJ, Balfour JA. Eprosartan. *Drugs* 1998;55:713–718.

106. Schwocho L, Masonson H. Pharmacokinetics of CS-866, a new angiotensin II receptor blocker, in healthy subjects. *J Clin Pharmacol* 2001;41:515–527.

107. Laies P, Puchler K, Kirch W. The pharmacokinetic and metabolic profile of olmesartan medoxomil limits the risk of clinically relevant drug interactions. *J Hypertens* 2001;19: S21–S32.

108. Ji H, Leung M, Zhang Y, et al. Differential structural requirements for specific binding on nonpeptide and peptide antagonists to the AT_1 angiotensin receptor: identification of amino acid residues that determine binding of the antihypertensive drug losartan. *J Biol Chem* 1994;269:1653–1656.

109. Azizi M, Chatellier G, Guyene T, et al. Additive effects of combined angiotensin converting enzyme inhibition and angiotensin II antagonism on blood pressure and renin release in sodium depleted normotensives. *Circulation* 1995;92:825–834.

110. Conlin P, Spence D, Williams B, et al. Angiotensin II antagonists for hypertension: are there differences in efficacy? *Am J Hypertens* 2000;13:418–426.

111. Fogari R, Zoppi A, Mugellini, et al. Comparative efficacy of losartan and valsartan in mild to moderate hypertension: results of 24-hour ambulatory blood pressure monitoring. *Curr Ther Res* 1999;60:195–206.

112. Burnier M, Maillard M. The comparative pharmacology of angiotensin II receptor antagonists. *Blood Press* 2001;1(Suppl):6–11.

113. Pitt B, Poole-Wilson PA, Segal R, et al. Effect of losartan compared with captopril on mortality in patients with symptomatic heart failure: randomised trial – the Losartan Heart Failure Survival Study ELITE II. *Lancet* 2000;355:1582–1587.

114. Julius S, Kjeldsen SE, Weber M, et al; for the VALUE trial group. Outcomes in hypertensive patients at high cardiovascular risk treated with regimens based on valsartan or amlodipine: the VALUE randomised trial. *Lancet* 2004;363:2022–2031.

115. Serebruany VL, Pokov AN, Malinin AI, et al. Valsartan inhibits platelet activity at different doses in mild to moderate hypertension: Valsartan Inhibits Platelets (VIP) trial. *Am Heart J* 2006;151:92–99.

116. Schupp M, Janke J, Clasen R, et al. Angiotensin type 1 receptor blockers induce proliferator-activated receptor-γ activity. *Circulation* 2004;109:2054–2057.

117. Cooper ME, Tikellis C, Thomas MC. Preventing diabetes in patients with hypertension: one more reason to block the renin-angiotensin system. *J Hypertens* 2006;24(Suppl 1): S57–S63.

118. Olsen MH, Fossum E, Høieggen A, et al. Long-term treatment with losartan versus atenolol improves insulin sensitivity in hypertension: ICARUS, A LIFE substudy. *J Hypertens* 2005;23:891–898.

119. Ridker PM, Danielson E, Rafai N, Glynn RJ; for the Val-MARC Investigators. Valsartan, blood pressure reduction, and C-reactive protein. Primary report of the Val-MARC trial. *Hypertension* 2006;48:73–79.

120. Koh KK, Quon MJ, Han SH, et al. Additive beneficial effects of losartan combined with simvastatin in the treatment of hypercholesterolemic, hypertensive patients. *Circulation* 2004;110:3687–3692.

121. Yasumari R, Maeda K, Watanabe T, et al. Comparative effect of valsartan versus amlodipine on left ventricular mass and reactive oxidative species formation by monocytes in hypertensive patients with left ventricular hypertrophy. *J Am Coll Cardiol* 2004;43:2116–2123.

122. Campbell DJ, Krum H, Esler MD. Losartan increases bradykinin in hypertensive humans. *Circulation* 2005;111:315–320.

123. Burke TA, Sturkenboom MC, Lu S, et al. Discontinuation of antihypertensive drugs among newly diagnosed hypertensive patients in UK general practice. *J Hypertens* 2006;24:1193–1200.

124. Pouleur HG. Clinical overview of irbesartan. *Am J Hypertens* 1997;10:S318–S324.

125. Ramsay L, Yeo W. ACE inhibitors, angiotensin II antagonists and cough. The losartan cough study group. *J Hum Hypertens* 1995;9(Suppl 5):S51–S54.

126. Acker CG, Greenberg A. Angioedema induced by the angiotensin II blocker losartan. *N Engl J Med* 1995;333:1572.

127. Frye C, Pettigrew T. Angioedema and photosensitivity rash induced by valsartan. *Pharmacotherapy* 1998;18:866–868.

128. Cicarde M, Zingale LC, Bergamaschini L, Agostoni A. Angioedema associated with angiotensin-converting enzyme use. Outcome after switching to a different treatment. *Arch Intern Med* 2004;164:908–913.

129. Tsuruoka S, Wakaumi M, Ioka T, et al. Angiotensin II receptor blocker-induces blunted taste sensitivity: comparison of candesartan and valsartan. *Br J Clin Pharmacol* 2005;60:204–207.

130. Morton J, Muir J, Lim D. Rash and acute nephritic syndrome due to candesartan. *BMJ* 2004;328:25.

131. Kaukonen K, Olkkola K, Neuvonen P. Fluconazole but not itraconazole decreases the metabolism of losartan to E-3174. *Eur J Clin Pharmacol* 1998;53:445–449.

132. De Smet M, Schoors D, De Meyer G, et al. Effect of multiple doses of losartan on the pharmacokinetics of single doses of digoxin in healthy volunteers. *Br J Clin Pharmacol* 1995;40:571–575.

133. Kong A, Tomasko L, Waldman S, et al. Losartan does not affect the pharmacokinetics and pharmacodynamics of warfarin. *J Clin Pharmacol* 1995;35:1008–1015.

134. Fossum E, Moan A, Kjeldsen SE, et al. The effect of losartan versus atenolol on cardiovascular morbidity and mortality in patients with hypertension taking aspirin. The Losartan Intervention For Endpoint reduction in hypertension (LIFE) study. *J Am Coll Cardiol* 2005;46:770–775.

135. Jonkman JHG, Van Lier JJ, Van Heiningen PNM, et al. Pharmacokinetic drug interaction studies with candesartan cilexetil. *J Hum Hypertens* 1997;11(Suppl 2):S31–S35.

136. Oparil S, Dyke S, Harris F, et al. The efficacy and safety of valsartan compared with placebo in the treatment of patients with essential hypertension. *Clin Ther* 1996;18:797–810.

137. Holwerda N, Fofari R, Angeli P, et al. Valsartan, a new angiotensin II antagonist for the treatment of essential hypertension: efficacy and safety compared with placebo and enalapril. *J Hypertens* 1996;14:1147–1151.

138. Oparil S, Barr E, Telkins M, et al. Efficacy, tolerability and effects on quality of life of losartan, alone or with hydrochlorothiazide, versus amlodipine, alone or with hydrochlorothiazide, in patients with essential hypertension. *Clin Ther* 1996;18:608–625.

139. Chrysant S, Weber M, Wang A, Hinman D. Evaluation of antihypertensive therapy with the combination of olmesartan medoxomil and hydrochlorothiazide. *Am J Hypertens* 2004;17:252–259.

140. Corvol P, Plouin P. Angiotensin II receptor blockers: current status and future prospects. *Drugs* 2002;62:53–64.

141. Andersson OK, Neldam S. The antihypertensive effect and tolerability of candesartan cilexetil, a new generation angiotensin II antagonist, in comparison with losartan. *Blood Pressure* 1998;7:53–59.

142. Oparil S, Guthrie R, Lewin A, et al. An elective-titration study of the comparative effectiveness of two angiotensin II-receptor blockers, irbesartan and losartan. *Clin Ther* 1998;20:398–409.

143. Gradman AH. AT_1-receptor blockers: differences that matter. *J Hum Hypertens* 2002;16:S9–S16.

144. Oparil S, Williams D, Chrysant S, et al. Comparative efficacy of olmesartan, losartan, valsartan and irbesartan in the control of essential hypertension. *J Clin Hypertens* 2001;3:283–291.

145. Tedesco MA, Ratti G, Aquino D, et al. The effectiveness and tolerability of losartan and effect on left ventricular mass in patients with essential hypertension. *Cardiologia* 1998;43:53–59.

146. Thurmann PA, Kenedi P, Schmidt A, et al. Influence of the angiotensin II antagonist valsartan on left ventricular hypertrophy in patients with essential hypertension. *Circulation* 1998;98:2037–2042.

147. Schneider MP, Klingbeil AU, Delles C, et al. Effect of irbesartan versus atenolol on left ventricular mass and voltage. Results of the CardioVascular Irbesartan Project. *Hypertension* 2004;44:61–66.

148. Ciulla MM, Puliotti R, Esposito A, et al. Different effect of antihypertensive therapies based on losartan or atenolol on ultrasound and biochemical markers of myocardial fibrosis. Results of a randomized trial. *Circulation* 2004;110:552–557.

149. Muller-Brunotte R, Edner M, Malmqvist K, Kahan T. Irbesartan and atenolol improve diastolic function in patients with hypertensive left ventricular hypertrophy. *J Hypertens* 2005;23:633–640.

150. Dahlöf B, Devereux RB, Kjeldson SE, et al; for the LIFE study group. Cardiovascular morbidity and mortality in the Losartan Intervention For Endpoint reduction in hypertension study (LIFE): a randomised trial against atenolol. *Lancet* 2002;359:995–1003.

151. Schrader J, Lüders S, Kulschewski A, et al. Morbidity and mortality after stroke, eprosartan compared with nitrendipine for secondary prevention. Principal results of a prospective randomised controlled study (MOSES). *Stroke* 2005;36:1218–1226.

152. The ONTARGET/TRANSCEND Investigators. Rationale, design, and baseline characteristics of 2 large, simple, randomized trials evaluating telmisartan, ramipril, and their combination in high-risk patients: The Ongoing Telmisartan alone and in Combination with Ramipril Global Endpoint Trial/Telmisartan Randomized Assessment Study in ACE Intolerant Subjects with Cardiovascular Disease (ONTARGET/TRANSCEND) trials. *Am Heart J* 2004;148:52–61.

153. Lindholm LH, Ibsen H, Dahlöf B, et al; for the LIFE study group. Cardiovascular morbidity and mortality in patients with diabetes in the Losartan Intervention For Endpoint reduction in hypertension study (LIFE): a randomised trial against atenolol. *Lancet* 2002;359:1004–1010.

154. Lindholm LH, Dahlöf B, Edelman JM, et al. Effects of losartan on sudden cardiac death in people with diabetes: data from the LIFE study. *Lancet* 2003;362:619–620.

155. Devereux RB, Dahlöf B, Gerdts E, et al. Regression of hypertensive left ventricular hypertrophy by losartan compared with atenolol. The Losartan Intervention for Endpoint reduction in hypertension (LIFE) trial. *Circulation* 2004;110:1456–1462.

156. Wachtell K, Lehto M, Gerdts E, et al. Angiotensin II receptor blockade reduces new-onset atrial fibrillation and subsequent stroke compared to atenolol. The Losartan Intervention for Endpoint reduction in hypertension (LIFE) study. *J Am Coll Cardiol* 2005;45:712–719.

157. Lindholm LH, Ibsen H, Borch-Johnsen K, et al; for the LIFE Study Group. Risk of new-onset diabetes in the Losartan Intervention For Endpoint reduction in hypertension study. *J Hypertens* 2002;20:1879–1886.

158. Kjeldsen SE, Dahlöf B, Devereux RB, et al; for the LIFE Study Group. Effects of losartan on cardiovascular morbidity and mortality in patients with isolated systolic hypertension and left ventricular hypertrophy : A Losartan Intervention for Endpoint Reduction (LIFE) substudy. *JAMA* 2002;288:1491–1498.

159. Kizer JR, Dahlöf B, Kjeldsen SE, et al. Stroke reduction in hypertensive adults with cardiac hypertrophy randomized to losartan versus atenolol. The Losartan Intervention For Endpoint reduction in hypertension study group. *Hypertension* 2005;45:46–52.

160. McInnes G, Burke TA, Carides G. Cost-effectiveness of losartan-based therapy in patients with hypertension and left ventricular hypertrophy: a UK-based economic evaluation of the Losartan Intervention For Endpoint reduction in hypertension (LIFE) study. *J Hum Hypertens* 2006;20:51–56.

161. Lithell H, Hansson L, Skoog I, et al; for the SCOPE Study Group. The Study on COgnition and Prognosis in the Elderly (SCOPE): outcomes in patients not receiving add-on therapy after randomization. *J Hypertens* 2004;22:1605–1612.

162. Papademetriou V, Farsang C, Elmfeldt D, et al; for the SCOPE Study Group. Stroke prevention with the angiotensin II type 1-receptor blocker candesartan in elderly patients with isolated systolic hypertension. The Study on Cognition and Prognosis in the Elderly (SCOPE). *J Am Coll Cardiol* 2004;44:1175–1180.

163. Schrader J, Lüders S, Kulschewski A, et al. Acute Candesartan Cilexetil Therapy in Stroke Survivors Study Group. The ACCESS study: evaluation of Acute Candesartan Cilexetil Therapy in Stroke Survivors. *Stroke* 2003;34:1699–1703.

164. Skoog I, Lithell H, Hansson L, et al; for the SCOPE Study Group. Effect of baseline cognitive function and antihypertensive treatment on cognitive and cardiovascular outcomes: Study on COgnition and Prognosis in the Elderly (SCOPE). *Am J Hypertens* 2005;18:1052–1059.

165. Weber M, Julius S, Kjeldsen SE, et al. Blood pressure dependent and independent effects of antihypertensive treatment on clinical events in the VALUE trial. *Lancet* 2004;363:2049–2051.

166. Julius S, Weber MA, Kjeldsen SE, et al. The Valsartan Antihypertensive Long-term Use Evaluation (VALUE) trial. Outcomes in patients receiving monotherapy. *Hypertension* 2006;48:385–391.

167. Strauss MH, Hall AS. Do angiotensin receptor blockers increase the risk of myocardial infarction? Angiotensin-receptor blockers may increase risk of myocardial infarction. Unravelling the ARB-MI paradox. *Circulation* 2006;114:838–854.

168. Verma S, Strauss M. Angiotensin receptor blockers and myocardial infarction. *BMJ* 2004;329:1248–1249.

169. McDonald MA, Simpson SH, Ezekowitz JA, et al. Angiotensin receptor blockers and risk of myocardial infarction: Systemic review. *BMJ* 2005;331:873–878.

170. Tsuyuki RT, McDonald MA, Strauss MH, Hall AS. Angiotensin receptor blockers do not increase risk of myocardial infarction. *Circulation* 2006;114:855–860.

171. Cheung BMY, Cheung GTY, Launder IJ, et al. Meta-analysis of large outcome trials of angiotensin receptor blockers in hypertension. *J Hum Hypertens* 2006;20:37–43.

172. Abuissa H, Jones PG, Marso SP, O'Keefe JH. Angiotensin-converting enzyme inhibitors or angiotensin receptor blockers for prevention of type 2 diabetes. A meta-analysis of randomized clinical trials. *J Am Coll Cardiol* 2005;46:821–826.

173. McMurray J, Solomon S, Pieper K, et al. The effect of valsartan, captopril, or both on atherosclerotic events after acute myocardial infarction. An analysis of the Valsartan in Acute Myocardial Infarction Trial (VALIANT). *J Am Coll Cardiol* 2006;47:726–733.

174. Pitt B, Segal R, Martinez FA, et al. Randomised trial of losartan versus captopril in patients over 65 with heart failure (Evaluation of Losartan in the Elderly Study, ELITE). *Lancet* 1997;349:747–752.

175. Carson P, Tognoni G, Cohn J. Effect of valsartan on hospitalization: results of Val-HeFT. *J Cardiac Fail* 2003;3:164–171.

176. Cohn JN, Tognoni G; for the Valsartan Heart Failure Investigators. A randomized trial of the angiotensin-receptor blocker valsartan in chronic heart failure. *N Engl J Med* 2001;345:1667–1675.

177. Granger C, McMurray J, Yusuf S, et al; for CHARM Investigators and Committees. Effects of candesartan in patients with chronic heart failure and reduced left ventricular systolic function intolerant of angiotensin converting enzyme inhibitors: the CHARM-Alternative trial. *Lancet* 2003;362:772–776.

178. McMurray J, Ostergren J, Swedberg K, et al; for CHARM Investigators and Committees. Effects of candesartan in patients with chronic heart failure and reduced left ventricular systolic function taking angiotensin-converting-enzyme inhibitors: the CHARM-Added trial. *Lancet* 2003;362:767–771.

179. Pfeffer MA, Swedberg K, Granger CB, et al; for CHARM Investigators and Committees. Effects of candesartan on mortality and morbidity in patients with chronic heart failure : the CHARM-Overall programme. *Lancet* 2003;362:759–766.

180. Yusuf S, Pfeffer MA, Swedberg K, et al; for CHARM Investigators and Committees. Effects of candesartan in patients with chronic heart failure and preserved left ventricular ejection fraction: the CHARM-Preserved trial. Lancet 3003; 362: 777–781.

181. Dickstein K, Kjekshus J; for the OPTIMAAL Steering Committee, for the OPTIMAAL Study Group. Effects of losartan and captopril on mortality and morbidity in high-risk patients after acute myocardial infarction: the OPTIMAAL randomised trial. *Lancet* 2002;360:752–760.

182. Pfeffer MA, McMurray JJ, Velazquez EJ, et al; for Valsartan in Acute Myocardial Infarction Trial Investigators. Valsartan, captopril, or both in myocardial infarction complicated by heart failure, left ventricular dysfunction, or both. *N Engl J Med* 2003;349:1893–1906.

183. Ducharme A, Swedberg K, Pfeffer MA, et al. Prevention of atrial fibrillation in patients with symptomatic chronic heart failure by candesartan in the Candesartan in Heart failure: Assessment of Reduction Mortality and morbidity (CHARM) program. *Am Heart J* 2006;151:985–991.

184. Healey JS, Baranchuk A, Crystal E, et al. Prevention of atrial fibrillation with angiotensin-converting enzyme inhibitors and angiotensin receptor blockers. A meta-analsysis. *J Am Coll Cardiol* 2005;45:1832–1839.

185. Wachtell K, Hornestan B, Lehto M, et al. Cardiovascular morbidity and mortality in hypertensive patients with a history of atrial fibrillation. The Losartan Intervention for EndPoint Reduction in Hypertension (LIFE) Study. *J Am Coll Cardiol* 2005;45:705–711.

186. Franklin SS, Wachtell K, Papademetriou V, et al. Cardiovascular morbidity and mortality in hypertensive patients with lower versus higher risk. A LIFE substudy. *Hypertension* 2005;46:492–499.

187. Madrid AH, Bueno MG, Rebello JM, et al. Use of irbesartan to maintain sinus rhythm in patients with long-lasting persistent atrial fibrillation: a prospective randomized study. *Circulation* 2002;106:331–336.

188. Brenner BM, Cooper ME, De Zeeuw D, et al; for the RENAAL Study Investigators. Effects of losartan on renal and cardiovascular outcomes in patients with type 2 diabetes and nephropathy. *N Engl J Med* 2001;345:861–869.

189. Lewis EJ, Hunsicker LG, Clarke WR, et al; for the Collaborative Study Group. Renoprotective effect of the angiotensin-receptor antagonist irbesartan in patients with nephropathy due to type 2 diabetes. *N Engl J Med* 2001;345:851–860.

190. Mogensen CE, Neldam S, Tikkanen I, et al. Randomised controlled trial of dual blockade of renin-angiotensin system in patients with hypertension, microalbuminuria, and non-insulin dependent diabetes: the candesartan and lisinopril microalbuminuria (CALM) study. *BMJ* 2000;321:1440–1444.

191. Parving HH, Lehnert H, Brochner Martensen J, et al. The effect of irbesartan on the development of diabetic nephropathy in patients with type 2 diabetes. *N Engl J Med* 2001;345:870–878.

192. Viberti G, Wheeldon NM; for the MicroAlbuminuria Reduction with VALsartan (MARVAL) Study Investigators. Microalbuminuria reduction with valsartan in patients with type 2 diabetes mellitus. A blood pressure-independent effect. *Circulation* 2002;106: 672–678.

193. Frascini LM, Van Vigier R, Pfister R, et al. Effectiveness and safety of the angiotensin II antagonist irbesartan in children with chronic kidney diseases. *Am J Hypertens* 2002;15:1057–1063.

194. Kurokawa K. Effects of candesartan on the proteinuria of chronic glomerulonephritis. *J Hum Hypertens* 1999;13:s57–s60.

195. Plum J, Bunten B, Grabense B. Effects of the angiotensin II antagonist valsartan on blood pressure, proteinuria, and renal hemodynamics on patients with chronic renal failure and hypertension. *J Am Soc Nephrol* 1998;9:2223–2234.

196. Carr AA, Kowey PR, Devereux RB, et al. Hospitalizations for new heart failure among subjects with diabetes mellitus in the RENAAL and LIFE studies. *Am J Cardiol* 2005;96:1530–1536.

197. Schmieder RE, Klingbeil AU, Fleischmann EH, et al. Additional antiproteinuric effect of ultrahigh dose of candesartan: a double-blind randomized, prospective study. *J Am Soc Nephrol* 2005;16:3038–3045.

198. Weir MR. Angiotensin II receptor blockers: the importance of dose in cardiovascular and renal risk reduction. *J Clin Hypertens* 2004;4:315–323.

199. Haller H, Viberti GC, Mimran A, et al. Preventing microalbuminuria in patients with diabetes: rationale and design of the Randomised Olmesartan and Diabetes Microalbuminuria Prevention (ROADMAP) Study. *J Hypertens* 2006;24: 403–408.

200. Casas JP, Chua W, Loukogeorgakis S, et al. Effect of inhibitors of the renin-angiotensin system and other antihypertensive drugs on renal outcomes: systemic review and meta-analysis. *Lancet* 2005;366:2026–2033.

201. Stergiou GS, Skeva II, Baibas NM, et al. Additive hypotensive effect of angiotensin converting enzyme inhibition and angiotensin receptor antagonism in essential hypertension. *J Cardiovasc Pharmacol* 2000;35:937–941.

202. Weir MR, Smith DH, Neutal JM, Bedigian MP. Valsartan alone or with a diuretic or ACE inhibitor as treatment for African-American hypertensives: relation to salt intake. *Am J Hypertens* 2001;14:665–671.

203. Stergiou GS, Makris T, Papavasiliou M, et al. Comparison of the antihypertensive effects of an angiotensin-converting enzyme inhibitor, a calcium antagonist and a diuretic in patients with hypertension not controlled by angiotensin receptor blocker monotherapy. *J Hypertens* 2005;23:883–889.

204. Taal MW, Brenner BM. Renoprotective benefits of RAS inhibition: from ACE inhibitors to angiotensin II antagonism. *Kidney Int* 2000;57:1803–1817.

205. Delles C, Jacobi I, John S. Effects of enalapril and eprosartan on the renal vascular nitric oxide system in human essential hypertension. *Kidney Int* 2002;61: 1462–1468.

206. Noris M, Remozzi G. ACE inhibitors and AT_1 receptor antagonists: is two better than one? *Kidney Int* 2002;61:1545–1547.

207. Campbell R, Sangalli F, Petricucci F, et al. Effects of combined ACE inhibitor and angiotensin II antagonist treatment in human chronic nephropathies. *Kidney Int* 2003;63:1094–1103.

208. Segura J, Praga M, Campo C, et al. Combination is better than monotherapy with ACE inhibitor or angiotensin receptor antagonist at recommended doses. *JRAAS* 2003;4: 43–47.

209. Nakao N, Yoshimura A, Morita H, et al. Combination treatment of angiotensin II receptor blockers and angiotensin converting enzyme inhibitor in non-diabetic renal disease (COOPERATE): a randomised controlled trial. *Lancet* 2003;361:117–124.

210. Andersen NH, Poulsen PL, Knudsen ST, et al. Long-term dual blockade with candesartan and lisinopril in hypertensive patients with diabetes: the CALM II study. *Diabetes care* 2005;28:273–277.

211. Chobanian AV, Bakris GL, Black HL, et al. Seventh report of the Joint National Committee on prevention, detection, evaluation, and treatment of high blood pressure. *Hypertension* 2003;42:1206–1252.

212. Guidelines Committee 2003. European Society of Hypertension – European Society of Cardiology guidelines for the management of arterial hypertension. *J Hypertens* 2003;21:1011–1053.
213. Williams B, Poulter NR, Brown MJ, et al. Guidelines for management of hypertension: report of the fourth working party of the British Hypertension Society, 2004 – BHS IV. *J Human Hypertens* 2004;18:139–185.

14 | Vasopeptidase inhibitors

Luis Miguel Ruilope

INTRODUCTION

Vasopeptidase inhibitors are a class of drugs which simultaneously inhibit both angiotensin-converting enzyme and neutral endopeptidase (NEP). Angiotensin-converting enzyme inhibitors (ACE inhibitors) have a well-established clinical role in hypertension and heart failure[1] (Chapter 12).

Neutral endopeptidase is a membrane-bound metalloprotease found principally in the brush-border membrane of renal tubules, in the lungs, intestine, adrenal, brain, heart, and peripheral blood vessels.[2,3] NEP plays a role in the initial enzymatic degradation of the bioactive carboxyterminal portions of the natriuretic peptides. These peptides are involved in the regulation of blood pressure and plasma volume.[4] The atrial and so-called brain-derived natriuretic peptides (A- and B-type natriutetic peptides) are produced principally in the myocardium in response to atrial distention. C-type natriuretic peptide, found in the kidney, heart, lung, and vascular endothelium, is released in response to shear stress.[3] Natriuretic peptides exert physiological effects at several sites, resulting in vasodilation, natriuresis, diuresis, decreased aldosterone release, decreased cell growth, and inhibition of the sympathetic nervous system and the renin–angiotensin–aldosterone system.[4] In addition, atrial (A-type) natriuretic peptide inhibits production of endothelin, a potent vasoconstrictor peptide with growth-promoting properties derived mainly from the endothelium.[5]

Beside the degradation of the natriuretic peptides, NEP has many other substrates including adrenomedullin, Ang I, Ang II, endothelin, bradykinin, substance P, chemotactic peptide, enkephalins, and the amyloid (beta) peptide.[6,7]

CLASSIFICATION: COMPOUNDS

The similarity of the structure of the active sites of NEP and ACE provided a theoretical basis for the development of single molecules that inhibit both enzymes, thus targeting multiple pathways of cardiovascular regulation.

Several agents have been synthesized; some have been assessed clinically while others have not undergone clinical assessment, because of low potency, short duration of action, and poor bioavailability or for other reasons.

This section provides a brief description of several vasopeptidase inhibitors including omapatrilat, the most intensively studied member of the group. A detailed account of the pharmacology and clinical use of omapatrilat is contained in later sections.

Sampatrilat

Sampatrilat is a dual inhibitor of neutral endopeptidase (NEP) and angiotensin converting enzyme (ACE), developed by Pfizer and Shire for the potential treatment of hypertension.[8] Sampatrilat reduces mean arterial pressure, enhances daily sodium excretion, increases renal blood flow and decreases left ventricular mass in a dog model of heart failure. In hypercholesterolaemic rabbits, sampatrilat suppresses atherogenesis and improves endothelial function.[9] In rats with coronary heart failure following left coronary artery ligation (CAL), sampatrilat 30 mg/kg per day administered orally from the first to the sixth week after surgery improves haemodynamic function and cardiac remodelling through a direct action on the failing heart.[10] Mortality was reduced (20% versus 57% for untreated rats). Sampatrilat did not affect arterial blood pressure, whereas the drugs attenuated the CAL-induced increases in the left ventricular end-diastolic pressure, heart weight, and collagen content of the viable left ventricle.

MDL 100,240

MDL 100,240 is a prodrug that, upon conversion to MDL 100,173, acts as a potent dual inhibitor of ACE and NEP with a balanced action on both enzymes. Studies in vivo in experimental models of hypertension and congestive heart failure confirmed the vasodilatory and natriuretic effects of MDL, which appear to be independent of the degree of activation of the renin–angiotensin–aldosterone system. In addition, MDL 100,240 was shown to be effective both in preventing and in regressing hypertension-induced vascular remodelling and cardiac hypertrophy.[11] In a transgenic rat model of hypertension[12] with severe cardiovascular damage due to enhanced tissue synthesis of angiotensin II (Ang II) MDL 100,240 (and ramipril) significantly lowered blood pressure compared with placebo. Both drugs attenuated left ventricular hypertrophy. MDL 100,240 also prevented aortic dilatation and hypertrophy of the mesenteric arterioles and lowered the tension responses to phenylephrine, and endothelin-1. Plasma aldosterone and creatinine levels were also decreased. Thus, severe hypertension and related cardiovascular disease were regressed by MDL 100,240.

Gemopatrilat

This azepinone derivative (BMS-189921) showed blood pressure-lowering properties in animal models of hypertension with activity similar to that of omapatrilat.[13] In normotensive Wistar nephrotic rats, the renoprotective actions of gemopatrilat were dependent on dietary sodium intake: during a low sodium diet, gemopatrilat was renoprotective, but less effective than lisinopril.

Fasidotril

This compound also proved to be effective in animal models of hypertension.[14] Fasidotril treatment (100 mg/kg twice daily for 3 weeks) resulted in a progressive and sustained decrease in systolic blood pressure (-20 to -30 mmHg) in spontaneously hypertensive and Goldblatt (renovascular) rats compared with vehicle-treated rats and prevented the progressive rise in blood pressure in DOCA-salt hypertensive rats.[14]

Mixanpril

Mixanpril is a benzotylthioacetate prodrug of S21402 which has been studied extensively in various rat rodent models.[15] S21402 decreased blood pressure similarly in DOCA-salt and renovascular rats indicating that the antihypertensive effect is independent of the renin–angiotensin system. In diabetic spontaneously hypertensive rats, mean systolic blood pressure (200 ± 5 mmHg) was reduced by mixanpril (176 ± 2 mmHg) by captopril (162 ± 5 mmHg), valsartan (173 ± 5 mmHg), and amlodipine (159 ± 4 mmHg), and was further reduced by the combination of captopril with valsartan (131 ± 5 mmHg). Only mixanpril and the combination of captopril and valsartan significantly reduced mesenteric weight. The mesenteric wall/lumen ratio was reduced by all drugs, but to a greater extent by the combination of captopril and valsartan.[16]

Z-13752A

This drug has been studied in a canine model of coronary-artery occlusion, where it proved to be effective.[17] Z-13752 reduced the consequences of coronary artery occlusion in a canine model. This protection was largely due to potentiation of released bradykinin.[17]

Omapatrilat

The most extensively investigated ACE/NEP inhibitor is omapatrilat (Bristol Myers Squibb). As reviewed by Weber[18] and more recently by Campbell,[19] multiple experimental studies have demonstrated that omapatrilat lowers blood pressure in animals. The major characteristic of omapatrilat is that it lowers blood pressure in all models of hypertension whatever the degree of activity of the renin–angiotensin system.[20] In salt-sensitive Dahl rats, a high-sodium diet significantly impaired endothelium-dependent relaxation. When such animals were treated with omapatrilat there was a far greater return towards normal responsiveness than there was with captopril.[21] Relaxation was reduced to 31% of baseline by the high-salt diet, and was then increased to 86% by omapatrilat and to only 56% by captopril. In spontaneous hypertensive rats, omapatrilat induced a sustained lowering of systolic blood pressure (-68 mmHg) without changes in cardiac rate. Blood pressure normalization was accompanied by increases in plasma Ang I, Ang II and Ang-(1-7) levels, with relevant increases in urinary excretion rates of Ang I and Ang-(1-7) but not Ang II.[22] In conscious dogs made hypertensive by bilateral renal wrapping, intravenous administration of omapatrilat reduced peak left ventricular pressure through arterial vasodilation and preload reduction. Omapatrilat increased plasma levels of adrenomedullin whereas levels of the natriuretic peptide and cGMP were unchanged.[23]

Omapatrilat has beneficial cardiorenal and humoral actions in different animal models of congestive heart failure.[18,19] In a cardiomyopathic hamster model, treatment with omapatrilat decreased left-ventricular end-diastolic pressure and left-ventricular systolic pressure. The changes were associated with a 40% increase in cardiac output, a 47% decrease in peripheral vascular resistance, and a decrease in mean arterial pressure. In rats, survival 24 hours after myocardial infarction (MI) improved with omapatrilat.[24] Besides, omapatrilat reduced infarct size 24 hours after MI and reduced ventricular arrhythmia score 1-12 hours after MI. The rats treated with the drug had reduced left ventricular diastolic and systolic dimensions and left and right ventricular weights compared with controls, indicating a decrease in reactive hypertrophy. Improvement in cardiac remodelling was accompanied by improved cardiac haemodynamics.[24] Cardiomyocyte apoptosis continues at a high level late after MI and contributes to adverse cardiac remodelling.[25] Myocardial apoptosis was reduced by angiotensin converting enzyme inhibition. However, vasopeptidase inhibition was more effective than selective angiotensin converting enzyme inhibition in preventing adverse cardiac remodelling after MI.[25]

In insulin-resistant Zucker fatty rats, omapatrilat resulted in a lower rate of endogenous glucose production compared with placebo at baseline and greater suppression of endogenous glucose production after insulin administration both at low and high doses. The insulin-sensitizing effects of omapatrilat were blocked by HOE-140 (a bradykinin, B2 receptor antagonist) and NG-nitro L-arginine methyl ester (a nitric oxide synthase inhibitor) in all tissues except myocardium. This insulin sensitizing effect was greater than that of ramipril.[26] Furthermore, greater attenuation of albuminuria was afforded by omapatrilat than by perindopril in diabetic spontaneously hypertensive rats. Omapatrilat led to a 33% reduction in renal NEP binding and this was associated with less albuminuria and prevention of renal structural injury (assessed by glomerulosclerotic index and tubulointerstitial area).[27]

MECHANISM OF ACTION

NEP inhibition

Since inhibition of NEP protects the natriuretic peptides and bradykinin from catabolism, it should be beneficial in the treatment of hypertension and congestive heart failure. However, discordant findings have been reported among hypertensive patients.[28–31] The variable effect of NEP inhibition on blood pressure and systemic vascular resistance is likely to be due to increased levels of some vasoconstrictors such as Ang II and endothelin and reduced levels of the vasodilator Ang-(1-7). Increased blood pressure during NEP inhibition in healthy volunteers was associated with an increase in plasma endothelin levels.[31] Both animal and clinical studies show that NEP inhibition increases plasma levels of Ang I, Ang II, aldosterone and catecholamines.[28,32]

Rationale for combining ACE and NEP inhibitors

Like NEP, ACE is a peptidase found in both endothelial and epithelial cells, mainly in the lungs, kidneys, and blood vessels,[2,3] but which blocks the renin–angiotensin system at different levels (see Chapter 12). Therefore, NEP inhibition protects natriuretic peptides from inactivation whereas ACE inhibition attenuates the formation of Ang II. Ang II acts as a physiological antagonist of atrial natriuretic peptide. ACE's inhibition[33,34] not only interrupts the renin–angiotensin system but also increases bradykinin, nitric oxide and prostacyclin. Potential benefits of bradykinin include natriuretic, vasodilator, and cardioprotective effects; antihypertrophic and antiarrythmogenic effects; and improved glucose uptake by myocites.[35]

Simultaneous inhibition of both ACE and NEP lowers blood pressure more than either of them alone in both animals and humans. For example, in patients given candoxatril (a NEP inhibitor) for a month the blood pressure was unchanged,[36] and in healthy volunteers candoxatril administration was followed by a rise in systolic pressure in association with an increase in the concentration of endothelin.[31] However, in spontaneously hypertensive rats, the combination of a NEP inhibitor (SCH 42495) and the ACE inhibitor captopril, as well as the dual NEP/ACE inhibitor S21402, reduced systolic blood pressure more effectively than the ACE inhibitor or the NEP inhibitor alone.[37] In human hypertension, although candoxatril alone has little influence on blood pressure, when administered in combination with lisinopril, the antihypertensive effect is of considerable magnitude: supine systolic BP 19 mmHg, diastolic BP 8 mmHg. Lisinopril alone: erect systolic BP 25 mmHg, diastolic BP 10 mmHg.[38] Favrat et al.[30] compared a NEP inhibitor (sinorphan), captopril, and the two drugs in combination in patients with essential hypertension. Neither agent alone produced significant day-long blood pressure changes, but there were substantial decreases in the combination treatment.

The inhibition of these enzymes (NEP and ACE) and the increased availability of natriuretic peptides result in vasodilatory effects and, possibly, tissue protective effects, and also in reduced formation of angiotensin II (Fig. 14.1). Since NEP and ACE are intimately concerned with regulating structural and functional properties of the heart and circulation, the term vasopeptidase inhibitor has been coined for this new drug class.

PHARMACOKINETICS/METABOLISM

Omapatrilat has a plasma half-life of 14–19 hours at doses 10–80 mg/day.[39] It is absorbed rapidly after oral administration, and peak concentrations are reached in only 0.5–2.0 hours. The drug has a prolonged elimination profile. Omapatrilat is metabolized primarily by the formation of disulphide linkages with endogenous thiols, amide hydrolysis, S-methylation, and S-oxidation. The main metabolites of omapatrilat include phenylmercaptopropionic acid (PMPA), the side chain acid derived from amide hydrolysis of omapatrilat; S-methyl omapatrilat; S-methyl PMPA; and cyclic S-oxide omapatrilat, an active metabolite. The ratio of the area under the curve for plasma concentrates on day 10 to that of day 1 when omapatrilat was given constantly during a 10-day period was 1.65. Thus, there is only a small tendency to accumulation, and accumulation does not appear to be increased in the presence of reduced renal function.[40]

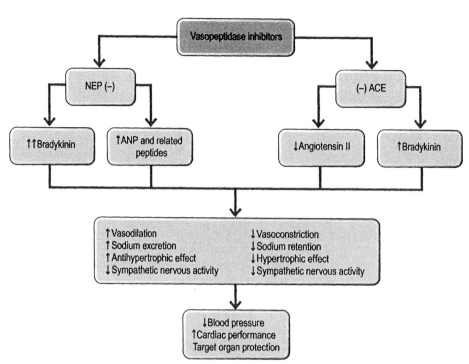

Fig. 14.1 Functional effects of vasopeptidase inhibition. NEP: neutral endopeptidase. ACE: angiotensin-converting enzyme. ANP: atrial natriuretic peptide.

PHARMACODYNAMICS

Omapatrilat inhibited NEP and ACE with inhibitory constants (Ki) of 9 nmol/L and 6 nmol/L, respectively. In a randomized, placebo-controlled trial, urinary and plasma ANP, cyclic guanosine 3¢, 5¢-monophosphate ([cGMP] a secondary messenger of NPs), serum ACE activity, and plasma renin activity were assessed after repeated omapatrilat administration in healthy subjects.[39] Increased urinary excretion of cGMP and elevated serum cGMP with increased urinary ANP indicated inhibition of NEP. Significant and sustained decreases in serum ACE activity were dose-related with omapatrilat. Small but consistent increases in plasma renin activity were also dose-related. Omapatrilat reduces serum ACE activity by more than 80% during the full 24-hour dosing interval at all doses.[39]

ADVERSE EFFECTS

Owing to overlapping pharmacological actions, some adverse effects commonly seen with ACE inhibitors are also seen with omapatrilat (Table 14.1). Common adverse effects include cough, hypotension, dizziness, increase in serum creatinine or blood urea nitrogen levels, and hyperkalaemia. Large clinical trials report similar frequencies of cough and hyperkalaemia to those seen with ACE inhibitors. However, significant increases in serum creatinine and blood

Table 14.1 Adverse effects of omapatrilat compared with lisinopril[53]

Adverse effect	Adverse effects [number (%)]		
	Omapatrilat N = 289	Lisinopril n = 284	p value
Dizziness	94 (33)	52 (18)	0.0001
Hypotension	29 (10)	17 (6)	NR
Cough	30 (10)	31 (11)	NS
Increased Scr	5 (1.8)	17 (6.1)	0.009
Increased BUN	7 (2.5)	19 (6.8)	0.016
Hyperkalaemia	6 (2.1)	10 (3.6)	NS
Diarrhoea	34 (12)	15 (5)	0.007
Visual disturbance	18 (6)	7 (3)	0.039
Tracheobronchitis	15 (5)	5 (2)	0.038
Study drug withdrawn	4 (1)	6 (2)	NS

NR = not reported; NS = not significant; Scr = serum creatinine; BUN = blood urea nitrogen.

urea nitrogen levels are less commonly reported compared with ACE inhibitors. Dizziness and hypotension seem to be more common with omapatrilat. This is likely the result of the large reduction in blood pressure seen with omapatrilat. Of greater concern is angio-oedema. Angio-oedema is believed to be a result of bradykinin accumulation. Based on pharmacodynamic studies in an animal model, omapatrilat appears to have the most potent inhibitory effect on bradykinin metabolism when compared with an ACE inhibitor and NEP inhibitor alone.[41,42] Among over 6000 patients exposed to the drug, 44 cases of angio-oedema were reported.[43] In four cases, intubation was required. Most cases were associated with a starting dose of omapatrilat 20 mg or higher, suggesting that this adverse effect is dose related. The Omapatrilat Cardiovascular Treatment Assessment Versus Enalapril (OCTAVE)[44] study randomized 25 302 hypertensive subjects to either omapatrilat titrated up to 80 mg daily or enalapril titrated up to 40 mg/day for a period of 24 weeks. The chief interest in this study was to assess the relative incidence of angio-oedema in the two treatment groups. Angio-oedema was reported in 2.17% of the subjects who received omapatrilat and in 0.68% of patients receiving enalapril. Furthermore, the individual episodes with omapatrilat were more severe and appeared earlier, the majority occurring within the first few hours after the initial dose. The relative risk for angio-oedema was 3.1 times higher in the omapatrilat group than in the enalapril group, but the risk for angio-oedema requiring hospitalization was 9.5 times higher. However, most cases did not require aggressive treatment; 59% and 76% of subjects experiencing angio-oedema with omapatrilat and enalapril, respectively, received either no treatment or were treated with antihistamines only. It was also possible to identify risk factors predisposing to angio-oedema, which was more common in black patients than in other ethnic groups and among smokers. In black patients, the rate of angio-oedema was increased approximately threefold with both omapatrilat and enalapril (5.54% and 1.62%, respectively). The rate of angio-oedema was also increased in current smokers receiving omapatrilat (3.93%) but not enalapril (0.81%).

DRUG INTERACTIONS

Drug and food interactions have not been observed with this drug. It is assumed that omapatrilat would share some of the drug interactions seen with ACE inhibitors. Some common drugs interacting with ACE inhibitors are allopurinol, aspirin, azathioprine, lithium, potassium supplements, potassium sparing diuretics, and trimethoprim.

CLINICAL USE

Due to the capacity to inhibit NEP and ACE, leading to potentiation of natriuretic peptide actions and suppression of the renin–angiotensin–aldosterone system, vasopeptidase inhibitors have potential for use in the management of hypertension and heart failure.

Preliminary human studies and clinical trials in hypertension

Preliminary studies demonstrated that omapatrilat lowers blood pressure dose-dependently[45,46] at doses ranging between 1 and 80 mg/day in normotensive subjects and in patients with mild to moderate hypertension, regardless of age, race or gender. In patients with hypertension, omapatrilat produces greater decreases in both systolic, diastolic, and pulse pressure than does ACE inhibition alone.[18,19,47] Omapatrilat (80 mg/d) was a more effective hypotensive agent than was enalapril (40 mg/d) over 12 weeks of therapy in hypertensive subjects studied 24 hours after the last administration. Comparison with the calcium channel blocker amlodipine also revealed more pronounced antihypertensive effects for omapatrilat.[48]

In OCTAVE[44] blood pressure reduction was greater with omapatrilat than with enalapril (systolic BP 3 mmHg, diastolic BP 2 mmHg). Subjects randomized to omapatrilat were more likely to reach BP target, regardless of demographics or comorbid conditions and whether omapatrilat was used as initial therapy, or in addition to existing therapy (Fig. 14.2). The OPERA (Omapatrilat in Persons with Enhanced Risk of Atherosclerotic Events) trial was a large international placebo-controlled trial intended to evaluate the effects of omapatrilat in elderly patients.[49] The plan was to study 12 600 participants in a 5-year multinational, randomized, double-blind, placebo-controlled trial. The primary objective of OPERA was to test the hypothesis that omapatrilat significantly enhances survival and reduces cardiovascular outcomes in older ($\geq$ 65 years) men and women with enhanced risk of atherosclerotic events due to stage 1 isolated systolic hypertension. OPERA would also determine whether or not treatment was justified in older patients with mild systolic hypertension where no clear evidence exists that any therapeutic intervention is of clinical value. The OPERA study was discontinued when the results of OCTAVE became available.

Clinical trials in congestive heart failure

In heart failure patients, omapatrilat produces an acute dose-related haemodynamic improvement that is maintained for at least 12 weeks.[50,51] Omapatrilat

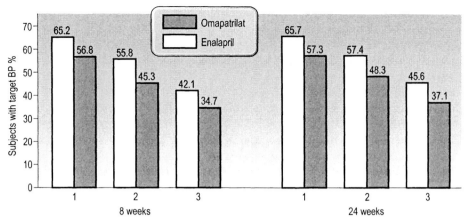

Fig. 14.2 Blood pressure control rates by study group at weeks 8 and 24: target blood pressure (BP) was < 140 mmHg systolic and < 90 mmHg diastolic. Group 1 included untreated hypertensive subjects (systolic BP ≥ 140 mmHg or diastolic BP ≥ 90 mmHg). Group 2 consisted of treated hypertensive patients with persistent mild hypertension (BP at randomization, stage I according to the Sixth Report of the Joint National Committee on Prevention, Detection, Evaluation, and Treatment of High Blood pressure (JNC-VI) criteria: trough SBP 140 to 159 mmHg and DBP < 100 mmHg, or trough DBP 90 to 99 mmHg and SBP < 160 mmHg) and replaced previous therapy with omapatrilat or enalapril at randomization. Group 3 comprised treated hypertensive subjects with persistent moderate to severe hypertension (BP at randomization in JNC-VI stage II: trough SBP 160 to 179 mmHg and DBP < 110 mmHg, or trough DBP 100 to 109 mmHg and SBP < 180 mmHg) who had omaptrilat or enalapril added to prior at randomization (from[43]).

not only reduced blood pressure in patients with heart failure but also reduced the augmentation index and increased post-obstructive brachial artery reactive hyperaemia.[52] In 48 patients in New York Heart Association functional class II or III, with left ventricular ejection fraction ≤ 40% and in sinus rhythm, omapatrilat improved functional status at 12 weeks. Dose-dependent improvements in left ventricular ejection fraction and left ventricular end-systolic wall stress (sigma), together with a reduction in systolic blood pressure were seen. There was evidence of a natriuretic effect, and total blood volume decreased. Omapatrilat induced an increase in post-dose plasma atrial natriuretic peptide levels in the high dose groups, with a reduction in pre-dose plasma brain natriuretic peptide and epinephrine levels after 12 weeks of therapy.[53]

IMPRESS (Inhibition of Metallo Protease by BMS-186716 in a Randomized Exercise and Symptoms Study in Subjects with Heart Failure)[54] compared 289 patients treated with omapatrilat (target dose 40 mg daily) and 284 patients given lisinopril (target dose 20 mg daily). All patients had previously been on an ACE inhibitor. Omapatrilat was more effective in improving outcomes in class III/IV patients. By the end of the 7-month observation period, omapatrilat had a significant advantage in the combined endpoint of mortality, admission for worsening heart failure, and discontinuation of study medication because of worsening heart failure. This promising finding led to a large clinical trial: Omapatrilat Versus Enalapril Randomized Trial of Utility in Reducing Events (OVERTURE). The OVERTURE study[55] assigned 5770 patients with New York Heart Association class II to IV heart failure to treatment with either enalapril (10 mg twice daily) or omapatrilat (40 mg once daily) for a mean of 14.5 months. Enalapril or omapatrilat were added to conventional therapy that included β-blockers in 50% of patients. The primary endpoint of combined risk of death or hospitalization for heart failure was not different for the two treatment groups, fulfilling prespecified criteria for non-inferiority but not for superiority. Analysis of secondary outcomes showed that the omapatrilat group had a 9% lower risk of cardiovascular death or hospitalization and a 6% lower risk of death. Post-hoc analysis showed an 11% lower risk for hospitalization for heart failure in patients treated with omapatrilat. Although angio-oedema was reported more commonly with omapatrilat than with enalapril, the absolute frequency, incremental risk, and severity in the OVERTURE study was lower than those reported in hypertensive patients and this was attributed to the possibility that patients with heart failure may be resistant to the ability of bradykinin to produce cutaneous exudation, as has been reported in dogs with experimental heart failure.[56] Of the other adverse events of the OVERTURE study, hypotension and dizziness were more frequent with omapatrilat (19.5% and 19.4%, respectively) than with enalapril (11.5% and 13.9%) but heart failure and renal impairment were less frequent with omapatrilat (22.6% and 6.8%) than with enalapril (25.6% and 10.1%). The incidence of cough was similar for omapatrilat and enalapril therapy (9.7% and 9.0%, respectively). In conclusion, the OVERTURE trial demonstrated that omapatrilat reduced morbidity and mortality in patients with moderate-to-severe heart failure but was not more effective than ACE inhibition alone in reducing the risk of a primary clinical event. However, secondary and post-hoc analysis focusing on all cardiovascular events suggested the possibility of between-group differences in favour of omapatrilat.

Sheth et al.[57] randomized 107 patients with ischaemic or dilated cardiomiopathy, NYHA functional class II to III, with left ventricular ejection < 40%, and on ACE inhibitor therapy either to omapatrilat 40mg daily or lisinopril 20 mg/day. C-terminal atrial natriuretic peptide levels decreased with lisinopril but not with omapatrilat. Endothelin-1 levels increased in both groups, but the increase reached statistical significance only with omapatrilat. Levels of the proinflammatory cytokine interleukin-6 tended to decrease, and the anti-inflammatory cytokine interleukin-10 increased in both groups but with statistical significance only for omapatrilat therapy. These effects of omapatrilat on endothelin-1 and anti-inflammatory cytokines may provide potential explanations for differences in clinical outcomes in heart failure patients.

CONCLUSIONS

The natriuretic peptides have actions that might be considered beneficial for hypertensive patients: vasodilation, natriuresis, and inhibition of the sympathetic nervous system and the renin–angiotensin–aldosterone system.[19,58] Several studies with omapatrilat have shown that it is a highly potent antihypertensive agent, and higher than some of the leading antihypertensives such as losartan, amlodipine and lisinopril.[18] However, the angio-oedema risk with omapatrilat has cast a shadow over the entire ACE/NEP inhibitor class.

The future of the vasopeptidase inhibitors will depend on the ability to improve the risk/benefit ratio either by developing agents that produce less angio-oedema, or by defining more precisely a high risk population that could take advantage of dual ACE/NEP inhibition. The NEP drug class probably does have a role in hypertension, although only in otherwise difficult-to-manage hypertensive patients, where the risk of angio-oedema is counterbalanced by having effected blood pressure control. Omapatrilat reduced albuminuria, prevented renal structural injury in diabetic spontaneously hypertensive rats[27] and has insulin sensitizing effect.[26] Today, patients with diabetic renal failure represent a rapidly growing population. These patients have a high cardiovascular and high renal risk. Whether vasopeptidase inhibitors would help in retarding the progression of renal failure in these patients is not known. Therefore, additional studies are warranted in this and other high risk populations.

References

1. Dzau VJ, Bernstein K, Celermajer D, et al. Pathophysiologic and therapeutic importance of tissue ACE: a consensus report. *Cardiovasc Drugs Ther* 2002;16:149–160.
2. Wilkins MR, Unwin RJ, Kenny AJ. Endopeptidase-24.11 and its inhibitors: potential therapeutic agents for edematous disorders and hypertension. *Kidney Int* 1993;43:273–285.
3. Gonzalez W, Soleilhac JM, Fournie-Zaluski MC, et al. Characterization of neutral endopeptidase in vascular cells, modulation of vasoactive peptide levels. *Eur J Pharmacol* 1998;345:323–331.
4. Levin ER, Gardner DG, Samson WK. Natriuretic peptides. *N Engl J Med* 1998;339:321–328.
5. Ruschitzka F, Corti R, Noll G, Luscher TF. A rationale for treatment of endothelial dysfunction in hypertension. *J Hypertens* 1999;17:S25–S35.
6. Burnett Jr. JC. Vasopeptidase inhibition. A new concept in blood pressure management. *J Hypertens* 1999;17:S37–S43.
7. Robl JA, Sun CQ, Stevenson J, et al. Dual metalloprotease inhibitors: mercaptoacetyl-based fused heterocyclic dipeptide mimetics as inhibitors of angiotensin-converting enzyme and neutral endopeptidase. *J Med Chem* 1997;40:1570–1577.
8. Allikmets K. Sampatrilat Shire. *Curr Opin Investig Drugs* 2002;3:578–581.
9. Kullo IJ, Miller VM, Lawson GM, Burnett JC. Jr. Dual inhibition of neutral endopeptidase (NEP) and angiotensin converting enzyme (ACE) suppresses atherogenesis and improved endothelial function in hypercholesterolemic rabbits. *J Am Coll Cardiol* 1996;272:164A.
10. Maki T, Nasa Y, Tanonaka K, et al. Beneficial effects of sampatrilat, a novel vasopeptidase inhibitor, on cardiac remodeling and function of rats with chronic heart failure following left coronary artery ligation. *J Pharmacol Exp Ther* 2003;305:97–105.
11. Rossi GP. Dual ACE and NEP inhibitors: a review of the pharmacological properties of MDL-100,240. *Cardiovasc Drug Rev* 2003;21:51–66.
12. Rossi GP, Bova S, Sacchetto A, et al. Comparative effects of the dual ACE-NEP inhibitor MDL-100,240 and ramipril on hypertension and cardiovascular disease in endogenous angiotensin II-dependent hypertension. *Am J Hypertens* 2002;15:181–188.
13. Robl JA, Sulsky R, Sieber-McMaster E, et al. Vasopeptidase inhibitors: incorporation of geminal and spirocyclic substituted azepinones in mercaptoacyl dipeptides. *J Med Chem* 1999;42:305–311.
14. Laurent S, Boutouyrie P, Azizi M, et al. Antihypertensive effects of fasidotril, a dual inhibitor of neprilysin and angiotensin-converting enzyme, in rats and humans. *Hypertension* 2000;35:1148–1153.
15. Gonzalez W, Beslot F, Laboulandine I, et al. Inhibition of both angiotensin-converting enzyme and neutral endopeptidase by S21402 (RB105) in rats with experimental myocardial infarction. *J Pharmacol Exp Ther* 1996;278:573–578.
16. Lassila M, Davis BJ, Allen TJ, et al. Cardiovascular hypertrophy in diabetic spontaneously hypertensive rats: optimizing blockade of the reninangiotensin system. *Clin Sci (Lond)* 2003;104:341–347.
17. Rastegar MA, Marchini F, Morazzoni G, et al. The effects of Z13752A, a combined ACE/NEP inhibitor, on responses to coronary artery occlusion: a primary protective role for bradykinin. *Br J Pharmacol* 2000;129:671–680.
18. Weber MA. Vasopeptidase inhibitors. *The Lancet* 2001;358:1525–1532.
19. Campbell DJ. Vasopeptidase inhibition: a double-edged sword? *Hypertension* 2003;41:383–389.
20. Trippodo NC, Robl JA, Asaad MM, et al. Effects of omapatrilat in low, normal, and high renin experimental hypertension. *Am J Hypertens* 1998;11:363–372.

14

VOL 25 CLINICAL PHARMACOLOGY AND THERAPEUTICS OF HYPERTENSION

21. Quaschning T, d'Uscio LV, Lüscher TF. Greater endothelial protection by the vasopeptidase inhibitor omapatrilat compared to the ACE-inhibitor captopril in salt induced hypertension. *J Am Coll Cardiol* 2000;35:248–249.

22. Ferrario CM, Averill DB, Brosnihan KB, et al. Vasopeptidase inhibition and Ang-(1-7) in the spontaneously hypertensive rat. *Kidney Int* 2002;62:1349–1357.

23. Maniu CV, Meyer DM, Redfield MM. Hemodynamic and humoral effects of vasopeptidase inhibition in canine hypertension. *Hypertension* 2002;40:528–534.

24. Lapointe N, Ngguyen QT, Desjardins JF, et al. Effects of pre-, peri-, and postmyocardial infarction treatment with omapatrilat in rats: survival, arrhytmias, ventricular function, and remodeling. *Am J Physiol Heart Physiol* 2003;285:H398–H405.

25. Backlund T, Palojoki E, Saraste A, et al. Effect of vasopeptidase inhibitor omapatrilat on cardiomyocite apoptosis and ventricular remodeling in rat myocardial infarction. *Cardiovasc Res* 2003;57:727–737.

26. Wang Ch, Leung N, Lapointe N, et al. Vasopeptidase inhibitor omapatrilat induces profound insulin sensitization and increases myocardial glucose uptake in Zucker fatty rats: Studies comparing a vasopepetidase inhibitor, angiotensin-converting enzyme inhibitor, and angiotensin II type I receptor blocker. *Circulation* 2003;107:1923–1929.

27. Davies BJ, Johnston CI, Burrell LM, et al. Renoprotective effects of vasopeptidase inhibition in an experimental model of diabetic nephropathy. *Diabetologia* 2003;46:961–971.

28. Richards AM, Wittert GA, Crozier IG, et al. Chronic inhibition of endopeptidase 24.11 in essential hypertension: evidence for enhanced atrial natriuretic peptide and angiotensin II. *J Hypertens* 1993;11:407–416.

29. McDowell G, Coutgie W, Shaw C, et al. The effect of the neutral endopeptidase inhibitor drug, candoxatril, on circulating levels of two of the most potent vasoactive peptides. *Br J Clin Pharmacol* 1997;43:329–332.

30. Favrat B, Burnier M, Nussberger J, et al. Neutral endopeptidase versus angiotensin converting enzyme inhibition in essential hypertension. *J Hypertens* 1995;13:797–804.

31. Ando S, Rahman MA, Butler GC, et al. Comparison of candoxatril and atrial natriuretic factor in healthy men. Effects on hemodynamics, sympathetic activity, heart rate variability, and endothelin. *Hypertension* 1995;26:1160–1166.

32. Campbell DJ, Anastasopulos F, Duncan AM, et al. Effects of neutral endopeptidase inhibition and combined angiotensin converting enzyme and neutral endopeptidase inhibition on angiotensin and bradykinin peptides in rats. *J Pharmacol Exp Ther* 1998;287:567–577.

33. Blais C, Drapeau G, Raymond P, et al. Contribution of angiotensin converting enzyme to the cardiac metabolism of bradykinin: an interspecies study. *Am J Physiol* 1997;273: H2263–H2271.

34. Ishida H, Scicli AG, Carretero OA. Role of angiotensin converting enzyme and other peptidases in in-vivo metabolism of kinins. *Hypertension* 1989;14:322–327.

35. Gavras I. Bradykinin mediated effects of ACE inhibition. *Kidney Int* 1992;42:1020–1029.

36. Bevan EG, Connell JM, Doyle J, et al. Candoxatril, a neutral endopeptidase inhibitor: efficacy and tolerability in essential hypertension. *J Hypertens* 1992;10:607–613.

37. Tikkanen T, Tikkanen I, Rockell MD, et al. Dual inhibition of neutral endopeptidase and angiotensin-converting enzyme in rats with hypertension and diabetes mellitus. *Hypertension* 1998;32:778–785.

38. Stergiou GS, Hannah JA, Bevan EG, et al. Combined atriopeptidase inhibition and angiotensin converting enzyme inhibition in hypertensive patients. *J Hypentens* 1994;12:1310–1311.

39. Liao WC, Vesterqvist O, Delaney C, et al. Pharmacokinetics and pharmacodynamics of the vasopeptidase inhibitor, omapatrilat in healthy subjects. *Br J Clin Pharmacol* 2003;56:395–406.

40. Sica DA, Liao W, Gehr TW, et al. Disposition and safety of omapatrilat in subjects with renal impairment. *Clin Pharmacol Ther* 2000;68:261–269.

41. Dumoulin MJ, Adam A, Rouleau JL, Lamontagne D. Comparison of a vasopeptidase inhibitor with neutral endopeptidase and angiotensin-converting enzyme inhibitors on bradykinin metabolism in the rat coronary bed. *J Cardiovasc Pharmacol* 2001;37: 359–366.

42. Blais Jr. C, Fortin D, Rouleau JL, et al. Protective effect of omapatrilat, a vasopeptidase inhibitor, on the metabolism of bradykinin in normal and failing human hearts. *J Pharmacol Exp Ther* 2000;295:621–626.

43. Messerli FH, Nussberger J. Vasopeptidase inhibition and angio-edema. *Lancet* 2000;356:608–609.

44. Kostis JB, Packer M, Black HR, et al. Omapatrilat and enalapril in patients with hypertension: The Omapatrilat Cardiovascular Treatment vs. Enalapril (OCTAVE) trial. *Am J Hypertens* 2004;17:103–111.

45. Massien C, Azizi M, Guyene TT, et al. Pharmacodynamic effects of dual neutral endopepdidase-angiotensin-converting enzyme inhibition in humans. *Clin Pharmacol Ther* 1999;65:448–459.

46. Azizi M, Lamarre-Cliché M, Labatide-Alanore A, et al. Physiologic consequences of vasopeptidase inhibition in humans: effect of sodium intake. *J Am Soc Nephrol* 2002;13:2454–2463.

47. Nathisuwan S, Talbert RL. A review of vasopeptidase inhibitors: a new modality in the treatment of hypertension and chronic heart failure. *Pharmacotherapy* 2002;22:27–42.

48. Ruilope LM, Plantini P, Grossman E, et al. Randomized, double-blind comparison of omapatrilat with amlodipine in mild-to-moderate hypertension. *Am J Hypertens* 2000;13:134A.

49. Kostis JB, Cobbe S, Johnston C, et al. Design of the Omapatrilat in Persons with Enhanced Risk of Atherosclerotic events (OPERA) trial. *Am J Hypertens* 2002;15:193–198.

50. Klapholz M, Thomas I, Eng C, et al. Effects of omapatrilat on hemodynamics and safety in patents with heart failure. *Am J Cardiol* 2001;88:657–661.

51. McClean DR, Ikram H, Mehta S, et al. Vasopeptidase inhibition with omapatrilat in chronic heart failure: acute and long-term hemodynamic and neurohumoral effects. *J Am Coll Cardiol* 2002;39:2034–2041.

52. McClean DR, Ikram H, Garlick AH, Crozier IG. Effects of omapatrilat on systemic arterial function in patients with chronic heart failure. *Am J Cardiol* 2001;87:565–569.

53. McClean DR, Ikram H, Garlick AH, et al. The clinical, cardiac, renal, arterial and neurohormonal effects of omapatrilat, a vasopeptidase inhibitor, in patients with chronic heart failure. *J Am Coll Cardiol* 2000;36:479–486.

54. Rouleau JL, Pfeffer MA, Stewart DJ, et al. Comparison of vasopeptidase inhibitor, omapatrilat, and lisinopril on exercise tolerance and morbidity in patients with heart failure: IMPRESS randomized trial. *Lancet* 2000;356:615–620.

55. Packer M, Califf RM, Konstam MA, et al. Comparison of omapatrilat and enalapril in patients with chronic heart failure: the Omapatrilat Versus Enalapril Randomized Trial of utility in Reducing Events (OVERTURE). *Circulation* 2002;106:920–926.

56. Rubinstein I, Muns G, Zucker IH. Plasma exudation in conscious dogs with experimental heart failure. *Basic Res Cardiol* 1994;89:487–498.

57. Sheth T, Parker T, Block A, et al. Comparison of the effects of omapatrilat and lisinopril on circulating neurohormones and cytokines in patients with chronic heart failure. *Am J Cardiol* 2002;90:496–500.

58. Zanchi A, Maillad M, Burnier M. Recent clinical trials with omapatrilat: new developments. *Current Hypertension Reports* 2003;5:346–352.

VII
Future prospects

15 | Novel agents in development

Giuseppe Mancia, Raffaella Dell'Oro, Fosca Quarti Trevano and Guido Grassi

INTRODUCTION

New drugs for hypertension treatment are synthetized and tested with several goals in mind. The first goal is to provide agents capable of directly interfering with the mechanisms involved in the regulation of blood pressure (BP) and thus partly responsible for the development, maintenance and progression of the hypertensive state. The second goal is to provide BP reduction as effective as traditional drugs, but more balanced throughout the 24 hours, even when monotherapy is adopted as the therapeutic strategy. The third goal is to couple antihypertensive efficacy with a non-harmful side-effect profile, thus improving patients' compliance with drug treatment. The fourth goal is to achieve, through an improvement in the pharmacokinetic properties and/or via the discovery of new mechanisms of action, greater cerebral, coronary, renal and vascular protection against the organ damage associated with hypertension. This goal should also embrace antihypertensive drugs used in daily clinical practice that are capable of effectively lowering blood pressure values to the targets recommended by current guidelines.[1,2] This key target of the antihypertensive pharmacological approach still remains unmet in current clinical practice, particularly in the high-risk patient, as documented by the disappointing data collected in different European and non-European countries on BP control in the hypertensive population (Fig. 15.1).[3]

New antihypertensive drugs should also exert neutral, or possibly favourable, effects on the metabolic profile, taking into account: (1) the relevance of drug-induced dyslipidaemic and glycaemic alterations to the cardiovascular risk profile of the hypertensive patient[4] and (2) the high prevalence of metabolic disturbances and the close association between high BP, dyslipidaemia, hypertrygliceridaemia, insulin resistance and diabetes.[4] Finally, in looking for new drugs that might more effectively prevent cardiovascular disease, it is important to underline that traditional antihypertensive agents have never been shown to reduce the cardiovascular risk of the treated hypertensive patient to the level of the normotensive individual. Traditional drugs have also been found to incompletely prevent or regress the structural and functional

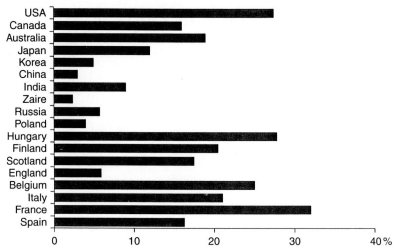

Fig. 15.1 The percentage of hypertensive patients with controlled blood pressure (≤140/90 mmHg) in different European and non-European countries.

alterations (so called 'end-organ damage') characterizing the high blood pressure state (Table 15.1).[5] This still unmet goal of antihypertensive treatment represents one of the main objectives of clinical pharmacology aimed at improving treatment-related cardiovascular protection.

The present chapter will focus on two classes of new cardiovascular drugs that will shortly be ready for therapeutic use in the clinical arena, i.e. the endothelin antagonists and the renin inhibitors. This will be pursued by highlighting, whenever possible, the advantages as well as the potential disadvantages of these 'new' drugs compared with traditional antihypertensive compounds.

Table 15.1 Intermediate endpoints in hypertension clinical trials

Heart
Left ventricular hypertrophy
Left ventricular systolic and/or diastolic dysfunction
Coronary artery calcium content

Vessels
Carotid artery thickness
Arterial stiffening
Arteriolar remodelling
Endothelial dysfunction

Brain
Silent cerebral lacunae
Silent cerebral ischaemia

Kidney
Microalbuminuria
High creatinine levels
Mild renal damage

ENDOTHELIN ANTAGONISTS

The past few years of basic and integrated cardiovascular research have been marked by increasing evidence that endothelial cells are not an inactive layer separating vessel wall from circulating blood, but rather the source of important humoral substances for both short- and long-term cardiovascular regulation. One of these factors has been characterized as nitric oxide and its role has been recognized both as a powerful local vasodilator and as a long-term inhibitor of cell growth and, thus, of vascular abnormalities, such as arteriolar remodelling and atherosclerosis.[6] Other substances have been characterized as endothelins, with cardiovascular effects largely opposite to those displayed by nitric oxide.[7,8] In physiological conditions exogenous or endogenous endothelin evokes marked vasoconstrictive effects mediated by both endothelin type-A and type-B receptor stimulation at the level of vascular smooth muscle cells (Fig. 15.2). However, this process is counterbalanced by endothelin-mediated stimulation of nitric oxide, via an involvement of type-B endothelin receptors. In contrast, in hypertensive patients the reduced bioavailability of nitric oxide potentiates the occurrence of systemic vasoconstriction (and thus of pressor effects), leaving endothelin type-B receptor stimulation almost unopposed by nitric oxide production.[7,8] The interaction between endothelin and its receptors appears to be complex. The receptors may interact with a second messenger, thereby contributing to the long-acting effects of endothelin both 'in vitro' and 'in vivo'. Repeated administration of endothelin may favour the occurrence of a down-regulation process, which appears to be more common for endothelin type-B than for type-A receptors.[7,8]

ENDOTHELIAL CELLS

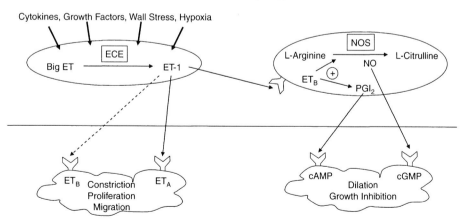

VASCULAR SMOOTH MUSCLE CELLS

Fig. 15.2 Schematic illustration of the physiopathological cascade of events related to endothelial cell activation. Several biochemical, humoral and haemodynamic factors lead to the synthesis of endothelin-1 (ET-1), which stimulates specific receptors (ETB and ETA) and through a variety of mechanisms leads to specific vascular effects. ECE = endothelin converting enzyme; NO = nitric oxide; PGI$_2$ = prostaglandin I$_2$; NOS = NO synthetase.

Endothelin receptor blockade: main features

Endothelin receptors are widely distributed in different organs that participate to a major extent in blood pressure regulation as well as in cardiovascular homeostatic control. These organs include vascular smooth muscle, the endothelium, the heart, the kidney, the adrenal gland and the brain.[7,8] Stimulation of vascular and cardiac endothelin receptors triggers a pressor response (accompanied by tachycardia), which appears to be linked to an increase in peripheral vascular resistance. At renal level, endothelin receptor agonism is usually accompanied by marked elevation in renal vascular resistance, with a concomitant and marked reduction of renal blood flow and glomerular filtration rate.[8]

Endothelin blockade can be achieved through three main mechanisms, via:[5] (1) the concomitant blockade of type-A and type-B endothelin receptors, (2) the selective blockade of type-A receptors and (3) the pharmacological blockade of endothelin-converting enzyme (ECE). Because the two endothelin receptor subtypes often display non-homogeneous cardiovascular effects (Table 15.2) only selective receptor antagonists may be useful in clinical practice. This recommendation is based on several sets of experimental and clinical data. For example, in experimental hypertension, while endothelin B receptor antagonists elicit a noticeable blood pressure elevation by directly increasing peripheral vascular resistance and by concomitantly reducing nitric oxide-mediated vasodilation, pharmacological blockade of type-A receptors triggers virtually the opposite effects.[9,10] However, these considerations should be balanced by the evidence that, as previously mentioned, endothelin type-B receptors often display up-regulation, thereby exerting unfavourable consequences, such as (1) a pro-hypertrophic effect on myocardial structure, (2) an increase in

Table 15.2 Biological effects mediated by type-A and type-B endothelin receptors

Effects	Type-A	Type-B
Vascular tissues		
Arterial smooth muscle (contraction)	+++	+
Venous smooth muscle (contraction)		++
Endothelial cell (release of EDRF)		+++
Cardiac muscle		
Postive inotropism	++	+
Positive chronotropism	++	+
Coronary vessel contraction	+++	+
Endocrine glands		
Adrenal cortex (release of aldosterone)	+	+++
Anterior pituitary (release of ACTH)	+	++
Kidney		
Afferent and efferent arterioles (contraction)	+++	++
Renal tubule (Na^+ excretion and diuresis)		+++
Central nervous system		
Mesencephalon (control of blood pressure)	+	+

EDRF = endothelial derived releasing factor; ACTH = adrenocorticotropin hormone coronary vascular resistance and (3) arterial and arteriolar vascular remodel-ling.[11,12] Part of these adverse cardiovascular effects appears to be reversible. For example, selective (type-B receptor) as well as unselective pharmacological blockade of endothelin receptors has been shown to trigger acute coronary vasodilation accompanied by BP reduction and a slight increase in heart rate. Interestingly, the increase in coronary diameter induced by bosentan, one of the recently synthesized endothelin receptor antagonists, was inversely related to plasma LDL-cholesterol both in vessels without and with angiographic lesions (Fig. 15.3).[12] This finding has been interpreted as an indirect demonstra-tion that LDL levels may faithfully mirror the degree of coronary vascular alterations.

Pharmacological profile

From a pharmacological viewpoint endothelin receptor antagonists can be clas-sified according to potency, selectivity of action and chemical structure.[13] The 'in-vitro' binding affinity for endothelin receptors can be expressed by indices (such as IC_{50}, 50% inhibitory concentration) used to assess antagonist potency. This is generally followed by the determination of the functional potency of these compounds on cells or tissue preparations, coupled by assess-ment of the ability of the receptor antagonist agents to block agonist-induced contractions in isolated vessels (so called 'selectivity of action'). From a chemi-cal/structural viewpoint, endothelin receptor antagonists can be classified as peptidic as well as non-peptidic compounds. Among the former are the modi-fied endothelin peptides, to which belong the first selective synthetic endothe-lin blocker (Fig. 15.4), the cyclic peptide antagonists, and the so-called modified peptides, such as those with a carboxy-terminal tryptophan structure or linear tripeptide ureas.[13] On the other hand, non-peptidic endothelin antagonists, to which belong a large number of chemical compounds, such as the so-called natural product-derived agents, the heterocyclic sulfonamides, the diarylino-lane carboxylic acids, the dihidropyridine anhydrides, the butenolides and

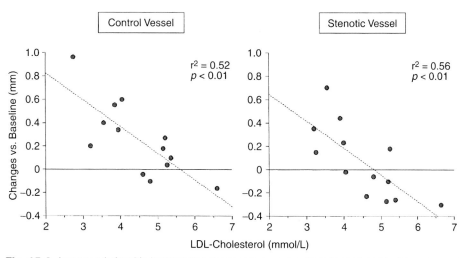

Fig. 15.3 Inverse relationship between the changes in coronary diameter induced by bosentan and plasma LDL-cholesterol. Data refer to coronary vessels without (control) and with (stenotic vessel) angiographic lesions. *(Modified from ref. (12).)*

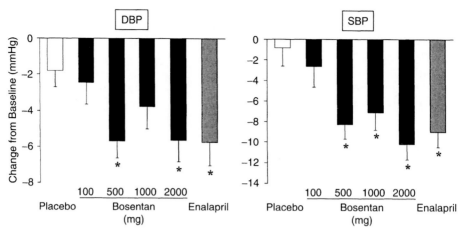

Fig. 15.4 Effects of placebo, bosentan (100, 500, 1000 and 2000 mg/day) and enalapril on 24-hour diastolic (DBP) and systolic (SBP) blood pressure in hypertensive patients. Data are shown as mean ($\pm$ SEM) differences from baseline values. Asterisks (*, $p < 0.01$) refer to the statistical significance of the differences over placebo. *(Modified from ref. (26).)*

the acylsulfonamides, represent interesting pharmacological approaches helpful for overcoming the unsatisfactory metabolic profile of peptidergic antagonists.[13] As mentioned above, these compounds differ from each other in the bioavailability, half-life and hepatic metabolism properties. For some agents there is metabolism to active moieties, and some cardiovascular (such as statins and warfarin) as well as non-cardiovascular drugs (e.g. ciclosporin or glibenclamide) may affect the pharmacokinetic properties of both peptidergic and non-peptidergic endothelin receptor antagonists.[13] Some of the above-mentioned agents are in the advanced phases of clinical investigation (Table 15.3).

Table 15.3 Unselective and selective endothelin receptor antagonists

Unselective receptor antagonists	Type-A receptor antagonists	Type-B receptor antagonists
A-182086	A-127722	A-192621
CGS-27830	ABT-627 (= atrasentan)	BQ-788
IRL3630	BE-18-572A/B	IRL-2500
L-753037	BMS-182874	K-8794
LU224332	BMS-193884	RES-701-1
LU302872	BQ-123	Ro-468443
PD-142-893	BQ-153	TBC-10894
PD-145-065	BQ-485	
Ro-46-2005	BQ-610	
Ro-46-0203 (= bosentan)	EMD-122946	
Ro-48-5695	EMD-94246	
Ro-61-0612	FR-139317	
(= tezosentan)	J-104121	
SB-209670	J-104132	
TAK-044	L-744453	
	L-749329	
	L-74142	
	LU-127043	
	LU-135252(= darusentan)	

Antihypertensive effects

Experimental studies

The role of endothelin receptors in the pathogenesis of hypertension and the effects of endothelin receptor blockers have been investigated in a number of experimental animal models.[14] The results obtained so far are conflicting however, and frequently the effects of endothelin receptor blockers differ according to the specific physiopathological background characterizing each experimental model of hypertension. In renovascular hypertension, for example, while the endothelin receptor blocker Ro-00203 has been shown to interfere with the development of the hypertensive state, neither bosentan nor the type-A receptor blocker BQ-123 was able to display any antihypertensive effect.[15,16] In contrast, in another experimental animal model of hypertension (Page model) and in other hypertensive states not linked to a renin–angiotensin stimulation, bosentan administration has displayed blood pressure lowering effects greater in magnitude than those of losartan.[17] These and other findings raise the question of whether the antihypertensive effects of endothelin receptor blockers are in some way antagonized by the stimulation of the renin–angiotensin system. Other evidence in Sprague-Dawley rats demonstrated that bosentan and other class-related compounds markedly antagonize the pressor effects of angiotensin II.[18] It is also possible that in experimental conditions characterized by a marked stimulation of the renin–angiotensin system endothelin receptor blockers, although displaying only modest antihypertensive effects, may be effective in attenuating the pro-hypertrophic action of angiotensin II at vascular level. This finding, although in need of future investigations, suggests selective interference via endothelin antagonism of the cardiovascular effects of angiotensin II. This speculation appears to be further strengthened by the evidence that in experimental animal models in which the hypertensive state is linked to an augmented secretion of mineralcorticoid hormones, endothelin receptor blockade exerts clearcut anti-hypertrophic effects both at cardiac and at peripheral vascular level, together with a reduction in blood pressure levels.[8,13] Similar interactions have been recently documented between endothelin receptors, the sympathetic nervous system and nitric oxide.[19,20] The results of studies published so far on endothelin receptor antagonists in experimental models of hypertension come from investigations that have been mainly focused on the assessment of the effects of this class of drugs on the end-organ damage rather than on the antihypertensive efficacy. This is probably a consequence of the use of endothelin antagonists as a tool to better clarify the pathophysiological role of the system on hypertensive complications, with special emphasis on vascular remodelling.[21]

Clinical studies

One of the experimental approaches more frequently employed in humans for evaluating the haemodynamic effects of antihypertensive drugs (and thus also of endothelin receptor antagonists) is plethysmographic measurement of blood flow in the forearm vascular bed, with assessment of the responses to stepwise intra-arterial local infusion of specific agonists and antagonists of a given receptor. Intra-arterial infusion of endothelin-I has been shown to trigger a dose-dependent vasoconstrictor response, which is abolished or even reversed by the concomitant administration of a type-A receptor endothelin antagonist, i.e. BQ-123.[22,23] When a non-selective antagonist is infused into the forearm circulation, a marked vasodilatory response is observed, with a magnitude of effect consistently greater in hypertensive than in normotensive subjects.[24] In contrast, intra-arterial administration of a type-B receptor endothelin antagonist is almost invariably associated with a forearm vasoconstriction.[25] Altogether these findings support the high selectivity of the endothelin receptor function.[7,8,21]

The most striking evidence for the antihypertensive effects of endothelin receptor antagonists, however, comes from the results of two studies.[26,27] The first,[26] performed in about 300 patients with uncomplicated mild-to-moderate essential hypertension, investigated the blood pressure lowering effects of bosentan at a dosage ranging from 100 to 1000 mg twice daily. Using a double-blind placebo-controlled design, the investigators compared the blood pressure lowering effects of bosentan to those of enalapril, 20 mg once daily. Antihypertensive efficacy was assessed by methods which included 24-hour ambulatory blood pressure monitoring. The study also included assessment of plasma renin and plasma norepinephrine levels, in order to provide some insights into the possible interplay between the level of the renin-angiotensin as well as sympathetic nervous system stimulation and the degree of the antihypertensive efficacy of these compounds. As shown in Figure 15.4, bosentan and enalapril displayed superimposable blood pressure lowering effects. For bosentan the antihypertensive effects: (1) reached a plateau at a daily dose of 500 mg, (2) were appreciable during the whole 24-hour period only during twice-a-day administration and (3) were not accompanied by any evidence of sympathetic stimulation both at cardiac (no increase in heart rate) and at peripheral vascular level (no change in plasma norepinephrine levels).

The second study evaluated the dose–response effects of darusentan (a type-A endothelin receptor antagonist) on BP in about 400 patients using a randomized, double-blind design.[27] Darusentan caused a dose-dependent reduction in both systolic and diastolic BP throughout the 2 months of the study and was unaccompanied by any heart rate change (Fig. 15.5). However, both at lower and higher dosage, the antihypertensive efficacy was more pronounced for systolic than for diastolic BP. If confirmed in future studies, these properties of the drug may help to address one of the unresolved issues concerning antihypertensive drug treatment, i.e. the poor systolic blood control.[1,2,28,29] This issue is of particular clinical relevance since systolic BP appears to be more important than diastolic BP in the development and progression of end-organ damage, as well as in determining the overall cardiovascular risk profile of the hypertensive patient.[30] Despite these promising results, no further work has been performed with endothelin receptor antagonists in the field of hypertension.

Other cardiovascular effects

Like other neurohumoral substances, circulating endothelin levels are increased in heart failure and also display an adverse impact on cardiovascular function as well as on prognosis.[31,32] This represents the rationale for the attempts made over the years to evaluate the clinical use of endothelin receptor antagonists in circumstances of low cardiac output. In both ischaemic and

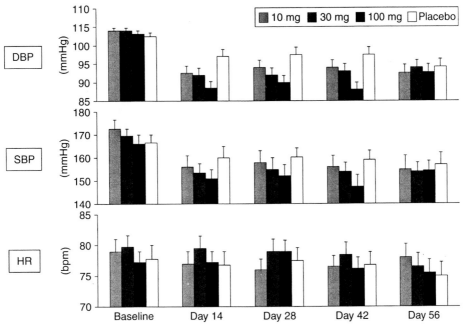

Fig. 15.5 Diastolic blood pressure (DBP), systolic blood pressure (SBP) and heart rate (HR) values measured before (baseline) and at different time periods during darusentan or placebo administration. Data are shown as mean (± SEM) absolute values. *(Modified from ref. (27).)*

non-ischaemic experimental models of heart failure, sustained blockade of endothelin receptors improves cardiac function by enhancing myocardial contractility and coronary flow reserve and by reducing left ventricular enlargement.[32,33] These findings have not been confirmed in humans (Table 15.4).[34–38] In the study by Sutsch et al. and in the Heart Failure ET-A receptor blockade (HEAT) Trial,[34,35] the unselective endothelin receptor antagonist bosentan and the type-A endothelin receptor antagonist darusentan improved cardiac function compared with placebo (Fig. 15.6),[34] but in other clinical trials, including the recently performed Randomized Intravenous Tezosentan (RITZ-D) trial,[36] no difference was found between the haemodynamic or the clinical effects of the active treatment based on an endothelin antagonist and placebo (Table 15.4). However, the data obtained so far only refer to: (1) short-lasting (from 72 hours to 30 days) effects of the drug and (2) heart failure syndrome of ischaemic aetiology. Since both the haemodynamic and the neurohumoral profile of acute and of chronic heart failure are different, the available data do not allow extrapolation to the therapeutic use of endothelin receptor antagonists in stable forms of heart failure or in hypertensive patients with chronic left ventricular dysfunction.[21,36]

In contrast, promising results have been obtained with the use of an endothelin receptor antagonist (bosentan) in the pulmonary hypertensive state associated with scleroderma, but without evidence of interstitial disease.[21,39] This was suggested by the results of a large-scale clinical trial, the BREATHE-1 Study,[40] and will be further evaluated in ongoing clinical investigations such as the STRIDE and the ARIES 1 and 2 studies.[21] Whether the

Table 15.4 Large-scale clinical studies performed with the use of endothelin receptor antagonists in heart failure patients

Trial	Treatment	Outcome
HEAT (Heart failure ETA receptor blockade Trial)	Darusentan vs. placebo for 3 weeks	Improvement in cardiac index
RITZ-1 (Randomized Intravenous Tezosentan Study 1)	Tezosentan 25 mg/hour IV for 72 or vs. placebo ($n = 669$)	No change
RITZ-2 (Randomized Intravenous Tezosentan Study 2)	Tezosentan 50 mg or 100 mg/hour IV vs. placebo ($n = 215$)	Improvement in cardiac index and reduction in wedge pressure
RITZ-4 (Randomized Intravenous Tezosentan Study 4)	Tezosentan 25–40 mg/h IV for 24–48 hours vs. placebo ($n = 193$)	No change
RITZ-5 (Randomized Intravenous Tezosentan Study 5)	Tezosentan 50–100 mg/hour IV for 24 hours ($n = 84$)	No change
REACH-1 (Resource Utilization Among Congestive Heart Failure)	Bosentan 250 mg × 2 vs. placebo ($n = 370$)	No change
ENABLE I/II (Endothelin Antagonist Bosentan for Lowering Cardiac Events in Heart Failure)	Bosentan 125 mg × 2 vs. placebo ($n = 1613$) for 9 months	No change
EARTH (Endothelin-A Receptor Antagonists Trial in Heart Failure)	Darusentan 10, 25, 50, 100, 300 mg vs. placebo for 24 weeks	No change

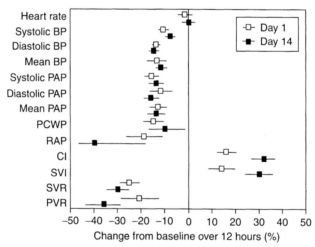

Fig. 15.6 Acute and subacute haemodynamic effects of bosentan administration (1000 mg × 2/day) on haemodynamic variables in patients with New York Heart Association class III heart failure. BP = blood pressure; PAP = pulmonary artery pressure; PCWP = pulmonary capillary wedge pressure; RAP = right atrial pressure; CI = cardiac index; SVI = stroke volume index; SVR = systemic vascular resistance; PVR = pulmonary vascular resistance. Data, collected after 1 and 14 days of treatment, are shown as per cent changes over baseline values. *(Modified from ref. (34).)*

favourable effects of the drug will also be observed in idiopathic pulmonary hypertension and in other conditions with increased pulmonary wedge pressure due to other mechanisms remains to be clarified. An overview of the clinical development status of endothelin receptor antagonists in cardiovascular disease is summarized in Table 15.5.

Table 15.5 Clinical development status of different endothelin receptor antagonists

Indication	Compound	Development status
Mild-to-moderate systemic hypertension	Bosentan Darusentan Sitaxentan	Discontinued after phase II
Resistant systemic hypertension	Darusentan	Phase IIb
Acute heart failure	Tezosentan	Discontinued during phase III
Chronic heart failure	Bosentan Darusentan Sitaxentan Enrasentan	Discontinued after phase III Discontinued after phase IIb Discontinued after phase II Discontinued after phase II
Pulmonary hypertension related to (auto) immune disorder	Bosentan	Phase III
Primary pulmonary artery hypertension	Bosentan Sitaxentan Ambrisentan	Approved Phase III Phase III

Side effects and tolerability profile

Accumulated clinical experience indicates that endothelin receptor antagonists have a satisfactory tolerability profile,[7,13] although in some studies several side effects closely related to the vasodilatatory properties of the compounds have been reported. In the HEAT study, among the most common side effects, peripheral oedema, headache and flushing appeared to be dose-dependent.[26] Endothelin receptor antagonists may also potentiate the BP lowering effects of ACE-inhibitors,[41] a finding that again underlines the close interrelationships between the endothelin and the renin–angiotensin systems.

RENIN INHIBITORS

Long-term regulation of BP as well as long-term control of cardiovascular homeostasis, to a large extent, depends on the renin–angiotensin system. As shown in Figure 15.7, the primary goal of the pharmacological blockade of the system is inhibition of the key hormone of the renin–angiotensin axis, i.e. angiotensin II, which exerts marked vasoconstrictive and sodium retaining properties in addition to a number of other unfavourable cardiovascular effects.[42] These include: (1) vascular and cardiac proliferative and pro-inflammatory properties, (2) activation of the thrombotic process, (3) increase in tissue fibrosis and mitogenesis, (4) stimulation of aldosterone, vasopressin and endothelin release and (5) potentiation of sympathetic neural discharge by stimulating the adrenergic function both at central and at peripheral neural sites.[42]

There are several pharmacological tools for blocking angiotensin II (Fig. 15.7). These include: (1) blockade of β-adrenergic receptor-mediated release of the renal enzyme renin from the juxtaglomerular cells via β-adrenergic blocking agents, (2) antagonism by renin inhibitors of the action of renin, which physiologically removes the amino-terminal decapeptide from

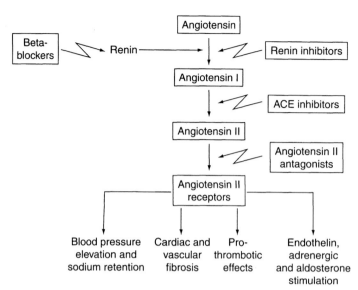

Fig. 15.7 Schematic illustration of the sites of action of different cardiovascular drugs acting on the renin–angiotensin system. The cardiovascular and metabolic effects mediated by angiotensin II receptors are also shown.

angiotensinogen to produce angiotensin I, (3) inhibition of the activation of angiotensin I to the biologically active angiotensin II by the decarboxypeptidase-converting enzyme via ACE-inhibitors and (4) antagonism of the cardiovascular and non-cardiovascular effects of angiotensin II, via angiotensin II receptor blockers. There are many reasons to explore new pharmacological tools capable of interfering with the renin–angiotensin axis.[43] For example, it has been clearly shown that β-adrenergic blockade of renin secretion from the juxtaglomerular apparatus has a major limitation, i.e. it is non-specific, being unable to interfere with enzyme production not mediated by β-adrenoreceptors. In addition, angiotensin-II-converting enzyme inhibition does not always: (1) produce long-term and stable blockade of angiotensin II generation and (2) display an optimal or near-optimal side-effect profile. Finally, angiotensin II receptor blockade, although effective in the long term, does not block other receptor subtypes, which may play an important role for determining the global effect of angiotensin II on cardiovascular structure and function. Current research on pharmacological interference with the renin–angiotensin system is aimed not only at improving and/or extending to other receptor subtypes the blockade of angiotensin II receptors, but also at obtaining full inhibition of renin enzyme activity by directly interfering via specific renin inhibitors with the first and rate-limiting enzyme of the renin–angiotensin axis. This latter approach is, for some compounds, at the late phases of clinical development. This approach would antagonize all the pathways involved in the generation or release of renin, at variance from ACE-inhibitors and angiotensin II receptor blockers (Table 15.6).

Renin inhibition: main features

Several attempts have been made to achieve complete and effective therapeutic inhibition of renin.[44] These attempts have been hampered by problems or

Table 15.6 Comparison of the effects of renin inhibitors, ACE-inhibitors (ACE inhibitors) and angiotensin receptor blockers (ARB) on the renin–angiotensin system

	Renin inhibitors	ACE inhibitors	ARB
Plasma renin levels	↓	↓	↑
Plasma angiotensin II levels	↓↓	↓	↑
Plasma bradykinin levels	→	↑	→
Stimulation of AT receptors other than AT1	↓	↓	↑

↓ = decrease; ↓↓ = marked decrease; → = no change; ↑ = increase

Table 15.7 Main specific renin inhibitor compounds

Renin-specific purified antibodies and antiserum for renin
Structural derivates of pepstatin
Angiotensinogen analogues
Prorenin peptidic prosegments
Transition state analogues
Non-peptidic renin-inhibitors

difficulties related to: (1) the low potency, (2) the limited duration of action and (3) the poor bioavailability or the unfavourable side effects profile of the newly synthetized drugs. There have been several approaches (Table 15.7). The first is an immunological approach based on the parenteral administration of renin-specific purified antibodies or of antiserum for renin (active immunization).[45,46] When these methods have been employed in experimental animal models of hypertension, blood pressure reduction has been obtained.[45] However, due to immunological reactions including induction of antigen-antibody precipitation, the clinical use of these drugs in humans has never been attempted. Nor has the second group of compounds, the so-called 'minimal substrate of renin', represented by structural derivates of pepstatin containing the renin inhibitory peptide[47,48] been evaluated in humans. The third approach is represented by the angiotensinogen analogues, i.e. by the renin inhibitor decapeptides (diteki-ren, enalkiren, remikiren, etc.), with peptidic structure that adversely affects bioavailability and prevents clinical use. Parenteral administration of angioten-sin analogues has been shown to reduce BP both in experimental animals and in human beings.[49,50] Two further approaches that interfere with renin are represented by prorenin peptidic prosegments,[51] abandoned several years ago, and the so-called 'transition-state analogues'.[52] The synthesis and develop-ment of these compounds avoids the cleavage process, thus obtaining the so-called 'hypothetical transition state conformation'[44,52] which guarantees a longer duration of action. This latter property has been confirmed by studies performed in humans, in which parenteral administration of H142 triggered a persistent blood pressure reduction.[53] However, despite excellent potency, these com-pounds cannot be administered orally due to peptidic structure. This limitation has been overcome by the synthesis of non-peptidic renin inhibitors.

Pharmacological profile

Among non-peptidic renin-inhibitors aliskiren represents the most advanced compound, with promising clinical applications. Synthesis originates from

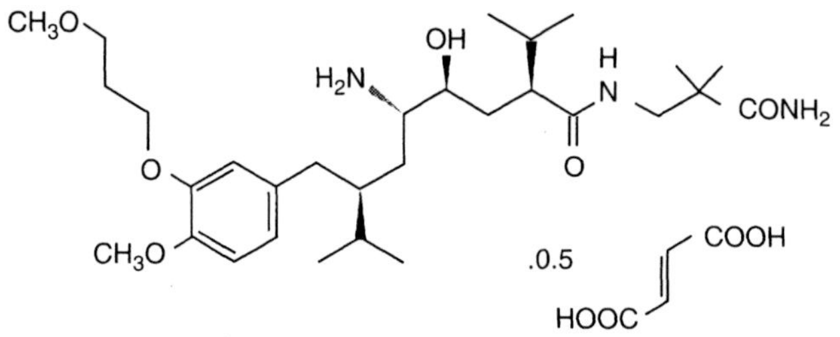

Fig. 15.8 Chemical octanamide-hemifumarate structure of aliskiren, a non-peptidic renin inhibitor.

the combination of molecular modelling techniques with crystal structure elucidation. From a chemical viewpoint the drug displays an octanamid-hemifumarate structure (Fig. 15.8) with a low-molecular weight, ensuring hydrophilic properties combined with potent inhibitory effects on renin (50% inhibitory concentration, $IC_{50} = 0.6$ mmol/L).[54] The plasma half-life of the drug is approximately 24 hours, meaning that once-a-day administration should be appropriate.

Antihypertensive effects

Experimental studies
A small number of studies has been performed in experimental animal models with use of the renin inhibitor aliskiren. The reason for this paucity of data is that the inhibitory properties of this drug are specific for the human renin-substrate and thus cannot be tested in other animal species. This limitation has been recently overcome by: (1) employing sodium-depleted marmosets and spontaneously hypertensive rats, i.e. animal models displaying a renin structure that can be inhibited by aliskiren and (2) the use of transgenic animals harbouring human renin and angiotensinogen genes. Aliskiren has been shown to lower BP in the long term in all the above animal species.[54–57] The magnitude of blood pressure reduction appears to be superimposable on that of other antihypertensive compounds, such as angiotensin I receptor blockers or angiotensin converting enzyme inhibitors.[55,56] Combination of aliskiren with these compounds markedly potentiates antihypertensive efficacy.[55]

Recent studies,[56,58] performed in rats transgenic for human renin and angiotensinogen genes, have added new information. First, aliskiren markedly attenuates the albuminuria and the myocardial fibrosis characterizing elevated blood pressure regimens in this animal model of hypertension. These tissue protective effects were: (1) more pronounced than those displayed by an angiotensin II receptor antagonist[56] and (2) accompanied by a reduction in complement expression.[58] Second, the reversibility of the organ damage associated with hypertension was paralleled by an increased survival rate of the diseased animals, a finding that again underlines the wide range of the cardiovascular protective effects derived from renin inhibition.

Clinical studies
In normotensive and otherwise healthy volunteers oral administration of aliskiren for 8 days caused a dose-dependent decrease in plasma renin activity, angiotensin I and angiotensin II, with maximal reduction in the latter humoral

substance of about 90% at the highest drug dosage.[59] The almost complete suppression of angiotensin II was coupled with a decrease in plasma and urinary aldosterone levels, a finding that further strengthens the potential of this drug to elicit a marked and sustained blockade of the renin–angiotensin system.

The antihypertensive efficacy of aliskiren was tested in two studies. In the first,[60] performed according to a randomized, double-blind active comparator trial design, essential hypertensive patients were randomly assigned to receive aliskiren at 4 different daily dosages (37.5, 75, 150 and 300 mg or losartan 100 mg) for 4 weeks. The blood pressure lowering effects of the drug treatment tested in the study were assessed not only via an automated sphygmomanometric device, but also via 24-hour ambulatory BP monitoring. The marked and sustained reduction in plasma renin levels induced by aliskiren (Fig. 15.9) resulted in daytime and night-time blood pressure reductions of magnitude directly related to the drug dosage (Fig. 15.10). This finding was confirmed by the analysis of the ambulatory blood pressure profiles (Fig. 15.11), which showed that aliskiren: (1) induced a dose-dependent reduction in 24-hour blood pressure values, (2) did not significantly affect heart rate and (3) at the daily dosage of 300 mg displayed antihypertensive effects superimposable on those of losartan 100 mg daily. These results have been confirmed by a multicentre, randomized, double-blind placebo-controlled study,[61] in which the antihypertensive effects of three progressively greater dosages of aliskiren (150, 300 and 600 mg/day) were compared with those of irbesartan 150 mg/day. As shown in Figure 15.12 both systolic and diastolic sitting BPs were significantly reduced by aliskiren 150–600 mg/day, the magnitude of the antihypertensive effects being: (1) equivalent for the 300 and 600 mg doses and (2) significantly greater than those displayed by the angiotensin II receptor antagonist. Several clinical studies are planned with the aim of investigating further the antihypertensive properties of aliskiren, particularly during long-term administration or when used as combination treatment with other antihypertensive drugs.

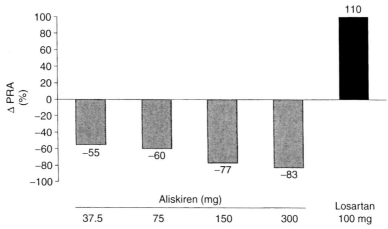

Fig. 15.9 Renin inhibitory effects of aliskiren (37.5 mg, 75 mg, 150 mg and 300 mg/day) in hypertensive patients. The increase in renin induced by losartan is also shown. Data are reported as per cent changes over baseline (no drug). *(Modified from ref. (60).)*

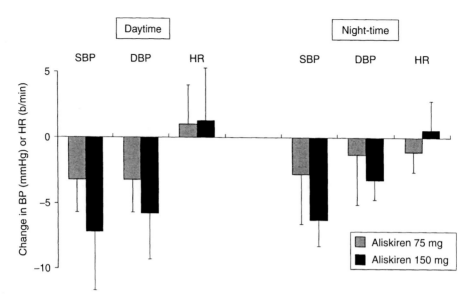

Fig. 15.10 Effects of aliskiren at 75 mg and 150 mg daily dosage on systolic blood pressure (SBP), diastolic blood pressure (DBP) and heart rate (HR) during the daytime and night-time period. Data are shown as means ± standard deviations. *(Modified from ref. (60).)*

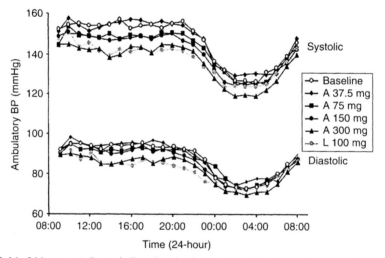

Fig. 15.11 24-hour systolic and diastolic blood pressure (BP) profile in the no-drug condition (baseline) and following different dosages of aliskiren (A) or losartan (L). Data are shown as mean hourly values. *(Modified from ref. (60).)*

Other cardiovascular effects

The marked activation of the renin–angiotensin system characterizing congestive heart failure, renal failure and acute myocardial infarction could represent a potential therapeutic target for the renin inhibitors and aliskiren in particular. No information is available on this issue either in animals or in humans.

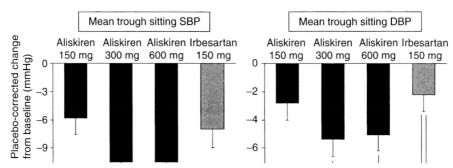

Fig. 15.12 Placebo-corrected changes in systolic (SBP) and diastolic (DBP) blood pressure induced by different doses of aliskiren or irbesartan. Data are shown as means ± standard errors. *(Modified from ref. (61).)*

Side effects and tolerability profile

From the limited clinical experience accumulated so far it appears that aliskiren treatment is well tolerated, the adverse event profile (represented more frequently by headache, dizziness and diarrhoea) being almost superimposable on that observed with placebo administration.

CONCLUSIONS

Investigation of new antihypertensive drugs represents a top priority in hypertension research. Success in this area will allow improvement in therapeutic interventions until the advent of pharmacogenomic approaches in the distant future.

References

1. Chobanian AV, Bakris GL, Black HR, et al. The Seventh Report of the Joint National Committee on Prevention, Detection, Evaluation and Treatment of High Blood Pressure: the JNC7 Report. *JAMA* 2003;289:2560–2572.
2. 2003 European Society of Hypertension-European Society of Cardiology guidelines for the management of arterial hypertension. Guidelines Committee. *J Hypertens* 2003;21:1011–1053.
3. Erdine S, Aran SN. Current status of hypertension control around the world. *Clin Exp Hypertens* 2004;26:731–738.
4. Mancia G. The association of hypertension and diabetes:prevalence, cardiovascular risk and protection by blood pressure reduction. *Acta Diabetol* 2005;42(Suppl 1):S17–S25.
5. Grassi G. Intermediate versus hard end points in clinical trials on hypertension. *Curr Hypertens Rep* 2005;7:294–297.
6. Shimokawa H, Vanhoutte PM. Endothelium and vascular injuries in hypertension and atherosclerosis. In: Zanchetti A, Mancia G, eds. *Handbook of hypertension*, Amsterdam: Elsevier; 1998:1006–1068.
7. Schiffrin EL. Endothelin and endothelin antagonists in hypertension. *J Hypertens* 1998;16:1891–1895.
8. Remuzzi G, Perico N, Benigni A. New therapeutics that antagonize endothelin: promises and frustrations. *Nat Rev Drug Discov* 2002;1:986–1001.
9. Ohuchi T, Kuwaki T, Ling GY, et al. Elevation of blood pressure by genetic and pharmacological disruption of the ETB receptor in mice. *Am J Physiol* 1999;276:R1071–R1077.
10. Verhaar MC, Strachan FE, Newby DE, et al. Endothelin-A receptor antagonist-mediated vasodilatation is attenuated by inhibition of nitric oxide synthesis and by endothelin-B receptor blockade. *Circulation* 1998;97:752–756.

11. Kaddoura S, Firth JD, Boheler KR, et al. Endothelin-1 is involved in norepinephrine induced ventricular hypertrophy in vivo: acute effects of bosentan, an orally active, mixed endothelin ETA and ETB receptor antagonist. *Circulation* 1998;93:2068–2079.

12. Wenzel RR, Fleisch M, Shaw S, et al. Hemodynamic and coronary effects of the endothelin antagonist bosentan in patients with coronary artery disease. *Circulation* 1998;98:2235–2240.

13. Williams DL, Walsh TF. Endothelin blockade in hypertension. In: Van Zwieten PA, Greenle WJ, eds. *Antihypertensive drugs*. Amsterdam: Harwood Academic Publishers; 1997:213–280.

14. Moreau P, Schiffrin EL. Role of endothelin in animal models of hypertension: focus on cardiovascular protection. *Can J Physiol Pharmacol* 2003;81:511–521.

15. Schricker K, Scholz H, Hamann M, et al. Role of endogenous endothelins in the renin system of normal and two-kidney, one clip rats. *Hypertension* 1995;25:1025–1029.

16. Hocher B, George I, Rebstock J, et al. Endothelin system-dependent cardiac remodelling in renovascular hypertension. *Hypertension* 1999;33:816–822.

17. Massart PE, Hodeige DG, Van Mechelen H, et al. Angiotensin II and endothelin-1 receptor antagonists have cumulative hypotensive effects in canine Page Hypertension. *J Hypertens* 1998;16:835–841.

18. Herizi A, Jover B, Bouriquet N, et al. Prevention of the cardiovascular and renal effects of angiotensin II by endothelin blockade. *Hypertension* 1998;31:10–14.

19. Liu JL, Pliquett RU, Brewer E, et al. Chronic endothelin-1 blockade reduces sympathetic nerve activity in rabbits with heart failure. *Am J Physiol Regul Integr Comp Physiol* 2001;280: R1906–R1913.

20. Taddei S, Grassi G. Angiotensin II as the link between nitric oxide and neuroadrenergic function. *J Hypertens* 2005;23:935–937.

21. Kirchengast M, Luz M. Endothelin receptor antagonists. Clinical realities and future directions. *J Cardiovasc Pharmacol* 2005;45:182–191.

22. Haynes WG, Strachan FE, Gray GA, et al. Forearm vasoconstriction to endothelin-1 is mediated by ET_A and ET_B receptors in vivo in humans. *J Cardiovasc Pharmacol* 1995;26: S40–S43.

23. Jougasaki M, Schriger JA, Simari RD, et al. Autocrine role for the endothelin-B receptor in the secretion of adrenomedullin. *Hypertension* 1998;32:917–922.

24. Taddei S, Virdis A, Ghiadoni L, et al. Vasoconstriction to endogenous endothelin-1 is increased in the peripheral circulation of patients with essential hypertension. *Circulation* 1999;100:1680–1683.

25. Strachan FE, Spratt JC, Wilkinson IB, et al. Systemic blockade of the ET_B receptor increases peripheral vascular resistance in healthy volunteers in vivo. *Hypertension* 1999;33:581–586.

26. Krum H, Vikoper RJ, Lacourciere Y, et al; for the bosentan Hypertension Investigators. The effect of an endothelin receptor antagonist, bosentan, on blood pressure in patients with essential hypertension. *N Engl J Med* 1998;338:784–790.

27. Nakov R, Pfarr E, Eberle S on behalf of the HEAT Investigators. Darusentan: an effective endothelin A receptor antagonist for treatment of hypertension. *Am J Hypertens* 2002;15:583–589.

28. Mancia G, Grassi G. Systolic and diastolic blood pressure control in antihypertensive drug trials. *J Hypertens* 2002;20:1461–1464.

29. Mancia G, Bombelli M, Lanzarotti A, et al. Systolic vs diastolic blood pressure control in the hypertensive patients of the PAMELA population. Pressioni Arteriosa Monitorate E Loro Associazioni. *Arch Intern Med* 2002;162:582–586.

30. Levy D. The role of systolic blood pressure in determining risk for cardiovascular disease. *J Hypertens* 1999;17(Suppl):S15–S18.

31. Kiowski W, Sutsch G, Hunziker P, et al. Evidence for endothelin 1-mediated vasocontriction in severe chronic heart failure. *Lancet* 1995;346:732–736.

32. Wei CM, Lerman A, Rodeheffer RJ, et al. Endothelin in human congestive heart failure. *Circulation* 1994;89:1580–1586.

33. Cowburn PJ, Cleland JGF. Endothelin antagonists for chronic heart failure: do they have a role. *Eur Heart J* 2001;22:1772–1784.

34. Sutsch G, Kiowski W, Yan XW, et al. Short term oral endothelin receptor antagonist therapy in conventionally treated patients with symptomatic severe chronic heart failure. *Circulation* 1998;98:2262–2268.

35. Luscher T, Enseleit F, Pacher R, et al. Hemodynamic and neurohumoral effects of selective endothelin A (ET_A) receptor blockade in chronic heart failure. The Heart Failure ETa receptor blockade trial (HEAT). *Circulation* 2002;106:2666–2672.

36. Rich S, McLaughlin V. Endothelin receptor blockers in cardiovascular disease. *Circulation* 2003;108:2184–2190.

37. Anand I, McMurray J, Cohn YN, et al on behalf of the EARTH investigators. Long-term effects of darusentan on left-ventricular remodelling and clinical outcomes in the Endothelin A Receptor Antagonist Trial in Heart Failure (EARTH): randomized, double blind, placebo-controlled trial. *Lancet* 2004;364:347–354.

38. Colletta A, Thackray S, Nikitin N, Cleland JG. Clinical trials update: highlights of the scientific sessions of the American College of Cardiology 2002: LIFE, DANAMI 2, MADIT-2, MIRACLE-ICD, OVERTURE, OCTAVE, ENABLE 1 and 2, CHRISTMAS, AFFIRM, RACE, WIZARD, AZACS, REMATCH, BNP trial and HARDBALL. *Eur J Heart Fail* 2002;4:381–388.

39. Budhiraja R, Tuder RM, Hassoun PM. Endothelial dysfunction in pulmonary hypertension. *Circulation* 2004;109:159–165.

40. Rubin LJ, Badesch DB, Barst RJ, et al. Bosentan therapy for pulmonary arterial hypertension. *New Engl J Med* 2002;346:896–903.

41. Donckier JE, Massart PE, Hodeige D, et al. Additional hypotensive effect of endothelin-1 receptor antagonism in hypertensive dogs under angiotensin-converting enzyme inhibition. *Circulation* 1997;64:1250–1256.

42. Dzau V. The cardiovascular continuum and renin-angiotensin-aldosterone system blockade. *J Hypertens* 2005;23(Suppl):S9–S17.

43. Stanton A. Potential of renin inhibition in cardiovascular disease. *J Renin Angiotensin Aldosterone Syst* 2003;4:6–10.

44. Nussberger J. Renin inhibitors. In: Oparil S, Weber MA, eds. *Hypertension*. Philadelphia: Elsevier Saunders; 2004:754–764.

45. Michel JB, Galen FX, Guettier C, et al. Immunological approach to blockade of the renin-substrate reaction. *J Hypertens* 1989;7(Suppl):S63–S70.

46. Johnson CA, Wakerlin GE. Antiserum for renin. *Proc Soc Exp Biol Med* 1940;44:277–281.

47. Boger J, Lohr NS, Ulm EH, et al. Novel renin inhibitors containing the amino acid statine. *Nature* 1983;303:81–84.

48. Hui K, Haber E. Renin inhibitors. In: Robertson JIS, Nicholls MG, eds. *The renin-angiotensin system*. New York: Raven Press; 1983:85.1–85.14.

49. Haber E. Peptide inhibitors of renin in cardiovascular studies. *Fed Proc* 1983;42:3155–3161.

50. Rongen GA, Lenders JWM, Smits P, et al. Clinical pharmacokinetics and efficacy of renin inhibitors. *Clin Pharmacokinet* 1995;29:6–14.

51. Cumin F, Evin G, Fehrentz JA, et al. Inhibition of human renin by synthetic peptides derived from its prosegment. *J Biol Chem* 1985;260:9154–9157.

52. Szelke M, Leckie B, Hallett A, et al. Potent new inhibitors of human renin. *Nature* 1982;299:555–557.

53. Webb DJ, Manhem PJO, Ball SG, et al. A study of the renin inhibitor H142 in man. *J Hypertens* 1985;3:653–658.

54. Wood JM, Maibaum J, Rahuel J, et al. Structure-based design of aliskiren, a novel orally effective renin inhibitor. *Biochem Biophys Res Commun* 2003;308:698–705.

55. Wood JM, Schnell CR, Cumin F, et al. Aliskiren, a novel, orally effective renin inhibitor, lowers blood pressure in marmosets and spontaneously hypertensive rats. *J Hypertens* 2005;23:417–426.

56. Pilz B, Shagdarsuren E, Wellner M, et al. Aliskiren, a human renin inhibitor, ameliorates cardiac and renal damage in double-transgenic rats. *Hypertension* 2005;46:569–576.

57. Kelly DJ, Wilkinson-Berka JL, Gilbert RE. Renin inhibition: new potential for an old therapeutic target. *Hypertension* 2005;46:471–472.

58. Shagdarsuren E, Wellner M, Braesen JH, et al. Complement Activation in Angiotensin II-Induced Organ Damage. *Circulation Res* 2005;97:716–724.

59. Nussberger J, Wuerzner G, Jensen C, et al. Angiotensin II suppression in human by the orally active renin inhibitor aliskiren (SPP100) comparison with enalapril. *Hypertension* 2002;39: e1–e8.

60. Stanton A, Jensen C, Nussberger J, et al. blood pressure lowering in essential hypertension with an oral renin inhibitor, aliskiren. *Hypertension* 2003;42:1137–1143.

61. Gradman AH, Schmieder RE, Lins RL, et al. Aliskiren, a novel orally effective renin inhibitor, provides dose-dependent antihypertensive efficacy and placebo-like tolerability in hypertensive patients. *Circulation* 2005;111:1012–1018.

VIII
Clinical trials

16 | Evidence-base for treatment of hypertension

William J. Elliott and Henry R. Black

INTRODUCTION

Epidemiological studies have clearly and convincingly established that elevated blood pressure (BP) is a powerful risk factor for cardiovascular disease, the most common cause of death in most countries across the world.[1] Compilation of data from nearly 1 million adults in 61 prospective studies shows that the risk of cardiovascular death doubles for each 20/10 mmHg increase in BP $\leq 115/75$ mmHg, and is essentially independent of age.[2] Although these and other similar data provide the background for lowering BP, many well-designed and properly-executed outcome-based clinical trials have been performed that demonstrate the benefits of different approaches to lowering BP. Details of many of the older (and now 'classic') studies are available in a recently published monograph.[3] The results from most of these trials have been combined and summarized in other forms (e.g. meta-analyses), which has helped to shape hypertension treatment guidelines across the world. It should be remembered that the results of clinical trials, analyzed by traditional 'intent-to-treat' methods, generally **underestimate** the true benefits of an effective therapy, since those who abandon their assigned treatments bias 'toward the null'. This chapter attempts to summarize some of the clinical trials and pivotal meta-analyses that have helped to shape thinking about how and to what extent BP should be lowered. Although placebo-controlled and other 'classic' studies are discussed, the focus is on more recent studies that have addressed more precise and more difficult questions.

BENEFITS OF TREATING ELEVATED DIASTOLIC BLOOD PRESSURE

In the 1920s–1950s, conventional wisdom (and a lack of well-tolerated antihypertensive medications) supported the notion that elevated BP was a natural response to ageing, was required to perfuse end organs, and probably should not be treated. In the 1950s, however, several oral antihypertensive drugs were shown to be effective in lowering BP in the short term. The clinical benefits of these drugs in the longer term were demonstrated in a series of placebo-controlled clinical trials, all of which showed benefit. Perhaps the most compelling of the early studies was the First Veterans' Affairs Cooperative Group Trial on Antihypertensive Agents, which was terminated early, and required no statistical analyses to show the benefits of lowering BP.[4] In the early 1960s, 143 male American veterans whose diastolic BPs were between 115 and 129 mm Hg after 6 days of a low-sodium diet in the hospital were randomized to placebo or combination antihypertensive therapy (hydrochlorothiazide 50 mg twice daily, reserpine 0.1 mg twice daily, and hydralazine 25 mg thrice daily). Antihypertensive drugs were provided to any patients who were hospitalized, had terminating events, or had diastolic BP of >130 mmHg and developed high-grade retinopathy during follow-up. During the first 12 months of observation, BPs didn't change in the placebo-treated group, but fell from 186/121 to 156/92 mmHg in the drug-treated group. When the oversight committee reviewed the data at 18 months of follow-up, 4 of the 70 randomized to placebo had died; no deaths were observed among the 73 in the drug-treated group. Furthermore, the distribution of terminating events was 27 vs. 2, respectively, with those in the drug-treated group being one non-disabling stroke and one adverse drug reaction. This was the first multicentre, randomized clinical trial to show a major long-term benefit of lowering diastolic BP.

Many other studies that randomized patients with lower diastolic BPs to active antihypertensive drugs or other strategies then followed. The two largest continue to be of interest today, even 20 years after their completion. The British Medical Research Council funded the largest clinical trial of hypertension then undertaken. They screened about 515 000 and enrolled 17 354 young (aged 35–64 years) and otherwise healthy British subjects with diastolic BPs between 90 and 109 mmHg, and systolic BP <200 mmHg. Randomization was to placebo (50%), bendrofluazide (25%), and propranolol (25%), followed by methyldopa or guanethidine (as required). Individuals whose BPs exceeded threshold limits (initially 210/115 mmHg) were provided with open-label antihypertensive treatment. After 5.5 years of follow-up, about 18% of those randomized to placebo had persistent diastolic BPs <90 mmHg, so the difference in BPs between groups was much less than expected. In the intention-to-treat analysis, death and myocardial infarction were not significantly reduced by either antihypertensive therapy. Stroke was significantly reduced, but the absolute risk reduction was small: 850 patients would require treatment for a year to prevent one stroke.[5] These bleak conclusions reflected the low risk and small potential benefit in that population, and were followed by many important reports of subgroups and other analyses that allowed other studies to be done more efficiently.

The largest study of diastolic BP in the US was the Hypertension Detection and Follow-up Program, which began in 1972. Its 14 clinical centres screened 159 566 and enrolled 10 940 individuals between 30 and 69 years of age with diastolic BP >95 mmHg at the first screen, and >90 mmHg at the second. Half were randomized to 'stepped care' in specialized clinics (SC): thrice yearly visits and stepwise treatment with chlorthalidone, reserpine or methyldopa, hydralazine, guanethidine, and then other drugs as needed, all free of charge. Newer antihypertensive agents could be added after being approved by the US FDA. The other half of the participants was referred back to their local physicians, to receive whatever therapy was deemed appropriate. As time progressed, the drugs given to these 'referred care' patients (seen in routine clinics) became similar to the antihypertensive regimen of 'stepped care' participants. Annual home visits were made to measure BP and ascertain outcomes. BPs and the proportion remaining untreated were significantly lower among the 'stepped care' group. Five years after randomization, there was a significant ($p = 0.006$) 17% reduction in death among those randomized to 'stepped care', which persisted and increased further even after the study closed.[6] Importantly, there was a highly significant reduction in death among black men (16%) and black women (24%) who were randomized to 'stepped care' (as opposed to 'referred care'). This study suggested a much larger benefit to lowering diastolic BP than the MRC trial, and paved the way for several community-based trials of hypertension in the USA.

Nearly all of the placebo-controlled clinical trials that involved patients with diastolic hypertension were collected in a meta-analysis published in 1990.[7] By that time, 14 unconfounded trials involving more than 37 000 patients compared antihypertensive drug therapy and placebo, with an observed diastolic BP difference of 5–6 mmHg between groups over 5 years. Vascular mortality was significantly reduced ($p = 0.0002$), and non-vascular mortality was not different between treated and untreated patients. Stroke was significantly ($p < 0.0001$) reduced by $42 \pm 6\%$ (mean $\pm$ standard deviation), essentially all the reduction predicted by epidemiological data. Coronary heart disease was reduced by only $14 \pm 5\%$, which, although significant at $p < 0.01$, was much less than the expected reduction predicted from epidemiological data.

It was, nonetheless, clear from these studies and their combination in meta-analysis that there are significant and substantial benefits to reducing diastolic BP. Later meta-analyses indicated that antihypertensive drug therapy also significantly prevented progression of hypertension, cardiovascular death (by about 21%) and heart failure (by 52%).[8]

BENEFITS OF TREATING ELEVATED SYSTOLIC BLOOD PRESSURE

During the last several decades, systolic BP has been shown to be a better predictor of cardiovascular and renal events than diastolic BP, especially in the sixth decade of life and beyond. In the Prospective Studies Collaborative database, systolic BP was a better predictor than diastolic BP for both stroke (89% vs. 83% of the >12 000 deaths) and especially coronary heart disease (93% vs. 73% for the >34 000 deaths).[2] Only in the last 20 years, however, have clinical trials enrolled patients with 'isolated systolic hypertension', which is the most common form of hypertension in older people.

The first of the three trials to demonstrate the benefits of lowering systolic BP was the Systolic Hypertension in the Elderly Program (SHEP).[9] In this landmark study, 4736 Americans aged 60 years or older with systolic BPs between 160 and 209 mmHg, but diastolic BPs of <90 mmHg were randomized to placebo or active antihypertensive drug therapy beginning with low-dose chlorthalidone (12.5 mg/day), which was titrated to 25 mg/day in those above goal BP. Atenolol, reserpine, or other drugs were then added sequentially, if needed. As in previous studies, active therapy was given to those who had an event or whose BPs exceeded pre-specified thresholds, or if the patient's physician thought it was appropriate. After 4.5 years of average follow-up, BPs changed from 171/77 to 143/68 mmHg in the actively-treated group, and from 170/76 to 154/72 mmHg in the placebo-treated group (perhaps because 44% in this group were taking antihypertensive medications). Even so, the actively-treated group had a significant ($p = 0.0003$) 36% reduction in fatal or non-fatal stroke (the primary endpoint), a significant ($p < 0.05$) 25% reduction in fatal or non-fatal myocardial infarction, a 25% reduction ($p < 0.05$) in coronary events, a 32% ($p < 0.01$) reduction in cardiovascular events, and a 49% ($p < 0.001$) reduction in heart failure.[10] All types of stroke were reduced, and there was no evidence that lowering BP was associated with an excess risk of stroke.[11]

The Systolic Hypertension in Europe (Syst-Eur) trial was begun before the results of SHEP were known, to compare an antihypertensive drug regimen beginning with a calcium antagonist against placebo for prevention of stroke in patients at least 60 years old with systolic BPs between 160 and 219 mmHg, and diastolic BP of <95 mmHg. After 8926 patients were screened, 4695 were randomized to either placebo or nitrendipine 10 mg, taken initially in the evening. Doses could be increased, and enalapril and then hydrochlorothiazide could be added, if necessary. The actively-treated patients had a fall in seated BP from 174/85 to 150/79 mmHg at 2 years of follow-up, as compared to 174/86 to 160/84 monthly for the placebo-group. The study was terminated prematurely at the second of four planned interim analyses.[12] After an average of 2 years of follow-up, there was already a 42% reduction in fatal or non-fatal stroke ($p = 0.003$), a 26% reduction in cardiac endpoints (heart failure or myocardial infarction, $p = 0.03$), and a 31% reduction in all cardiovascular endpoints ($p < 0.001$). Many other results, based on extended follow-up, subgroups, per-protocol analyses, and secondary endpoints have subsequently been published. One of the more interesting of these was a 50% reduction in dementia (as assessed by Mini-Mental Status Examination screening, and further testing if abnormal) seen in those randomized to active drug therapy.[13]

The primary results of Syst-Eur were verified in a very similar trial (using the same drug treatment strategy, but substituting captopril for enalapril) in China, where local custom did not use randomization; instead treatment allocations were made by sequential assignment. In this study, 2394 older Chinese patients with an average BP of 170/86 mmHg were treated for 3 years. BP was significantly lower in the actively-treated group (by 9/3 mmHg). Compared to placebo, antihypertensive drug therapy was associated with a significant 38% reduction in stroke ($p = 0.01$), 39% reduction in mortality ($p = 0.003$), and a 37% reduction in all cardiovascular endpoints ($p = 0.004$).[14] This study is not usually included in meta-analyses, as treatment allocation was not randomized.

A large effort was made to collect outcomes data about older patients with isolated systolic hypertension who were randomized in eight clinical trials (including both SHEP and Syst-Eur), to assess the global benefits of lowering systolic BP.[15] Data were gathered from 15 693 patients with baseline BP of 174/83 mmHg who were treated for a mean of 3.8 years with either placebo or active antihypertensive drug therapy. The average difference in BP was 10/4 mmHg between the two groups. In meta-analysis, this relatively small reduction in BP was associated with a significant 30% reduction in fatal or non-fatal stroke ($p < 0.0001$), a 23% reduction in fatal or non-fatal coronary heart disease ($p < 0.001$), a 26% reduction in all cardiovascular events ($p < 0.001$), and a 13% reduction in all-cause mortality ($p = 0.02$), fulfilling epidemiological predictions. There was no evidence of an increase in non-cardiovascular deaths with antihypertensive drug therapy. These data provide strong evidence in favour of lowering systolic BP with antihypertensive drugs.

BENEFITS OF DRUG THERAPY FOR HIGH BLOOD PRESSURE (SYSTOLIC OR DIASTOLIC)

A recent network meta-analysis has attempted to summarize the benefits of **any** active drug therapy vs. no treatment in 25 trials, irrespective of whether the elevation in BP was systolic or diastolic, and irrespective of what antihypertensive drug was used initially.[16] Analogous results from a similar meta-analysis[17] of all 37 available clinical trials are shown in Figure 16.1. Generally, all examined endpoints benefited significantly from drug treatment. There was significant heterogeneity across trials for all endpoints, probably because early studies gave placebo and no antihypertensive drugs, whereas more recent 'placebo-treated' patients also received active antihypertensive drug therapy that was different from that in the other randomized arm of the study. Overall, however, stroke was reduced by $29 \pm 3\%$ (mean ± standard deviation), coronary heart disease events by $19 \pm 3\%$, heart failure by $29 \pm 5\%$, major cardiovascular events by $22 \pm 2\%$, cardiovascular mortality by $17 \pm 3\%$, and total mortality by $9 \pm 2\%$. These results clearly indicate that antihypertensive drug therapy, in the aggregate, has many benefits across all types of major cardiovascular events.

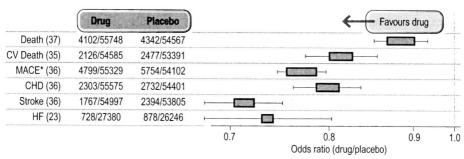

Fig. 16.1 Results of a traditional meta-analysis (using the Mantel-Haenszel technique) showing outcomes for 37 long-term trials involving 110 315 patients comparing any initial antihypertensive drug therapy vs. placebo or no treatment. These results are similar to those reported by Psaty et al., based only on 28 trials;[16] both ignore potentially important differences across trials, i.e. heterogeneity. CV = cardiovascular; MACE* = major adverse cardiovascular events (stroke, myocardial infarction, or cardiovascular death, estimated for some trials that did not report this endpoint directly); CHD = coronary heart disease (fatal or non-fatal myocardial infarction); HF = heart failure. The number of trials reporting each type of event is given in parentheses; the upper and lower limits of the 95% confidence interval are denoted by the horizontal bars; the rectangles are proportional to the total number of events.

BENEFITS OF TREATING TO DIFFERENT TARGET BLOOD PRESSURES

Although the studies cited above indicate that lowering elevated BP is, in general, beneficial, there has long been concern that lowering diastolic BP 'too far' could be harmful, especially for cardiac endpoints, since the coronary arteries fill during diastole. Epidemiological studies have suggested that a target BP of 140/90 mmHg is not only useful for the cutoff for diagnosis among untreated people, but that it should also be the target for treated hypertensives. Even lower BPs have been recently recommended for high-risk hypertensive patients, including those with diabetes and chronic kidney disease. We now have clinical trial data that support recent national and international guidelines on this topic.

In the US in 1997, the Sixth Report of the Joint National Committee recommended a lower-than-usual target BP for diabetics (<130/85 mmHg), but had no data to support it at that time. A year later, the results of the United Kingdom Prospective Diabetes Study #38 were reported.[18] In the late 1980s, 1148 British type 2 diabetic patients with hypertension were randomized in a 1:2 ratio to BP targets of <180/105 or <150/85 mmHg. During 8.4 years of average follow-up, those treated to the lower target had 24% fewer diabetes-related endpoints (the primary endpoint, $p = 0.0046$), 32% fewer deaths ($p < 0.02$), 44% fewer strokes ($p < 0.02$), and 37% fewer microvascular endpoints ($p < 0.01$) than those assigned to the higher goal. The achieved BP difference between groups was 10/5 mmHg (154/87 vs. 144/82 mmHg), which when subtracted from the usual BP target for non-diabetics (140/90 mmHg), gives a target for diabetics that is **identical** to that recommended in the USA a year earlier: 130/85 mmHg!

Concerns have been raised that the lower-than-usual BP goal now recommended for diabetics would be expensive, as it requires more antihypertensive pills and more visits to healthcare providers. A cost analysis of the UKPDS clinical trial did **not** support this hypothesis: despite higher drug and provider costs, the strategy of the lower BP goal SAVED lives, strokes, limbs, *and money*. The cost-effectiveness ratio for the lower BP goal was −£720 per year of life saved, and an even more impressive −£1049 year of life without diabetic complications.[19] A similar conclusion was derived from an economic analysis of US epidemiological and clinical trial data for older (≥60 years) diabetics treated to a goal of <130/85 mmHg (recommended in 1997 in the USA), compared to leaving the target BP at <140/90 mmHg.[20] Because the lower BP goal impressively reduces the risk of expensive cardiovascular events, including stroke, heart attack, heart failure, and renal replacement therapy, the incremental cost-effectiveness ratio for the lower BP goal is negative (meaning more intensive treatment SAVES money!), just as in UKPDS. Another cost-analysis of treatment of diabetics, based on the US population, showed that the cost per quality-adjusted year of life saved by lowering BP is −$1959 (i.e. a prolongation of life by half a year, and a cost-savings), whereas lowering cholesterol and treating hyperglycaemia each cost between $41 000 and $52 000 to add a quality-adjusted year of life to a diabetic.[21] These calculations translate the clinical benefits of the lower-than-usual BP target into economic terms that everyone can understand: overall, lowering BP in very high-risk hypertensives saves not only lives and cardiovascular events, but also money.

The BP target for diabetics was refined further by a pre-specified subgroup analysis from the Hypertension Optimal Treatment (HOT) study. In this 3.8-year trial, there were 1501 type 2 diabetics randomized to diastolic BP targets of ≤80, ≤85 or ≤90 mmHg. In the intention-to-treat analysis, there was a 51% lower risk of the primary endpoint (stroke, myocardial infarction, or cardiovascular death) among those randomized to ≤80 mmHg, compared to those at ≤90 mmHg; the risk was intermediate for those at the middle goal.[22] These data have helped to convince all authorities that the appropriate BP target for type 2 diabetics is <130/80 mmHg.

A lower-than-usual BP target has sometimes been recommended for patients with chronic kidney disease. An analysis from the Modification of Diet in Renal Disease study suggested that a target of <125/75 mmHg was beneficial in delaying the progression toward renal failure.[23] This target was directly compared with the usual and customary goal (<140/90 mmHg) in the African American Study of Kidney disease and hypertension. In a randomization scheme that involved three initial drugs and two BP targets, 1094 hypertensive US blacks with hypertensive nephrosclerosis showed only a non-significant 2% difference in the composite secondary outcome of decline in glomerular filtration rate (by 50% compared to baseline, or by 25 mL/minute/1.73 m^2), end-stage renal disease, or death, with slightly fewer events in the higher BP group (167 vs. 173, $p = 0.85$).[24] Similar non-significant differences were found for all other composite clinical endpoints in AASK, suggesting that the lower BP target leads only to more expenditures for drugs and clinic visits, without improved clinical outcomes. A somewhat different conclusion was reached in a 'patient-level' *post-hoc* meta-regression analysis of 11 trials comparing angiotensin converting enzyme (ACE)-inhibitors with placebo in 1860 patients with non-diabetic renal disease.[25] For patients with more than 1 gm of proteinuria/day, maintaining a usual systolic BP between 110 and 129 mmHg was associated with significant protection against doubling serum creatinine or end-stage renal disease. Overall, therefore, the data regarding the lower BP target for chronic kidney disease patients are not as homogeneous or as compelling as the data regarding type 2 diabetics. As a result, the Seventh Report of the Joint National Committee on Prevention, Detection, Evaluation and Treatment of High Blood Pressure (JNC 7) recommended the same target for both groups: <130/80 mmHg.[26,27]

The largest clinical trial that investigated the potential benefits or harm of a lower-than-usual BP in uncomplicated hypertensive patients was the HOT study. It enrolled 18 790 patients treated with the sequence of dihydropyridine calcium antagonist, ACE-inhibitor or β-blocker and then a diuretic, to achieve the randomized targets of ≤80, ≤85, or ≤90 mmHg.[22] In the intention-to-treat analysis of the primary endpoint (stroke, myocardial infarction, or cardiovascular death), there was no significant difference ($p = 0.50$) across the three randomized groups, although the separation in achieved diastolic BPs across the three groups was less than planned (2 vs. 5 mmHg). In the 'on-treatment analysis', the BP that was associated with the lowest cardiovascular risk was 138.5/82.6 mmHg. Since this number is, in fact <140/90 mmHg, some claim these data validate this traditional target for antihypertensive drug therapy in uncomplicated patients. The HOT data at least show that there was no significant **increase** in risk by lowering BP to a diastolic target of ≤80 mmHg, but there was no further benefit either.[22] Because the probability of drug-related side effects often increases as the doses are increased, it is likely that the target BP of <140/90 mmHg for uncomplicated hypertensive patients will be defensible for some time to come.

A meta-analysis of four outcome-based clinical trials that compared more intensive vs. less intensive BP lowering has been reported by the Blood Pressure Lowering Trialists' Collaborative.[28] In addition to HOT, AASK, and UKPDS 38 (discussed above), this analysis included both subgroups of the Appropriate Blood pressure Control in Diabetes (ABCD) study, which randomized either 480 normotensive or 470 hypertensive diabetics, and followed them for 5.3 years. The observed difference in BPs across these four studies was only 4/3 mmHg; only AASK was successful in achieving its planned BP difference, but it has so far only reported the numbers of patients who died and had major cardiovascular events.[24] The results of the meta-analysis showed no significant differences (over all studies) for total mortality, cardiovascular mortality, coronary heart disease events, or heart failure, although the trends all favoured the more intensively over the less intensively treated group. In contrast, significant 15% reductions were seen for both stroke and major cardiovascular events among those treated to the lower BP target. The conclusions of these meta-analyses were tempered somewhat by meta-regression analyses that plotted the observed differences in systolic BP in trials comparing various types of antihypertensive drugs (or placebo) vs. the relative risk of outcome events.[29,30] These analyses suggested that, with the exception of heart failure, all types of events showed a significant and linear relationship: the higher the achieved systolic BP difference, the greater the prevention of the event.

BENEFITS OF DIFFERENT INITIAL DRUG THERAPIES

Trials of active drug therapy vs. placebo/no treatment

For historical and ethical reasons, the number of trials that compared active antihypertensive drugs with placebo/no treatment is limited. Most of these studies were done when the benefits of antihypertensive drug therapy were uncertain, and long-term outcome-driven studies using placebo or no treatment could be morally justified. Most of the larger studies of this type used diuretics or β-blockers, simply because these drugs were developed first. By the time newer drugs were introduced, large-scale studies comparing them with placebo or no treatment to prevent cardiovascular events would have been ethically indefensible. Thus the amount of direct evidence to support the long-term safety and efficacy of the newer antihypertensive drug classes is small, compared to the now-classic studies of diuretics and/or β-blockers. The results of a meta-analysis of the results from existing trials comparing each of the initial classes of drugs vs. placebo or no treatment are shown in Table 16.1.

Diuretics
Some of the more important studies that compared cardiovascular outcomes with diuretics vs. placebo or no treatment have been discussed above. Some of the European trials used an 'either/or' strategy for the initial drug used in

Table 16.1 Results of traditional meta-analyses (using the Mantel-Haenszel method) of clinical trials comparing antihypertensive drugs of different classes with placebo or no treatment

Event (no. of studies)	No. of events	No. of patients	Odds ratio (95% CI)	p-value*
Low-dose diuretic				
All-cause mortality (5)	1531	15 086	0.88 (0.79–0.99)	0.03
Cardiovascular mortality (5)	627	15 086	0.77 (0.76–0.89)	0.0006
Fatal or non-fatal coronary heart disease (5)	578	15 086	0.69 (0.59–0.82)	<0.0001
Fatal or non-fatal stroke (5)	886	15 086	0.67 (0.58–0.77)	<0.0001
Major cardiovascular events (5)	1764	15 086	0.69 (0.62–0.77)	<0.0001
Heart failure (2)	168	5287	0.52 (0.38–0.72)	<0.0001
High-dose diuretic				
All-cause mortality (12)	1304	30 785	0.95 (0.86–1.06)	0.33
Cardiovascular mortality (12)	788	30 785	0.80 (0.70–0.93)	0.003
Fatal or non-fatal coronary heart disease (12)	885	30 785	0.95 (0.83–1.10)	0.49
Fatal or non-fatal stroke (12)	580	30 785	0.54 (0.46–0.67)	<0.0001
Major cardiovascular events (12)	1538	30 785	0.73 (0.66–0.82)	<0.0001*
Heart failure (10)	39	6894	0.28 (0.18–0.83)	<0.0001
β-blocker				
All-cause mortality (6)	1316	21 076	0.94 (0.84–1.06)	0.32
Cardiovascular mortality (6)	771	21 076	0.91 (0.71–1.07)	0.22*
Fatal or non-fatal coronary heart disease (6)	852	21 076	0.93 (0.81–1.08)	0.32
Fatal or non-fatal stroke (6)	752	21 076	0.78 (0.67–0.91)	0.001
Major cardiovascular events (5)	1491	20 192	0.87 (0.78–0.98)	0.02
Heart failure (2)	116	2511	0.56 (0.38–0.83)	0.003
Calcium antagonist				
All-cause mortality (6)	682	11 508	0.80 (0.68–0.94)	0.005
Cardiovascular mortality (5)	340	10 682	0.72 (0.58–0.90)	0.002
Fatal or non-fatal coronary heart disease (6)	392	11 508	0.73 (0.60–0.90)	0.003
Fatal or non-fatal stroke (6)	351	11 508	0.60 (0.49–0.75)	<0.0001
Major cardiovascular events (6)	906	11 508	0.72 (0.63–0.84)	<0.0001*
Heart failure (5)	373	10 682	1.03 (0.84–1.31)	0.78
ACE-inhibitor				
All-cause mortality (7)	3233	35 359	0.91 (0.85–0.98)	0.02
Cardiovascular mortality (7)	1840	35 359	0.84 (0.77–0.92)	0.0004
Fatal or non-fatal coronary heart disease (7)	2357	35 359	0.77 (0.70–0.84)	<0.0001
Fatal or non-fatal stroke (7)	1567	35 359	0.77 (0.70–0.86)	<0.0001*
Major cardiovascular events (7)	4563	35 359	0.79 (0.74–0.84)	<0.0001*
Heart failure (4)	690	27 044	0.78 (0.67–0.90)	0.002
Angiotensin receptor blocker				
All-cause mortality (4)	1035	7937	0.96 (0.84–1.10)	0.53
Cardiovascular mortality (3)	410	6424	0.95 (0.78–1.16)	0.60
Fatal or non-fatal coronary heart disease (3)	341	7598	0.92 (0.74–1.15)	0.46
Fatal or non-fatal stroke (3)	290	6424	0.79 (0.63–1.00)	0.06
Major cardiovascular events (4)	1082	7937	0.91 (0.80–1.04)	0.15
Heart failure (2)	348	2661	0.72 (0.57–0.90)	0.003

*Significant (p<0.05) heterogeneity (by Breslow-Day test) across the trials

the treatment algorithm, both in studies against placebo, e.g. Swedish Trial of Older Patients with Hypertension (STOP-Hypertension), and in studies against other antihypertensive drug classes (e.g. Nordic Diltiazem [NORDIL] study). The results of these trials have been reported only as randomized, and in the aggregate, so the number of patients with outcomes who were initially given a diuretic, for example, is unknown.

If these concerns are ignored and all 17 studies are combined (see below for details) initial diuretic (compared to placebo or no treatment) is associated with a 9% (95% CI: 1–16%, p for heterogeneity $= 0.57$) reduction in all-cause mortality, a 21% (95% CI: 13–29%, p for heterogeneity $= 0.68$) reduction in cardiovascular mortality, a 16% (95% CI: 6–24%, p for heterogeneity $= 0.58$) reduction in coronary heart disease, a 46% (95% CI: 33–54%, p for heterogeneity $= 0.34$) reduction in stroke, a 29% (95% CI: 23–34%, p for heterogeneity $= 0.14$) reduction in major cardiovascular events, and a 54% (95% CI: 33–63%, p for heterogeneity $= 0.74$) reduction in heart failure.[16]

There are five studies comparing low-dose diuretics with placebo: EWPHE, SHEP-pilot, SHEP, MRC-Elderly, and PATS. The results of a traditional meta-analysis (using the Mantel-Haenszel method) of these five studies involving 15 086[17] patients are shown in the top section of Table 16.1. The results of a 'network meta-analysis' of the same data from these trials were only slightly different from these estimates.[16] In the traditional meta-analysis of the data,[17] there were no significant heterogeneities across the trials for any endpoint. All six endpoints of interest were significantly reduced by low-dose diuretic therapy: 12% for all-cause mortality, 23% for cardiovascular mortality, 31% for coronary heart disease, 33% for stroke, 31% for major cardiovascular events (non-fatal stroke, non-fatal myocardial infarction or cardiovascular death), and 48% for heart failure (based on 168 events in two studies).

In contrast, 12 earlier studies involving 30 785 patients compared high doses of diuretics with placebo or no treatment.[17] When these are combined in a meta-analysis using the traditional Mantel-Haenszel method, significant heterogeneity ($p < 0.05$) if found for major cardiovascular events studies (as noted by the asterisks in the last column in the second section of Table 16.1). The heterogeneity may be due to mixing of studies that used 'no treatment', as opposed to placebo followed by active treatment thereafter, as the control group. With high-dose diuretics, the reductions in all-cause mortality and fatal or non-fatal coronary heart disease are not significant (compared to placebo or no treatment). The point estimates of the reductions in both stroke and heart failure are greater for high-dose than low-dose diuretics, but the number of heart failure episodes was only 39 and the confidence interval for this comparison is quite wide. These data support the current practice of using only low-dose diuretics in the treatment of hypertension.

β-blockers

Six clinical trials involving 21 076 patients compared an initial β-blocker with placebo or no treatment: MRC-1, Coope and Warrender, STOP-Hypertension, MRC-E, Dutch TIA study, and TEST. The results of a traditional meta-analysis of the events observed in these trials[17] are shown in the third section of Table 16.1. In addition to significant heterogeneity for cardiovascular mortality, there was no significant reduction in all-cause mortality, cardiovascular mortality, and coronary heart disease events with an initial β-blocker (compared to placebo or no treatment). These data confirm and extend a prior meta-analysis of two studies in the elderly with identical conclusions.[31]

Calcium antagonists

Six studies have compared outcomes with an initial calcium antagonist or placebo: Syst-Eur, PREVENT, STONE, Syst-China, and IDNT. All of these studies used dihydropyridine calcium antagonists; there are no placebo-controlled outcomes studies with diltiazem, verapamil, or any other non-dihydropyridine calcium antagonist. Neither STONE nor Syst-China was randomized, for cultural reasons discussed above, so they have not been included in prior meta-analyses of randomized clinical trials. As shown in the third section of Table 16.1, there is heterogeneity in the results for heart failure and major cardiovascular events and coronary heart disease.[17] With the exception of heart failure, the initial calcium antagonist was associated with a significant prevention of all endpoints, compared with placebo or no treatment.

ACE-inhibitors

Seven clinical trials compared outcomes in patients randomized to an ACE-inhibitor or placebo: HOPE, PART2, QUIET, SCAT, PROGRESS, EUROPA and DIABHYCAR. Although there was heterogeneity for stroke and major cardiovascular events,[17] over all the studies, all endpoints were significantly reduced (Table 16.1). Heart failure was a reported endpoint in only four of the seven studies, limiting the power of the meta-analysis of this endpoint. It was, nonetheless, significantly reduced, supporting the use of ACE-inhibitors in not only the treatment, but also prevention of heart failure.

Angiotensin II receptor blockers (ARBs)

There have so far been four studies comparing outcomes in patients treated with angiotensin II receptor blockers or placebo: IDNT, RENAAL, SCOPE, and ACCESS. In each case, placebo was soon followed (by design) with other effective antihypertensive drugs, leaving a much smaller difference in achieved systolic BPs across the two randomized groups (0–2 mmHg) than had been the case in placebo-controlled trials of other drug classes (typically 6–30 mmHg). The studies involving angiotensin II receptor blockers were also shorter in duration than other trials (range 1–3.75 years). The first two were designed primarily to compare renal outcomes, rather than cardiovascular events. Despite these differences, the last section of Table 16.1 shows no heterogeneity across studies with significant protection of angiotensin II receptor blockers against only heart failure (based on only IDNT and RENAAL, but consistent with both Val-HeFT, CHARM, and VALIANT).[17] This meta-analysis suffers from a smaller number of trials and events, compared to those discussed above, limiting statistical power.

In general, most of the drug classes used in the above trials are reasonably effective in preventing most of the cardiovascular events with which hypertension is associated. The differences across the various active treatments appear, in most cases, to be smaller than the effectiveness of each drug vs. placebo or no treatment. However, comparing different classes of initial drug therapy to each other when each was pitted against placebo or no treatment obviously is only indirect and somewhat imprecise. Other major confounders include the different doses used (e.g. high- vs. low-dose diuretics), different secular trends during the execution of the different trials (e.g. later trials have much wider use of aspirin and lipid-lowering therapies), and inconsistent definitions of some endpoints (e.g. 'major cardiovascular events' in some trials includes heart failure and amputations). Clearly more meaningful and consistent comparisons result from head-to-head trials comparing different classes of drugs, which has been done only in the last 15 years.

Review of outcomes-based clinical trials by class of initial drug

The emergence in the early 1980s of two relatively well-tolerated antihypertensive drug classes with few contraindications created a conundrum for their developers. When diuretics and β-blockers were introduced, the competition included only reserpine, hydralazine, methyldopa, and guanethidine. In very early clinical trials against placebo, these other drugs were demonstrated to be effective in lowering BP and reducing cardiovascular risk in individuals who could take them, but each had major disadvantages, particularly at high doses, which many patients did not tolerate. As a result, it was appropriate to test initial diuretics and/or β-blockers against placebo in long-term clinical trials, rather than against the few active drugs then available. These trials (summarized above) were quite impressive, and resulted in overwhelming acceptance of the concept that lowering BP with drug therapy (typically diuretics and/or β-blockers) was a worthwhile intervention.

With the introduction of dihydropyridine calcium antagonists and ACE-inhibitors in 1981, the diuretics and β-blockers were well established as the 'standard of care' for hypertension, and it was not generally considered ethical to do large-scale outcome-based clinical trials of these drugs in unselected hypertensive people against placebo. Because the bar had been raised (consistent with the Declaration of Helsinki), it was recognized that trials of the newer drug classes would require many more patients or a much longer duration of follow-up, because the comparator would be an active control, rather than placebo. As a result, few large-scale clinical trials in unselected hypertensive patients of the newer vs. older drugs were launched until concerns were raised about the long-term safety of calcium antagonists and until studies in other cardiovascular conditions (e.g. heart failure, high-risk hypertensives) suggested a very large benefit of ACE-inhibitors.

Diuretics and/or β-blockers

From 1985 to 1992, the results of five outcome-based clinical trials comparing an initial diuretic with an initial β-blocker were published: MRC-1, IPPPSH, HAPPHY, MAPPHY, MRC-E; only the last used a low-dose diuretic. The two Medical Research Council trials (in younger and older patients) were discussed above, as they included placebo as a third randomized arm (to which half the patients were allocated). IPPPSH, HAPPHY, and MAPPHY were European trials; their interpretation and relevance to current clinical practice have been questioned, as HAPPHY and MAPPHY were not carried out independently, and IPPPSH used oxprenolol, which is now little used. Although the overall benefits of a diuretic and β-blocker were not different, an advantage for the diuretic was seen in the MRC trial in the elderly, but the analysis was complicated by a high dropout rate among those originally assigned to the β-blocker.

α-blockers

Although α-blockers had been approved antihypertensive agents since the late 1970s, very few clinical trials included these agents. Prazosin was inferior to enalapril in the first V-HeFT trial in heart failure,[32] and it was superior to placebo and captopril only in lowering BP in the long term in the Veterans' Administration Trial of monotherapy.[33] Doxazosin was associated with the fewest sexual side effects and a slight long-term improvement in both lipids and glucose in the Trial of Mild Hypertension Study (TOMHS), but cardiovascular events were not reported separately by drug class for this trial.[34] Perhaps because the risk of orthostatic hypotension associated with use in older individuals tended to outweigh potential improvement in symptoms of benign prostatic hyperplasia, α-blockers had never been commonly used as initial (or even second-step) drugs in most algorithms for therapy of hypertension.

The outcome-based clinical trial that solidified this position and, indeed, recommended **against** the use of α-blockers as initial treatment for hypertension was the Antihypertensive and Lipid Lowering [to prevent] Heart Attack Trial (ALLHAT). This trial, which figures prominently and predominantly in any discussion of outcomes with antihypertensive drugs, randomized 42 448 hypertensive patients in North America to one of four different initial therapies, two of which were doxazosin (representing α-blockers) and chlorthalidone (representing thiazide-like diuretics). Although the mean follow-up was initially planned for 6 years, the doxazosin arm of the trial was terminated after about 3 years of follow-up on the recommendation of the original ALLHAT Data Safety and Monitoring Board (DSMB), and an Ad Hoc group convened to reconsider the data.[35] Two major reasons were cited: the futility of finding doxazosin superior to chlorthalidone (if the arm had been carried to completion), and because doxazosin was associated with a significant 25% increased risk of combined cardiovascular disease, a secondary endpoint. One component of this composite endpoint was heart failure, which was seen at a highly significant 2.04-times higher rate with doxazosin than chlorthalidone.[35] Some objected to the early termination of this arm of ALLHAT, and to the implication that the adverse effects were related to the drug, rather than to the 3.3 mmHg higher systolic BP in the doxazosin group on average (compared to the chlorthalidone group), but many subsequent analyses have tended to support the view of the ALLHAT Collaborative Research Group. Their position, simply stated, is that if a randomized treatment provides better BP control **and** is associated with improved outcomes (as was the case with chlorthalidone), it should be used preferentially and recommended by guideline committees. Since 2000, the popularity of α-blockers has declined,[36] and their use has shifted to mostly being fourth- or fifth-line agents, where they are quite effective in lowering BP.[37]

ACE-inhibitors

Three major long-term outcome-based clinical trials have demonstrated impressive benefits of ACE-inhibitors, although only one trial enrolled only hypertensive patients. The first, and most important for changing prescribing habits, was the Heart Outcomes Prevention Evaluation (HOPE) study.[38] This international study enrolled 9297 subjects, 55 years of age or older, with either current evidence of vascular disease, or diabetes and one other cardiovascular risk factor, but without heart failure or a history of a subnormal left-ventricular ejection fraction. Two randomized treatments (either ramipril, an ACE-inhibitor [up to 10 mg/day], or placebo; or vitamin E 400 IU/day or placebo) were provided, in addition to any other appropriate drug therapy (including antihypertensive agents) thought to be indicated by the treating physician. The ramipril vs. placebo part of the study was halted prematurely by the DSMB, because subjects given ramipril had a significant 22% lower risk of the composite primary endpoint (MI, stroke, or cardiovascular death). These benefits were alleged to be independent of BP lowering, but this view is not universally shared. The authors claimed that the 3/2 mmHg average difference in BP between randomized groups during nearly 5 years of treatment could account for perhaps 40% of the observed reduction in stroke and a quarter of the reduction in myocardial infarction. These estimates are based on meta-analyses of previous hypertension trials (none of which used ACE-inhibitors) and epidemiological information about low-risk hypertensives. Neither of these databases may be pertinent to the enrolled subjects in HOPE, since the benefit of this degree of BP lowering is likely to be greater in high-risk individuals. Ambulatory BP measurements have been reported from 38 HOPE participants with peripheral arterial disease; all received ramipril at bedtime, and their BPs at 1 year after randomization were much lower (17/8 mmHg difference at night, for instance) than reported for the entire HOPE cohort.[39] Nonetheless, these data provide strong evidence that interfering with the RAAS prevents cardiovascular events in high-risk patients. In HOPE, ramipril was associated with a highly significant 34% reduction in the risk of new-onset diabetes, but the 3577 known diabetics in HOPE also benefited from treatment. A separate publication showed even greater benefits among diabetics regarding cardiovascular event reduction than in the cohort as a whole. Although ramipril was associated with significant prevention (by 24%) of the incidence of proteinuria (>300 mg/day), there were only 18 patients who required dialysis: eight in the ramipril group vs. 10 given placebo; this difference was not statistically significant. Some have cited this finding as a reason why subsequent studies of angiotensin II receptor blockers for renoprotection in type 2 diabetics were ethical.

The second study showing major benefits of an initial ACE-inhibitor was PROGRESS (Perindopril pROtection aGainst REcurrent Stroke Study).[40] This clinical trial was done largely in Australasia and Europe, and involved 6105 patients with a stroke or transient ischaemic attack in the preceding 5 years. They were randomized to perindopril, an ACE-inhibitor (with or without indapamide, a diuretic) or matching placebo(s); the diuretic was recommended as part of the initial treatment strategy, but could be withheld at the discretion of the investigator. The mean BP across groups over 4 years was lower in the group receiving active antihypertensive drugs by 9/4 mmHg, and was accompanied by a 28% reduction in the risk of recurrent stroke, and a 26% reduction in major cardiovascular events. The benefit in secondary stroke prevention was seen across all levels of both systolic and diastolic BPs. However, as discussed below, the reduction in recurrent stroke and cardiovascular events was significant only for those who received both perindopril and indapamide.

The African American Study of Kidney diseases and hypertension (AASK) trial also supported the use of an ACE-inhibitor over (first) a dihydropyridine calcium antagonist, and (later) a β-blocker.[24,41] In AASK, 1094 non-diabetic

African Americans with hypertensive nephrosclerosis were randomized to ramipril, amlodipine, or metoprolol succinate, to which could be added any other antihypertensive agent except an ACE-inhibitor, ARB, calcium antagonist, or β-blocker. Although the primary endpoint was decline in glomerular filtration rate (GFR, measured directly by iothalamate clearance), the amlodipine arm was stopped prematurely because of major differences in clinical events (reduction in GFR, end-stage renal disease, or death).[41] Similar, but not quite as striking conclusions were later provided for the comparison of the ACE-inhibitor to the β-blocker.[42] These data gave strong support to using an ACE-inhibitor (along with diuretics appropriate to the individual patient's level of renal function) to prevent progressive renal deterioration in African Americans with chronic kidney disease, despite the greater risk of cough and angio-oedema in this racial/ethnic group.

Calcium antagonists

Beginning in 1995, calcium antagonists were implicated by several epidemiological and cohort studies as being associated with significantly higher rates of myocardial infarction and other adverse outcomes. These allegations were buttressed by the initial report from the Appropriate Blood pressure Control in Diabetes (ABCD) study, claiming a 9.5-fold increase in risk of acute myocardial infarction with nisoldipine, compared to enalapril.[42] Individuals who supported the view that calcium antagonists were inferior generally dismissed STONE and Syst-China (because they were not randomized clinical trials), and claimed that Syst-Eur was unethical (as SHEP had previously shown active antihypertensive drug therapy beginning with a low-dose diuretic to be superior to placebo in treating isolated systolic hypertension). In 2000, they published a meta-analysis, which compared outcomes for patients randomized to calcium antagonists compared to **any** other initial therapy, which concluded that an initial calcium antagonist was associated with a significant 25% increased risk of myocardial infarction and a 26% increased risk of heart failure.[43] Little media attention was given to the next pages in *The Lancet*, which summarized all the prospectively-gathered individual-patient-level data from these and other clinical trials, and concluded that both ACE-inhibitors and calcium antagonists were more effective than placebo in reducing cardiovascular events, and that the few small differences noted would be overwhelmed in the next few years when the results of ongoing comparative trials were revealed (see below).[44]

Although not a direct comparative trial of calcium antagonists against another class of drugs, the Hypertension Optimal Treatment (HOT) Study was important, since it compared long-term outcomes in hypertensive patients treated initially with a dihydropyridine calcium antagonist to three different target diastolic BPs.[22] One interpretation of the results of HOT argues that those who received more intensive treatment, using higher doses of the calcium antagonist, did **not** have more major cardiovascular events, demonstrating long-term safety of the drug. The counterargument is that those treated more intensively **also** received other antihypertensive drugs that may have **protected** them from the adverse effects of the high-dose calcium antagonist. In any case, the HOT study enrolled the greatest number of patients who received calcium antagonists in a long-term study, and in most of them, there appeared to be mostly benefit, with little evidence of harm.

Angiotensin II receptor blockers

Four outcome-based clinical trials comparing angiotensin II receptor blockers and either a placebo or a β-blocker have been published. All involved specific, high-risk patient groups; none were conducted in a broad range of hypertensive patients (like most of the studies discussed above and below). The first three were presented on the same day (and later published in the same issue of the *New England Journal of Medicine*) and involved diabetic hypertensives.

The Irbesartan Diabetic Nephropathy Trial (IDNT) enrolled 1715 type 2 diabetics with renal impairment and proteinuria (average = 2.9 gm/day). They were randomized to irbesartan (150 mg initially, 269 mg/day + 3.0 other drugs at conclusion), amlodipine (5 mg initially, 9.1 mg/day + 3.0 other drugs at conclusion), or placebo (+4.0 other drugs at conclusion). Any antihypertensive drug except an ACE-inhibitor, angiotensin II receptor blocker, or calcium antagonist could thereafter be added. The primary endpoint was doubling of serum creatinine, end-stage renal disease, or death. Although stopped prematurely because of external data from other trials, IDNT was able to show a significant benefit of irbesartan over both placebo and amlodipine in the composite endpoint and in doubling of serum creatinine, despite no significant differences in cardiovascular events across the randomized groups. BP control was quite similar for the irbesartan-amlodipine comparison as opposed to the irbesartan-placebo pair, leading to the possible conclusion that the angiotensin II receptor blocker had renal benefits 'beyond BP control'.

The Reduction of Endpoints in Non-Insulin Dependent Diabetes Mellitus with the Angiotensin II Antagonist Losartan (RENAAL) study used the same primary endpoint, but randomized 1513 patients to only two arms. Calcium antagonists were used in about 80% of the participants, since they were randomized to either losartan (50 mg initially, 86 mg/day + about 3.1 other drugs during treatment) or placebo (+about 3.3 other drugs during treatment). Despite stopping after about 3.4 years because of external data showing cardiovascular benefits for ACE-inhibitors, the group receiving losartan had a significant benefit on the primary endpoint, doubling of serum creatinine, and the incidence of end-stage renal disease (ESRD). These data have resulted in **both** losartan and irbesartan being approved by the US FDA to retard the progression of type 2 diabetic nephropathy.

In the IRbesartan MicroAlbuminuria (IRMA-2) trial, 590 European type 2 hypertensive diabetics who had only microalbuminuria (defined by overnight timed urine collections containing between 20 and 2000 µg/minute of protein) were randomized to treatment with placebo, irbesartan 150 mg/day or irbesartan 300 mg/day.[45] The target doses were reached after 2 weeks at half the final dose. Only ACE-inhibitors, ARBs, and dihydropyridine calcium antagonists were forbidden. After 2 years of observation, the proportion of subjects reaching the primary endpoint (>200 µg/minute of protein in an overnight urine collection of at least 30% higher than baseline rate on two consecutive occasions) occurred in 10 of 194 people receiving 300 mg/day, 19 of 195 receiving 150 mg/day, and 30 of 201 receiving placebo. Only the high-dose group was significantly different from placebo ($p < 0.001$), although the low-dose group became so after adjustment for baseline level of microalbuminuria and achieved BP. These data confirmed in the long-term what several previous studies had shown: that interruption of the renin–angiotensin–aldosterone system in diabetics reduces protein excretion, a surrogate for 'harder' cardiovascular and renal events.

In contrast to the Losartan Intervention For Endpoint (LIFE) reduction trial (discussed below), the Valsartan Antihypertensive Long-term Use Evaluation (VALUE) trial did not achieve equivalent or better BP control or demonstrate cardiovascular benefits with the tested angiotensin receptor blocker.[46] Investigators from 31 countries randomized 15 245 high-risk hypertensive patients aged 50 years and older to valsartan 80 mg or amlodipine 5 mg. Doses could be doubled and hydrochlorothiazide (to 25 mg/day) and other drugs (except angiotensin receptor blockers) added, if needed to achieve the target BP of <140/90 mmHg. ACE-inhibitors or calcium antagonists were allowed only if clearly indicated for reasons besides hypertension. BPs were significantly lower, particularly during the early months of the 4.2-year-long study, in the amlodipine group. The primary endpoint was a composite of cardiac morbidity and mortality; each component of the primary endpoint, stroke, all-cause mortality, and new-onset diabetes were secondary endpoints. Follow-up was terminated at an average of 4.2 years (as planned) after 1450 patients suffered a primary endpoint. Although slightly more common in the valsartan-treated group (810 vs. 789 patients), the primary endpoint was not significantly different across the groups. An analysis of temporal trends of the primary and each of the secondary cardiovascular endpoints, however, suggested that valsartan treatment was associated with a significantly higher risk of each endpoint during the first 3 months of the study, paralleling the differences in observed BPs between the groups. At the conclusion of the trial, myocardial infarction was significantly less common among those randomized to amlodipine; in this group, new-onset diabetes was significantly more common. The authors performed several other analyses attempting to overcome the differences in achieved BP control, but the results did not favour valsartan, as originally hypothesized.[47] The investigators thus concluded that early BP control is an important predictor of future cardiovascular events, and recommended its prompt reduction, rather than favouring valsartan over amlodipine as initial therapy.

Comparisons of newer vs. older drug classes

For reasons discussed above, results from outcome-based clinical trials pitting ACE-inhibitors and calcium antagonists against diuretics and/or β-blockers were non-existent before 1996. Since then, however, a large number of such trials have been published. Unfortunately, results from many subgroups about some endpoints have not appeared; in several important Scandinavian studies, for example, patients were randomized to initial therapy with either a diuretic or a β-blocker, and the choice was left to the clinical judgment of the treating physician. In CAPPP, STOP-2, NORDIL (but unlike CONVINCE), the endpoints observed in the group receiving each type of initial therapy have not been reported. This means that meta-analyses that attempt to combine the results of trials that used, for example, an initial diuretic cannot use the data from CAPPP, STOP-2 and NORDIL. Only if one compares outcomes with either a diuretic or a β-blocker can these important studies be included. This approach is justified since direct comparison showed no overall difference and is the method chosen by most recent meta-analysts.[28,41,29,30,44]

ACE-inhibitor vs. diuretic/β-blocker

The first study to report the results of a randomized comparison between an initial ACE-inhibitor and a β-blocker was the United Kingdom Prospective Diabetes Trial.[48] After 8.4 years of average follow-up, the 400 type 2 diabetics randomized to initial captopril had no significant differences in any of the microvascular or macrovascular endpoints compared with the 358 randomized to initial atenolol. BPs were similarly reduced (144/83 vs. 143/81 mmHg, respectively). More patients stayed on the captopril than atenolol during follow-up (78% vs. 65%, $p < 0.0001$), with slightly more in the atenolol group requiring three or more antihypertensive drugs (27% vs. 31%). The authors, therefore, reported that the BP target for type 2 diabetics is more important for avoiding cardiovascular outcomes than the initial drug selected to begin the BP lowering process.[18]

The second study to compare an ACE-inhibitor with either a diuretic or β-blocker as initial treatments for hypertension was the Captopril Primary Prevention Project (CAPPP). In a PROBE (Prospective, Randomized, Open-label, Blinded Endpoint) design, 10 985 hypertensive Swedes or Finns between 25 and 66 years of age, with a diastolic BP of >100 mmHg, were treated for 6.1 years (on average) and followed-up for major cardiovascular events. The captopril-treated group had higher BPs (by about 3/1 mmHg) at both randomization and during follow-up, so (unlike many other trials) the statistical model that calculated the study results included baseline systolic BP. The captopril group had more strokes (189 vs. 149, $p = 0.044$), but slightly fewer cardiovascular deaths (76 vs. 95, $p = 0.092$). In a pre-planned subgroup analysis of the 572 diabetics, those assigned to captopril had fewer major cardiovascular events (35 vs. 47, $p = 0.018$) and deaths (20 vs. 34, $p = 0.03$). Overall, CAPPP concluded that the two treatment regimens did not differ in efficacy in preventing cardiovascular morbidity and mortality.[49] CAPPP was the first of several clinical trials to observe a lower rate of new-onset diabetes in the group randomized to an ACE-inhibitor. However, concerns about the randomization procedure in CAPPP casts doubt on the veracity of the results.[50]

The third study to report no major differences between an initial ACE-inhibitor and a diuretic or β-blocker was the Swedish Trial in Older Patients with Hypertension #2 (STOP-Hypertension 2). This was a larger and more ambitious undertaking, as it compared three antihypertensive drug regimens and also used a PROBE design. Hypertensive Swedes between 70 and 84 years of age were randomized to initial treatment with either 'conventional therapy' (atenolol 50 mg/day, metoprolol 100 mg/day, pindolol 5 mg/day, or hydrochlorothiazide 25 mg + amiloride 5 mg/day, $n = 2213$), a calcium antagonist (felodipine 2.5 or isradipine 2.5 mg/day, $n = 2196$) or an ACE-inhibitor (enalapril 10 or lisinopril 10 mg/day, $n = 2205$). BP was controlled similarly in all groups by adding either a diuretic (if the initial therapy was either an ACE-inhibitor or a β-blocker) or a β-blocker (if the initial therapy was either a diuretic or calcium antagonist). After an average of 5 years of follow-up, there was no significant difference between newer and older drugs in any endpoint, leading the authors to conclude that calcium antagonists and ACE-inhibitors have similar effects to 'conventional therapy' in preventing major cardiovascular events in older hypertensive patients.[51]

The African American Study of Kidney diseases and hypertension (AASK) trial (discussed above) differs in a number of ways from other comparative trials of ACE-inhibitors and diuretics or β-blockers. It compared ramipril, metoprolol succinate, and amlodipine, and used diuretics appropriate to the level of renal function in **all** patients. Its primary and most of its secondary endpoints were renally-driven, so it has so far only reported the percentage of subjects who died and had major cardiovascular events during follow-up. Although the numbers of affected patients are small compared to other trials, the renal benefits of an ACE-inhibitor (compared to an initial β-blocker) became evident over the entire 4.1 years of follow-up.[23]

Two arms of ALLHAT compared lisinopril (which became the best-selling ACE-inhibitor) with chlorthalidone (the best studied thiazide-like diuretic) in more than 24 000 hypertensive patients, including 8592 blacks (the largest such experience ever). By design, other ACE-inhibitors, angiotensin II receptor blockers, and diuretics were not to be prescribed during follow-up, which is unlike current clinical practice. In ALLHAT, lisinopril was associated with the lowest proportion of patients who continued on the original or equivalent drug treatment, the highest proportion of patients who required additional drugs, and the poorest control of BP, which was even worse among blacks. Although after 4.9 years of average follow-up, there were no significant differences between those assigned chlorthalidone or lisinopril in the primary endpoint, fatal or non-fatal coronary heart disease, stroke and combined cardiovascular disease were both higher with lisinopril (and especially among blacks). Heart failure was also 19% higher among those originally given lisinopril; the Kaplan-Meier curves diverged quickly in the first few years of follow-up (when BPs were much different), but grew closer toward the end of the study when BP differences were smaller, as additional drugs were added to the initial therapies. The only advantage for the lisinopril-treated group was a 44% relative risk reduction for the incidence of diabetes mellitus (8.1% vs. 11.6% at 4 years), although those who developed diabetes during the trial were said not to be at increased risk for cardiovascular events during the ensuing few years of observation in ALLHAT.[52] These observations and their relevance to clinical practice have been debated extensively in the recent literature, but the ALLHAT results have been temporally linked with a decrease in prescribing of ACE-inhibitors, at least in Ontario.[53]

Less than 2 months after the publication of ALLHAT, the results of the Second Australian National Blood Pressure Study were published. In this PROBE study, 6083 Australians between 65 and 84 years of age were followed for 4.1 years after being randomly assigned to enalapril or hydrochlorothiazide; the study committee recommended these agents, but the actual treatment decision was left to the individual practitioner. Only 83% of subjects actually received the recommended treatment at randomization, and only 58% or 62% were taking the recommended treatment at the end of the study. The change in BP was nearly exactly equal across randomized groups (a decrease of 26/12 mmHg). The primary outcome measure was a composite of the number of cardiovascular events or mortality in each group, regardless of the number of patients affected or the time to the event(s). This endpoint was more common among those assigned to the diuretic (736 of 3039 vs. 695 of 3044, $p = 0.05$). The first secondary outcome was the more traditional 'number of first cardiovascular events or deaths', but this did not achieve traditional levels of significance (529 vs. 490 patients, $p = 0.06$). Event rates (especially myocardial infarctions) and their prevention by the ACE-inhibitor appeared to be better only among men. In view of the unusual methods and since this trial enrolled fewer subjects than ALLHAT had patients with combined cardiovascular disease **events** the debate about the relative merits of these two studies with similar overall objectives, has been limited.

The other trial in which an initial ACE-inhibitor was compared with an initial diuretic is the HYpertension in Very Elderly Trial (HYVET), for which some results have been reported.[54] In a PROBE design, 847 European men and women aged 80 years and older were randomized to the physician's choice of bendroflumethiazide (or a different thiazide-type diuretic) or perindopril (or a different ACE-inhibitor) and followed for 1.1 years (on average). There was no significant difference between all-cause and cardiovascular mortality across randomized groups.

Calcium antagonist vs. diuretic/β-blocker

The first reported randomized clinical trial to compare an initial calcium antagonist with an initial diuretic or β-blocker was the Swedish Trial in Older Patients with Hypertension #2 (STOP-Hypertension 2) discussed above.[51] Physicians had a multiple-choice: felodipine or isradipine for the 2196 Swedes randomized to the calcium antagonist, enalapril or lisinopril for the 2205 assigned to the ACE-inhibitor arm, or atenolol, metoprolol, pindolol or hydrochlorothiazide + amiloride for the 2213 randomized to 'conventional therapy'. Although the groups did not differ significantly in any endpoint after an average of 5 years of follow-up, *post-hoc* analyses did find differences, with a 23% lower risk of acute myocardial infarction and a 22% lower risk of heart failure among patients randomized to ACE-inhibitors, as compared to those randomized to calcium antagonists.

The International Nifedipine [GITS] Study: Intervention as a Goal in Hypertension Treatment (INSIGHT) study compared a calcium antagonist and a diuretic.[55] In this study, 6321 hypertensive patients from Europe and Israel with an additional cardiovascular risk factor were randomized to once-daily 30 mg of nifedipine GITS or hydrochlorothiazide 25 + amiloride 2.5 mg. Doses were doubled, if necessary, and atenolol 25–50 mg or enalapril 5–10 mg could be added to achieve goal BP. With nearly identical BP control, the primary outcome (cardiovascular death, myocardial infarction, stroke, or heart failure) was found in 200 patients in the nifedipine group and 182 in the diuretic group (relative risk 1.10, 95% CI: 0.91–1.34, $p = 0.35$). There were similarly no significant differences between randomized groups in all-cause mortality, non-fatal endpoints, combined primary and secondary endpoints, or in stratified analyses according to baseline risk factors (e.g. diabetes). Only in fatal myocardial infarction (16 vs. 5) and non-fatal heart failure (24 vs. 11) did the results achieve putative statistical significance ($p = 0.017$ or 0.028 respectively) favouring nifedipine, but these were not pre-specified analyses, and could have arisen by chance. About 40% of those randomized to nifedipine switched to another treatment by the end of the study, as compared to 33% given the diuretic. A further *post-hoc* analysis[55] suggested that the two regimens were 'equivalent' in preventing major cardiovascular events. Peripheral oedema was significantly more common with nifedipine (725 vs. 518 patients, $p < 0.0001$), but significantly more serious adverse events occurred in those given the diuretic (880 vs. 796, $p = 0.02$). The authors suggested that, as the primary results were so similar, the proportion of patients afflicted by side effects of the drugs may be more important than their effects on cardiovascular morbidity and mortality.

The primary results of the Nordic Diltiazem (NORDIL) study were published immediately following the INSIGHT results.[56] Using a PROBE design, 10 881 previously-untreated hypertensive Norwegians or Swedes aged 50–74 years with a diastolic BP > 100 mmHg were randomized to 180 mg/day of diltiazem or the physician's choice of a diuretic or β-blocker. An ACE-inhibitor was added if either diltiazem at 360 mg/day or both a diuretic and β-blocker did not achieve a diastolic BP of <90 mmHg. During a mean follow-up of 4.5 years, a primary event (stroke, myocardial infarction or cardiovascular disease-related death) was found in 403 patients initially given diltiazem and 400 patients given the diuretic or β-blocker (relative risk 1.00, 95% CI: 0.87–1.15, $p = 0.97$). Diltiazem was associated with about 3 mmHg higher systolic BP throughout follow-up, $p < 0.001$. Stroke was less common with diltiazem than with the diuretic/β-blocker (159 vs. 196, respectively, $p = 0.04$), whereas myocardial infarction was slightly (but not significantly) more common with diltiazem (183 vs. 157, $p = 0.17$). Many patients required more than monotherapy (50% for diltiazem, 55% for the diuretic/β-blocker), but more patients abandoned diltiazem (23%) than the diuretic/β-blocker (7%) during the study. A follow-up publication indicated that strokes were especially less common among patients randomized to diltiazem who had higher baseline systolic or diastolic BPs, or a relative bradycardia (heart rate <66 beats/minute).[57]

In ALLHAT, the longest-acting calcium antagonist, amlodipine (which is the most widely-used dihydropyridine), was compared directly with chlorthalidone (the longest-acting and best studied of the thiazide-like diuretics), with the hypothesis that the newer drug would fare better than the traditional diuretic. After randomization, fewer participants abandoned their original class of assigned drug or required additional therapy with amlodipine; it also lowered diastolic (but not systolic) BP better than chlorthalidone (by about 1 mmHg). Compared to the 15 255 given chlorthalidone, the 9048 subjects given amlodipine had a 2% lower risk of the primary outcome (fatal or non-fatal coronary heart disease), a 7% reduction in stroke risk, a 4% reduction in mortality, and a 4% **increase** in combined cardiovascular events; none of these comparisons was significant. The increase in combined cardiovascular events could be traced to a highly-significant 38% increase in the risk of heart failure; this was significant in all pre-specified subgroups.[51] These results and their interpretation have been hotly debated, but they are the primary reason why JNC 7 recommended 'a thiazide-type diuretic should be first-line drug therapy for most hypertensive patients'. Some ALLHAT investigators have recommended that **all** hypertensive patients should be taken off their current antihypertensive therapy (regardless of its effectiveness in lowering BP) and switched to a low-dose of a thiazide-like diuretic, as that is what was done with the volunteers in ALLHAT.

A completely different study objective was planned in the Controlled ONset Verapamil INvestigation of Cardiovascular Endpoints (CONVINCE) trial.[58] This head-to-head comparison of the physician's choice of hydrochlorothiazide or atenolol vs. controlled-onset extended-release verapamil was intended as an 'equivalence trial' from the very beginning. As such, 2024 primary events (stroke, myocardial infarction, or cardiovascular death) were originally required to establish 'equivalence'; this was expected to take 5 years of follow-up. Despite enrolling 16 602 hypertensive subjects with at least one additional risk factor for cardiovascular events (including obesity), the study was stopped prematurely by the sponsor 'for business reasons'. Nonetheless, 729 primary events were observed, and they were split between the two randomized treatment regimens in a nearly equal proportion. Unfortunately, the upper limit of the 95% confidence interval for the hazard ratio was 1.18, just 0.02 (or 2%) higher than the pre-specified definition of 'equivalence', and thus CONVINCE failed to meet its objective. Heart failure and bleeding were both significantly more common in the group randomized to verapamil. The test agent had been developed specifically to deliver verapamil during the early morning hours (when the BP and risk of cardiovascular events is higher). Despite this the number of primary events was higher in the group given verapamil at bedtime than in the other group (who received either hydrochlorothiazide or atenolol in the morning).

The International VErapamil SR/Trandolapril (INVEST) Study was performed in 22 576 subjects with both hypertension and coronary artery disease, and compared a regimen starting with verapamil SR (followed by trandolapril) with a more traditional regimen starting with atenolol (followed by hydrochlorothiazide). This study randomized the largest number of patients to an initial calcium antagonist. More than 17 000 eligible individuals were recruited from the USA, with the majority of the remainder coming from other countries in North America. After an average of 2.7 years of open-label treatment, BPs were equally well-controlled in both randomized groups (despite discontinuation of study medication in about 43% in both groups): this was the first study to incorporate the new, lower BP goal for diabetics into the calculation of 'controlled BPs'. There was no significant difference between the primary endpoint (non-fatal myocardial infarction, non-fatal stroke, or all-cause mortality) and its components across the randomized treatments; thus the claim of 'equivalence' was made for the two regimens. The primary outcome results were homogeneous across a wide variety of baseline parameters (e.g. age, gender, race/ethnicity), but a *post-hoc* analysis showed a significant reduction in the risk of new-onset diabetes in the verapamil/trandolapril group.[59]

Angiotensin receptor blocker vs. β-blocker

The only long-term trial clearly indicating cardiovascular endpoint benefits in hypertensive patients treated with an initial angiotensin receptor blocker was the Losartan Intervention For Endpoint reduction (LIFE) trial, presented and published simultaneously in March 2002.[60] Because of the important role of left ventricular hypertrophy (LVH) as a risk factor for cardiovascular events in hypertensive patients, 9193 patients fulfilling very strict electrocardiographic criteria for LVH were enrolled and randomized initially to losartan or atenolol, each at 50 mg/day. Doses could be doubled and hydrochlorothiazide and then other drugs (excluding β-blockers, ARBs, or ACE-inhibitors) added in each arm, if needed, to control BP. The primary endpoint was a composite of myocardial infarction, stroke or cardiovascular death. After 4.8 years (on average), BP was reduced slightly more (1.3/0.4 mmHg) in the losartan group. Even after adjustment for baseline degree of LVH and Framingham risk score, the losartan group had a significantly lower risk of the primary endpoint (by 13%, $p = 0.021$), which was entirely driven by a 25% reduction in stroke ($p < 0.001$). The 533 blacks had fewer primary endpoints in the atenolol group, a disparity that was not explained by different achieved BPs. Although the losartan group as a whole had a non-significant higher risk of myocardial infarction (7%, $p = 0.49$), there was also a lower risk of new diabetes (26%, $p < 0.001$), adverse events ($p < 0.0001$), and an improvement in LVH ($p < 0.0001$) with losartan. Subgroup analyses have also shown the benefits of losartan among diabetics,[61] and individuals with 'isolated systolic hypertension'.[62] This analysis was possible only because of the placebo run-in period, which was not part of VALUE, ALLHAT, INVEST, or CONVINCE. The LIFE diabetic substudy was the first to show that an angiotensin receptor blocker reduces cardiovascular morbidity and/or mortality. The LIFE study was the first to show the benefits of reducing BP to improve left ventricular hypertrophy and concomitantly prevent cardiovascular events.

Meta-analyses

The results of many of the studies discussed above have been combined in meta-analyses, in an attempt to overcome the possibility of a type 2 statistical error that can result when small numbers of endpoints are observed in any one study. Some believe that this provides a better estimate of the relative efficacy of a given type of treatment, although others point out that such 'gross lumping' of data tends to obscure potentially important differences across combined studies in design, execution and endpoint definitions.

The largest and most comprehensive recent meta-analysis combined data from 42 clinical trials that included 192 478 patients randomized to seven major treatment strategies, including placebo.[16] By a complex statistical scheme that allows internal comparisons, interpolations, extrapolations and indirect calculations of relative risks for treatments, the 'network meta-analysis' method allows estimates to be made for comparisons that are not based on head-to-head studies. For example, this technique can infer a relative risk for a diuretic alone as first-line therapy in such studies as CAPPP, NORDIL and STOP-Hypertension 2, although the actual number of endpoints in this subgroup (as opposed to those who received a β-blocker first) has never been published or presented. The technique also allows the authors to calculate estimates of relative risks from studies that have disparate definitions of endpoints. For instance, in ALLHAT, the 'combined cardiovascular disease' endpoint included coronary heart disease death, non-fatal myocardial infarction, stroke, coronary revascularization procedures, hospitalized or treated angina, treated or hospitalized heart failure, and peripheral arterial disease, either hospitalized or outpatient revascularization (event rate/3 years = 43.5%). For CONVINCE, the definition of 'major cardiovascular events' included only non-fatal myocardial infarction, non-fatal stroke, or cardiovascular death (event rate/3 years = 7.2%).

As might be expected, the results of the meta-analysis are driven by the results of ALLHAT. Low-dose diuretics were determined to be significantly better than placebo for any cardiovascular outcome, and no other initial therapy was superior to a low-dose diuretic for any outcome. Low-dose diuretics were superior in the prevention of heart failure to calcium antagonists, ACE-inhibitors and α-blockers. They were also superior in prevention of cardiovascular events to calcium antagonists, ACE-inhibitors, β-blockers and α-blockers. The authors, therefore, concluded that low-dose diuretics are the most effective first-line treatment for preventing cardiovascular morbidity and mortality, and that a low-dose diuretic should hereinafter serve alone as the 'gold standard' initial therapy in any future clinical trials of antihypertensive drugs.

For this chapter, we have updated the traditional meta-analyses performed by both Staessen et al. and the Blood Pressure Lowering Trialists' Collaboration, to include trials reported since these publications.[28,30] The results are discussed below. We attempted to standardize all definitions of events across trials; for example, 'major cardiovascular events' included only myocardial infarction, stroke or cardiovascular death. This required estimation of the numbers of events in each arm of several trials (e.g. INSIGHT, ALLHAT, INVEST), since each of these included other endpoints in their definitions of 'major cardiovascular events'. These discrepancies have been largely eliminated in the meta-analyses based on patient-level data performed by the Blood Pressure Lowering Treatment Trialists' Collaboration.[28] The results of our meta-analyses indicate that heart failure events are significantly more common with calcium antagonists or ACE-inhibitors, compared to a diuretic or β-blocker. The effect of calcium antagonists on stroke is just barely significantly better than an initial diuretic or β-blocker, whereas an ACE-inhibitor is just slightly worse ($p = 0.04$ in each case). These estimates may change after ongoing trials [e.g. Anglo Scandinavian Cardiac Outcomes Trial (ASCOT)] are completed and reported.

Diuretic vs. β-blocker

Published meta-analyses summarizing results in trials comparing an initial diuretic with an initial β-blocker showed few significant differences between the drugs, but none included all five studies. This may be either because MRC-E was not yet published,[7,63] the meta-analysis focused only on older people[31] or a subgrouping according to the dose of diuretic used had already been performed.[16] Figure 16.2 shows the results of a traditional meta-analysis of all five studies that compared an initial diuretic vs. an initial β-blocker: none of the tabulated endpoints shows a significant difference across initial treatments. In contrast, the 'network meta-analysis' of Psaty et al.[90] (based on only one direct comparative trial) concluded that an initial low-dose diuretic was significantly superior to an initial β-blocker only for preventing cardiovascular events (by 11%, $p = 0.02$). The differences for other endpoints were not significant: coronary heart disease events (by 13%, $p = 0.10$), heart failure

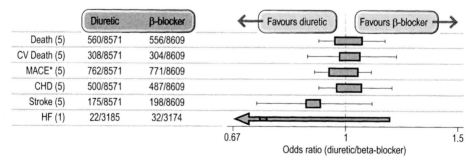

	Diuretic	β-blocker
Death (5)	560/8571	556/8609
CV Death (5)	308/8571	304/8609
MACE* (5)	762/8571	771/8609
CHD (5)	500/8571	487/8609
Stroke (5)	175/8571	198/8609
HF (1)	22/3185	32/3174

Odds ratio (diuretic/beta-blocker)

Fig. 16.2 Results of a traditional meta-analysis (using the Mantel-Haenszel technique) showing outcomes for five long-term, randomized, clinical trials involving 17 180 patients, comparing an initial diuretic vs. an initial β-blocker. Presumed obstacles to the publication of these relatively old data are summarized in the text. Other abbreviations and formatting details are as in Figure 16.1.

(by 17%, $p = 0.07$), stroke (by 10%, $p = 0.20$), cardiovascular mortality (by 7%, $p = 0.34$), and all-cause mortality (by 1%, $p = 0.73$). In these meta-analyses, significant heterogeneity was found across trials for the endpoints of stroke ($p < 0.05$, largely due to MRC-1 and HAPPHY), CHD events ($p = 0.004$, largely due to MRC-E), and major CV events ($p < 0.02$, largely due to MRC-E and HAPPHY).

ACE-Inhibitor vs. diuretic/β-blocker

Except for AASK (which provides only small numbers of cardiovascular events and deaths), the meta-analysis of Staessen et al. includes all seven currently-available studies comparing an initial ACE-inhibitor vs. a diuretic or β-blocker.[46] When the AASK results are added, the results reported by Staessen et al. change very little (see Fig. 16.3): the diuretic/β-blocker prevents stroke and heart failure slightly more (each by 10.2%, $p = 0.03$ and $p = 0.04$, respectively). With the exception of coronary heart disease endpoints (-3%, $p = 0.42$), other endpoints favoured the diuretic/β-blocker; none were significantly different (mortality: 0%, $p = 0.97$; cardiovascular mortality: 3%, $p = 0.48$; major cardiovascular events: 1.5%, $p = 0.59$). In the meta-analysis of these trials no endpoint shows significant heterogeneity.

Calcium antagonist vs. diuretic/β-blocker

The meta-analysis of Staessen et al. does not include AASK, SHELL or INVEST.[46] When the results of these three studies are included (see Fig. 16.4),

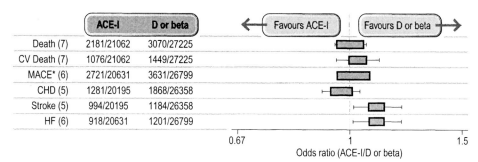

	ACE-I	D or beta	Favours ACE-I	Favours D or beta
Death (7)	2181/21062	3070/27225		
CV Death (7)	1076/21062	1449/27225		
MACE* (6)	2721/20631	3631/26799		
CHD (5)	1281/20195	1868/26358		
Stroke (5)	994/20195	1184/26358		
HF (6)	918/20631	1201/26799		

0.67   1   1.5
Odds ratio (ACE-I/D or beta)

Fig. 16.3 Results of a traditional meta-analysis (using the Mantel-Haenszel technique) showing outcomes for seven long-term trials involving 48 287 patients, comparing an initial ACE-inhibitor with an initial diuretic or β-blocker. The numbers of patients in AASK who had stroke, myocardial infarction, and heart failure are not yet published, so these endpoints include the results of only six trials. Other abbreviations and formatting details are as in Figure 16.1.

	CCB	D or beta	Favours CCB	Favours D or beta
Death (12)	3389/42957	4327/49609		
CV Death (11)	1605/42105	1977/48669		
MACE* (12)	3610/42957	4602/49609		
CHD (11)	1868/42740	2388/49168		
Stroke (11)	1182/42740	1568/49168		
HF (10)	1323/41563	1408/48011		

0.67   1   1.5
Odds ratio (CCB/D or beta)

Fig. 16.4 Results of a traditional meta-analysis (using the Mantel-Haenszel technique) showing outcomes for 12 long-term trials involving 92 036 patients, comparing an initial calcium antagonist with an initial diuretic or β-blocker. Other abbreviations and formatting details are as in Figure 16.3.

only stroke (8% lower with a calcium antagonist, $p = 0.03$) and heart failure (29% higher with a calcium antagonist, $p < 0.0001$) achieve statistical significance. All-cause mortality (-1%, $p = 0.65$), and major cardiovascular events (-1%, $p = 0.63$) were slightly less common with the calcium antagonist, whereas cardiovascular mortality (3%, $p = 0.49$) and coronary heart disease events (2%, $p = 0.54$) were slightly more common with the calcium antagonist. These estimates will change when ongoing studies (e.g. ASCOT) are completed. In the meta-analyses of these trials no endpoints show significant heterogeneity.

ACE-inhibitor vs. calcium antagonist

The list of six trials that directly compared outcomes with an initial ACE-inhibitor vs. calcium antagonist has not changed since the 2003 review by the Blood Pressure Trialists' Collaboration.[28] They reported significant differences between the two initial therapies for heart failure (18% lower with an ACE-inhibitor, $p = 0.002$, although only four trials reported the numbers of patients affected) and stroke (12% lower with a calcium antagonist, $p = 0.03$). The group with initial ACE-inhibitor had slightly higher all-cause mortality (by 4%, $p = 0.18$) and cardiovascular mortality (by 3%, $p = 0.49$), but the calcium antagonist had slightly more major cardiovascular events (by 3%, $p = 0.59$) and coronary heart disease events (by 4%, $p = 0.17$). Staessen et al. did not include this comparison in their summary, presumably because the results would have been quite similar.[30] In the meta-analyses of these trials, only CHD events show significant heterogeneity ($p < 0.004$, largely due to ABCD).

Angiotensin receptor blocker vs. any other initial therapy

Neither meta-analysis published in 2003 included the results of the VALUE trial. Staessen et al. included only LIFE and SCOPE, whereas the Blood Pressure Lowering Trialists' Collaborative added the results of RENAAL and IDNT (omitting the amlodipine results).[28,30] The Trialists' Collaborative noted significant benefit with the angiotensin receptor blocker for the endpoints of stroke, heart failure, and major cardiovascular events. However, when the VALUE data are added in a traditional meta-analysis to those already summarized in the Trialists' Collaborative (Fig. 16.5), none of the endpoints except heart

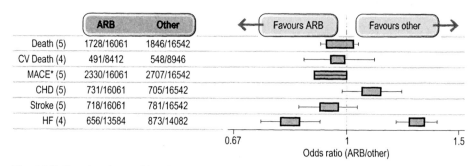

	ARB	Other
Death (5)	1728/16061	1846/16542
CV Death (4)	491/8412	548/8946
MACE* (5)	2330/16061	2707/16542
CHD (5)	731/16061	705/16542
Stroke (5)	718/16061	781/16542
HF (4)	656/13584	873/14082

Odds ratio (ARB/other)

Fig. 16.5 Results of a traditional meta-analysis (using the Mantel-Haenszel technique) showing outcomes for five long-term trials involving 32 603 patients, comparing an initial ARB (angiotensin receptor blocker) with any other initial antihypertensive drug. Other abbreviations and formatting details are as in Figure 16.4.

failure is significantly different between the angiotensin receptor blocker and the control treatment(s). This may be partly explained by the larger blood pressure advantage for amlodipine in VALUE. Significant heterogeneity across treatments exists in stroke ($p < 0.0003$), largely because LIFE and VALUE disagreed about this endpoint. It is impossible to estimate a summary odds ratio for a standard definition of major cardiovascular events across all ARB trials, since the trials used different definitions, and have not published the numbers of patients with each of the components of the composite endpoint. If one accepts the published numbers, as has been done for the meta-analysis of Psaty et al.,[16] the meta-analysis changes from highly favouring the angiotensin receptor blocker (15%, $p < 0.0001$) before VALUE, to being no longer significant (6%, $p = 0.06$, with significant heterogeneity $p < 0.04$) after addition of the VALUE data. These estimates will likely change as further trials using angiotensin receptor blockers are completed.

Combination therapy

A few recent trials have been designed to explore the potential benefits of combination therapy, i.e. several drugs from different pharmacological classes being used in the same patient. Although perhaps scientifically more difficult to evaluate than trials that randomize to different initial single-drug therapy, it appears that the majority of patients with hypertension will eventually require more than one drug.[26] Even in ALLHAT, which denied enrollment to those with initial BPs of >180/110 mmHg, by the end of the trial the average number of drugs used per patient was 2.0.[64] The potential benefits of combination therapy (as opposed to monotherapy) often use PROGRESS as the illustration.[40] In this study, monotherapy with ACE-inhibitor alone was associated with a 4.9/2.8 mmHg reduction in BP compared to placebo, whereas the combination of the ACE-inhibitor + diuretic reduced BP by 12.3/5.0 mmHg. Monotherapy was associated with a reduction in stroke of only 5% (95% CI: −19–23%) and in cardiovascular events by only 4% (95% CI: −15–20%). The combination, however, showed a 43% reduction (95% CI: 30–54%) in stroke and a 40% reduction in cardiovascular events (95% CI: 29–49%). Both of the latter were highly statistically significant ($p < 0.001$), whereas neither of the monotherapy comparisons was even close. These data suggest that the diuretic was quite important, both in lowering BP and preventing events.

The only trial so far to compare results of two add-on therapies (after an initial low-dose diuretic) is the Study of COgnition and Prognosis in the Elderly (SCOPE) trial.[65] It enrolled 4937 mainly European people aged 70–89 years with a mini-Mental Status Examination score higher than 24, with BP between 160 and 179 mmHg systolic or 90 and 99 mmHg diastolic while taking 12.5 mg/day of hydrochlorothiazide. They were then randomized to either candesartan or any other antihypertensive drug of the investigator's choosing (but not an ACE-inhibitor or another angiotensin receptor blocker). After about 3.5 years, BPs were lower in the candesartan group (drop of about 22/11 vs. 18/9 mmHg, $p < 0.0001$). The primary endpoint (stroke, myocardial infarction, or cardiovascular death) was not significantly different across randomized groups, but there was a slight (and significant) 24% reduction in stroke in those initially given candesartan ($p = 0.04$). Cardiovascular death was about the same, but myocardial infarction was slightly more common in those given candesartan. Although formal assessments of cognition were not significantly different across groups at the end of the study, two of three measures of quality of life favoured candesartan.

The potential benefits of combining an ACE-inhibitor and an angiotensin II receptor blocker were explored in the Candesartan And Lisinopril Microalbuminuria (CALM) trial.[66] It was designed according to classical pharmacological principles that indicate that the maximum chance of finding an additive effect is to use both drugs at half-maximal doses. As a result, 199 European type 2 diabetics were given either 16 mg/day of candesartan or 20 mg/day of lisinopril for 12 weeks, and their BP and urinary protein excretion rates were measured. Thereafter, half were randomized to the combination of half-maximal doses of both drugs. After 12 weeks of further therapy, those receiving the combination had significantly lower BP than those continuing on half-maximal doses of either lisinopril or candesartan. Proteinuria was significantly reduced (from baseline) by each monotherapy during the first 12 weeks, but after the second 12-week period, those receiving the combination had significantly lower protein excretion than with candesartan; the difference between the combination and the ACE-inhibitor was not quite significant ($p = 0.20$). This comparison may have been underpowered statistically, because only about 25 patients received the combination after receiving lisinopril first and the study did not explore the effect of increased dose of either drug class. This study nonetheless suggested that there might be some benefit to giving both kinds of antagonists of the renin–angiotensin–aldosterone system to the same patient.

A somewhat more ambitious study was undertaken in 263 Japanese patients with non-diabetic renal impairment.[67] Prior to randomization, increasing doses of an ACE-inhibitor (trandolapril) were given, each for 3 weeks, that determined that 3 mg/day was the dose beyond which proteinuria was maximally reduced. Thereafter, patients were randomized to trandolapril (3 mg/day), losartan (100 mg/day), or the combination and followed for about 36 months. BPs were not different across the treatments (perhaps due to the addition of other drugs), and reduction in proteinuria was about the same (42 or 44%) in each monotherapy group. There was, however, a further reduction in proteinuria (by about 76%) when both drugs were used together at full doses ($p = 0.01$ for trend). The primary endpoint for this study, however, was doubling of serum creatinine or end-stage renal disease. The trial was stopped early because there was a significantly lower risk of the primary endpoint with the combination (about 11%) than with either monotherapy (22% or 23%) at about 36 months ($p = 0.017$). These data indicate that there are benefits to full-dose ACE-inhibitor + full-dose ARB, although even this therapy is not totally effective in preventing deterioration in renal function.

Recently, a trial comparing two popular combination therapies has been launched. In the ACCOMPLISH (Avoiding Cardiovascular events through COMbination therapy in Patients LIving with Systolic Hypertension) study, 12 600 hypertensive patients will be randomized to treatment with either benazepril + hydrochlorothiazide or benazepril + amlodipine in a double-blind, parallel group design. Two primary endpoints are planned, involving cardiovascular morbidity or mortality, along with a wide variety of secondary endpoints. Study completion is expected in about 2008.

DIFFERENT DRUGS FOR DIFFERENT HIGH-RISK CONDITIONS ('COMPELLING INDICATIONS')

Unfortunately, many patients with hypertension come to medical attention with existing target organ damage, following a clinical event that is often a consequence of hypertension or with other major risk of factors. JNC VI was the first set of guidelines to formally recommend treating such patients with an antihypertensive drug that has also been shown to improve prognosis in a different condition. In JNC VI, however, only five 'compelling indications' for specific antihypertensive drug therapy were recognized; in 2004, the literature supports many more (Table 16.2).

Heart failure

Heart failure is a common consequence of untreated or undertreated hypertension.[68] Fortunately, many of the drugs used to treat hypertension now have outcomes trials showing their effectiveness in heart failure for preventing death and/or hospitalization for heart failure. This was first and most impressively shown for ACE-inhibitors, and more recently benefits have been shown with β-blockers, aldosterone antagonists,[69] and angiotensin receptor blockers.

The last group has been extensively studied, with controversial results. Two early clinical trials (ELITE and ELITE-2) directly comparing captopril with low-dose losartan in heart failure did not show significant differences in long-term prognosis.[70,71] Nonetheless, the Valsartan in Heart Failure (Val-HeFT) trial randomized 5010 heart failure patients to receive either placebo or valsartan (target dose 160 mg twice daily), in addition to an ACE-inhibitor and/or whatever 'standard' heart failure treatment was warranted. After approximately 24 months of follow-up, only one of two 'primary' endpoints was significant: there was a 13.3% reduction in heart failure-related morbidity or mortality with valsartan, most of which was due to a 27.5% reduction in hospitalization for heart failure.[72] In *post-hoc* subgroup analyses, valsartan had a significantly higher risk of death in patients receiving both an ACE-inhibitor and a β-blocker (which are now routinely recommended as first- and second-line agents for chronic heart failure). These fears were largely allayed by the much larger experience in CHARM-Added, in which those treated with 'triple therapy' had significant prevention of cardiovascular death or hospitalization for CHF, compared to those who did not receive candesartan.[73] Angiotensin receptor blockers were first approved in the USA for patients with heart failure who cannot or will not take an ACE-inhibitor, based originally on a subgroup of 366 patients in the Val-HeFT trial.[74] This interesting, but unusual, subgroup had a 41% reduction in mortality ($p = 0.017$), 49% reduction in morbidity ($p = 0.002$), and 57% reduction in heart failure hospitalization ($p = 0.0006$) with valsartan, compared to placebo. CHARM-Alternative arrived at a similar conclusion, based on 2028 patients.[75]

Post-myocardial infarction

β-blockers have become a 'quality of care indicator' for patients after a myocardial infarction, as they reduce the risk of death and recurrent infarction, as well as lowering BP.[76] ACE-inhibitors have also shown impressive benefits in this

Table 16.2 Compelling conditions for which specific antihypertensive drug therapy has reduced morbidity and mortality in clinical trials

'Compelling indication'	Treatment prevents/ delays	Recommended in 1997	Recommended in 2004
Heart failure (systolic type)	Cardiovascular (CV) events	ACE-I (CONSENSUS, SAVE, etc.)	β-blocker (MERIT-HF, etc.); spironolactone (RALES); ARB (Val-HeFT)
After recent myocardial infarction (MI)	Recurrent infarction or death	β-blocker (ISIS, etc.)	
Diminished left ventricular (LV) function after recent MI	Recurrent infarction, coronary heart failure (CHF) hospitalization	ACE-I (SAVE, AIRE, TRACE)	Eplerenone (EPHESUS)
Known CV disease	CV events		ACE-I (HOPE, EUROPA)
Coronary heart disease	CV events	β-blocker	Verapamil (INVEST)
Type 1 diabetes mellitus	Deterioration in renal function	ACE-I (CCSG)	
Type 2 diabetes	CV events		ACE-I (MICRO-HOPE)
Type 2 diabetic nephropathy	Deterioration in renal function		ARBs (IDNT, RENAAL)
Type 2 diabetes	Progression of microalbuminuria		ACE-I (MICRO-HOPE); ARB (IRMA-2)
Older hypertensive persons	CV events	Diuretic (SHEP); DHP-CA (Syst-Eur)	ACE-I or DHP-CA (STOP-2); DHP-CA (Syst-China); ARB (SCOPE, second-line)
Non-diabetic renal impairment	Deterioration in renal function		ACE-I (REIN, AIPRI, AASK); ARB + ACE-I (COOPERATE)
Prior stroke/TIA	Stroke and CV events		ACE-I (PROGRESS); ARB (ACCESS)
LVH (using strict criteria)	CV events (perhaps limited to stroke?)		ARB (LIFE)

ACE-I= angiotensin converting enzyme-inhibitor; ARB= angiotensin receptor blocker; DHP-CA= dihydropyridine calcium antagonist
CONSENSUS= COoperative North Scandinavian ENalapril SUrvival Study (*N Engl J Med*.1987;316:1429-1435); SAVE = Survival And Ventricular Enlargement study (*N Engl J Med.*, 1992;327:669–677); MERIT-HF = MEtoprolol Randomized Intervention Trial in congestive Heart Failure (*JAMA*, 2000;283:1295–1302); RALES = Randomized ALdactone Evaluation Study (*N Engl J Med.* 1999;341:709–717); Val-HeFT = Valsartan Heart Failure Trial (*N Engl J Med.* 2001;345:1667–1675); ISIS = International Study of Infarct Survival (*Lancet*, 1986;2:57–66); AIRE = Acute Infarction Ramipril Efficacy (*Lancet*, 1993;342:821) TRACE = TRAndolapril Cardiac Evaluation (*N Engl J Med.*, 1995;333:1670–1676); EPHESUS = Eplerenone Post-myocardial infarction Heart Failure Efficacy and Survival Study (*N Engl J Med.*, 2003;348:1309–1321); HOPE = Heart Outcomes Prevention Evaluation (*N Engl J Med.*, 2000;342:145–153); INVEST = INternational VErapmil/trandolapril STudy (*JAMA*, 2003;290:2805–2816); EUROPA = EUropean Reduction Of cardiac events with Perindopril in stAble coronary disease (*Lancet*, 2003;362:782–788); CCSG = Captopril Cooperative Study Group (*N Engl J Med.*, 1993; 323:1456–1462); MICRO-HOPE = MIcroalbuminuria, Cardiovascular and Renal Outcomes substudy of the Heart Outcomes Prevention Evaluation (*Lancet*, 2000;355:253–259); IDNT = Irbesartan Diabetic Nephropathy Trial (*N Engl J Med.* 2001;345:841–860); RENAAL = Reduction of Endpoints in Non-Insulin Dependent Diabetes Mellitus with the Angiotensin II Antagonist Losartan (*N Engl J Med.* 2001;345:861–869); IRMA-2 = Irbesartan Microalbuminuria study #2 (*N Engl J Med.*, 2001;345:870–878); SHEP = Systolic Hypertension in the Elderly Program (*JAMA*, 1991;265:3255–3264); Syst-Eur = Systolic Hypertension in Europe trial (*Lancet*. 1997;360:757–764); STOP-2 = Swedish Trial in Old Patients with hypertension #2 (*Lancet*, 1999;354:1751–1756); Syst-China = Systolic Hypertension in China trial (*J Hypertens*. 1998;16:1823–1829); SCOPE = Study on COgnition and Prognosis in the Elderly (*J Hypertens.* 2003;21:875–886); REIN = Ramipril Evaluation In Nephropathy trial (*Lancet*, 1998;352:1252–1256); AIPRI = Angiotensin-converting-enzyme Inhibition in Progressive Renal Insufficiency (*Kidney Int.*, 1997;Suppl. 63:S63-S67); AASK = African American Study of Kidney disease and hypertension (*JAMA*. 2002;288:2421–2431); COOPERATE = Combination treatment of angiotensin-II receptor blocker and angiotensin-converting enzyme inhibitor in non-diabetic renal disease (*Lancet*. 2003;361:117–124); PROGRESS = Perindopril pROtection aGainst REcurrent Stroke Study (*Lancet*, 2001;358:1033–1041); ACCESS = Acute Candesartan Cilexitil Evaluation in Stroke Survivors (*Stroke*. 2003;34:1699–1703); LIFE = Losartan Intervention for Endpoint Reduction (*Lancet*, 2002;359:995–1003).

population, particularly among individuals with reduced left ventricular function during hospitalization.[77] Subgroups in HOPE and the EUropean Reduction Of cardiac events with Perindopril in stAble coronary disease (EUROPA) trial have also shown significant benefits of an ACE-inhibitor, even when given well after the index infarction.[38,78] In the Eplerenone Post-myocardial infarction Heart failure Efficacy and SUrvival Study (EPHESUS), selective aldosterone blockade significantly reduced mortality and morbidity in post-myocardial infarction patients with diminished left ventricular function.[79]

The role of angiotensin receptor blockers after myocardial infarction is more controversial. OPTIMAAL showed non-significant trends, favouring captopril over low-dose losartan in patients with a recent myocardial infarction and left-ventricular dysfunction, although losartan was better tolerated.[80] The VAL-IANT trial established 'equivalence' of valsartan or an ACE-inhibitor for patients with diminished left ventricular function or heart failure after an acute myocardial infarction, but the combination was not more effective in preventing cardiovascular morbidity and mortality than either drug alone.[81]

Diabetes

The proper choice of antihypertensive agent(s) in diabetics is controversial. There are, however, some 'compelling indications' for drugs other than a diuretic, although usually the diuretic is required to achieve the lower BP target (<130/80 mmHg). The 3577 diabetics in the HOPE trial had significant prevention of most types of cardiovascular events when given high-dose ramipril atop whatever other cardiovascular medications were thought by the investigator to be appropriate;[82] low-dose ramipril had no such benefits.[83]

For type 1 diabetics with proteinuria and chronic kidney disease, an ACE-inhibitor has demonstrated significant renoprotection, with a 50% reduction in the composite endpoint of death, dialysis or kidney transplantation,[84] although to what extent this reflects better blood pressure control is uncertain. Renoprotection for type 2 diabetics (although not to such a degree) has been shown in both IDNT and RENAAL, discussed above.[85,86] For type 2 diabetics with microalbuminuria, either an ACE-inhibitor or an angiotensin receptor blocker can be recommended to prevent the progression to frank proteinuria.[45,87]

Older people

Hypertension in older individuals is particularly important, since the majority of hypertensives are older than 55 years, and because age is the largest single predictor of cardiovascular events. The cost-effectiveness of therapy is, therefore, much greater in older than younger individuals, although current treatment paradigms in the USA do not have different recommendations based on age. No age-adjustment is required for target BP; it is the same for all hypertensives, regardless of age. Nor are there different recommendations for those with 'isolated systolic hypertension', which was found in 57% of male and 65% of female hypertensives between 65 and 84 years old in the Framingham Heart Study.

The evidence-base for treatment of hypertension in older individuals is robust,[83] even in those with isolated systolic hypertension,[15,88] or above the age of 80 years.[89] Chlorthalidone has been proven effective in older individuals in several NIH-sponsored trials (SHEP, MRFIT, TOMHS, and ALLHAT); the evidence-base for other diuretics is not as extensive in this age group.[90] Calcium antagonists have been used successfully in Syst-Eur and Syst-China, but amlodipine was not as effective in preventing heart failure as chlorthalidone in ALLHAT. This finding has special public health importance, as heart failure continues to be the most common reason patients above age 65 are admitted to hospital in the USA. The importance of prompt control of BP to prevent heart failure and other cardiovascular events was confirmed by both ALLHAT and VALUE.[46]

Chronic kidney disease

As noted above, diabetics with kidney disease have compelling indications for either an ACE-inhibitor or an angiotensin receptor blocker. ACE-inhibitors have been more extensively studied in non-diabetic renal disease, and the results summarized in several meta-analyses.[25,91] These compilations of data from 11 randomized clinical trials show the importance of blocking the renin–angiotensin–aldosterone system and achieving and maintaining a systolic BP between 110–129 mmHg. Formal guidelines about delaying the progression of chronic kidney disease have been issued by the National Kidney Foundation; BP control to <130/80 mmHg is again recommended.[92]

Post-stroke/transient ischaemic attack

PROGRESS (discussed above) was the first clinical trial to show the benefits of BP reduction in patients with a relatively remote history of a neurological event. Significant reductions in BP, recurrent stroke, and cardiovascular events were seen only in those given both the ACE-inhibitor and the diuretic.[40] More recently, the angiotensin receptor blocker, candesartan, was beneficial in a small study in acute stroke patients.[93] Larger studies of similar design are in progress (see: www.moses-study.com). These will presumably confirm that it is not only safe, but also important to lower BP in stroke survivors.

Left ventricular hypertrophy

Epidemiological studies have shown that electrocardiographic or echocardiographic evidence of an enlarged left ventricle reveals a very large risk of future cardiovascular events, presumably because it reflects a long duration of uncontrolled hypertension. The Losartan Intervention For Endpoint reduction (LIFE) study was designed to compare two antihypertensive regimens on cardiovascular endpoints in patients with very strict definitions of electrocardiographic left ventricular hypertrophy, based on the Cornell voltage-duration criteria.[60] This study, summarized above, was the first to show that lowering BP with an angiotensin receptor blocker led to significant reduction of left ventricular hypertrophy and was associated with a reduced cardiovascular event rate. Based on these results, the US FDA has approved the use of losartan to prevent stroke in hypertensive individuals with left ventricular hypertrophy.

SUMMARY AND CONCLUSIONS

There can be little doubt, based on the clinical trial results gathered to date and summarized above, that the evidence-base for treatment of hypertension is overwhelmingly positive. BP lowering is a very powerful means of reducing cardiovascular events. One of the bigger challenges has been to identify any benefit of antihypertensive drug therapy **over and above** the confounding issue of differential BP lowering that occurred during the trial with the regimens used. Multiple economic analyses also indicate that, in addition to being effective in preventing cardiovascular events, antihypertensive drug therapy is also extremely cost-effective, compared to other commonly employed treatment strategies used in medicine today.[94] BP lowering with antihypertensive drugs can, therefore, be embraced as a very large potential benefit to humankind, and correctly deserving its place as the most common reason for consultation with a healthcare provider.

References

1. Ezzati M, Lopez AD, Rodgers A, et al, and the Comparative Risk Assessment Collaborating Group. Selected major risk factors and global and regional burden of disease. *Lancet* 2002;360:1347–1360.
2. Age-specific relevance of usual blood pressure to vascular mortality. A meta-analysis of individual data for one million adults in 61 prospective studies. Prospective Studies Collaborative. *Lancet* 2002;360:1903–1913.
3. Black HR.*Clinical trials in hypertension*. New York: Marcel Dekker, Inc., 2001:659 pp.
4. Veterans Administration Cooperative Study Group on Antihypertensive Agents. Effects of treatment on morbidity in hypertension: results in patients with diastolic blood pressure averaging 115 through 129 mmHg. *JAMA* 1967;202:1028–1034.
5. MRC Trial of treatment of mild hypertension: principal results. Medical Research Council Working Party. *Brit Med J (Clin Res)* 1985;291:97–104.
6. Hypertension Detection and Follow-up Cooperative Group. Persistence of reduction in blood pressure and mortality in participants in the Hypertension Detection and Follow-up Program. *JAMA* 1988;259:2113–2122.
7. Collins R, Peto R, MacMahon S, et al. Blood pressure, stroke, and coronary heart disease: Part 2, Short-term reductions in blood pressure: overview of randomised drug trials in their epidemiological context. *Lancet* 1990;335:827–838.
8. Moser M, Hebert PR. Prevention of disease progression, left ventricular hypertrophy and congestive heart failure in hypertension treatment trials. *J Am Coll Cardiol* 1996;27:1214–1218.
9. The SHEP Cooperative Study Group. Prevention of stroke by antihypertensive drug treatment in older persons with isolated systolic hypertension. *JAMA* 1991;265:3255–3264.
10. Kostis JB, Davis BR, Cutler J, et al; for the SHEP Cooperative Research Group. Prevention of heart failure by antihypertensive drug treatment in older persons with isolated systolic hypertension. *JAMA* 1997;278:212–216.
11. Perry Jr. HM, Davis BR, Price TR, et al. Effect of treating isolated systolic hypertension on the risk of developing various types and subtypes of stroke. The Systolic Hypertension in the Elderly Program (SHEP). *JAMA* 2000;284:465–471.
12. Staessen JA, Fagard R, Thijs L, et al; for the Systolic Hypertension in Europe (Syst-EUR) Trial Investigators. Morbidity and mortality in the placebo-controlled European Trial on Isolated Systolic Hypertension in the Elderly. *Lancet* 1997;360:757–764.
13. Forette F, Seux ML, Staessen JA, et al. Prevention of dementia in randomised double-blind placebo-controlled Systolic Hypertension in Europe (Syst-Eur) trial. *Lancet* 1998;352:1347–1351.
14. Liu L, Wang J, Gong L, et al; for the Systolic Hypertension in China (Syst-China) Collaborative Group. Comparison of active treatment and placebo in older Chinese patients with isolated systolic hypertension. *J Hypertens* 1998;16:1823–1829.
15. Staessen JA, Gasowski J, Wang JG, et al. Risks of untreated and treated isolated systolic hypertension in the elderly: meta-analysis of outcome trials. *Lancet* 2000;355:865–872.
16. Psaty BM, Lumley T, Furberg CD, et al. Health outcomes associated with various antihypertensive therapies used as first-line agents: A network meta-analysis. *JAMA* 2003;289:2534–2544.
17. Elliott WJ. Cardiovascular events in clinical trials of antihypertensive drugs vs. placebo/no treatment: a meta-analysis [abstract]. *J Hypertens* 2005;23(Suppl. 2): S273.
18. Tight blood pressure control and risk of macrovascular and microvascular complications in type 2 diabetes: UKPDS 38. UK Prospective Diabetes Study Group. *BMJ* 1998;317:703–713.

19. Raikou M, Gray A, Briggs A, et al. Cost-effectiveness analysis of improved blood pressure control in hypertensive patients with type 2 diabetes: UKPDS 40. U.K. Prospective Diabetes Study Group. *BMJ* 1998;317:720–726.

20. Elliott WJ, Weir DR, Black HR. Cost-effectiveness of lowering treatment goal of JNC VI for diabetic hypertensives. *Arch Intern Med* 2000;160:1277–1283.

21. CDC Diabetes Cost-effectiveness Group. Cost-effectiveness of intensive glycemic control, intensified hypertension control, and serum cholesterol level reduction for Type 2 diabetes. *JAMA* 2002;287:2542–2551.

22. Hansson L, Zandretti A, Carruthers SG, et al. Effects of intensive blood pressure lowering and low-dose aspirin in patients with hypertension: principal results of the Hypertension Optimal Treatment (HOT) randomised trial: The HOT Study Group. *Lancet* 1998;351:1755–1762.

23. Lazarus JM, Bourgoignie JJ, Buckalew VM, et al. Achievement and safety of a low blood pressure goal in chronic renal disease: The Modification of Diet in Renal Disease Study Group. *Hypertension* 1997;29:641–650.

24. Wright Jr. JT, Bakris GL, Greene T, et al. Effect of blood pressure lowering and antihypertensive drug class on progression of hypertensive kidney disease: Results from the AASK Trial. *JAMA* 2002;288:2421–2431.

25. Jafar TH, Stark PC, Schmid CH, et al. Progression of chronic kidney disease: The role of blood pressure control, proteinuria, and angiotensin-converting enzyme inhibition: A patient-level meta-analysis. *Ann Intern Med* 2003;139:244–252.

26. Chobanian AV, Bakris GL, Black HR, et al. The Seventh Report of the Joint National Committee on Prevention, Detection, Evaluation, and Treatment of High Blood Pressure: The JNC 7 Report. *JAMA* 2003;289:2560–2572.

27. Seventh Report of the Joint National Committee on Prevention, Detection, Evaluation and Treatment of High Blood Pressure. National High Blood Pressure Education Program Coordinating Committee. *Hypertension* 2003;42:1206–1252.

28. Blood Pressure Lowering Treatment Trialists' Collaboration. Effects of different blood-pressure-lowering regimens on major cardiovascular events: results of prospectively-designed overviews of randomised trials. *Lancet* 2003;362:1527–1535.

29. Staessen JA, Wang JG, Thijs L. Cardiovascular protection and blood pressure reduction: A meta-analysis. *Lancet* 2001;358:1305–1315.

30. Staessen JA, Wang J-G, Thijs L. Cardiovascular prevention and blood pressure reduction: A quantitative overview updated until 01 March 2003. *J Hypertension* 2003;21:1005–1076.

31. Messerli FH, Grossman E, Goldboourt U. Are beta-blockers efficacious as first-line therapy for hypertension in the elderly: A systematic review. *JAMA* 1998;279:1903–1907.

32. Cohn JN, Archibald DG, Ziesche S, et al. Effect of vasodilatory therapy on mortality in chronic congestive heart failure. Results of a Veterans Administration Cooperative Study. *N Engl J Med* 1986;314:1547–1552.

33. Materson BJ, Reda DJ, Cushman WC. Department of Veterans Affairs Single-Drug Therapy of Hypertension Study. Revised figures and new data. Department of Veterans Affairs Cooperative Study Group on Antihypertensive Agents. *Am J Hypertension* 1995;8:189–192.

34. Neaton JD, Grimm RH, Prineas RJ, et al. Treatment of mild hypertension study: Final results. *JAMA* 1993;270:713–724.

35. The ALLHAT Collaborative Research Group. Major cardiovascular events in hypertensive patients randomized to doxazosin vs. chlorthalidone: The Antihypertensive and Lipid-Lowering Treatment to Prevent Heart Attack Trial (ALLHAT). *JAMA* 2000;283:1967–1975.

36. Stafford RS, Furberg CD, Finkelstein SN, et al. Impact of clinical trial results on national trends in alpha-blocker prescribing, 1996–2002. *JAMA* 2004;291:54–62.

37. Singer GM, Izhar M, Black HR. Goal-oriented hypertension management: Translating clinical trials to practice. *Hypertension* 2002;40:464–469.

38. The Heart Outcomes Prevention Evaluation (HOPE) Study Investigators. Effects of an angiotensin-converting-enzyme inhibitor, ramipril, on death from cardiovascular causes, myocardial infarction, and stroke in high-risk patients. *N Engl J Med* 2000;342:145–153.

39. Svensson P, de Faire U, Sleight P, et al. Comparative effects of ramipril on ambulatory and office blood pressures: A HOPE Substudy. *Hypertension* 2001;38:E28–E32.

40. PROGRESS Collaborative Group. Randomised trial of a perindopril-based blood-pressure-lowering regimen among 6105 individuals with previous stroke or transient ischaemic attack. *Lancet* 2001;358:1033–1041.

41. Agodoa LY, Appel L, Bakris GL, et al. Effect of ramipril vs. amlodipine on renal outcomes in hypertensive nephrosclerosis: A randomized controlled trial. African American Study of Kidney Disease and Hypertension (AASK) Study Group. *JAMA* 2001;285:2719–2728.

42. Estacio R, Jeffers B, Hiatt W, et al. The effect of nisoldipine as compared with enalapril on cardiovascular outcomes in patients with non-insulin dependent diabetes and hypertension. *N Engl J Med* 1998;338:645–652.
43. Pahor M, Psaty BM, Alderman MH, et al. Health outcomes associated with calcium antagonists compared with other first-line antihypertensive therapies: A meta-analysis of randomised controlled trials. *Lancet* 2000;356:1949–1951.
44. Blood Pressure Lowering Treatment Trialists' Collaborative. Effects of ACE-inhibitors, calcium antagonists, and other blood-pressure-lowering drugs: Results of prospectively designed overviews of randomised trials. *Lancet* 2000;356:1955–1964.
45. Parving H-H, Lehnert H, Brochner-Mortensen J, et al. The effect of irbesartan on the development of diabetic nephropathy in patients with type 2 diabetes. The Irbesartan in Patients with Type 2 Diabetes and Microalbuminuria Study Group. *N Engl J Med* 2001;345:870–878.
46. Julius S, Kjeldsen S, Weber M, et al. Outcomes in hypertensive patients at high cardiovascular risk treated with regimens based on valsartan or amlodipine: The VALUE randomised trial. *Lancet* 2004;363:2022–2031.
47. Weber M, Julius S, Kjeldsen KE, et al. Blood pressure dependent and independent effects of antihypertensive treatment on clinical events in the VALUE trial. *Lancet* 2004;363:2049–2051.
48. UK Prospective Diabetes Study Group. Efficacy of atenolol and captopril in reducing the risk of macrovascular and microvascular complications in type 2 diabetes: UKPDS 39. *BMJ* 1998;317:713–720.
49. Hansson L, Lindholm LH, Niskanen L, et al. Effect of angiotensin-converting-enzyme inhibition compared with conventional therapy on cardiovascular morbidity and mortality in hypertension: The Captopril Prevention Project (CAPPP) randomised trial. *Lancet* 1999;353:611–616.
50. Peto R. Failure of randomization by 'scaled' envelope. *Lancet* 1999;354:73.
51. Hansson L, Lindholm LH, Ekbom T, et al. Randomised trial of old and new antihypertensive drugs in elderly patients: Cardiovascular mortality and morbidity. The Swedish Trial in Old Patients with Hypertension-2 study. *Lancet* 1999;354:1751–1756.
52. The ALLHAT Officers and Coordinators for the ALLHAT Collaborative Research Group. Major outcomes in high-risk hypertensive patients randomized to angiotensin-converting enzyme inhibitor or calcium channel blocker vs. diuretic: The Antihypertensive and Lipid Lowering Treatment to Prevent Heart Attack Trial (ALLHAT). *JAMA* 2002;288:2981–2997.
53. Austin P, Mamdan MM, Tu K, Zwarenstein M. Changes in prescribing patterns following publication of the ALLHAT trial [research letter]. *JAMA* 2004;291:44–45.
54. Bulpitt CJ, Beckett NS, Cooke J, et al. Results of the pilot study for the Hypertension in the Very Elderly Trial. Hypertension in the Very Elderly Working Group. *J Hypertens* 2003;21:2409–2417.
55. Brown MJ, Palmer CR, Castaigne A, et al. Morbidity and mortality in patients randomised to double-blind treatment with a long-acting calcium-channel blocker or diuretic in the International Nifedipine GITS study: Intervention as a Goal in Hypertension Treatment (INSIGHT). *Lancet* 2000;356:366–372.
56. Hansson L, Hedner T, Lund-Johansen P, et al; for the NORDIL Study Group. Randomised trial of effects of calcium antagonists compared with diuretics and beta-blockers on cardiovascular morbidity and mortality in hypertension. The Nordic Diltiazem (NORDIL) Study. *Lancet* 2000;356:359–365.
57. Kjeldsen SE, Hedner T, Syvertsen JO, et al. Influence of age, sex, and blood pressure on the principal endpoints of the Nordic Diltiazem (NORDIL) Study. *J Hypertension* 2002;20:1231–1237.
58. Black HR, Elliott WJ, Grandits G, et al; for the CONVINCE Research Group. Principal results of the Controlled ONset Verapamil INvestigation of Cardiovascular Endpoints (CONVINCE) Trial. *JAMA* 2003;289:2073–2082.
59. Pepine CJ, Handberg EM, Cooper-DeHoff RM, et al. A calcium antagonist vs. a non-calcium antagonist hypertension treatment strategy for patients with coronary artery disease: The International Verapamil-Trandolapril Study (INVEST): A randomized controlled trial. The INVEST Investigators. *JAMA* 2003;290:2805–2816.
60. Dahlöf B, Devereux RB, Kjeldsen SE, et al; for the LIFE study group. Cardiovascular morbidity and mortality in the Losartan Intervention For Endpoint reduction in hypertension study (LIFE): A randomised trial against atenolol. *Lancet* 2002;359:995–1003.
61. Lindholm L, Ibsen H, Dahlöf B, et al; for the LIFE study group. Cardiovascular morbidity and mortality in patients with diabetes in the Losartan Intervention For Endpoint reduction in hypertension study (LIFE): A randomised trial against atenolol. *Lancet* 2002;359:1004–1010.
62. Kjeldsen SE, Dahlöf B, Devereux RB, et al. LIFE (Losartan Intervention for Endpoint reduction) Study Group. Effects of losartan on cardiovascular morbidity and mortality in

patients with isolated systolic hypertension and left ventricular hypertrophy: A Losartan Intervention for Endpoint Reduction (LIFE) Substudy. *JAMA* 2002;288:1491–1498.

63. Shinton RA, Beevers DG. A meta-analysis of mortality and coronary prevention in hypertensive patients treated with beta-receptor blockers. *J Human Hypertens* 1990;4(Suppl 2):31–34.

64. Cushman WC, Ford CE, Cutler JA, et al. Success and predictors of blood pressure control in diverse North American settings: The Antihypertensive and Lipid-Lowering Treatment to Prevent Heart Attack Trial (ALLHAT). *J Clin Hypertension* 2002;4:393–404.

65. Lithell H, Hansson L, Skoog I, et al. The study on cognition and prognosis in the elderly (SCOPE): Principal results of a randomized double-blind intervention trial. *J Hypertension* 2003;21:875–886.

66. Mogensen CE, Neldam S, Tikkanen I, et al. Randomised controlled trial of dual blockade of renin-angiotensin system in patients with hypertension, microalbuminuria, and non-insulin dependent diabetes: the candesartan and lisinopril microalbuminuria (CALM) study. *BMJ* 2000;321:1440–1444.

67. Nakao N, Yoshimura A, Morita H, et al. Combination treatment of angiotensin-II receptor blocker and angiotensin-converting-enzyme inhibitor in non-diabetic renal disease (COOPERATE): a randomised controlled trial. *Lancet* 2003;361:117–124.

68. Levy D, Larson MG, Vasan RS, et al. The progression from hypertension to congestive heart failure. *JAMA* 1996;275:1557–1562.

69. Pitt B, Zannad F, Remme WJ, et al; for the Randomized Aldactone Evaluation Study (RALES) Investigators. The effect of spironolactone on morbidity and mortality in patients with severe heart failure. *N Engl J Med* 1999;341:709–717.

70. Pitt B, Segal R, Martinez FA, et al; for the ELITE Investigators. Results of the Evaluation of Losartan In The Elderly (ELITE) trial. *Lancet* 1997;349:757–762.

71. Pitt B, Poole-Wilson PA, Segal R, et al. Effect of losartan compared with captopril on mortality in patients with symptomatic heart failure: randomised trial. The Losartan Heart Failure Survival Study ELITE II. *Lancet* 2000;355:1582–1587.

72. Cohn JN, Tognoni G; for the Val-HeFT Investigators. A randomized trial of the angiotensin-receptor blocker valsartan in chronic heart failure. *N Engl J Med* 2001;345:1667–1675.

73. McMurray JJV, Östergren J, Swedberg K, et al. Effects of candesartan in patients with chronic heart failure and reduced left-ventricular systolic function taking angiotensin-converting-enzyme inhibitors: The CHARM-Added trial. CHARM Investigators and Committees. *Lancet* 2003;362:767–771.

74. Maggioni AP, Anand I, Gottlieb SO, et al. Effects of valsartan on morbidity and mortality in patients with heart failure not receiving angiotensin-converting enzyme inhibitors. Val-HeFT Investigators (Valsartan Heart Failure Trial). *J Am Coll Cardiol* 2002;40:1414–1421.

75. Granger CB, McMurray JJV, Yusuf S, et al. Effects of candesartan in patients with chronic heart failure and reduced left-ventricular function intolerant to angiotensin-converting-enzyme inhibitors: The CHARM-Alternative trial. CHARM Investigators and Committees. *Lancet* 2003;362:772–776.

76. Freemantle N, Cleland J, Young P, et al. Beta-blockade after myocardial infarction: systematic review and meta-regression analysis. *BMJ* 1999;318:1730–1737.

77. Flather MD, Yusuf S, Kober L, et al. Long-term ACE-inhibitor therapy in patients with heart failure or left ventricular dysfunction: an overview of data from individual patients. ACE-Inhibitor Myocardial Infarction Collaborative Study Group. *Lancet* 2000;355:1575–1581.

78. Fox KM, and the EUROPA investigators. Efficacy of perindopril in reduction of cardiovascular events among patients with stable coronary artery disease: randomised, double-blind, placebo-controlled, multicentre trial (The EUROPA study). *Lancet* 2003;362:782–788.

79. Pitt B, Remme W, Zannad F, et al; for the Eplerenone Post-acute myocardial infarction HEart Failure Efficacy and SUrvival Study investigators. Eplerenone, a selective aldosterone blocker, in patients with left ventricular dysfunction after myocardial infarction. *N Engl J Med* 2003;348:1309–1321.

80. Dickstein K, Kjekshus J; for the OPTIMAAL Steering Committee. Effects of losartan and captopril on mortality and morbidity in high-risk patients after acute myocardial infarction: The OPTIMAAL randomised trial. OPTIMAAL Study Group. *Lancet* 2002;360:752–760.

81. Pfeffer MA, V MJJ, Velazquez EJ, et al. Valsartan, captopril, or both in myocardial infarction complicated by heart failure, left ventricular dysfunction, or both. VALIANT Investigators. *N Engl J Med* 2003;349:1893–1906.

82. Heart Outcomes Prevention Evaluation (HOPE) Study Investigators. Effects of ramipril on cardiovascular and microvascular outcomes in people with diabetes mellitus: The HOPE study and MICRO-HOPE substudy. *Lancet* 2000;355:253–259.

83. Marre M, Lievre M, Chatellier G, et al. Effects of low dose ramipril on cardiovascular and renal outcomes in patients with type 2 diabetes and raised excretion of urinary albumin:

randomised, double blind, placebo controlled trial (The DIABHYCAR study). DIABHYCAR Study Investigators. *BMJ* 2003;328:495(doi:10.1136/bmj.37970.629537.0D, published 11 February 2004).

84. Lewis EJ, Hunsicker LG, Bain RP, Rohde RD. The effect of angiotensin converting enzyme inhibition in diabetic nephropathy. *N Engl J Med* 1993;323:1456–1462.

85. Lewis EJ, Hunsicker LG, Clarke WR, et al. Renoprotective effect of the angiotensin-receptor antagonist irbesartan in patients with nephropathy due to Type 2 diabetes. Collaborative Study Group. *N Engl J Med* 2001;345:841–860.

86. Brenner BM, Cooper ME, de Zeeuw D, et al. Effects of losartan on renal and cardiovascular outcomes in patients with Type 2 diabetes and nephropathy. Reduction of Endpoints in Non-Insulin Dependent Diabetes Mellitus with the Angiotensin II Antagonist Losartan (RENAAL) Study Group. *N Engl J Med* 2001;345:861–869.

87. Elliott WJ, Black HR. Treatment of hypertension in the elderly. *Am J Geriatr Cardiol* 2002;11:11–22.

88. Chaudhry SI, Krumholz HM, Foody JM. Systolic hypertension in older persons. *JAMA* 2004;292:1074–1080.

89. Gueyffier F, Bulpitt C, Boissel J-P, et al; for the INDANA Group. Antihypertensive drugs in very old people: a subgroup meta-analysis of randomised controlled trials. *Lancet* 1999;353:793–796.

90. Psaty BM, Lumley T, Furberg CD. Meta-analysis of health outcomes of chlorthalidone-based vs nonchlorthalidone-based low dose diuretic therapies. *JAMA* 2004;292:43–44.

91. Jafar TH, Schmid CH, Landa M, et al. Angiotensin-converting enzyme inhibitors and progression of nondiabetic renal disease: A meta-analysis of patient-level data. *Ann Intern Med* 2001;135:73–87.

92. Abosaif NY, Arije A, Atray NK, et al. K/DOQI clinical practice guidelines on hypertension and antihypertensive agents in chronic kidney disease. *Am J Kidney Dis* 2004;43(5 Suppl 1): S1–S290.

93. Schrader J, Luders S, Kulschewski A, et al. The ACCESS Study: Evaluation of Acute Candesartan Cilexetil Therapy in Stroke Survivors. *Stroke* 2003;34:1699–1703.

94. Elliott WJ. Economic Considerations in the Management of Hypertension. In: Izzo Jr. JL, Black HR, eds. *Hypertension primer, 3rd edn.* Baltimore, MD: Lippincott, Williams & Wilkins; 2003:317–319.

IX

Therapeutic strategies

17 | Combination therapy

John Webster and Sarah Ross

INTRODUCTION

For several decades there has been intense discussion about which drugs should be used as 'first line' monotherapy for hypertension. Even the most recently published guidelines lay much store by this, and, indeed, give a somewhat inconsistent least patchy message about first-line therapy. For example, in the UK two guidelines published within months of each other advise a slightly different approach. The British Hypertension Society (BHS) guidelines[1] recommend the use of an algorithm that accommodates one of four drug groups as first line, whereas the National Institute of Clinical Excellence (NICE) has made a firm recommendation[2] of low-dose thiazide to be used as first line in most circumstances. The relative merits and disadvantages of these strategies will undoubtedly be the cause of continuing debate. To some extent that debate is justified as a number of patients will be controlled on monotherapy and the particular choice is important not only for the individual patient, but also in respect of the pharmacoeconomics of treating hypertension. For example, the ABCD algorithm[1] promulgated in the most recent BHS guidelines is based on a renin-profiling paradigm,[3] and tends to be aligned to individual patient characteristics, whereas the 'thiazide first' approach favoured by the NICE guidelines adopts a broader view by also taking account of cost-effectiveness within the resource limitations of the National Health Service in the UK.

The International Society of Hypertension (ISH) Guidelines[4] had previously indicated a somewhat more liberal approach to first-line therapy, which acknowledged a place for combination therapy, but did not really address the full implication of this for antihypertensive management. A subsequent statement by the ISH[5], specifically in respect of stroke prevention, however, clearly advocates thiazide diuretics for initiation of therapy and for inclusion in combination regimens.

The Seventh Report of the Joint National Committee on Prevention, Detection, Evaluation and Treatment of High Blood Pressure (JNC7)[6] also advocates thiazide-type diuretics as preferred initial agent, reasoning that these are 'virtually unsurpassed' in preventing the cardiovascular complications of hypertension. However, this report also emphasizes that more than two-thirds of hypertensive individuals are inadequately controlled on one drug and makes the case for combination therapy in many patients, even from the time of initiation of treatment. JNC7 differs importantly from BHS and ISH Guidelines in advocating therapy at much lower levels of blood pressure (BP), and, indeed, introduces for the first time the concept of 'prehypertension' for individuals with BPs between 120 to 139 mmHg systolic and/or 80 to 89 mmHg diastolic. Patients in this category with diabetes or kidney disease should be considered for appropriate drug treatment.

It has become increasingly apparent in recent years that in order to achieve optimal target BPs, a very large proportion of patients require to be on more than one drug. This implies that an increasingly relevant question is not so much 'what is the best first-line therapy?' but 'which combinations are likely to provide the most effective/cost-effective strategy?' Several aspects of this question will be explored in this chapter: Which combinations have been formally evaluated? How important is it to achieve blood pressure targets? Are certain combinations more potent/more effective than others? Are some combinations more prone to adverse effects than others?

Monotherapy has undoubted attractions – the convenience of a single medication, the ability to match a single drug to a particular patient, the potential for careful dose-titration, cost containment and, perhaps most important to many prescribers, a sense of 'therapeutic precision'. However, recent years have seen a very pronounced move away from treating hypertension as a discrete entity in isolation, towards a broader cardiovascular risk-prevention approach. This has seen the adoption of polypharmacy as a norm for many hypertensive patients in a move towards comprehensive cardiovascular risk reduction. Such a strategy is further supported by the results of specific major studies demonstrating, in hypertensive subjects, the benefits of co-treatment with both aspirin[7] and statins.[8] It is no longer unusual for patients to be prescribed a number of antihypertensives, plus aspirin plus a statin. Furthermore, it should be understood that very few, if any, antihypertensives have a single specific mode of action – most lower BP by a number of mechanisms. Thiazides for example, have been used for nearly half a century yet their antihypertensive mode of action is imperfectly understood – sodium depletion, attenuation of effects of vasoconstrictor agents and alteration in prostanoid biosynthesis may all play a part.[9] Depletion of extracellular volume may be relatively more important during the early days and weeks of treatment, whereas once treatment has been established for a few weeks the main haemodynamic property of thiazides is a reduction in total peripheral resistance. β-blockers alter baroreflex sensitivity, inhibit renin release and may alter presynaptic neurotransmitter release.[10] Blood pressure lowering propensity is shared by most drugs in the group, whereas ancillary properties, including lipid solubility and ability to penetrate the central nervous system, may have important, though as yet unquantified effects on overall outcome. Even the most recently introduced antihypertensive drugs – the angiotensin receptor blocking drugs – while perhaps more clearly associated with antagonism of the direct vascular effects of angiotensin II, may have other important mechanisms of action.[11] The implication of this is that if a single antihypertensive drug has multiple modes of action, there is no inherent reason not to use drugs in combination if necessary in order to lower BP. The 'magic bullet' concept in hypertension no longer carries much conviction.

The treatment of hypertension has been greatly assisted in recent years by a huge body of evidence from a series of major outcome trials. So substantial is this body of evidence that it has been possible to amalgamate these data in a series of meta-regression analyses conducted by the Blood Pressure Trialists Collaboration[12,13,14] and others.[2,15] That lowering of BP prevents stroke, myocardial infarction, heart failure and progressive renal impairment cannot be disputed. What is also apparent from these meta-analyses is that over the time course of most of these trials – generally 5–6 years – there is little to choose between the major drug groups in respect of potency and efficacy. As a general rule lowering BP is the key to success and lowering BP per se is at least as important as the choice of individual agent. That general statement does need to be qualified, however, in the light of a recent meta-analysis that suggests that β-blockers may not fully protect against stroke.[16] Furthermore, the outcome of apparently optimal therapy within a 5-year time frame may not apply in the longer term – particularly if metabolic disturbances related to the medication accumulate over time. The only really long-term randomized trial in hypertension is the UK Prospective Diabetes Study (UKPDS) – in which patients with type 2 diabetes were followed for up to 20 years.[17] There may have been some design weaknesses in this trial, including lack of statistical power, but it suggested that atenolol was at least as effective as captopril. This may seem a slightly incongruous result in the light of subsequent data from larger studies, but it does have the distinction of long-term follow-up. It might be wise not to extrapolate results beyond the duration of the trials.

Moreover, virtually all the studies reported to date have evaluated different forms of monotherapy, either versus placebo (in the earlier trials) or versus another monotherapy. Although 'add on' therapy has been permitted in these studies in all limbs of the trials, it is difficult to tease out the effects of combination therapy in such studies because of constraints of either the design or inadequate power, or both. Only one major outcome trial [Anglo Scandinavian Outcomes Trial (ASCOT)][18] has evaluated the effect of two different combination strategies (see below).

A further stimulus to the concept of combination therapy has come from the report of Law et al.[19] The authors' hypothesis is based on three key observations. First, the blood pressure lowering effect of combining the major groups of antihypertensives is strictly additive. Second, halving the standard dose of these medications results in a relatively smaller (perhaps 20%) loss of efficacy. Third, the adverse effect profile of most individual agents is very substantially diluted by reducing the dose. The authors make a persuasive case for starting therapy with a combination of three antihypertensives in half the standard dose, rather than higher doses of individual drugs. Such a combination, by reducing mean diastolic BP by approximately 10 mmHg, could be expected to reduce the risk of stroke by over 60% and of coronary events by 46%. The concept of starting combination therapy de novo in all eligible patients thus has a good deal to commend it, but is so completely at odds with current guidelines that it is unlikely to be widely adopted in the near future. All the main guidelines advocate starting with monotherapy in the majority of patients. Furthermore, they advocate combinations on the basis of theoretical synergism rather than simply additive efficacy.

A further limitation to implementation of the Law et al. approach is the lack of suitable combination products. Numerous combinations of two products in standard dosage are available (for example thiazide plus β-blocker, thiazide plus ACE inhibitor, β-blocker plus dihydropyridine). These may aid compliance with therapy, but the advantage in respect of combining two drugs is limited. Imagine the unfortunate patient with type 2 diabetes and hypertension, in whom ambitious targets are set for BP, serum cholesterol and blood glucose control. Such an individual may well be required to take four antihypertensives, metformin, a thioglitazone, a statin and aspirin, not to mention medication for obesity, gout, arthritis and depression! What would really help that patient might be a combination antihypertensive with three or four components at substandard dosages – that concept seems some way off yet. However, this is undoubtedly a strategy that is worthy of attention and further pragmatic evaluation.

Wald & Law extend their concept of a 'Polypill' by suggesting the addition to triple antihypertensive drug therapy of low-dose aspirin, folic acid and a statin in a six-component cardioprotective cocktail, estimating that this combined formulation might reduce the risk of stroke and coronary disease by over 80%.[20] The authors go even further, arguing that BP per se is a poor discriminant of death from coronary disease and that the 'Polypill' should be rather targeted on the basis of cardiovascular risk, focusing on secondary prevention, diabetes and the over 50s. The concept requires refinement and formal testing, and may take some time to be accepted, particularly among hypertension traditionalists, but has stimulated a great deal of interest in combination therapy. JNC7 eschews the risk-stratification approach and advocates that antihypertensive therapy be based on blood pressure criteria.[6] There is thus some way to go before these somewhat divergent approaches are reconciled.

IMPORTANCE OF TARGET BLOOD PRESSURE

Most of the major antihypertensive drug trials have specified a target for BP lowering. The more recent trials have tended to set a target of <140/90 mmHg, with tighter limits in diabetes. The Hypertension Optimal Treatment (HOT) study explored this in a formal way[7] by testing the hypothesis that in moderate hypertension lowering BP to a 'tighter' target would result in fewer major endpoints. The HOT study randomized 18 790 patients to three treatment groups: the first to achieve a target of ≤90 mmHg, the second to achieve a target of ≤85 mmHg, and the third to achieve a target of ≤80 mmHg. First-line therapy was felodipine, to be supplemented by ACE inhibitor, β-blocker and diuretic if necessary. At baseline mean BP was 170/105 mmHg. The original study design aimed to achieve a separation in target BP of 5 mmHg between each of the three groups. In practice a separation of only 2 mmHg was achieved (144/85, 141/83 and 140/81 respectively). Possibly as a result of this, the overall study results did not show an overwhelming advantage in lowering diastolic BP below 90 mmHg. It was clearly demonstrated, however, that large reductions in BP could be achieved by combination therapy, the mean differences from baseline in the groups being 26/20, 28/22 and 30/24 mmHg, respectively. An important message appeared to be that the initial reduction in BP from 170/105 to 145/90 mmHg avoided most of the morbidity and mortality. Reductions below this may have been of further value, but a law of diminishing returns may apply.

In an important subgroup analysis of the HOT study, a convincing case is made that in hypertensive patients with diabetes, a significant advantage in respect of major outcomes was achieved in those patients in the group achieving the lowest BPs. This has been used to support the strategy of rigorous blood pressure lowering in such patients. To achieve the impressive reductions in BP observed in this trial, by the end of the study 78% of patients were still taking felodipine as originally allocated, while 41% were taking an ACE inhibitor, 28% a β-blocker, and 22% a diuretic, reflecting the need for combination therapy. Overall, this study supports the observation that, in general, people with lower BP have a lower risk of coronary heart disease and stroke.[21] It remains possible that differences between drugs may yet emerge in respect of cause-specific outcomes, but these will only emerge from much larger meta-analyses than have hitherto been undertaken.

UKPDS[17,22] was designed to investigate the benefits of treating patients with type 2 diabetes in respect of macro- and microvascular outcomes. The study lasted the best part of 20 years (median follow up 8.4 years) and suffered from a number of design weaknesses and enforced protocol changes during the prolonged course of the trial. Nevertheless, few have disputed one of the main conclusions of the study – that lowering BP has a major favourable impact on outcomes. In the 'tight control' group, only 56% of patients achieved both systolic <150 mmHg and diastolic <85 mmHg. It was also apparent in this trial that in order to achieve satisfactory levels of 'target' BPs, a very large proportion of patients required combination antihypertensive drug therapy – 29% of patients in the 'tight control' group were on three drugs and 33% on two drugs at 9 years. First-line therapy was randomized to atenolol or captopril. The sequence of additional drug therapy was furosemide, followed by nifedipine, followed by methyldopa, followed by prazosin. Although the study suggested that the atenolol-based regimen was marginally superior (not statistically significant) to a captopril-based regimen, it did not have the statistical power to prove superiority. The main messages in respect of BP were that lower was better and that combination therapy was frequently required. In a secondary analysis of the Systolic Hypertension European (Syst-eur) trial,[23] it was shown that for a similar degree of blood pressure reduction, the outcomes in diabetic patients appeared to be relatively greater than in non-diabetic patients. Only about 40% of patients in this trial reached target BP on monotherapy. Thus, there is evidence both that diabetics should be treated more rigorously and also that they benefit relatively more from treatment of BP.

The concept of 'tight' blood pressure control in diabetes is now widely accepted (if not always implemented). At least one guideline[6] clearly highlights the advice that antihypertensive medication should start with combination therapy in such patients.

SELECTED OTHER TRIALS

It is not our remit to undertake a comprehensive or systematic review of all major trials in hypertension. We have chosen rather to present a number of the more prominent and more recent trials to illustrate the degree to which combinations of drugs, rather than the individual components, may have influenced both the outcome and the interpretation of results.

The Systolic Hypertension in the Elderly Program (SHEP)[24] and SYST-EUR[25] investigated the role of antihypertensive therapy in treating isolated systolic hypertension in the elderly. Both reached the conclusion that active therapy was superior to placebo in respect of all major cardiovascular outcomes. In SHEP first-line therapy was chlorthalidone supplemented by atenolol or reserpine. By the end of the 5-year study period, 46% of patients in the active therapy group were on step 1 monotherapy, 23% of patients required two drugs, and 21% of patients were receiving other active antihypertensive drugs in an attempt to reach the goal BP (systolic <160 mmHg, or a reduction of 20 mmHg). Even so, the placebo-adjusted reduction in mean systolic BP was modest (approximately 12 mmHg) and was achieved in approximately 70% of patients. In SYST-EUR, first-line therapy was nitrendipine, supplemented by enalapril, followed by hydrochlorothiazide if necessary. At 4 years, approximately 40% of the patients were on monotherapy with nitrendipine, 36% of patients in the active treatment group had required the addition of enalapril and 24% had required triple therapy in an attempt to achieve the target systolic BP of <150 mmHg or a reduction in systolic pressure of at least 20 mmHg. Approximately 50% of patients had achieved target systolic pressure. The mean placebo-corrected reduction in BP was 10/4 mmHg. These studies confirmed that less than half of patients with systolic hypertension were controlled on monotherapy, but did not identify the optimal combination to achieve target BP (they were not designed to do so).

The Valsartan Antihypertension Long-term Evaluation (VALUE)[26] compared the effects of valsartan with an amlodipine-based regimen in high-risk patients with hypertension. Hydrochlorothiazide was added to 24% of patients in both groups per protocol, and other drug combinations in a further 23% of the valsartan group and 17% of the amlodipine group in an attempt to achieve the target BP of <140/90 mmHg. In addition large numbers of patients on both groups received concomitant β-blockers (48% valsartan, 44% amlodipine), α-blockers (24% valsartan, 18% amlodipine) and ACE inhibitors (21% valsartan, 20% amlodipine). By the end of the trial valsartan was being used as monotherapy in 27% of patients, and amlodipine as monotherapy in 35.3% of patients. Thus, this trial is essentially a comparison of combination therapy based on the two primary drugs rather than a direct comparison of the individual first-line agents. The primary composite outcome measure (time to first cardiac event) did not differ between treatment groups. Amlodipine-based treatment was rather more effective in controlling BP. Among the secondary outome measures, myocardial infarction was significantly more frequent in the valsartan group (OR 1.19) and stroke marginally more frequent (OR 1.15), whereas new-onset diabetes was significantly less frequent (OR 0.77). Numerous statistical manipulations of the results of this trial have been performed,[27] debated and disputed,[28] but the overall conclusion is that blood pressure control is of paramount importance over the 5-year timescale of such studies, and probably over-rides the influence of the specific pharmacological properties of individual drugs or combinations.

The PROGRESS trial[29] was designed to evaluate the effects of lowering BP (even from levels usually considered normal) in patients with a history of stroke or transient cerebral ischaemic attack. Active treatment consisted of perindopril 4 mg daily with or without the addition of the diuretic indapamide. Mean reduction in BP in patients on the combination treatment (58% of total) was 12/5 mmHg. In this subgroup the relative risk of stroke was reduced by 43%. In the subgroup on perindopril alone (42% of total) the reduction in BP was 5/3 mmHg. In this subgroup active treatment had no discernible effect on the relative risk of recurrent stroke. Participants were not randomized between single drug or combination therapy and direct comparisons must be made with caution. However, the data from PROGRESS, viewed in the context of other trials, strongly supports the hypothesis that outcomes are directly related to the magnitude of BP reduction and that combination therapy is generally desirable.

In contrast to the PROGRESS trial, in which most, if not all of the benefit appeared to derive from combination therapy and in which perindopril alone appeared to have little effect on outcome despite a reduction in BP of 5/3 mmHg, the Heart Outcomes Prevention Evaluation (HOPE)[30] reached a diametrically opposite conclusion. This study was conducted in patients with a wide spectrum of increased vascular risk. Using ramipril titrated to 10 mg daily a mean reduction in BP from baseline of merely 3.8/2.8 mmHg was observed in the active treatment group. Unfortunately, the measurement of BP was not documented robustly in this trial and the interpretation of the BP data from this trial is of limited value. Nevertheless, despite the apparent meagre mean reduction in BP (in contrast to virtually every other major outcome trial), active treatment was associated with a highly significant reduction in major outcomes, including a 32% reduction in the relative risk of stroke. In HOPE, the benefit appeared to be independent of baseline BP. There has been much speculation about whether ramipril may have some protective effect against vascular events independent of BP lowering, but that remains entirely conjectural. Significant numbers of patients in HOPE were also receiving β-blockers (28%), diuretics (20%) or calcium channel blockers (44%), but the effects of various permutations of drugs have not been disentangled. This trial is thus both an outlier (in respect of effects on BP) and a trial of formative importance in the strategic management of cardiovascular disease (demonstrating a 'broad-spectrum' benefit of ramipril). Its conclusion that ramipril monotherapy conveys singular benefit sits in sharp contrast to the conclusion of PROGRESS, which implies that combination therapy with perindopril and indapamide is necessary to derive the most favourable outcome. An interesting addendum to the HOPE trial is a small substudy in 38 patients of 24-hour ambulatory BP monitoring.[31] This shows clearly that the 24-hour mean, particularly the overnight blood pressure control, on ramipril was much better compared with placebo. In the HOPE trial ramipril was administered in the evening and it is possible that the maximal effect on BP may have occurred overnight and may have been underestimated by the 'casual' outpatient pressures recorded in the main study. While not detracting from the overall conclusions on primary and secondary outcomes, it is a confounder in respect of interpretation of the data, and is entirely consistent with the view that blood pressure control is the key determinant of outcomes.

The Antihypertensive and lipid-lowering treatment to prevent heart attack trial (ALLHAT)[32,33] was one of the largest randomized trials ever undertaken. Over 40 000 patients with hypertension and increased risk of cardiovascular disease were randomized to receive one of four first-line antihypertensive strategies based on chlorthalidone, amlodipine or lisinopril and doxazosin respectively. Atenolol, reserpine or clonidine could be added to each limb as second-line therapy and hydralazine as third line. The choice of 'add on' drugs is remarkable – and reflects the cultural idiosyncrasies that characterize antihypertensive drug prescribing. Clonidine, hydralazine and reserpine are seldom used now in a European context. (The authors of this chapter have not prescribed clonidine for over 30 years and have never prescribed reserpine.) Nonetheless, in ALLHAT at least one second- or third-line drug was used in 26–33% of patients by year one and in 40–43% of patients by year 5. Systolic and diastolic BP was lowest in the chlorthalidone group. In 2000 the doxazosin treatment arm was prematurely discontinued because of a 25% increase in the relative rate of combined cardiovascular events (largely heart failure) in that group compared to chlorthalidone, and the futility of being able to find a difference in the primary outcome measure. The incidence of primary outcome events (fatal and non-fatal coronary heart disease) was indistinguishable in the other three groups. Amlodipine was marginally more effective at preventing stroke and chlorthalidine was marginally more effective at reducing combined cardiovascular events, particularly heart failure. At 4 years the incidence of diabetes was 11.6% in the chlorthalidone group, 9.8% in the amlodipine group and 8.1% in the lisinopril group. Metabolic differences were not reflected in a difference in cardiovascular outcomes over the course of the trial, but this may have been of too short a timescale to translate into major events, and uncertainty remains about the clinical significance of this observation.

Although ALLHAT was a very large study, questions persist over quality control and some important details have not been disclosed. It is not, for example, strictly a trial of monotherapy, as a substantial proportion of patients received combination therapy – it is unclear exactly what these combinations were, although we are given to believe that the same proportions of second- and third-line therapies were used in the three groups. Furthermore, it appears that by year 4 less than 80% of patients were on their original step 1 therapy or drug from a similar therapeutic group. By the same time, 'crossover' had occurred in 5–10% of patients. For example, 9% of patients in the chlorthalidone group had discontinued chlorthalidone and were taking a calcium channel antagonist or an ACE inhibitor, 6.9% of patients in the amlodipine group were taking a diuretic without a calcium channel antagonist and 8.5% of patients in the lisinopril group were taking a diuretic without an ACE inhibitor. There was thus considerable 'contamination' within this study that would tend to diminish the discriminating power of the intention to treat analysis. A reasonable conclusion would be that a combination of drugs based on a diuretic as first line is hard to beat over a 5-year timescale. In contemporary practice most practitioners would tend to use combinations based on the first-line drugs amlodipine, atenolol, chlorthalidone or lisinopril (or their within-class equivalents) rather than the combinations used in the study. However, if chlorthalidone can more than hold its own with other first-line agents, perhaps it is also time to look again at some of our less fashionable second-line agents!

The Losartan Intervention for Endpoint reduction (LIFE) study[34] reported that in hypertensive patients with left ventricular hypertrophy (LVH) losartan was superior to atenolol in the prevention of stroke. Regression of LVH was also greater in the losartan group, as was the incidence of new-onset atrial fibrillation and new-onset diabetes. These effects were achieved with a near-identical reduction in BP in the two groups. It has since been noted that hydrochlorothiazide was added in significantly more patients (44%) on losartan than on atenolol (38%).[35] In this study patients were on supplementary diuretics for about 70% of the total follow-up time. Whereas slightly more frequent use of hydrochlorothiazide may have contributed to the more favourable outcomes in the losartan group, this effect was probably small, according to a post-hoc analysis.[36] However, the clear message is again, that achieving target BP requires combination therapy in a significant proportion of patients.

ASCOT recruited 20 000 mild-to-moderate-risk hypertensive patients in the UK and Ireland and the Scandinavian countries. A factorial design allowed evaluation of both antihypertensive strategies and a comparison of atorvastatin against placebo, the lipid-lowering arm was stopped early because of a substantial benefit from atorvastatin over placebo.[8] The BP-lowering arm was also stopped prematurely, in December 2004. This trial differs from many other antihypertensive drug trials in being primarily a comparison of two combination treatment strategies. One arm consisted of a combination of amlodipine supplemented by perindopril, the other a combination of atenolol supplemented by bendroflumethiazide. Third-, fourth- and even fifth-line drugs were allowed in the form of doxazosin, moxonidine, and spironolactone, but strenuous efforts were made to avoid 'crossing over' while at the same time encouraging staff to push hard to attain the target pressures. This trial, therefore, provides robust data for the comparison of an 'established' (some would say 'outdated') combination of β-blocker/diuretic, with a 'contemporary' (some would say 'expensive and unproven') combination of ACE inhibitor/Calcium Channel Blockers (CCB). The factorial design will also yield data on the interaction between antihypertensive and lipid-lowering therapy, although these are likely to be substantially diluted as a result of the early curtailment of the lipid-lowering arm.

The study was stopped because a planned interim analysis found that all-cause mortality was lower in the amlodipine/perindopril arm. Final results have now been disclosed.[17] The reduction in the primary endpoint of fatal and non-fatal myocardial infarction was not statistically significant (OR 0.90, 95% CI: 0.79–1.02, $p = 0.105$). However, the 'headline' result is that the amlodipine/perindopril combination was associated with a significant reduction in most major prespecified secondary major endpoints compared with atenolol/bendrofluazide-K. Significant risk reductions were seen in respect of fatal and non-fatal stroke (HR 0.77, 0.66–0.89, $p = 0.0003$), total cardiovascular events and revascularization procedures (HR 0.84, 0.78–0.90, $p = 0.0001$). Unusually for an antihypertensive drug trial, all-cause mortality was also lower in the amlodipine/perindopril group (HR 0.89, 0.81–0.99, $p = 0.025$), almost all of this effect relating to cardiovascular deaths. Unstable angina, new-onset peripheral arterial disease, and new onset of renal impairment were all less frequent in the amlodipine/perindopril arm. New-onset diabetes was significantly less frequent in the amlodipine/perindopril arm (HR 0.70, 0.63–0.78, $p = 0.0001$). The mean blood pressure difference throughout the trial in favour of amlodipine/perindopril was 2.7/1.9 mmHg, but there was a much larger difference in favour of the amlodipine/perindopril arm early in the trial. Dual therapy was sufficient to achieve blood pressure targets throughout the trial in just over half of patients. Initial analyses have suggested a major favourable interaction with atorvastatin. The relative risks of both coronary disease and stroke were reduced by approximately half in the amlodipine/perindopril group randomized to atorvastatin compared with the atenolol/bendrofluazide group randomized to placebo statin. It has been suggested that much of the benefit in respect of prevention of stroke accrued through the difference in BP achieved, whereas the difference in respect of coronary events was significantly influenced by the differential effect of the two drug combinations on HDL cholesterol.[37] The results of ASCOT show a reassuring degree of internal consistency, demonstrating a broad spectrum of added cardiovascular protection from the amlodipine/perindopril combination. External consistency is also impressive, supporting a growing body of evidence linking the combination of β-blocker and thiazide with impaired glucose tolerance and blockade of the renin–angiotensin system with some protection against the same effect. It is worth noting, however, that all of these differential effects in ASCOT are small in absolute terms. Avoidance of one stroke required 500 patient treatment years, although if all cardiovascular events and new-onset diabetes are considered together the number needed to treat per year is nearer 100. A more detailed pharmacoeconomic analysis will be required to assess the relative cost-effectiveness of the two strategies.

The results of ASCOT provide, for the first time, robust data to support a preferred strategy for combination therapy in hypertension. The findings strongly suggest that a combination based on β-blocker plus thiazide should not be preferred as first choice, at least in a substantial proportion of patients.

The ONgoing Telmisartan Alone and in combination with Ramipril Global Endpoint Trial (ONTARGET) is an even larger study in 25 620 high-risk patients.[38] The baseline characteristics are very similar to those included in the HOPE trial, and include a very broad spectrum of prior vascular disease, as well as traditional risk factors – 49% have a previous history of myocardial infarction, 21% stroke or transient ischaemic attack, 17% peripheral vascular disease. Recruitment was completed in July 2003 and follow-up is scheduled to run until 2007/08. It is a three-way comparison of therapy with ramipril versus telmisartan and the combination. Other drugs are used extensively – 75% are on aspirin, 60% are on statins, 57% on β-blocker, 28% on diuretics and 33% on calcium channel antagonists. Thus, the outcome will reflect the influence of the trial drugs over and above these. Although designed as a trial of cardiovascular protection rather than blood pressure lowering, 68% of patients recruited had prior hypertension and the main interests will be whether combined sequential inhibition of the renin–angiotensin system will add to the effect of the individual drugs and how closely outcomes will be related to blood pressure lowering. Ramipril blocks the conversion of angiotensin I to angiotensin II, but it is known that 'escape' pathways exist to allow continued formation of angiotensin II even in the presence of a competitive inhibitor of converting enzyme. Telmisartan is a competitive blocker at angiotensin type I receptors. The two drugs in combination at consecutive steps in the angiotensin pathway should produce a more complete blockade. In effect, this is a study designed to extend the findings of HOPE, but with more robust measurement of BP. An equally important outcome will be whether benefits can be achieved without a penal increase in the risk of hypotension, hyperkalaemia or impaired renal function.

BENEFICIAL AND ADVERSE EFFECTS WITH COMBINATION THERAPY

Knowledge of the basic mode of action of individual antihypertensive agents coupled with clinical experience, supports the use of a number of combinations that will undoubtedly make life more bearable for patients. Similarly, certain combinations can be reasonably predicted to be less desirable, though detailed exploration of the lower dosages now drifting back into favour may minimize the risk of adverse reactions.

Thiazides and β-blockers

Perhaps the biggest current issue in respect of antihypertensive combination therapy relates to the use of β-blockers with thiazides. For decades it has been recognized that both groups of drugs may have adverse metabolic consequences. Diuretics in particular can cause hypokalaemia, hyperuricaemia and dyslipidaemia. These effects are dose-related, however,[39] and it has been assumed that low doses of thiazides are relatively innocuous and that metabolic effects are insufficiently large to translate into adverse cardiovascular outcomes. The striking benefits of thiazide, in many clinical trials and their favourable performance in comparison to other major antihypertensive drug groups have been used to make a case for the metabolic effects being of little consequence. These conclusions generally relate to outcome trials conducted over 5 years or so and some concerns remain about the potential cumulative effects over a much longer time frame. More recently, a longer shadow has been cast on this aspect of treatment with a meta-analysis suggesting that the combination of low-dose thiazide with β-blocker therapy may increase the risk of type 2 diabetes.[2,40] It has been estimated that this risk amounts to one incident case per 250 patients treated for 1 year. Unfortunately, despite three decades of widespread use of combination therapy with thiazides and β-blockers, very few trials have looked prospectively at the emergence of new diabetes in randomized trials with diabetes as a clear and well-defined endpoint. There is much uncertainty about possible dose-response and about interindividual variation in respect of individual drugs. It is not at all clear what the impact of this effect will be on major vascular outcomes. A recent report[41] suggested that new-onset diabetes in hypertensive patients (half of whom were on a diuretic) carries a similar risk for subsequent cardiovascular disease as established diabetes, but that study was subject to considerable baseline confounders and is difficult to interpret. Remarkably little is known about the reversibility of drug-related diabetes and the real impact of this effect on major outcomes. For the moment it seems reasonable to adhere to the BHS guidance that advocates avoidance of this combination in patients at particularly high risk of type 2 diabetes. A further stimulus to this debate has been the observation in a number of recent trials (Captopril Primary Prevention Project CAPPP,[42] HOPE,[30] LIFE,[34] VALUE[26]) that blockade of the renin–angiotensin system (RAS) with ACE inhibitors/Angiotensin Receptor Blockes (ARB) may result in a reduced incidence of type 2 diabetes. The results of ASCOT[37] are compatible with a dual effect – enhancement of risk with β-blocker/thiazide, and attenuation of risk from ACE inhibitors, but data from International Nifedipine GITS Study: Intervention as a goal in hypertension treatment (INSIGHT),[43] Controlled Onset Verapamil Investigation of Cardiovascular Endpoints (CONVINCE)[44] and International Verapamil-Trandolapril Study (INVEST),[45] where β-blockers were compared to metabolically neutral calcium antagonists, suggest that the problem lies mainly with a higher risk of new diabetes when β-blockers are combined with diuretics. The findings of VALUE[26] where valsartan was compared with CCB-based therapy, provides robust evidence that blockage of the RAS has antidiabetogenic potential. These observations support the notion that the real balance of risk vs. benefit in respect of antihypertensive medication can only be assessed over a much longer timescale than has been the norm in trials to date. A 10–20 year perspective may be necessary in order adequately to judge the impact of relatively minor metabolic disturbances. Pending such information, however, it does seem reasonable to take account of the metabolic effects of these drugs, along with other factors, when making decisions in individual patients.

Thiazides and ACE inhibitors/ARBs

Adding ACE inhibitors/ARBs to patients receiving diuretics may result in exaggerated 'first-dose' hypotension. This may be less of a problem with the use of long-acting ACE inhibitors/ARBs and is seldom a serious clinical problem unless the patient is severely volume depleted or has systolic dysfunction – such as in heart failure. In uncomplicated hypertension it is seldom necessary to adopt precautions other than advising that a first dose be taken at bedtime. Diuretics may also exaggerate the nephrotoxicity associated with ACE inhibitors/ARBs if patients become severely volume depleted. In contrast hypokalaemia secondary to diuretic use may be ameliorated with concurrent ACE inhibitors/ARB therapy.

At one stage it was thought that combining an ACE inhibitor with a diuretic resulted in a uniquely effective antihypertensive combination. However, that myth has effectively been exploded by the demonstration by Law & Wald[19] that all the major groups of antihypertensive drugs have a strictly additive effect.

Thiazides and calcium channel blockers

Peripheral oedema is the most troublesome limiting feature of vasodilator drugs including CCBs and accounts for a significant withdrawal rate from treatment. In clinical trials with CCBs, withdrawal rates of up to 5% per year are not uncommon.[26,43] Diuretics are commonly co-prescribed in the mistaken belief that they will reduce this side effect, but this is almost always unsuccessful, because the problem is not due to fluid retention per se but to a local vascular effect. With the very powerful vasodilator drug minoxidil, reserved for the most refractory hypertension, it is virtually impossible for patients to tolerate the resultant reflex tachycardia and peripheral oedema without the concomitant use of both a β-blocker and a loop diuretic.

Thiazides and potassium sparing diuretics

Thiazide and loop diuretics not infrequently cause hypokalaemia with or without hypomagnesaemia. These metabolic complications can be avoided by the addition of potassium sparing diuretics such as amiloride, spironolactone or triamterene. This is a more efficient method of conserving/restoring potassium levels than the addition of potassium chloride. A combination of hydrochlorothiazide/amiloride was used to good effect in the MRC Hypertension in the Elderly Trial[46] that demonstrated benefit in respect of cardiovascular protection with negligible risk of hypokalaemia. This same combination was used in INSIGHT.[43] Though showing equivalence in respect of major outcomes, INSIGHT showed an excess of biochemical/metabolic abnormalities in the combined diuretic group. Hydrochlorothiazide was combined with triamterene in the European Working Party on High blood pressure in the Elderly (EWPHE) trial[47] that first demonstrated the benefits of antihypertensive medication in an elderly population.

Adverse biochemical effects of thiazides, including hypokalaemia, are clearly dose-dependent.[39] Treating hypertension with high doses of thiazides may increase the risk of ventricular extrasystoles[48] and possibly serious arrythmias, thereby partly negating the beneficial effect of thiazides on cardiovascular outcomes. This has been further investigated in a population based case-controlled study where it was found that not only was the risk of primary cardiac arrest related to the dose of thiazide used, but also that the addition of a potassium-sparing drug to low-dose thiazide was associated with a reduced risk of cardiac arrest.[49] It is now difficult to assess the clinical significance of this effect of thiazides as the trend has been to use low doses, thereby diminishing any such risk. In these circumstances the need for adjunctive potassium sparing therapy as a routine is less obvious. Nevertheless there is a good case to be made for using such combination therapy if patients show evidence of hypokalaemia.

Diuretic-induced hypokalaemia may be a manifestation of underlying primary aldosteronism. Recent observations have suggested that as many as 15% of the adult hypertensive population may have a form of primary aldosteronism.[50] This remains controversial and its distinction from low-renin hypertension is a subject of much debate. Irrespective of the precise nomenclature, there has been a growing awareness of this phenomenon and a corresponding trend towards the use of potassium sparing agents as an adjunct to therapy when hyperaldosteronism is suspected.

β-blockers and vasodilators

The combination of β-blockers with rate-limiting CCBs, such as verapamil and diltiazem, increases the risk of bradycardia and heart block and is thereby contraindicated. Such combinations may also reveal the propensity of these drugs to cause negative inotropic effects and heart failure may develop.

Adding a β-blocking drug will suppress the reflex tachycardia that accompanies the use of vasodilators, such as hydralazine, minoxidil and dihydropyridines – particularly a problem with the shorter-acting dihydropyridines. This may minimize the feeling of palpitation and, to some degree, the vascular headache that such drugs may engender. The dihydropyridines may reduce the severity of beta-blocker-induced Raynaud's phenomenon. The combination of β-blocker and a dihydropyridine is frequently used in the management of patients with angina.

β-blockers and ACE inhibitors/ARBs

This combination has not been formally evaluated in major outcome trials. The renin/angiotensin paradigm might suggest that this is not a logical combination to enhance blood pressure response, and some early reports did suggest that the combination of β-blocker with ACE inhibitor resulted in a BP-lowering response that might be less than the sum of the individual effects.[51] However, a formal study has suggested an additive effect when β-blockers are combined with ACE inhibitor plus diuretic.[52]

Vasodilators

It should seldom be necessary to combine two or more peripheral vasodilator drugs, but when this is practised, it can be expected that there will be an increased risk of vasodilator side effects, such as peripheral oedema, flushing and headache. The authors have encountered these problems on a number of occasions in obstetric practice when short-acting parenteral hydralazine has been added to patients already on a dihydropyridine to control episodes of elevated BP. This has the unfortunate, though entirely predictable, outcome of causing symptoms such as severe headache, palpitation and malaise that can mimic the symptoms of pre-eclampsia, thereby exacerbating anxiety about progression of the underlying disease and confounding assessment of progress. This combination is very seldom used now outwith pregnancy-associated hypertension, although some patients with renal failure may still receive such combination therapy. A more common combination in everyday practice is that of dihydropyridine with an α-blocking drug. This is not a particularly poorly tolerated combination, but does run the risk of an increased incidence of peripheral oedema.

ACE inhibitors and ARBs

Individually, ACE inhibitors and ARBs may cause renal impairment in susceptible individuals – particularly patients with bilateral renovascular disease or renovascular disease in a solitary kidney. The most common circumstance is an elderly smoker with pre-existing peripheral vascular disease and widespread atheroma, although patients with vasculitis may also be at risk. This form of nephrotoxicity is exacerbated by the co-administration of either diuretics or non-steroidal anti-inflammatory drugs, or both. The current fashion of adding potassium sparing drugs, such as spironolactone, for refractory hypertension may further exacerbate this problem and certainly increases the risk of hyperkalaemia, so that particularly careful biochemical monitoring is required.

There is considerable interest in the possibility of combining ACE inhibitor with ARB in the management of refractory hypertension or of high-risk individuals.[38] It is very likely that this will result in some additional cases of hypotension, hyperkalaemia and renal impairment, as was seen in the CHARM series of studies with candesartan in heart failure,[53] but it will be the balance of these effects measured against any improvement in outcomes that will determine the place of this particular combination in hypertension.

Centrally acting drugs

Centrally acting drugs, such as clonidine, methyldopa, moxonidine or reserpine, are used more sparingly now than in former years, largely because these drugs tend to share a number of central side effects, such as drowsiness, dry mouth, nasal stuffiness and depression. They are very seldom used in combination with each other because the central side effects tend to be additive. However, with other groups of antihypertensives combined use is possible. The main limitation is in combination with lipid-soluble β-blockers, such as propranolol and labetalol, when central effects, such as vivid dreams, nightmares and hallucinations, may be greatly exaggerated. Methyldopa is often used in pregnancy and labetalol is also favoured by some obstetricians. There is reasonably good evidence for efficacy and safety when each is used alone, but the combination is particularly prone to give adverse central effects.

Fixed-dose combinations

Several are available for prescription. In very general terms the potential merits of these need to be weighed against the potential disadvantages. The main advantage is convenience which may also improve compliance with therapy. If this were truly the case it would be a significant advantage. There are persuasive data to support the view that once-daily dosage improves adherences rates with prescribed medication.[54] There are no corresponding data to show that fixed combination therapy has similar advantages over the use of individual constituents. The potential benefit of fixed combination therapy needs to be set against the lack of flexibility in dose titration and dose adjustment and the potential increase in cost that may arise from the prescription of some proprietary combinations rather than the use of individual constituents. Some combinations may include unnecessarily high dosage of the individual constituents – many of the β-blocker/diuretic combinations, for example, contain doses of diuretics that may be unnecessary and inappropriate. There is nothing wrong in principle in the use of fixed combination therapy, particularly if it is recognized that even individual agents may have numerous modes of action, but the lowest effective doses should be chosen. Another very important issue is that both patient and prescriber should be aware of the individual constituents. It is often the case that the proprietary name bears little resemblance to the individual drugs. Prescribers need to use their own judgement according to local formularies and pricing arrangements, but we recommend that at the very least they should use approved names.

CONCLUSIONS

No single antihypertensive drug trial published to date has been a trial exclusively of monotherapy. To a greater or lesser extent all the major outcome trials have permitted add-on therapy. In some trials this has been on a relatively strict stepped care basis, in others the add-on drugs have been largely at the discretion of prescribers. While mimicking, to some extent, what happens in everyday practice, this has had the effect of making interpretation of the contribution of specific combinations rather problematic. What is clear is that the use of combination therapy can result in substantial reductions in BP. Overall the data to date suggest that cardiovascular outcome is very largely determined by achieved BP rather than by the properties of individual agents. Exceptions to this rule have been claimed. Ramipril is reputed to have cardiovascular protective properties over and above the meagre blood pressure lowering seen in HOPE, although doubts have been expressed about this interpretation. Recent analyses have claimed that β-blockers may perform less well than their blood pressure lowering properties would suggest, particularly in respect of stroke prevention.[16,55] Additional meta-analyses may cast some further light on this.

Claims of exaggerated benefits of one drug or suboptimal performance of another would be less likely to be important if it were more widely recognized that low-dose combination therapy is the way forward for most patients. What is then needed is a somewhat more complex analysis of the relative benefits of different combinations. Unfortunately, because of the scale of study required, and the absence of a major commercial interest in evaluating low-dose, off-patent medications, it is unlikely that all permutations will be fully tested.

The ASCOT trial provides the first such evidence by evaluating a traditional versus a more contemporary combination strategy and strongly favours the more contemporary regimen. The combination of a dihydropyridine calcium antagonist with an ACE inhibitor runs a low risk of biochemical and metabolic effects and may offer favourable outcome in respect of major cardiovascular events. It is likely that the trend towards contemporary drugs in combination will be hard to resist.

Declaration of interest

JW has been principal local investigator for the following multicentre trials: EWPHE, SYST-EUR, PROGRESS, VALUE, ASCOT and ONTARGET. This has been associated with institutional funding for those trials, as well as numerous other research studies funded by pharmaceutical companies. Current funding sources include Pfizer, MSD and Boehringer-Ingelheim. JW is a full-time NHS physician and all grants are processed via the hospital Medicines Assessment Research Unit.

References

1. Williams B, Poulter NR, Brown MJ, et al. Guidelines for management of hypertension: report of the fourth working party of the British Hypertension Society, 2004 – BHS IV. *J Human Hypertension* 2004;18:139–185.
2. North of England Hypertension Guideline Development Group. Essential Hypertension: managing adult patients in primary care. National Institute of Clinical Excellence, August 2004. Online. Available: *http://www.nice.org.uk/* 1 August 2004.
3. Brown MJ, Cruickshank JK, Dominiczak AF, et al. Better blood pressure control: how to combine drugs. *J Human Hypertension* 2003;17:81–86.
4. Guidelines Subcommittee. 1999 World Health Organization – International Society of Hypertension Guidelines for the Management of Hypertension. *J Hypertension* 1999;17:151–183.
5. International Society of Hypertension Writing Group. International Society of Hypertension (ISH): statement on blood pressure lowering and stroke prevention. *J Hypertension* 2003;21:651–663.
6. Chobanian AV, Bakris GL, Black HR, et al. The National High Blood Pressure Education Program Coordinating Committee. *Hypertension* 2003;42:1206–1252.
7. Hansson L, Zanchetti A, Carruthers SG, et al; for the HOT Study Group. *Lancet* 1998;351:1755–1762.
8. Sever PS, Dahlof B, Poulter NR, et al; for the ASCOT investigators. Prevention of coronary and stroke events with atorvastatin in hypertensive subjects who have average or lower-than-average cholesterol concentrations, in the Anglo-Scandinavian Cardiac Outcomes Trial-Lipid Lowering Arm (ASCOT-LLA). *Lancet* 2003;361:1149–1158.
9. Webster J, Hensby CN, Dollery CT, Friedman LA. The antihypertensive action of bendroflumethiazide – increased prostacyclin production? *Clin Pharmacol Ther* 1980;28:751–758.
10. Cruickshank JM, Pritchard BNC. *Beta-blockers in clinical practice.* Edinburgh: Churchill Livingstone; 1988.
11. Balt JC, Mathy M-J, Pfaffendorf M, van Zwieten PA. Sympatho-inhibitory properties of various AT_1 receptor antagonists. *J Hypertension* 2002;20(Suppl 5):S3–S11.

12. World Health Organization – International Society of Hypertension Blood Pressure Lowering Treatment Trialists' Collaboration. Protocol for prospective collaborative overviews of major randomised trials of blood pressure lowering treatments. *J Hypertension* 1998;16:127–137.

13. Blood Pressure Lowering Treatment Trialists' Collaboration. Effects of ACE inhibitors, calcium-antagonists and other blood pressure lowering drugs: results of prospectively designed overviews of randomised trials. *Lancet* 2000;355:1955–1964.

14. Blood Pressure Lowering Treatment Trialists' Collaboration. Effects of different blood-pressure-lowering regimens on major cardiovascular events: results of prospectively-designed overviews of randomised trials. *Lancet* 2003;362:1527–1535.

15. Staessen JA, Wang JG, Thijs L. Cardiovascular prevention and blood pressure reduction. *Lancet* 2001;358:1305–1315.

16. Lindholm LH, Carlberg B, Samuelsson O. Should beta blockers remain first choice in the treatment of primary hypertension? A meta-analysis. *Lancet* 2005;366:1545–1553.

17. UK Prospective Diabetes Study Group. Efficacy of atenolol and captopril in reducing risk of macrovascular and microvascular complications in type 2 diabetes: UKPDS 39. *BMJ* 1998;317:713–720.

18. Dahlof B, Sever PS, Poulter NR, et al; the ASCOT investigators. Prevention of cardiovascular events with an antihypertensive regimen of amlodipine adding perindopril as required versus atenolol adding bendrofluazide as required, in the Anglo-Scandinavian Cardiac Outcomes Trial – Blood Pressure Lowering Arm (ASCOT-BPLA): a multicentre randomized controlled trial. *Lancet* 2005;366:895–906.

19. Law MR, Wald NJ, Morris JK, Jordan RE. Value of low dose combination treatment with blood pressure lowering drugs: analysis of 354 randomised trials. *BMJ* 2003;326: 1427–1435.

20. Wald NJ, Law MR. A strategy to reduce cardiovascular disease by more than 80%. *BMJ* 2003;326:1419–1425.

21. Prospective Studies Collaboration. Age-specific relevance of usual blood pressure to vascular mortality: a meta-analysis of individual data for one million adults in 61 prospective studies. *Lancet* 2002;360:1903–1913.

22. UK Prospective Diabetes Study Group. Tight blood pressure control and risk of macrovascular and microvascular complications in type 2 diabetes: UKPDS 38. *BMJ* 1998;317:703–713.

23. Tuomilehto J, Rastentye D, Birkenhager WH, et al. Effects of calcium channel blockade in older patients with diabetes and systolic hypertension. *N Engl J Med* 2999; 340: 677–684.

24. SHEP Cooperative Research Group. Prevention of stroke by antihypertensive drug treatment in older patients with isolated systolic hypertension. *JAMA* 1991;265:3255–3264.

25. Staessen JA, Fagard R, Thijs L, et al; for the Systolic Hypertension in Europe (Syst-Eur) Trial Investigators. Randomised double-blind comparison of placebo and active treatment for older patients with isolated systolic hypertension. *Lancet* 1997;350:757–764.

26. Julius S, Kjeldsen SE, Weber M, et al; for the VALUE trial group. Outcomes in hypertensive patients at high cardiovascular risk treated with regimens based on valsartan or amlodipine: the VALUE randomized trial. *Lancet* 2004;363:2022–2031.

27. Weber MA, Julius S, Kjeldsen SE, et al. Blood pressure dependent and independent effects of antihypertensive treatment on clinical events in the VALUE trial. *Lancet* 2004;363:2049–2051.

28. Staessen JA, Thijs L, Birkenhager WH. VALUE: analysis of results. *Lancet* 2004;364:931.

29. PROGRESS Collaborative Group. Randomised trial of a perindopril-based blood pressure lowering regimen among 6105 individuals with previous stroke or transient ischaemic attack. *Lancet* 2001;358:1033–1041.

30. HOPE (Heart Outcomes Prevention Evaluation) Study Investigators. Effects of an angiotensin-converting-enzyme inhibitor, ramipril, on cardiovascular events in high-risk patients. *N Engl J Med* 2000;342:145–153.

31. Svenssen P, de Faire U, Sleight P, et al. Comparative effects of ramipril on ambulatory and office blood pressures. A HOPE substudy. *Hypertension* 2001;38:e28.

32. ALLHAT Officers and Coordinators for the ALLHAT Collaborative Research Group. Major cardiovascular events in hypertensive patients randomized to doxazosin vs chlorthalidone: the Antihypertensive and Lipid-Lowering Treatment to Prevent Heart Attack Trial (ALLHAT). *JAMA* 2000;283:1967–1975.

33. ALLHAT Officers and Coordinators for the ALLHAT Collaborative Research Group. Major outcomes in high-risk hypertensive patients randomized to angiotensin-converting enzyme inhibitor or calcium channel blocker vs diuretic. *JAMA* 2002;288:2981–2997.

34. Dahlof B, Devereux RB, Kjeldsen SE, et al. Cardiovascular morbidity and mortality in the Losartan Intervention For Endpoint reduction in hypertension study (LIFE): a randomized trial against atenolol. *Lancet* 2002;359:995–1003.

35. Kato J, Eto T. Diuretics in the LIFE study. *Lancet* 2004;364:413.

36. Dahlof B, Devereux RB, Kjeldsen SE. Diuretics in the LIFE study. *Lancet* 2004;364:413.

37. Poulter NR, Wedel H, Dahlof B, et al; for the ASCOT investigators. Role of blood pressure and other variables in the differential cardiovascular event rates noted in the Anglo-Scandinavian Cardiac Outcomes Trial – Blood Pressure Lowering Arm (ASCOT-PBLA). *Lancet* 2005;366:907–913.

38. The ONTARGET/TRANSCEND Investigators. Rationale, design, and baseline characteristics of 2 large, simple, randomized trials evaluating telmisartan, ramipril, and their combination in high-risk patients: The Ongoing Telmisartan Alone and in Combination with Ramipril Global Endpoint Trial/Telmisartan Randomized Assessment Study in ACE Intolerant Subjects with Cardiovascular Disease (ONTARGET/TRANSCEND) trials. *Am Heart J* 2004;148:52–61.

39. Carlsen JE, Kober L, Torp-Pedersen C, Johansen P. Relation between dose of bendrofluazide, antihypertensive effect, and adverse biochemical effects. *BMJ* 1990;300:975–978.

40. Mason JM, Dickinson HO, Nicolson DJ, et al. The diabetogenic potential of thiazide-type diuretic and beta-blocker combinations in patients with hypertension. *J Hypertension* 2005;23:1777–1781.

41. Verdecchia P, Reboldi G, Angeli F, et al. Adverse prognostic significance of new diabetes in treated hypertensive subjects. *Hypertension* 2004;43:963–969.

42. Hansson L, Lindholm LH, Niskanen L, et al; for the Captopril Prevention Project (CAPPP) study group. Effect of angiotensin-converting-enzyme inhibition compared with conventional therapy on cardiovascular morbidity and mortality in hypertension: the Captopril Prevention Project (CAPPP) randomized trial. *Lancet* 1999;353:611–616.

43. Brown MJ, Palmer CR, Castaigne A, et al. Morbidity and mortality in patients randomized to double-blind treatment with a long-acting calcium channel blocker or diuretic in the International Nifedipine GITS Study; Intervention as a Goal in Hypertension Treatment (INSIGHT). *Lancet* 2000;356:366–372.

44. Black HR, Elliot WJ, Grandits G, et al. Principal results of the Controlled Onset Verapamil Investigation of Cardiovascular End Points (CONVINCE) trial. *JAMA* 2003;289:2073–2082.

45. Pepine CJ, Handberg EM, Cooper-DeHoff RM, et al. A calcium antagonist vs a non-calcium antagonist hypertension treatment strategy for patients with coronary artery disease. The International Verapamil-Trandolapril Study (INVEST): a randomized controlled trial. *JAMA* 2003;290:2805–2816.

46. MRC Working Party. Medical Research Council trial of treatment of hypertension in older adults: principal results. *BMJ* 1992;304:405–412.

47. Amery A, Birkenhager W, Brixko P, et al. Mortality and morbidity results from the European Working Party on High Blood Pressure in the Elderly trial. *Lancet* 1985;325:1349–1354.

48. Medical Research Council Working Party on Mild to Moderate Hypertension. Ventricular extrasystole during thiazide treatment: substudy of MRC mild hypertension trial. *BMJ* 1983;287:1249–1253.

49. Siscovick DS, Raghunathan TE, Psaty BM, et al. Diuretic therapy for hypertension and the risk of primary cardiac arrest. *N Engl J Med* 1994;330:1852–1857.

50. Kaplan NM. The current epidemic of primary aldosteronism: causes and consequences. *J Hypertension* 2004;22:863–869.

51. MacGregor GA, Markandu ND, Banks RA, et al. Captopril in essential hypertension; contrasting effects of adding hydrochlorothazide or propranolol. *BMJ* 1982;284:693–696.

52. Webster J, Petrie JC, Robb OJ, et al. Atenolol or propranolol in hypertensive patients poorly controlled on captopril and frusemide. *J Hum Hypertension* 1987;1:121–126.

53. Pfeffer MA, Swedberg K, Grayer CB, et al. Effects of candesartan on mortality and morbidity in patients with chronic heart failure: the CHARM Overall programme. *Lancet* 2003;362:759–766.

54. Iskedjian M, Einarson TR, MacKeigan LD, et al. Relationship between daily dose frequency and adherence to antihypertensive pharmacotherapy: evidence from a meta-analysis. *Clin Ther* 2002;24:302–316.

55. Carlberg B, Samuelsson O, Lindholm LH. Atenolol in hypertension: is it a wise choice? *Lancet* 2004;364:1684–1689.

18 | Sequential monotherapy

Bernard Waeber, François Feihl and Lucas Liaudet

INTRODUCTION

During the last few decades considerable efforts have been directed to screen for hypertension and treat patients with high blood pressure (BP). It is now well established that pharmacological treatment of hypertension is effective in decreasing cardiovascular morbidity and mortality.[1,2] However, hypertension remains a worldwide health problem.[3] The main reason is the poor BP control achieved in the community, even in countries where patients have easy access to health care.[4,5] This is partially due to the low target BPs recommended today (<140/90 mmHg in most patients, and <130/80 mmHg in patients with selected disease such as renal insufficiency and/or diabetes).[6–8] Normalization of systolic BP appears crucial to improve outcome,[9,10] but is clearly more difficult to achieve than diastolic BP control.[11–13]

Almost all hypertensive patients require lifelong treatment. In order to facilitate compliance with therapy, the prescribed drug regimen ought to be at the same time efficacious and well tolerated. To achieve this, five main classes of BP-lowering drugs are available, i.e thiazide diuretics, β-blockers, calcium antagonists, angiotensin converting enzyme (ACE) inhibitors and angiotensin II antagonists (AT$_1$-receptor blockers).[6–8] The aim of the present chapter is to compare the overall efficacy and tolerability of these antihypertensive agents administered as monotherapy. Because of the heterogeneous character of essential hypertension, any antihypertensive drug is expected to normalize BP in only a fraction of hypertensive patients.[14,15] A patient unresponsive to a given medication may normalize his or her BP in response to a drug acting by a different mechanism.[16] Switching from one to another type of antihypertensive agent represents a rational therapeutic strategy. This chapter will also focus on the advantages and the limitations of such a so-called 'sequential monotherapy' approach.

COMPARATIVE ANTIHYPERTENSIVE EFFICACY OF MONOTHERAPIES

Monotherapies in long-term placebo-controlled trials

A number of randomized placebo-controlled trials have been performed to compare monotherapies. In most the treatment period lasted only a few weeks or a few months, making it difficult to estimate the potential of single drug therapy for the long-term management of hypertensive patients. Two trials with a 1-year follow-up are worthy of mention.

The first was carried out to assess in untreated patients with mild hypertension the relative efficacy and safety of representatives of various classes of antihypertensive agents together with lifestyle changes (weight loss, reduction of sodium and alcohol intake, and increased physical activity) compared with a similar nutritional-hygienic intervention alone.[17] A total of 849 men and women aged 45 to 69 years completed the study. They all received counselling about nutritional-hygienic measures at both group and individual sessions. In addition they were randomly allocated to double-blind 1-year treatment with a diuretic (chlorthalidone, 15 mg/day), a β-blocker (acebutolol, 400 mg/day), a calcium antagonist (amlodipine, 5 mg/day), an ACE inhibitor (enalapril, 5 mg/day), an α_1-blocker (doxazosin, 2 mg/day), or placebo. The medication dosage could be doubled if diastolic BP remained $\geq$ 95 mmHg. In the placebo group BP was lowered during the course of the study by an average of 10.6/8.1 mmHg. The corresponding fall in BP was significantly greater ($p < 0.01$) when the nutritional-hygienic intervention was associated with an active compound (chlorthalidone : −21.8/−13.1 mmHg; acebutolol: −20.1/−13.7 mmHg; amlodipine: −17.5/−12.9 mmHg; enalapril: −17.6/−12.2 mmHg; doxazosin: −16.1/−12.0 mmHg). No consistent differences in BP responses were observed between the active treatments (Fig. 18.1).

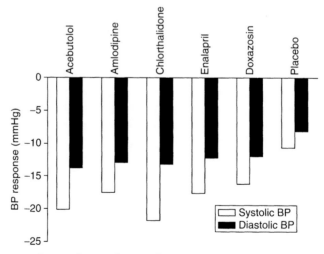

Fig. 18.1 Average changes in systolic and diastolic blood pressure (BP) observed during the 1-year follow-up in the placebo group (nutritional-hygienic intervention alone) and the active treatment groups (nutritional-hygienic intervention combined with an antihypertensive agent). *(Modified from ref. (17).)*

The second double-blind trial involved 1292 untreated men with diastolic BPs of 95 to 109 mmHg. They were randomly assigned to receive one of six drugs or placebo.[18,19] The active compounds consisted of the diuretic hydrochlorothiazide (12.5 to 50 mg/day), the β-blocker atenolol (25–100 mg/day), the ACE inhibitor captopril (25–100 mg/day), a sustained-release preparation containing the calcium antagonist diltiazem (120–360 mg/day), the α_1-blocker prazosin (4–20 mg/day), and the centrally acting sympatholytic agent clonidine (0.2–0.6 mg/day). The drug doses were titrated until a diastolic BP of less than 90 mmHg was reached. This was followed by a 1-year maintenance phase. Treatment success was defined as a diastolic BP of less than 90 mmHg at the end of the titration period and of less than 95 mmHg at completion of the maintenance phase. The fraction of patients with treatment success was 72.4% in the diltiazem group, followed by 62.4%, 59.6%, 54.8%, 53.7%, 50.0% and 31.0% in the clonidine, atenolol, hydrochlorothiazide, prazosin, captopril and placebo groups, respectively. Race and age were found to have an important effect on the response to single-drug therapy for hypertension. The success rate according to race and age is illustrated in Figure 18.2, which shows only the results obtained with placebo and the four classes of antihypertensive agents currently recommended as first-line therapy. Younger patients were <60 years old and older patients >60 years old. A difference between groups of more than 15% was considered clinically relevant. The calcium antagonist ranked first for younger and older African Americans, the ACE inhibitor for younger non-African Americans and the β-blocker for older non-African Americans.

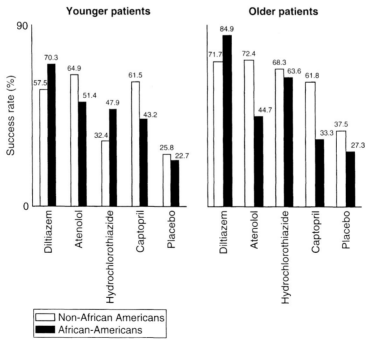

Fig. 18.2 Percentage of patients with treatment success (diastolic BP <90 mmHg at the end of the titration period and <95 mmHg at the end of the 1-year maintenance phase) when treated with an active compound or placebo. *(Modified from refs (18,19).)*

Unfortunately no information was provided on the systolic BP responses to the different study drugs.

Meta-analysis of clinical trials including monotherapies

The average reductions in BP induced by the five main categories of BP-lowering drugs according to dose were compared in a meta-analysis of 354 randomized, double-blind placebo-controlled trials, which included 40 000 active-treated patients and 16 000 patients given placebo.[20] There was a dose-dependent relationship for both systolic and diastolic BP, as illustrated in Figure 18.3. The placebo-corrected systolic and diastolic BP responses to the different classes of drugs were very similar. This was consistent for each of the dose categories.

Another meta-analysis of antihypertensive drug trials compared the BP responses to monodrug therapy in African-Americans and non-African Americans.[21] Table 18.1 summarizes the observations made with thiazides, β-blockers, calcium antagonists and ACE inhibitors. ACE inhibitors and β-blockers were less effective in African-Americans than in non-African Americans, the converse being true for thiazide diuretics and calcium antagonists.

Monotherapies in controlled morbidity-mortality trials

Until recently, randomized interventional trials designed to assess the effects of various therapies on cardiovascular and/or renal outcome used diastolic BP as target, accounting for the unsatisfactory control of systolic BP observed in these trials.[11] However, the protection afforded by BP normalization is at least as

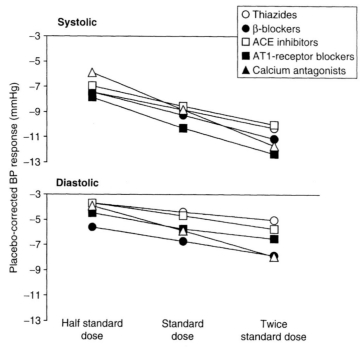

Fig. 18.3 Average reductions (placebo-corrected) in systolic and diastolic blood pressure (BP) according to dose for the five main classes of antihypertensive agents. *(Modified from ref. (20).)*

Table 18.1 Average changes in blood pressure (BP, mmHg) induced by different classes of antihypertensive agents in African and non-African Americans with hypertension

	African-Americans			Non-African Americans		
	No. of trials	No. of patients	Changes in BP	No. of trials	No. of patients	Changes in BP
Thiazides	3	342	−17.5/−11.6	4	409	−14.7/−9.7
β-blockers	1	81	−8.2/−11.2	9	442	−15.3/−12.9
Calcium blockers						
• dihydropyridine	3	286	−20.2/−13.0	10	1.993	−17.1/−10.5
• non-dihydropyridine	2	148	−15.5/−13.1	1	90	−11.6/−13.6
ACE inhibitors	8	272	−6.8/−5.6	10	696	−12.5/−9.2

(Modified from ref. (21).)
BP=blood pressure

great and may be greater for systolic than diastolic.[9,10] It has also become clear that it is more difficult to control systolic than diastolic BP.[11–13]

During the last few years a few event-based trials have been conducted with the goal to normalize both systolic ($\leq$140 mmHg or <140 mmHg) and diastolic ($\leq$90 mmHg or <90 mmHg) BP.[22–27] The BP control rates achieved in those trials ranged from 50 to 70%, percentages which are higher than those usually observed in studies of community care industrialized countries.[5] In these trials all patients received initially a single antihypertensive agent, but thereafter had their treatment intensified if needed to reach the target BP. Adding two or more antihypertensive agents was necessary in the majority of patients. Combination therapy was required in up to 80% of patients to achieve a BP normalization rate of about 70%.[26] It may be tempting to consider the results of these event-based trial as reflecting the impact of different monotherapies. In reality, however, these trials represent comparisons between drug regimens based initially on different monotherapies, but eventually consisting mainly of combination therapies.

TOLERABILITY OF MONOTHERAPIES

The incidence of adverse effects of most antihypertensive agents is dose-dependent. This is true for diuretics, β-blockers and calcium antagonists, as confirmed in a meta-analysis of placebo-controlled trials.[20] Attempting to normalize BP in each patient by titrating the dose of these agents is not appealing, as such an approach is often associated with reduced tolerability. However, this is not the case for ACE inhibitors and AT_1-receptor blockers: increasing the dose of these agents to achieve full blockade of the renin–angiotensin system does not compromise tolerability. This is illustrated in Figure 18.4.

RATIONALE OF SEQUENTIAL MONOTHERAPY

For many years, hypertensive patients have been treated according to the classic stepped-care approach, a second drug being added to the first-line therapy

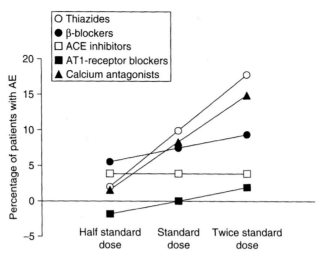

Fig. 18.4 Incidence of side effects according to dose for the 5 main classes of antihypertensive agents. *(Modified from ref. (20).)*

whenever the latter is insufficient to normalize BP.[16] More recently, the concept of sequential monotherapy has emerged. It is derived directly from the inability to predict the BP response to antihypertensive drugs in an individual patient. The purpose of this approach is to establish for each patient the drug that will most adequately control BP when administered as monotherapy. The concept is based on the following observation: most antihypertensive agents of the different therapeutic classes exhibit similar overall BP response rates. However, not every drug normalizes BP in exactly the same fraction of patients. It is, therefore, possible to normalize BP in more patients by switching one drug to another, acting by a different mechanism. This does not mean that every patient should receive consecutively a diuretic, a β-blocker, a calcium antagonist and a blocker of the renin–angiotensin system. The presence of associated diseases may preclude the administration of some classes of drug. In some patients, agents may have to be avoided in order to preserve the patient's lifestyle. For example, β-blockers might not be chosen for a young patient involved in heavy athletic activities. One important aspect of sequential monotherapy is that drugs must be administered for several weeks in order to evaluate their efficacy appropriately. Thus, antihypertensive therapy should ideally not be modified at intervals of less than 4 to 6 weeks. In general, this does not represent a major limitation in patients with moderate uncomplicated hypertension. Such an approach may be time consuming in the individual patient, potentially raising the fear of having a drug-resistant form of hypertension, with the consequent negative impact on the motivation to adhere with the prescribed preparation.

What can be expected from the sequential monotherapy approach in terms of BP control? To answer this question it is imperative to conduct drug trials according to a cross-over design. Two trials are of special interest in this context:

(1) The first included 56 white patients, aged 22–51 years, with mild essential hypertension (systolic BP $\geq$140 mmHg and/or diastolic BP $\geq$90 mmHg).[28] These patients underwent a systematic cross-over rotation of a diuretic

(hydrochlorothiazide + triamterene, 25 mg + 50 mg), a β-blocker (bisoprolol, 5 mg), a calcium antagonist (long-acting formulation of nifedipine, 30 mg) and an ACE inhibitor (lisinopril, 20 mg). Each drug was administered once daily for 1 month, with a 1 month wash-out phase between each treatment phase. The sequence of the monthly cycles of treatment was the same for all patients, with a randomized allocation of the initial drug to start the rotation. Thirty-six patients received the four classes of agents, 22 (39%) achieved BP <140/90 mmHg with the first drug, and 41 (73%) on any of the four antihypertensive agents. The only significant correlations found between the BP responses involved the diuretic and the calcium antagonist on one hand and the β-blocker and the ACE inhibitor on the other hand. It was concluded that rotation through different monotherapies represents an effective approach to treat hypertension. In routine practice it seems possible to abbreviate the rotation by selecting a β-blocker or an ACE inhibitor when a diuretic or a calcium antagonist fails to normalize BP, and a diuretic or a calcium antagonist if BP remains high despite the administration of a β-blocker or an ACE inhibitor as initial therapy.

(2) The second was aimed at comparing different treatment strategies in patients with uncomplicated essential hypertension (systolic BP ≥160 mmHg and/or diastolic BP ≥95 mmHg).[29] The goal was to normalize BP (<140/90 mmHg) within 6 to 9 months. The patients were randomized to double-blind treatments representative of different therapeutic approaches: (1) a sequential monotherapy strategy (atenolol 50 mg, followed by losartan 50 mg, and amlodipine 5 mg as needed [$n = 151$]); (2) a fixed low-dose combination strategy (perindopril-indapamide, 2 mg/0.625 mg, increased first to 3 mg/0.937 mg and later, if required, to 4 mg/1.25 mg [$n = 162$]); (3) a stepped-care strategy (valsartan 40 mg, increased if necessary to 80 mg, then to valsartan 80 mg plus hydrochlorothiazide 12.5 mg if the target pressure was still not achieved [$n = 157$]). The three groups did not differ significantly in baseline age, body mass index or BP. All study tablets were encapsulated to conceal their identity and were taken once daily. The final visit took place at the end of month 9, or end of month 6 if the target BP had been reached. The primary endpoint, i.e. the blood pressure normalization rate at the final visit, was achieved significantly more often in the 'low-dose combination' (62%) than in the 'sequential monotherapy' (49%, $p = 0.01$) or the 'stepped-care' group (47%, $p = 0.005$). No difference in tolerability was found between the different treatments. These data confirm the efficacy of a sequential monotherapy strategy allowing the use in a row of three classes of antihypertensive medications, but also demonstrate that starting therapy with a preparation containing a diuretic and an ACE inhibitor at low doses is even more effective in normalizing BP.

The importance of controlling systolic BP is now well recognized and elderly patients with isolated systolic hypertension benefit greatly from antihypertensive therapy.[30] A trial has been performed according to a crossover design to compare the antihypertensive efficacy of four main groups of antihypertensive drugs in previously untreated elderly patients with elevated systolic BP.[31] Seventy-four subjects aged 65–86 years (mean = 77 years) with systolic BP >150 mmHg received daily a low and high dose of a diuretic (hydrochlorothiazide, 25–50 mg), a β-blocker (atenolol, 25–50 mg), a calcium antagonist (felodipine or amlodipine, 5–10 mg), an ACE inhibitor (enalapril, 20–40 mg, or perindopril, 4–8 mg), and placebo. The sequence of phases was randomly allocated. The patients received consecutively each therapy for 1 month first at the lower dose, and then in the higher dose, unless the titration was considered contraindicated because of unacceptable side effects or excessively low BP during the low-dose phase. β-blockers could not be given in 15 patients because of asthma or bronchospasm. The fraction of patients who achieved the target systolic BP of less than 140 mmHg was 12% on placebo, 18% on ACE inhibitor, 17% on β-blocker, 23% on diuretic and 27% on calcium antagonist therapy. The percentage of patients with a normal systolic BP during any of the treatment phases was 41%. Side effects prevented the progression from the lower to the higher dose in 20% of patients on β-blocking drugs, in 6% of those on calcium entry blockade or diuretic therapy, and in 1.6% in patients during ACE inhibition.

Taken together the experience accumulated in the trials discussed above indicates the relative ineffectiveness of monotherapies to bring systolic and diastolic BP to <140 and 90 mmHg, respectively. The sequential switch from one to another type of antihypertensive agent extends importantly the probability of reaching these targets, but even better BP results can be achieved more easily with preserved tolerability by initiating treatment using a combination of two antihypertensive drugs acting by different mechanisms.

IS THERE A BEST CHOICE TO START A SYSTEMATIC ROTATION THROUGH SEVERAL MONOTHERAPIES?

Blood pressure control as a priority

In the individual patient it is possible to predict with some confidence the BP response to a given antihypertensive drug. If the priority is to normalize BP at the first attempt the best drug may be a diuretic or a calcium antagonist in older patients and in African-Americans, and a β-blocker or a blocker of the renin–angiotensin system in younger patients and in non-African Americans. This approach was recommended in 2004 by the British Hypertension Society guidelines for hypertension management (Fig. 18.5).[32] The experts of the European Society of Hypertension and the European Society of Cardiology leave it to the prescriber to initiate treatment with either a single drug belonging to any of the main classes, but at a low dose in order to minimize the occurrence of side effects, or to initiate with a two-drug combination, also at low dose.[6] In the United States of America, the selection of the initial drug depends on the severity of hypertension:[7] preference is given to a thiazide diuretic in patients with stage 1 hypertension, whereas the value of two-drug combinations to start therapy is recognized for patients with stage 2 hypertension.

Renin profiling may serve to match the right initial drug to the right patient. Diuretics tend to be more effective in patients with low rather than in those with high renin levels, the converse being true for blockers of the renin–angiotensin system and β-blockers. Selection based on age/race subgroup is, however, much simpler and better predicts BP responses to monotherapies.[33]

The sequential monotherapy approach represents a valuable option only in patients with uncomplicated essential hypertension. High-risk conditions

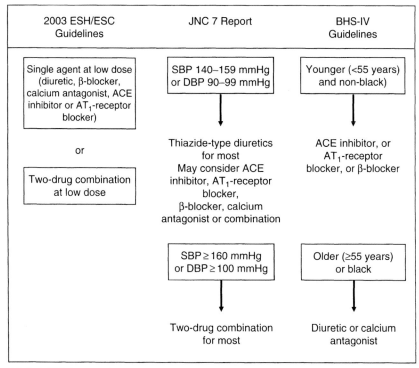

Fig. 18.5 Initial drug choices according to the 2003 European Society of Hypertension-European Society of Cardiology Guidelines for the Management of Arterial Hypertension (2003 ESH/ESC Guidelines), the Seventh Report of the Joint National Committee on Prevention, Detection, Evaluation, and Treatment of High Blood Pressure (JNC7 Report), and the British Hypertension Society guidelines for hypertension management 2004. *(Modified from refs (6,7,32).)*

(such as heart failure, coronary heart disease, cardiac hypertrophy, postmyocardial infarction, diabetes, chronic renal disease or albuminuria) represent compelling indications for specific antihypertensive drug classes, and combination therapy is required in many cases to achieve strict BP control.[6-8,32]

Preserved tolerability as a priority

In order to promote long-term compliance with antihypertensive therapy it is necessary to tailor the drug regimen to the individual patient, the goal being to normalize BP in each patient without interfering adversely with quality of life. The class of agents used to initiate treatment is in this respect very important because of more or less favourable side effect profiles. Among patients with newly diagnosed hypertension, the persistence with treatment may depend on different factors, in particular the patients' satisfaction with the efficacy and the tolerability of the prescribed drug. Analysis of prescriptions has been performed to assess whether there exist differences in continuation with therapy between the main classes of antihypertensive agents. Taken together the percentage of patients still on the same medication after a 12-month follow-up was highest for blockers of the renin–angiotensin system and lowest for diuretics.[34,35] Observations made over 4 years have confirmed the superiority of the blockers of the renin–angiotensin system in terms of probability of staying on the same medication for a prolonged period (Fig. 18.6).[36]

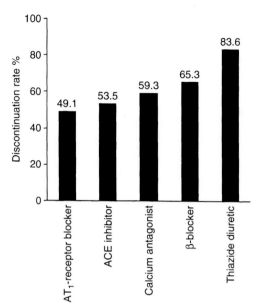

Fig. 18.6 Discontinuation rates at 12 and 48 months by initial antihypertensive drug class. *(Modified from ref (36).)*

Low cost as a priority

The cost-benefit of treating hypertension is well established.[37] When applying the sequential monotherapy strategy it may be tempting to use in every patient the least expensive drugs, i.e. thiazide diuretics and β-blockers. Whether such an approach would really decrease the cost per life year saved is, however, doubtful. Newer, more expensive classes of agents might afford better cardiovascular and renal protection when taken for years. In persistence studies, more patients are expected to remain on treatment when the initial drug is a blocker of the renin–angiotensin system rather than a thiazide diuretic or a β-blocker.[34–36] The latter two agents also have potentially harmful metabolic effects, which might translate into an adverse impact on outcome after years of treatment. Moreover, it must be recognized that there exists no event-based trial comparing monotherapies. Wherever possible the cost of the initial drug should, therefore, not drive the treatment strategy.

CONCLUSION

Sequential monotherapy is a conceptually valid, but limited approach to the treatment of hypertension. Rotation from one class to another class of antihypertensive agents allows normalization of BP in a large fraction of patients, but not all types of medications can be administered to everyone. In everyday practice, if a monotherapy is used as initial step, it is often more efficacious to add a second drug when needed rather than to titrate the initial agent. The increased antihypertensive efficacy obtained by combination therapy is usually not gained at the expense of a reduced tolerability. Sequential monotherapy is time consuming and is appropriate only in patients with uncomplicated essential hypertension. The probability of normalizing BP using monotherapies in older patients and African-Americans is somewhat greater with thiazide diuretics and calcium antagonists than with blockers of the renin–angiotensin system and β-blockers, whereas the latter agents tend to be more effective in younger patients and non-African Americans. These differential effects on BP may serve to guide choice of initial therapy, but other factors might be even more important, notably long-term tolerability.

References

1. Staessen JA, Wang JG, Thijs L. Cardiovascular prevention and blood pressure reduction: a quantitative overview updated until 1 March 2003. *J Hypertens* 2003;21:1055–1076.
2. Williams B. Recent hypertension trials: implications and controversies. *J Am Coll Cardiol* 2005;45:813–827.
3. Ezzati M, Lopez AD, Rodgers A, et al. Selected major risk factors and global and regional burden of disease. *Lancet* 2002;360:1347–1360.
4. Marques-Vidal P, Tuomilehto J. Hypertension awareness, treatment and control in the community: is the 'rule of halves' still valid? *J Hum Hypertens* 1997;11:213–220.
5. Wolf-Maier K, Cooper RS, Kramer H, et al. Hypertension treatment and control in five European countries, Canada, and the United States. *Hypertension* 2004;43:10–17.
6. 2003 European Society of Hypertension-European Society of Cardiology guidelines for the management of arterial hypertension. *J Hypertens* 2003;21:1011–1053.
7. Chobanian AV, Bakris GL, Black HR, et al. Seventh report of the Joint National Committee on Prevention, Detection, Evaluation, and Treatment of High Blood Pressure. *Hypertension* 2003;42:1206–1252.
8. Whitworth JA. 2003 World Health Organization (WHO)/International Society of Hypertension (ISH) statement on management of hypertension. *J Hypertens* 2003;21:1983–1992.
9. Benetos A, Safar M, Rudnichi A, et al. Pulse pressure: a predictor of long-term cardiovascular mortality in a French male population. *Hypertension* 1997;30:1410–1415.
10. Wang JG, Staessen JA, Franklin SS, et al. Systolic and diastolic blood pressure lowering as determinants of cardiovascular outcome. *Hypertension* 2005;45:907–913.
11. Mancia G, Grassi G. Systolic and diastolic blood pressure control in antihypertensive drug trials. *J Hypertens* 2002;20:1461–1464.
12. Lloyd-Jones DM, Evans JC, Larson MG, et al. Differential impact of systolic and diastolic blood pressure level on JNC-VI staging. Joint National Committee on Prevention, Detection, Evaluation, and Treatment of High Blood Pressure. *Hypertension* 1999;34:381–385.
13. Swales JD. Current clinical practice in hypertension: the EISBERG (Evaluation and Interventions for Systolic Blood pressure Elevation-Regional and Global) project. *Am Heart J* 1999;138:231–237.
14. Sever P. The heterogeneity of hypertension: why doesn't every patient respond to every antihypertensive drug? *J Cardiovasc Pharmacol* 1998;31(Suppl. 2):S1–S4.
15. Staessen JA, Wang J, Bianchi G, Birkenhager WH. Essential hypertension. *Lancet* 2003;361:1629–1641.
16. Brunner HR, Menard J, Waeber B, et al. Treating the individual hypertensive patient: considerations on dose, sequential monotherapy and drug combinations. *J Hypertens* 1990;8:3–11.
17. The Treatment of Mild Hypertension Research Group. The treatment of mild hypertension study. A randomized, placebo-controlled trial of a nutritional-hygienic regimen along with various drug monotherapies. *Arch Intern Med* 1991;151:1413–1423.
18. Materson BJ, Reda DJ, Cushman WC, et al; for The Department of Veterans Affairs Cooperative Study Group on Antihypertensive Agents. Single-drug therapy for hypertension in men. A comparison of six antihypertensive agents with placebo. The Department of Veterans Affairs Cooperative Study Group on Antihypertensive Agents. *N Engl J Med* 1993;328:914–921.
19. Materson BJ, Reda DJ. Correction: single-drug therapy for hypertension in men. *N Engl J Med* 1994;330:1689.
20. Law MR, Moris JK, Jordan RE. Value of low dose combination treatment with blood pressure lowering drugs: analysis of 354 randomized trials. *BMJ* 2003;326:1427–1431.
21. Wu J, Kraja AT, Oberman A, et al. A summary of the effects of antihypertensive medications on measured blood pressure. *Am J Hypertens* 2005;18:935–942.

22. The ALLHAT Collaborative Research Group. Major outcomes in high-risk hypertensive patients randomized to angiotensin-converting enzyme inhibitor or calcium channel blocker vs diuretic: The Antihypertensive and Lipid-Lowering Treatment to Prevent Heart Attack Trial (ALLHAT). *JAMA* 2002;288:2981–2997.

23. Cushman WC, Ford CE, Cutler JA, et al. Success and predictors of blood pressure control in diverse North American settings: the antihypertensive and lipid-lowering treatment to prevent heart attack trial (ALLHAT). *J Clin Hypertens* 2002;4:393–404.

24. Dahlöf B, Devereux RB, Kjeldsen SE, et al. Cardiovascular morbidity and mortality in the Losartan Intervention For Endpoint reduction in hypertension study (LIFE): a randomised trial against atenolol. *Lancet* 2002;359:995–1003.

25. Julius S, Kjeldsen SE, Weber M, et al. Outcomes in hypertensive patients at high cardiovascular risk treated with regimens based on valsartan or amlodipine: the VALUE randomised trial. *Lancet* 2004;363:2022–2231.

26. Pepine CJ, Handberg EM, Cooper-DeHoff RM, et al. A calcium antagonist vs a non-calcium antagonist hypertension treatment strategy for patients with coronary artery disease. The International Verapamil-Trandolapril Study (INVEST): a randomized controlled trial. *JAMA* 2003;290:2805–2816.

27. Dahlöf B, Sever PS, Poulter NR, et al. Prevention of cardiovascular events with an antihypertensive regimen of amlodipine adding perindopril as required versus atenolol adding bendroflumethiazide as required, in the Anglo-Scandinavian Cardiac Outcomes Trial-Blood Pressure Lowering Arm (ASCOT-BPLA): a multicentre randomised controlled trial. *Lancet* 2005;366:895–906.

28. Dickerson CJE, Hingorani AD, Ashby MJ, et al. Optimisation of antihypertensive treatment by crossover rotation of four major classes. *Lancet* 1999;353:2008–2013.

29. Mourad JJ, Waeber B, Zannad F, et al. Comparison of different therapeutic strategies in hypertension: a low-dose combination of perindopril/indapamide versus a sequential monotherapy or a stepped-care approach. *J Hypertens* 2004;22:2379–2386.

30. Staessen JA, Gasowski J, Wang JG, et al. Risks of untreated and treated isolated systolic hypertension in the elderly: meta-analysis of outcome trials. *Lancet* 2000;355:865–872.

31. Morgan TO, Anderson AI, MacInnis RJ. ACE inhibitors, beta-blockers, calcium blockers, and diuretics for the control of systolic hypertension. *Am J Hypertens* 2001;14:241–247.

32. Williams B, Poulter NR, Brown MJ, et al. British Hypertension Society guidelines for hypertension management 2004 (BHS-IV): summary. *BMJ* 2004;328:634–640.

33. Preston RA, Materson BJ, Reda DJ, et al. Age-race subgroup compared with renin profile as predictors of blood pressure response to antihypertensive therapy. Department of Veterans Affairs Cooperative Study Group on Antihypertensive Agents. *JAMA* 1998;280:1168–1172.

34. Bloom BS. Continuation of initial antihypertensive medication after 1 year of therapy. *Clin Ther* 1998;20:671–681.

35. Hasford J, Mimran A, Simons WR. A population-based European cohort study of persistence in newly diagnosed hypertensive patients. *J Hum Hypertens* 2002;16:569–575.

36. Conlin PR, Gerth WC, Fox J, et al. Four-year persistence patterns among patients initiating therapy with the angiotensin II receptor antagonist losartan versus other antihypertensive drug classes. *Clin Ther* 2001;23:1999–2010.

37. Elliott WJ. The economic impact of hypertension. *J Clin Hypertens* 2003;5(Suppl. 3):3–13.

X
Special patient groups

19 | Pregnancy

Catherine Calderwood and Catherine Nelson-Piercy

Hypertension is the commonest medical problem encountered in pregnancy, complicating up to 15% of pregnancies. The effects of hypertension in pregnancy range from the very mild to serious morbidity with the development of pre-eclampsia and eclampsia. There are also significant consequences for the fetus. Hypertensive disorders of pregnancy remain one of the commonest causes of maternal death in the UK and pre-eclampsia is the commonest cause of iatrogenic prematurity in the UK. Hypertensive disorders were responsible for 14 deaths in the most recent Confidential Enquiry into Maternal Deaths 2000–2002, published in 2004.[1]

INTRODUCTION

Much is now known about the processes which lead to an apparently healthy woman who becomes pregnant becoming so unwell with a hypertensive condition that she is at risk of death. Pregnancy is a physiological process which involves many adaptations. It is the failure of some of these adaptations which leads to the development of pregnancy-induced hypertension, pre-eclampsia and eclampsia. The unique setting of pregnancy calls for an insightful approach to the diagnosis and management of these conditions.

The approach to hypertension in the non-pregnant setting involves the management of hypertension to prevent sequelae over many years. However, in pregnancy the consequences of hypertension become apparent in days or weeks and affect two patients: the woman and her fetus. Understanding of the physiological adaptations to pregnancy, the processes involved in the development of hypertensive disorders during pregnancy and the necessary considerations in the treatment of these disorders, with the altered response of the pregnant woman to therapeutic interventions, is vitally important for the obstetrician and those practising internal medicine from whom advice is often sought when complications arise.

NORMAL PHYSIOLOGICAL CHANGE IN BLOOD PRESSURE DURING PREGNANCY

The changes in blood pressure during pregnancy begin early in the first trimester with a gradual fall in blood pressure which continues until 22–24 weeks gestation. This fall is caused by active vasodilatation, via the action of local mediators such as prostacyclin and nitric oxide. The diastolic blood pressure is primarily affected. After 24 weeks gestation blood pressure begins to rise and this trend continues until term. By this time the blood pressure has returned to pre-pregnancy levels. Immediately after delivery blood pressure usually falls, then increases over the first five postnatal days. This rise is independent of breastfeeding.

Definition of hypertension in pregnancy and blood pressure measurement

There are many definitions of hypertension in pregnancy. These are not uniform and can lead to confusion. The European Guidelines for Management of Hypertension published in 2003[2] have endeavoured to define 3 categories of hypertension in pregnancy (Table 19.1). Much antenatal care, particularly in the third trimester, is directed towards the detection of pre-eclampsia. Pre-existing hypertension may cause a diagnostic dilemma as undiagnosed women may be normotensive at their first visit because of the normal physiological fall in blood pressure and subsequent hypertension may be interpreted as gestational. The woman may then only be diagnosed post partum when her blood pressure continues to be elevated. Pre-eclampsia may rarely present prior to 20 weeks gestation and can be mistaken for pre-existing hypertension.[3] The risks of subsequent problems in pregnancy can be predicted to some extent at the first antenatal visit.

Pre-existing hypertension approximately doubles the risk of developing pre-eclampsia and also increases the risk of placental abruption and intrauterine growth restriction. Severe pre-existing hypertension carries a risk of developing pre-eclampsia of up to 50%.

The risk of gestational hypertension evolving into pre-eclampsia is 15–26%[4] but this risk is dependent on the gestation at which the hypertension is

Table 19.1 Hypertension in pregnancy

Pre-existing hypertension	BP > 140/90 mmHg ± proteinuria, predating pregnancy or noted before 20 weeks gestation. It normally persists more than 42 days post partum.
Gestational hypertension	Pregnancy-induced hypertension without proteinuria.
Pre-eclampsia	Gestational hypertension + significant proteinuria (>300 mg/L or >500 mg/24 h or dipstick 2+ or more) >20 weeks gestation, most commonly in the third trimester. Usually resolves within 42 days post partum.
Pre-existing hypertension plus superimposed gestational hypertension with proteinuria	Pre-existing hypertension associated with further worsening of blood pressure and protein excretion>3 g/day in 24 h urine collection > 20 weeks gestation.

diagnosed. If diagnosed prior to 32 weeks gestation, new-onset hypertension will progress to pre-eclampsia in 50%. The average duration of new hypertension before progression is 33 days (median). If gestational hypertension is diagnosed after 36 weeks gestation the risk of developing pre-eclampsia falls to 10%.

PRE-ECLAMPSIA AND ECLAMPSIA

Pre-eclampsia has classically been defined as hypertension in pregnancy combined with oedema and proteinuria. More recent definitions have concentrated on a gestational elevation in blood pressure together with >0.3 g proteinuria in 24 hours. Oedema is no longer included because of lack of specificity.[5]

Pre-eclampsia usually occurs after 20 weeks gestation and is a multi-system disorder. It may involve the renal, hepatic, cardiovascular, central nervous and coagulation systems. There can be enormous variation in the presentation, severity, timing and progression of different clinical features. Eclampsia is defined as the occurrence of a grand mal seizure in association with pre-eclampsia, although it may be the first presentation of the condition.

Pre-eclampsia complicates 5–6% of pregnancies[6] but this figure increases to up to 25% in women with pre-existing hypertension.[7,8] Other risk factors for pre-eclampsia include primigravidity, chronic medical conditions e.g. diabetes, renal disease, and family history or previous pre-eclampsia (Table 19.2).

Eclampsia complicates 1–2% of pre-eclamptic pregnancies in the UK. An estimated 50 000 women die each year from pre-eclampsia worldwide[10] and morbidity includes placental abruption, intracerebral haemorrhage, cardiac failure, and multi-organ failure. The risks to the fetus from pre-eclampsia include growth restriction secondary to placental insufficiency and premature delivery. Indeed, pre-eclampsia is the commonest cause of iatrogenic prematurity (accounting for 25% of all infants of very low birth weight < 1500 g). Pre-eclampsia may also manifest, with few maternal symptoms and signs, as isolated intrauterine growth retardation.

PATHOLOGY AND PATHOPHYSIOLOGY OF PRE-ECLAMPSIA

The three stages of the pathophysiological process in pre-eclampsia

The pathogenesis and manifestations of pre-eclampsia can be considered in a three stage model.[11] The first stage or primary pathology is placental in origin.

Table 19.2 Factors which increase the likelihood of pre- eclampsia. (Pre-eclampsia Community Guideline)[9]

1st pregnancy	Multiparous + previous pre-eclampsia
10 years or more since last baby	Multiple pregnancy
Age > 40	Hypertension or booking diastolic BP > 90 mmHg
BMI > 35 at booking	Renal disease or booking proteinuria + or quantified at 300 mg/24 h or more
Family history (mother, sister)	Diabetes
Booking diastolic BP 80–89 mmHg	Antiphospholipid antibody syndrome

Pre-eclampsia requires the presence of the placenta and can occur in conditions such as hydatidiform mole where there is no fetus. It is cured by delivery of the placenta although recovery may not be immediate. It is thought that the placental trigger may arise from either placental mass such as in twin pregnancy or by placental dysfunction with ischaemia such as in growth restriction. The secondary pathology is the maternal response to the placenta and involves abnormal placentation. In the first trimester, in a healthy pregnancy, the trophoblast invades the uterine decidua and reaches the inner layer of the myometrium. This migration transforms the small, musculo-elastic spiral arteries into large (4-fold increase in diameter) sinusoidal vessels, resulting in a high capacitance, low resistance blood supply to the intervillous space. Although commencing in the first trimester, the change is completed in the second trimester when another wave of trophoblast migration alters the myometrial segments of the arteries.[12] In pre-eclampsia these alterations do not occur or they are limited to vessels in the decidua.[13,14] In addition to the failure of demuscularization, the arteries maintain their response to vasomotor influences[15] and undergo accelerated atherosclerosis, which further impairs perfusion of the intervillous space. The third stage of the pathogenesis of pre-eclampsia involves the conversion of the uteroplacental maladaptation to the maternal systemic syndrome, which has protean manifestations such as eclampsia, cerebral haemorrhage, hepatic haematoma or rupture, renal failure, disseminated intravascular coagulation (DIC), pulmonary oedema and acute respiratory distress syndrome (ARDS).

Failure of the normal cardiovascular changes of pregnancy to take place results in hypertension, reduction in plasma volume and impaired perfusion of virtually every organ of the body. There is vasospasm and activation of platelets and the coagulation system, resulting in multiple-thrombi formation. The link between the placenta and the systemic disorder appears to involve endothelial dysfunction and oxidative stress.[16,17]

Women can present with a widely differing range of symptoms, from the very severe as described in Table 19.3, to mild, non-specific symptoms. The timing of the onset of clinical signs and abnormalities in blood results is also very variable (Table 19.4) and indeed an eclamptic seizure will pre-empt the development of hypertension and proteinuria in more than one-third of

Table 19.3 Symptoms and signs of severe pre-eclampsia

Maternal
- Headache and visual symptoms with 'flashing lights' (cerebral oedema)
- Nausea/vomiting
- Rapidly increasing swelling of face, fingers or legs
- Epigastric/right upper quadrant pain (liver oedema +/− hepatic haemorrhage)
- Hyperreflexia +/− clonus
- Oliguria
- Occipital lobe blindness
- Convulsions-eclampsia (cerebral oedema)
- Placental abruption

Fetal
- Intrauterine growth restriction/intrauterine death

Table 19.4 Investigations in the diagnosis of pre-eclampsia. Some, all or none of these abnormalities may be present

---

Maternal
- 24 hour urinary protein excretion > 0.3 g
- Raised serum creatinine and urea levels
- Raised serum uric acid level
- Thrombocytopenia – platelets < 100×10^9
- Prolonged clotting times
- Increased haematocrit and haemoglobin levels
- Abnormal liver function tests
- Abnormal maternal uterine artery Doppler (bilateral notching at 24 weeks may predict the development of later pre-eclampsia)

Fetal
- Reduced fetal growth, oligohydramnios
- Abnormal umbilical artery Doppler (shows fetal compromise)

---

women. The management of pre-eclampsia essentially focuses on recognition of the condition and ultimately delivery of the placenta, which is curative.

Since pre-eclampsia may arise with few symptoms, all women are screened during pregnancy through regular antenatal care. Those women who are recognised to be at increased risk have additional screening and more intensive monitoring.

MEASUREMENT OF HYPERTENSION IN PREGNANCY

Hypertension in pregnancy may be diagnosed either from an absolute rise in BP or from a relative rise above measurements obtained at booking. Previously an elevation in BP during the second trimester from a baseline reading in the first trimester, or compared to pre-pregnancy levels was used, but a definition based on absolute BP values (systolic BP > 140 mmHg or diastolic BP > 90 mmHg) is now preferred. Hypertension in pregnancy is considered severe if BP exceeds 170/110 mmHg.

A Royal College of Obstetricians and Gynaecologists Study Group on Pre-eclampsia published recommendations on the measurement of hypertension in pregnancy in September 2003.[18] Sphygmomanometry is labour intensive once more than a few readings are required and prone to inaccuracy – observer, mercury sphygmomanometer and stethoscope. Blood pressure variability can add to these errors. Blood pressure varies throughout the day and night, largely in association with activity. Levels are generally lower at night. Such variation occurs during normotensive and hypertensive pregnancies but there is a decreased fall in blood pressure during the night in women with pre-eclampsia.[19] Variability in blood pressure in an individual and between individuals can lead to errors in classification.

Postural changes in blood pressure are well described: an increase in diastolic pressure often occurs when standing. Exercise increases particularly systolic blood pressure. Many ordinary activities such as micturition, defecation, eating and drinking have significant effects on the blood pressure.

'White coat hypertension' is probably due to conditioning caused by the measurement of blood pressure itself or by the environment in which it is taken. This effect persists on repeated measurement. Some investigators have found 'white coat hypertension' to be more common in women.[20] Clinic blood pressure readings are significantly different from home readings in nearly 50% of pregnant women, the vast majority of readings being lower at home.[21]

It is essential to confirm high blood pressure readings on two occasions. Measurements should be made with the woman lying at a 45-degree angle or seated with an appropriately-sized cuff positioned at heart level. Lying supine, particularly in the third trimester, can cause a profound fall in blood pressure, due to compression of the inferior vena cava by the gravid uterus. The length and width of the bladder within the occluding cuff are important and incorrect cuff size can lead to errors. If the cuff is too small the pressure will not be fully transmitted to the artery; a standard cuff (with a 13×23 cm bladder) overestimates diastolic blood pressure by 5–10 mmHg and the systolic by 7–13 mmHg in obese patients.[22] The bladder length should be at least 80% and the width 40% of the circumference, measured around the middle of the upper arm. In a thin patient, a large cuff underestimates diastolic BP by 3–5 mmHg.

Sphygmomanometry relies on the auscultation of Korotkoff sounds over the brachial artery distal to a deflating cuff. Korotkoff Phase IV (K4) describes the 'muffling of sound' heard during this deflation, described by Ettinger in 1907, while Korotkoff Phase V (K5) is the 'disappearance of sound'. Phase V is universally recognised to be the diastolic identification point in non-pregnant subjects. In 1969 MacGillivray et al.[23] noted an unspecified but 'large number of very low and zero values' for diastolic BP when they were investigating BP changes in pregnancy and concluded that the disappearance of sound as an endpoint for determining diastolic BP was unsuitable. The reduced peripheral resistance in pregnancy may account for the sounds being heard when approaching, or at, zero cuff pressure. The phenomenon appears to be less common than originally thought and the ability to reproduce measurements using the muffling of sound is poor, while K5 is invariably heard.[24] There is lack of reproducibility in pregnancy of Korotkoff Phase IV as measured by mercury sphygmomanometry and K5 is now preferred.

Automated systems for BP measurement have been shown to be unreliable in severe pre-eclampsia[25,26] and tend to under-record the true value. A meta-analysis of studies relating to validation of automated devices in pregnancy and pre-eclampsia has shown that, overall, average errors were not large and, although these devices do under-record in pre-eclampsia, the degree of error does not preclude use in clinical practice. It is recommended that the equipment must be evaluated against a mercury sphygmomanometer before it can be assumed to be accurate. This was highlighted in the latest report of the Confidential Enquiry into Maternal Deaths[1] and a key recommendation was avoidance of inaccurate automated BP devices. The Association for the Advancement of Medical Instrumentation and the British Hypertension Society have published protocols which include details on how to evaluate device accuracy.[27]

Aneroid sphygmomanometers are often used especially in the community since these devices are more portable and may become more common as mercury sphygmomanometers are phased out. These devices become less accurate with time and should be checked regularly for accuracy.

CONSIDERATIONS FOR PRESCRIBING IN THE PREGNANT WOMAN

(1) Safety and side effects of the drug for the woman and safety of the drug for the fetus.
(2) Changes of pregnancy affecting the pharmacokinetics of the drug.

Those clinicians faced with a woman who has been prescribed a drug and who subsequently becomes pregnant or who requires drug treatment for the first time in pregnancy will most commonly be asked the question 'Is it safe for my baby?' The word teratology, derived from the Greek teras meaning 'monster', is the study of abnormal development or the production of defects in the fetus.[28] These defects can be due to deformation, disruption, dysplasia, or malformation.[29] Teratogenesis was previously used to describe structural defects in the fetus caused by drugs but this definition has been broadened (Table 19.5). Serious birth defects affect 2–3% of neonates.[28] Teratogens cause approximately 10% of birth defects, thus affecting 0.2–0.3% of all births.

Drugs can affect the fetus throughout the pregnancy, after the risk of structural defects has passed. Almost all drugs cross the placenta to a greater or lesser extent, notable exceptions being insulin and heparin because of high molecular weight.[30]

The Food and Drug Administration (FDA) introduced a drug classification system in 1979, the purpose of which was to discourage non-essential use of medication during pregnancy.[31] There is concern that reliance on the FDA classification by patients and health care providers can lead to maternal anxiety and unnecessary terminations. Since 1997, the FDA has been developing a new regulation that will revamp the pregnancy labelling system. The proposed regulation would replace the letter categories with more detailed, narrative descriptions. Information on fertility, pregnancy, and breastfeeding would be included.

Table 19.5 Teratogenesis

- Failure to implant, and miscarriage
- Major and minor structural defects
- Intrauterine growth restriction
- Fetal death
- postnatal effects e.g. neurobehavioural problems secondary to sodium valproate.

At present drugs are classified into 5 groups:

Current categories for drug use in pregnancy

Category	Description
A	Adequate, well-controlled studies in pregnant women have not shown an increased risk of fetal abnormalities.
B	Animal studies have revealed no evidence of harm to the fetus; however, there are no adequate and well-controlled studies in pregnant women. **or** Animal studies have shown an adverse effect, but adequate and well-controlled studies in pregnant women have failed to demonstrate a risk to the fetus.
C	Animal studies have shown an adverse effect and there are no adequate and well-controlled studies in pregnant women. **or** No animal studies have been conducted and there are no adequate and well-controlled studies in pregnant women.
D	Studies, adequate well-controlled or observational, in pregnant women have demonstrated a risk to the fetus. However, the benefits of therapy may outweigh the potential risk.
X	Studies, adequate well-controlled or observational, in animals or pregnant women have demonstrated positive evidence of fetal abnormalities. The use of the product is contraindicated in women who are or may become pregnant.

For developmental defects in particular, the timing of drug exposure in relation to conception is important. During the pre-embryonic period (until 17 days post conception), the all-or-nothing principle is currently favoured. If a chemical insult is inflicted, the result will either be total failure of the pregnancy or else the blastocyst will survive, any damaged cells will be replaced, and the pregnancy will continue without observable effects. The embryonic period (18–55 days post conception) is when most organogenesis occurs. Within this period more specific 'windows of opportunity' can be defined, during which given systems can be said to be vulnerable to teratogenic effects. Later in pregnancy, drug exposure is less likely to cause structural defects but can cause serious functional abnormalities or impairment.

CLINICAL PHARMACOLOGY CONCEPTS AND THE PREGNANT PATIENT

For a drug to be therapeutically effective, it must reach the site of its intended pharmacological activity within the body at a sufficient rate and in sufficient amounts to yield an effective concentration. Factors that are important in drug concentrations attained in serum and eventually at receptor sites include absorption, distribution, biotransformation, elimination, genetic factors and drug interactions.

Only a few studies have examined the pharmacokinetics of drugs during pregnancy. Dosing alterations during pregnancy have been published for only a few medications. Therefore most dosage recommendations are borrowed from the non-pregnant population. This lack of data on pharmacokinetics in pregnancy is problematic. Older, more established drugs have more published data on their use during pregnancy and clinicians have amassed experience with them. It is not always correct to assume that data from animal studies can be extrapolated to humans. It is also important to use a drug with which an individual clinician/department is familiar as this decreases the chance of drug errors.

Absorption

Absorption occurs via the gastrointestinal tract, skin, lungs and muscles, and after intravenous administration. The normal physiological changes of pregnancy alter absorption in many instances. During pregnancy, and particularly in the third trimester, progesterone prolongs gastric emptying time.[32] This may increase the time of peak plasma concentration (T_{max}) and reduce the peak plasma concentration (C_{max}) of orally administered drugs, although effects on overall bioavailability are relatively minor. Absorption and onset of action are delayed for some drugs, e.g. paracetamol,[33] whereas increased dissolution time helps increase the absorption of poorly water soluble drugs, e.g. digoxin.[34] In contrast, increased exposure to gut flora or mucosa decreases availability of other drugs. The composition of intestinal secretions may change – there is a reduction in gastric acid secretion, especially in the first and second trimesters. However, there is an increase in mucus secretion. This results in extended exposure of absorbable drug to the intestinal lumen, but appears to be of little clinical significance even for slowly absorbable drugs such as digoxin. Similarly, the rise in gastric pH has little impact on absorption.

Lung absorption is altered as cardiac output and minute volume respiration increase, thus decreasing the dose requirements for inhaled drugs. Skin and muscle perfusion increases, altering transdermal, subcutaneous and intramuscular absorption.

Distribution

The apparent volume of distribution (Vd) for most agents will increase during pregnancy due to increases in body water – intravascular (plasma volume) and extravascular (uterus, breasts and peripheral oedema). Total body water increases progressively during the pregnancy, creating a larger space within which hydrophilic drugs may distribute and by the $30^{th} - 34^{th}$ week of gestation, the circulatory plasma volume is increased by about 50%.

Highly water soluble drugs are particularly affected since the relative increase in body water is so marked and the C_{max} is thus reduced. Clinically, higher initial doses may be required in order to achieve therapeutic levels. Maintenance dose requirements are determined by the relationship between volume of distribution and clearance, both of which may be altered in pregnancy. As a result of the major expansion of the extracellular volume during pregnancy, concentrations of plasma proteins such as albumin tend to fall. Therefore during pregnancy plasma protein binding capacity decreases.

There is also some evidence that the drug binding capacity of plasma proteins is also reduced. Reduced protein binding leads to an increase in the unbound fraction and consequently greater availability for therapeutic activity. However, as elimination will also increase, levels of free drug are usually unchanged despite reduced total plasma levels. The major significance of this is in therapeutic drug monitoring where allowances must be made when interpreting results e.g. phenytoin levels, as most laboratories report total (rather than free) drug concentration.

Body fat increases by approximately 4 kg, creating a larger volume of distribution for lipophilic drugs. This has little practical importance.

Metabolism

Overall, the influence of pregnancy on metabolic elimination is often small and can involve an increase, decrease or no apparent effect. The activity of many metabolic processes is increased during pregnancy but these increases in drug clearance must be considered in conjunction with the increased volumes of distribution.

The metabolism of drugs primarily occurs in the liver. Although, during pregnancy, circulatory plasma volume increases by 50% and cardiac output by 30%, hepatic blood flow does not appear to be altered substantially. Therefore the magnitude of the first-pass metabolism, which is flow dependent, is not expected to differ from that in the non-pregnant woman.

Oestrogen and progesterone alter hepatic enzyme activity. Oestrogen competitively inhibits enzyme activity while progesterone inhibits some of the P-450 enzymes.[35] The former can result in drug accumulation while the latter can decrease elimination of drugs such as caffeine. Other P-450 enzyme activity is also increased so drugs like phenytoin are more rapidly cleared. Exceptions to the general absence of major change include metoprolol and sotalol, for which elimination is markedly increased, while labetalol, atenolol and propranolol require no dose alteration.

Elimination

The gradual increase in glomerular filtration rate, which rises by 50%, and the increase in renal blood flow by 60–80% during pregnancy, coupled with a reduction in protein binding, lead to increased renal clearance, particularly by simple filtration. Despite the increased volume of distribution, renal elimination rates are typically higher during pregnancy. It is possible that increased frequency of dosing may be required to ensure therapeutic efficacy of some drugs.

FETAL EXPOSURE TO DRUGS

The placenta is essentially a lipid barrier between the maternal and fetal circulations and the majority of drugs cross the placenta by passive diffusion. Thus, the movement of lipophilic drugs is favoured and the rate limiting step is placental blood flow.

Protein bound drugs and drugs with a high molecular weight e.g. heparin and insulin do not cross the placenta.[30] Both the immature fetal liver and the placenta can metabolize drugs; metabolism occurs in the fetus from 8 weeks post conception. However, metabolic enzyme activity is low, and 50% of the fetal circulation from the umbilical vein bypasses the fetal liver. Both these factors contribute to the problem of fetal drug accumulation. Elimination from the fetus is by diffusion back to the maternal compartment. As most drug metabolites are polar, this favours accumulation of metabolites within the fetus, although, as the fetal kidney develops, more drug metabolites are excreted into the amniotic fluid. Another process leading to accumulation of drugs within the fetus is the phenomenon of 'ion trapping'.[36] The basis for this is the slightly more acidic nature of fetal plasma pH compared to maternal plasma. Weak bases which are mainly non-ionized (lipophilic) diffuse across the placental barrier and become more ionized in the more acidic fetal blood, leading to a net movement from maternal to fetal systems.

In some instances, active transport mechanisms may exist. Virtually all maternally administered drugs will reach the fetus to some degree and all drugs can exert at least indirect effects.

Maternal dosing close to delivery can result in a newborn delivered with a quantity of the administered drug still present in its circulation. The loss of maternal and placental support may expose the infant's own very limited elimination capacity and result in adverse effects.

IMPLICATIONS FOR DRUG ADMINISTRATION IN PREGNANCY

The physiological changes in pregnancy influencing pharmacokinetics are complex. In general, volume of distribution is increased and drug clearance is increased, tending to reduce maternal plasma concentrations. To what extent this requires an alteration in dose schedule will depend on the size of the effect for individual drugs and also how critically therapeutic efficacy/toxicity relates to plasma concentrations. Specific data on how pharmacological parameters such as Vd and drug clearance vary in pregnancy for individual drugs are very limited. This is partly because of the ethical and practical considerations required when designing pharmacokinetic studies. Pharmacokinetic clinical trials do not often use pregnant women and women of reproductive age because of safety fears.

SPECIFIC INFORMATION REGARDING THE USE OF ANTIHYPERTENSIVE MEDICATION IN PREGNANT AND BREAST-FEEDING WOMEN

There is ever-increasing evidence regarding the safety and efficacy of many drugs in pregnancy, both antihypertensive drugs and drugs of other classes. When a drug is commenced de novo in pregnancy clinicians will generally prescribe from a small number of drugs with which they are familiar. Although there is some evidence of a need to adjust dosages and dose regimens in pregnant women, as discussed below, this is not often done in a clinical setting.

Beta-blockers and calcium channel blockers are used frequently during pregnancy. Elimination of nifedipine has been found to be faster during the immediate post partum period in patients with pre-eclampsia compared with non-pregnant women with hypertension.[37] Similarly, labetalol has been shown to have a shorter half-life in women with pregnancy-induced hypertension compared with non-pregnant women, suggesting the need for more frequent doses.[38] However, other studies have shown no difference between pregnant women and controls in plasma concentrations of labetalol.[39,40] This lack of consistency is perhaps due to confounding factors such as gestational age, sample size and different drug assays.

A review of studies of the pharmacokinetics during pregnancy of all classes of drugs was published by Little in 1999.[41] This included the above studies of labetalol and data for other beta-blockers. Metoprolol was hypothesised to induce enzymatic clearance during the third trimester because area under the curve, plasma levels, and half-lives were decreased compared with non-pregnant controls.[42] Plasma concentrations, clearance and half-life of propranolol during pregnancy were not different from those in non-pregnant controls.[43] Clearance of sotalol was increased during pregnancy, but half life and plasma concentrations were not different from non-pregnant levels.[44]

AIMS OF TREATING HYPERTENSION IN PREGNANCY

In the non-pregnant state the treatment of hypertension aims to reduce cardiovascular risk over many years, whereas in the pregnant woman the time frame for the treatment of hypertension in pregnancy is contracted. While the treatment of severe hypertension to prevent maternal complications is necessary and non-controversial, there is more controversy regarding the treatment of mild to moderate hypertension.

The rationale for treating hypertension in pregnancy may be divided into known and possible benefits.

(1) The prevention of serious maternal complications, particularly cerebral haemorrhage, multi-organ failure, HELLP syndrome and eclampsia.

The treatment of hypertension is indicated on the basis of the knowledge of potential cerebrovascular disease in the woman and in the case of women with renal disease or cardiac disease antihypertensive treatment will be indicated to minimize end-organ damage. However, the effect of antihypertensive medication on the risk of developing the HELLP syndrome, eclampsia or maternal death has not been subjected to randomized studies.

(2) The progression of pre-eclampsia and the risk of superimposed pre-eclampsia in women with hypertension.

Intensive antihypertensive treatment has been shown to reduce the risk of developing proteinuria.[45,46] This effect has not been confirmed by other studies.[47,48] Sibai et al. in two studies[49,50] found no effect of two different antihypertensive agents on the progression of pre-eclampsia or on the length of pregnancy. Superimposed pre-eclampsia has not been shown to be prevented by antihypertensive treatment.[51,52,53]

(3) Perinatal outcome – perinatal mortality, fetal distress, neonatal complications and birthweight.

There are a number of small studies which have looked at perinatal outcome but the power of these studies has been insufficient to demonstrate small differences in e.g. birth weight or neurological development of the child. Studies with oxprenolol did not find any reduction in birthweight of babies whose mothers had been treated in pregnancy.[47,48] In a recent review of nifedipine as an antihypertensive agent in pregnancy no adverse effects on perinatal outcome parameters were found.[54]

(4) Long-term prognosis of the children of hypertensive mothers.

Very few studies have followed up children born to mothers who have been treated with antihypertensive agents during pregnancy. Children of mothers treated with methyldopa followed up to school age had no detected adverse effects.[55]

(5) Long-term cardiovascular risks of the mother.[56]

Recent data on the long-term consequences of hypertension in pregnancy for the mother conflict with earlier studies which suggested that women with pregnancy-induced hypertension and eclampsia did not develop later chronic hypertension.[57,58,59] Sibai et al. found an increase in risk of later hypertension, especially when the hypertension in pregnancy began before 30 weeks gestation.[60] There does seem to be agreement that women whose pregnancies were not complicated by hypertension have a lower incidence of subsequent hypertension than does the female population of similar age and race.

The changes in the lipid profile in pre-eclampsia mimic those seen in ischaemic heart disease and there is also endothelial dysfunction. The specific vascular lesion of pre-eclampsia, acute atherosis in the placental bed, is similar to that observed in atherosclerosis, including foam cells loaded with lipid. There is also evidence that women with a history of pre-eclampsia may be at increased risk of ischaemic heart disease later in life.[61,62]

CHOICE OF ANTIHYPERTENSIVE AGENTS

First-line agent

Centrally acting dopamine antagonists

Methyldopa is the most frequently used antihypertensive agent in the UK and USA as there has been long clinical experience with the drug. This is the only drug for which children born to women treated for hypertension in pregnancy have been subjected to long-term follow up. No adverse effects were found up to the age of seven years.[55]

Women should be warned that methyldopa may cause sedation when first used but that they will become tolerant to this effect. The drug may cause elevation of liver transaminases in up to 5%. A positive Coomb's test may occur although haemolytic anaemia is uncommon. As depression is a side effect of methyldopa this drug should be avoided in women with a prior history of this condition including postnatal depression.

Second-line agents

Calcium channel blockers

Nifedipine is being used increasingly for the treatment of hypertension in pregnancy. This drug is safe at any gestation. A prospective cohort study showed no increased risk of teratogenicity.[63] Sibai et al[50] compared nifedipine with bed rest alone in pre-eclampsia remote from term. Nifedipine reduced the BP but had no effect on maternal hospitalization or perinatal outcome.

Slow release calcium channel blockers are used as second line antihypertensive treatment and some clinicians continue nifedipine or amlodipine if the woman is already taking the drug when she presents in pregnancy. Sublingual nifedipine should be avoided due to the risk of sudden hypotension which has a profound effect on placental perfusion.

Oral hydralazine

This drug is safe throughout pregnancy.[64] This drug can also be used by intravenous boluses or by infusion for the treatment of severe hypertension intrapartum.

Beta receptor antagonists

Atenolol has been studied by Rubin et al. in 1983[65] who found beneficial effects on fetal morbidity and respiratory distress. Treatment during the second and third trimesters was associated with reduced birthweight compared with the placebo group.[66] Thus atenolol is not recommended as a first line antihypertensive although this beta-blocker is used in women with Marfan's syndrome with dilatation of the aortic root to reduce the risk of further dilatation.

Labetalol is used widely for treatment of hypertension in pregnancy and is regarded as a safe and effective drug.[67] However, there has been a report of reduced birthweight in the babies of women with pre-eclampsia treated with labetalol.[49] A further study of the perinatal effects of long-term treatment (from late first trimester) with labetalol in women with mild chronic hypertension showed no difference in outcome when compared with methyldopa or no drug.[58] In a more recent meta-analysis of published data from randomized trials the presence of growth restriction appeared not to be related to the antihypertensive used.[69]

Due to the concerns raised in some of these studies it is usual for beta receptor antagonists to be reserved for use as a first-line antihypertensive in the 3rd trimester and to be used in the first and second trimesters only as a third-line agent (Table 19.6).[70] There are of course circumstances where beta-blockers are indicated in pregnancy and where benefit outweighs risk.

Table 19.6 Drugs used to treat hypertension in pregnancy

Drug	Indication	Starting dose	Maximum dose	Contraindications	Safe when breastfeeding?
Methyldopa	1st line	250 mg b.d.	1g t.i.d.	Depression	Yes
Nifedipine	2nd line	10 mg slow release b.d.	40 mg slow release b.d.		Yes
Hydralazine	2nd line	25 mg t.i.d.	75 mg q.i.d.		Yes
Labetalol	3rd line/1st or 2nd line in 3rd trimester	100 mg b.d.	500 mg t.i.d.	Asthma	Yes
Doxazosin	3rd line	1 mg o.d.	8 mg o.d.		Yes but prazosin preferred

Propranolol has been shown in several reports to reduce birthweight, increase fetal distress and perinatal mortality.[71-73] This beta-blocker is not ideal as a first line antihypertensive in pregnancy but can be used for selected diagnoses such as thyrotoxicosis and migraine prophylaxis.

Alpha antagonists

Prazosin has been shown to be safe and effective in pregnancy.[74] Doxazosin is also used as a third or fourth line antihypertensive and appears to be safe.

Angiotensin converting enzyme inhibitors

A recent study has shown these can cause major congenital malformations when used in the first trimester.[75,76] Women who conceive on an ACE inhibitor can be reassured, but a variety of malformations and adverse effects have been reported following second and third trimester use including: oligohydramnios, fetal renal tubular dysplasia and neonatal renal failure, IUGR, pulmonary hypoplasia, joint contractures and hypocalvaria (incomplete ossification of the fetal skull).[64,77] Women should therefore be informed of the need for discontinuation in the first trimester and substitution with another antihypertensive agent. Due to the similar mode of action of angiotensin II receptor antagonists and lack of data regarding their use in pregnancy these agents are currently not recommended.

PRESCRIBING FOR THE WOMAN WHO IS BREAST-FEEDING

Transfer of drugs into breast milk is a complex process determined by: maternal plasma concentrations, lipid solubility of the drug and fat content of milk, milk pH, half-life of the drug, molecular weight of the drug, and protein binding of the drug in maternal plasma. The baby's ability to metabolize drugs should also be considered, particularly if the baby is premature.

The most important determinant of the degree of drug penetration into breast milk is plasma protein binding. Drugs circulate in maternal plasma either bound to albumin or remaining freely soluble in the plasma. The protein-bound fraction stays in the maternal circulation, while the unbound fraction can be transferred into breast milk. Since more than half of maternal plasma protein is albumin, high protein binding effectively restricts many drugs to maternal plasma and prevents their transfer into breast milk. Thus highly protein-bound drugs e.g. warfarin are excreted into the breast milk in low amounts and this reduces the infant's exposure.

Maternal plasma concentrations are also important. Drug entry into and in most cases exit from breast milk is related directly to the concentration of the medication in maternal plasma.

The pKa of a drug is the pH at which a drug exists equally in ionic and non-ionic states. Drugs that have a pKa higher than 7.2 may be sequestered in breast milk to a slightly higher degree than those with a lower pKa. When the non-ionized molecule of a high pKa (ie weakly basic) drug enters breast milk, the molecule is quickly ionized and then is prevented from diffusing out of breast milk back into the maternal circulation. Thus the drug is 'trapped' in its ionized form and accumulates in the breast milk. Therefore medications with a lower pKa (acidic) are favoured when treating lactating women.

Since the mean pH of breast milk is 7.2 (lower than the plasma pH 7.4) drugs that are weakly basic tend to concentrate to a greater extent in the more weakly acidic breast milk. Furthermore, weak bases are non-ionized in the maternal plasma. Antihistamines and erythromycin, which are weakly basic, would be more likely to cross cell membranes from maternal plasma into breast milk than would penicillins, which are weakly acidic.

Lipid solubility of the drug and fat content of milk

Lipid soluble drugs readily diffuse across cell membranes by dissolving in the lipid bilayer. A medication that is more lipid soluble will transfer into breast milk more quickly and in greater amounts than one that is less lipid soluble. Water soluble drugs must pass through pores to cross cell membranes, a process that slows diffusion.

Colostrum is low in lactose and fat and high in protein. The reverse is true of mature milk. However, even mature milk has a low proportion of fat to total milk volume and allows a small amount of a drug to reach the infant.

Molecular weight of the drug

The semi-permeable lipid membrane of the mammary epithelium contains small pores that allow medications with a low molecular weight (less than 200 kDaltons) to traverse into breast milk. Drugs with a high molecular weight can only enter milk by being dissolved in the lipid membrane, which significantly reduces milk concentrations. Drugs with molecular weights greater than 200 kD e.g. heparin and insulin pass through at such low concentrations that they are virtually excluded from breast milk.

Drug half-life

Short half-life drugs are preferred as they usually reach peak concentration and are eliminated rapidly. Half-life can be used to determine whether the mother can successfully breastfeed by taking the medication immediately after feeding or before the infant's longest sleep period. If the half-life is short enough (i.e. 1–3 hours) then the drug level will have declined by the time the infant feeds. Long-acting or sustained release preparations should be avoided as they potentially expose the infant to a higher concentration for a longer period. Drugs with long half-lives (over 12 hours) may accumulate in the infant's plasma over time (e.g. barbiturates, benzodiazepines, pethidine).

Oral bioavailability to the infant

Once a drug enters the mother's milk and is ingested by the infant, it must traverse through the infant's highly acidic GI tract prior to absorption. Drugs such as aminoglycosides and omeprazole are denatured. The infant's short gastric emptying time and metabolism by the liver reduces exposure to the drug. The frequency and volume of feeding must also be considered as there will be less exposure to the drug if the infant is receiving supplementary feeds and/or other liquids.

Evaluation of the infant

The premature and newborn infants have immature hepatic and renal systems. Older infants have more mature organs and are larger and thus have a greater volume of distribution. Further reassurance can be gained if a particular drug has approval for use by the paediatric population in therapeutic doses and if there is a history of long-term safety in children.

Few large studies have addressed the excretion of drugs in breast milk. A systematic review of literature was carried out by Beardmore, Morris and Gallery in 2002.[78] There were 42 studies on the excretion of antihypertensive medication into breast milk. All studies had small numbers and were very varied in the stage of breastfeeding and in the indications for drug administration.

Beta-blockers are the most studied antihypertensive medications during lactation. The level of transfer into breast milk differs markedly among beta-blockers. All are weak bases but differ in lipid solubility and protein binding. Metoprolol, nadolol, acebutolol, sotalol and atenolol have the highest milk: plasma ratios of the beta-blockers, each averaging > 1. This indicates that these drugs are freely excreted into breast milk. However, there are only two reports of clinical effects on a breastfed infant and the majority of studies indicates that the dose of beta- blocker delivered to the infant would have no effect.[79, 80] As other beta-blockers have lower milk: plasma ratios these drugs are likely to be safer.

Calcium channel blockers

Knowledge about the excretion into breast milk of these drugs is much more limited. Evidence for nifedipine and diltiazem excretion is insufficient, with studies reporting only one subject for each drug.

There are also only case reports available for verapamil. The milk:plasma ratio varied from undetectable.[81,82] to a concentration of 2.1 ng/mL in the breastfed infant's serum.[83]

Methyldopa

This drug is traditionally avoided post partum due to the known side effect of depression. However, the studies which have included women who are breastfeeding while taking methyldopa have found low concentrations of methyldopa in the urine of one infant[84] and in the serum of another[85] with no adverse effects reported in the breastfed infants. As other antihypertensive drugs are known to have a good safety record most clinicians would not prescribe methyldopa post partum due to its high level of side effects.

Angiotensin converting enzyme inhibitors

ACE inhibitors display the lowest milk:plasma ratio of any of the groups of antihypertensive medications based on the limited data available.[86] There have been no reports of adverse effects in the breastfed infants of mothers being treated with a short-acting ACE inhibitor (captopril) or the longer-acting enalapril. The evidence thus far suggests that these are a safe choice of antihypertensive medication during breastfeeding. Whether the same will be true for even longer-acting ACE inhibitors is not known.

MANAGEMENT OF POST PARTUM HYPERTENSION

Many women with pre-eclampsia will continue to require treatment for hypertension following delivery. As noted previously, blood pressure falls in most women immediately following delivery and then rises for the first five days post partum. Although the cause of pre-eclampsia is removed by the delivery of the fetus and placenta the manifestations, particularly hypertension, may take many weeks to resolve.

Methyldopa should be avoided in the postnatal period due to the known side effect of depression and substitution with a beta-blocker such as atenolol is appropriate. Atenolol has the advantage over labetalol of once-daily dosing. Those taking labetalol or nifedipine can continue on their medication or change to atenolol. If a single drug is not sufficient the addition of a calcium channel blocker and/or an ACE inhibitor such as enalapril can be considered. All of these drugs are safe for use while breastfeeding. Women with known hypertension prior to pregnancy can change back to their original medication, although due to the increased fluid intake required for breastfeeding diuretics are not ideal.

Blood pressure is routinely measured daily in all women by midwives in the community for 10 days post partum. If necessary these checks can be continued by the health visitor. A follow-up clinic visit should be made for women with pre-eclampsia diagnosed during the pregnancy to ensure that hypertension and proteinuria have resolved. Antihypertensives should be able to be withdrawn within 6 weeks of delivery and resolution of proteinuria would be expected by 3 months post partum. Appropriate referral for investigation should be made if this is not the case.

The treatment of hypertension in the pregnant woman brings a unique series of challenges to the clinician. Two patients must be considered, the woman and her fetus, and a detailed understanding of the adaptive physiology of pregnancy and breastfeeding is required in order to choose the optimal management. An understanding of the disease processes surrounding hypertension in pregnancy, the potential outcomes for the woman and her fetus and the striking differences when compared with the management of hypertension in the context of the non-pregnant patient is very important. Promotion of this understanding between obstetricians and physicians is central to the achievement of the best possible outcome for the woman and her baby. There is increasing evidence of long-term sequelae in women who have been hypertensive in pregnancy and this opportunity for an insight into their future health must not be underestimated.

References

1. Lewis G, Drife J, eds. *Why Mothers Die 2000–2002. The sixth Report of the Confidential Enquiries into Maternal Deaths in the United Kingdom.* London: RCOG Press; 2004.
2. European Society of Hypertension. European Society of Cardiology guidelines for the management of arterial hypertension. *J Hypertens* 2003;21(6):1039–1041.
3. Walker JJ. Pre-eclampsia. *Lancet* 2000;356(9237):1260–1265.
4. Saudan P, Brown MA, Buddle ML, et al. Does gestational hypertension become pre-eclampsia? *Br J Obstet Gynaecol* 1998;105(11):1177–1184.
5. Brown MA, Hague WM, Higgins J, et al. The detection, investigation and management of hypertension in pregnancy: full consensus statement. *Aus N Z J Obstet Gynaecol* 2000;40:139–155.

6. Sibai BM, Caritis SN, Thom E, et al. Prevention of pre-eclampsia with low dose aspirin in healthy, nulliparous pregnant women. *N Engl J Med* 1993;329:1213–1218.
7. Caritis S, Sibai BM, Hauth J, et al. Low dose aspirin to prevent pre-eclampsia in those at risk. *N Engl J Med* 1998;338:701–705.
8. Sibai BM, Abdella TN, Anderson GD. Pregnancy outcome in 211 patients with mild chronic hypertension. *Obstet Gynecol* 1983;61:571–576.
9. Redman C, Walker J, eds. *Pre-eclampsia Community Guideline*. 2004. Action on Pre-eclampsia *www.apec.org.uk*.
10. Broughton Pipkin F. Risk factors for pre-eclampsia. *N Engl J Med* 2001;344:925–926.
11. Redman CWG. Hypertension in pregnancy. In: Chamberlain G, ed. *Turnbull's Obstetrics*. Edinburgh: Churchill Livingstone; 1995:441–469.
12. Robertson WB, Khong TY, Brosens I, et al. The placental bed biopsy: Review from 3 European centers. *Am J Obstet Gynecol* 1986;155:401–412.
13. Meekins JW, Pijnenborg R, Hanssens M, et al. A study of placental bed spiral arteries and trophoblast invasion in normal and severe pre-eclamptic pregnancies. *Br J Obstet Gynaecol* 1994;101:669–674.
14. Matijvic R, Johnston T. In vivo assessment of failed trophoblastic invasion of the spiral arteries in pre-eclampsia. *Br J Obstet Gynaecol* 1999;106:78–82.
15. Bernheim J. Hypertension in pregnancy. *Nephron* 1997;76:254–263.
16. Roberts J. Endothelial dysfunction in pre-eclampsia. *Semin Reprod Endocrinol* 1998;16:5–15.
17. Dekker GA, Sibai BM. Etiology and pathogenesis of pre-eclampsia: current concepts. *Am J Obstet Gynecol* 1998;179:1359–1375.
18. Critchley H, MacLean A, Poston P, Walker J, eds. *Pre-eclampsia*. RCOG Press; 2003.
19. Halligan A, Shennan A, Lambert PC, et al. Diurnal blood pressure difference in the assessment of pre-eclampsia. *Obstet Gynecol* 1996;87:205–208.
20. Khoury S, Yarows SA, O'Brien TK, et al. Ambulatory blood pressure monitoring in a non academic setting. Effects of age and sex. *Am J Hypertens* 1992;5:616–623.
21. Rayburn WF, Zuspan FP, Piehl EJ. Self monitoring of blood pressure during pregnancy. *Am J Obstet Gynecol* 1984;148:159–162.
22. Maxwell MH, Waks AU, Schroth PC, et al. Error in blood-pressure measurement due to incorrect cuff size in obese patients. *Lancet* 1982;ii:33–36.
23. MacGillivray I, Rose GA, Rowe B. Blood pressure survey in pregnancy. *Clin Sci* 1969;37:395–407.
24. Shennan AH, Gupta M, Halligan A, et al. Lack of reproducibility in pregnancy of Korotkoff phase IV as measured by mercury sphygmomanometry. *Lancet* 1996;347:139–142.
25. Gupta M, Shennan AH, Halligan A, et al. Accuracy of oscillometric blood pressure monitoring in pregnancy and pre-eclampsia. *Br J Obstet Gynaecol* 1997;104:350–355.
26. Penny J, Shennan AH, Halligan AW, et al. Blood pressure measurement in severe pre-eclampsia. *Lancet* 1997;349:1518.
27. O'Brien E, Petrie J, Littler W, et al. An outline of the revised British Hypertension Society protocol for the evaluation of blood pressure measuring devices. *J Hypertens* 1993;11:677–679.
28. Sever LE, Mortensen ME. Teratology and the epidemiology of birth defects: Occupational and environmental perspectives. In: Gabbe SG, Niebyl JR, Simpson JL, eds. *Obstetrics: Normal and Problem Pregnancies, third ed*. New York: Churchill Livingstone; 1996:185–213.
29. Aase JM, ed. *Diagnostic dysmorphology*. New York: Plenum; 1990.
30. Melissari E, Parker CJ, Wilson NV, et al. Use of low molecular weight heparin in pregnancy. *Thromb Haemost* 1992;68:652–656.
31. Teratology Society Public Affairs Committee. FDA Classification of drugs for teratogenic risk. *Teratology* 1994;49:446–447.
32. Mucklow JC. The fate of drugs in pregnancy. *Clin Obstet Gynecol* 1986;13:161–175.
33. Simpson KH, Stakes AF, Miller M. Pregnancy delays paracetamol absorption and gastric emptying in patients undergoing surgery. *Br J Anaesth* 1988;60:24–27.
34. Luxford AM, Kellaway GS. Pharmacokinetics of digoxin in pregnancy. *Eur J Clin Pharmacol* 1983;25:117–121.
35. Harris RZ, Benet LZ, Schartz JB. Gender effects in pharmacokinetics and pharmacodynamics. *Drugs* 1995;50:222–239.
36. Koren G. Changes in drug disposition in pregnancy and their clinical implications. In: Koren G, ed. *Maternal-fetal toxicology, second ed*. New York: Marcel Dekker Inc.; 1994:1–13.
37. Barton JR, Prevost RR, Wilson DA, et al. Nifedipine pharmacokinetics and pharmacodynamics during the immediate post partum period in patients with pre-eclampsia. *American J of Obstet Gynecol* 1991;165:951–954.
38. Rogers RC, Sibai BM, Whybrew WD. Labetalol pharmacokinetics in pregnancy-induced hypertension. *Am J Obstet Gynecol* 1990;162:362–366.
39. Rubin PC, Butters L, Kelman AW, et al. Labetalol disposition and concentration-effect relationships during pregnancy. *J Clin Pharm* 1983;15:465–470.

40. Saotome T, Minoura S, Terashi K, et al. Labetalol in hypertension during the third trimester of pregnancy; its antihypertensive effect and pharmacokinetic-dynamic analysis. *J Clin Pharm* 1993;33:979–988.
41. Little BB. Pharmacokinetics during pregnancy: evidence based maternal dose formulation. *Obstet Gynecol* 1999;93(5,Part 2S):858–868.
42. Hogstedt S, Lindberg B, Peng DR, et al. Pregnancy-induced increase in metoprolol metabolism. *Clin Pharmacol Ther* 1985;37:688–692.
43. O'Hare MF, Kinney CD, Murnaghan GA, et al. Pharmacokinetics of propranolol during pregnancy. *Eur J Clin Pharmacol* 1984;27:583–587.
44. O'Hare MF, Leahey W, Murnaghan GA, et al. Pharmacokinetics of sotalol during pregnancy. *Eur J Clin Pharmacol* 1983;24:521–524.
45. Blake S, MacDonald D. The prevention of maternal manifestations of pre-eclampsia by intensive antihypertensive treatment. *Br J Obstet Gynaecol* 1991;98:244–248.
46. Rubin PC, Butters L, Clark DM, et al. Placebo controlled trial of atenolol in treatment of pregnancy associated hypertension. *Lancet* 1983;I:431–434.
47. Fidler J, Smith Fayers P, deSwiet M. Randomized controlled comparative study of methyldopa and oxprenolol in treatment of hypertension in pregnancy. *Br Med J* 1983;286:1927–1930.
48. Plouin P-F, Breart G, Llado J, et al. Randomized comparison of early with conservative use of hypertensive drugs in the management of pregnancy-induced hypertension. *Br J Obstet Gynaecol* 1990;97:134–141.
49. Sibai BM, Gonzalez AR, Mabie WC, et al. A comparison of labetalol plus hospitalization versus hospitalization alone in the management of pre-eclampsia remote from term. *Obstet Gynecol* 1987;70:323–327.
50. Sibai BM, Barton JR, Sherif A, et al. A randomized prospective study of nifedipine and bed rest versus bed rest alone in the management of pre-eclampsia remote from term. *Am J Obstet Gynecol* 1992;167:879–884.
51. Redman CWG, Roberts JM. Management of pre-eclampsia. *Lancet* 1993;341:145–154.
52. Redman CWG. Treatment of hypertension in pregnancy. *Kidney Int* 1980;18:267–278.
53. Sibai BM, Mabie WC, Shamsa F, et al. A comparison of no treatment versus methyldopa or labetalol in chronic hypertension during pregnancy. *Am J Obstet Gynecol* 1990;162:960–967.
54. Levin AC, Doering PL, Hatton RC. Use of nifedipine in the hypertensive diseases of pregnancy. *Ann Pharmacother* 1994;28:1871–1878.
55. Cockburn J, Moar VA, Ounsted M, et al. Final report of study on hypertension during pregnancy: the effects of specific treatment on the growth and development of the children. *Lancet* 1982;1:647–649.
56. Sattar N, Greer IA. Pregnancy complications and maternal cardiovascular risk: opportunities for intervention and screening? *BMJ* 2002;325:157–160.
57. Chesley LC, Annitto JE, Cosgrove RA. The remote prognosis of eclamptic women: sixth periodic report. *Am J Obstet Gynecol* 1976;124:446–459.
58. Bryans CI. The remote prognosis in toxaemia of pregnancy. *Clin Obstet Gynecol* 1966;9:973–980.
59. Fisher KA, Luger A, Spargo BH, et al. Hypertension in pregnancy: clinical-pathological correlations and remote prognosis. *Medicine* 1981;60:267.
60. Sibai B, el-Nazer A, Gonzalel-Ruiz A. Severe pre-eclampsia in young primigravid women: subsequent pregnancy outcome and remote prognosis. *Am J Obstet Gynecol* 1986;155:1011–1016.
61. Jonsdottir LS, Arngrimsson R, Geirsson RT, et al. Death rates from ischaemic heart disease in women with a history of hypertension in pregnancy. *Acta Obstet Gynecol Scand* 1995;74:772–776.
62. Smith GCS, Pell JP, Walsh D. Pregnancy complications and maternal risk of ischaemic heart disease: a retrospective cohort study of 129 290 births. *Lancet* 2001;357:2002–2006.
63. Magee LA, Schick B, Donnenfeld AE, et al. The safety of calcium channel blockers in human pregnancy: a prospective, multicenter cohort study. *Am J Obstet Gynecol* 1996;174:823–828.
64. Briggs GG, Freeman RK, Yaffe SJ. In: Mitchell CW, ed. *Drugs in pregnancy and lactation: a reference guide to fetal and neonatal risk, 6[th]ed.* Philadelphia: Lippincott Williams and Wilkins; 2002.
65. Rubin PC, Butters L, Clark DM, et al. Placebo-controlled trial of atenolol in treatment of pregnancy-associated hypertension. *Lancet* 1983;1:431–434.
66. Butters L, Kennedy S, Rubin PC. Atenolol in essential hypertension during pregnancy. *BMJ* 1990;301:587–589.
67. Michael CA. The evaluation of labetalol in the treatment of hypertension complicating pregnancy. *Br J Clin Pharm* 1982;13(1 Suppl):127S–131S.
68. Sibai BM, Sarinoglu C, Mercer BM. Eclampsia. VII. Pregnancy outcome after eclampsia and long term prognosis. *Am J Obstet Gynecol* 1992;166:1757–1763.

69. Von Dadelszen P, Ornstein MP, Bull SB, et al. Fall in mean arterial pressure and fetal growth restriction in pregnancy hypertension: a meta-analysis. *Lancet* 2000;355:87–92.

70. Nelson-Piercy C. *Handbook of Obstetric Medicine, second ed.* Martin Dunitz: London; 2002.

71. Pruyn SC, Phelan JP, Buchanan G. Long term therapy in pregnancy: Maternal and fetal outcome. *Am J Obstet Gynecol* 1979;135:485–489.

72. Leiberman BA, Stirrat GM, Dohen SL, et al. The possible adverse effect of propranolol on the fetus in pregnancy complicated by severe hypertension. *Br J Obstet Gynaecol* 1978;85:678–683.

73. Habib A, McArthy JS. Effects on the neonate of propranolol administered in pregnancy. J Paediatr 177;91:808–811.

74. Rubin PC, Butters L, Low RA, et al. Clinical pharmacological studies with prazosin during pregnancy complicated by hypertension. *Brit J Clin Pharmacol* 1983;16:543–547.

75. Burrows RF, Burrows EA. Assessing the teratogenic potential of angiotensin-converting enzyme inhibitors in pregnancy. *Aust New Zeal J Obstet Gynecol* 1998;38:306–311.

76. Cooper WO, Hernandez-Diaz S, Arbogast PG, et al. Major congenital malformations after first trimester exposure to ACE inhibitors. *N Engl J Med* 2006; 354(23): 2443–2451.

77. Saji H, Yamanaka M, Hagiwara A, et al. Losartan and fetal toxic effects. *Lancet* 2001;357:363.

78. Beardmore KS, Morris JM, Gallery ED. Excretion of antihypertensive medication into human breast milk: a systematic review. *Hypertension in pregnancy* 2002; 21(1): 85–95.

79. Scheme MS, Sideman AI, Wilschanski MA, et al. Toxic effects of atenolol consumed during breast feeding. *J Paediatr* 1989;114(3):476–478.

80. Boutroy MJ, Bianchetti G, Dubruc C, et al. To nurse when receiving acebutolol: Is it dangerous for the neonate? *Eur J Clin Pharmacol* 1986;30:737–739.

81. Anderson P, Bondesson U, Mattiasson I, et al. Verapamil and norverapamil in plasma and breast milk during breast feeding. *Eur J Clin Pharmacol* 1987;31(5):625–627.

82. Miller MR, Withers R, Bhamra R, et al. Verapamil and breast feeding. *Eur J Clin Pharmacol* 1986;30(1):125–126.

83. Andersen HJ. Excretion of verapamil in human milk. *Eur J Clin Pharmacol* 1983;25(2):279–280.

84. Hauser GJ, Almog S, Tirosh M, et al. Effect of alpha-methyldopa excreted in human milk on the breast fed infant. *Helv Paediatr Acta* 1985;40(1):83–86.

85. White WB, Andreoli JW, Cohn RD. Alpha-methyldopa disposition in mothers with hypertension and in their breast fed infants. *Clin Pharmacol Ther* 1985;37(4):387–390.

86. Redman CW, Kelly JG, Cooper WD. The excretion of enalapril and enalaprilat in human breast milk. *Eur J Clin Pharmacol* 1990;38(1):99.

20 | The elderly

Sverre E. Kjeldsen, Aud Stenehjem, Ivar Aursnes and Ingrid Os

ELDERLY AND OLD PATIENTS

With the continued ageing of the general population, hypertension in the elderly (i.e. over age 65 years) is an increasingly important public health concern.[1] Raised blood pressure (BP), especially systolic pressure, confers significant risk and should be actively treated in elderly patients, at least until the age of 80 years. The prevalence of hypertension approaches or even exceeds 50% in people aged 70 years and above.[2] Hypertension is thus the dominant risk factor for cardiovascular disease in elderly persons. Much of the same could be said regarding the very old, i.e. people above the age of 80 years. However, it is still unclear whether treatment of hypertension in the very old prolongs life although it prevents stroke and heart failure.

HYPERTENSION – EPIDEMIOLOGY IN THE ELDERLY

Most elderly people with hypertension have isolated systolic hypertension, defined as a systolic pressure ≥ 140 mmHg and a diastolic pressure less than 90 mmHg, or more conservatively, defined as systolic BP greater than 160 mmHg with diastolic pressure less than 95 mmHg.[3–7] Increased systolic BP associated with ageing is not benign; systolic hypertension is a risk factor more potent than increases in diastolic pressure. Fewer than one-third have combined systolic and diastolic hypertension and the remainder, a decidedly small proportion of either sex, have isolated diastolic hypertension.

HYPERTENSION – PATHOPHYSIOLOGY IN THE ELDERLY

The increase in systolic BP with age is due to progressive vascular stiffening attributable to thickening of the arterial media and to changes in the nature and content of collagen and elastin that occur with advancing age.[8–10] Sluggish baroreceptor function and reduced cardiovascular sensitivity to catecholamines make the elderly more sensitive to natural or drug-induced falls in BP.

DIAGNOSTIC WORK-UP OF HYPERTENSION IN THE ELDERLY AND TARGET-ORGAN DAMAGE

There may be diagnostic problems in the elderly and very old people. 'Pseudo-hypertension' should be suspected in older patients who, despite high BP measurements, have vessels that feel rigid, have minimal vascular damage in the retina or elsewhere, and who experience inordinate postural dizziness despite cautious therapy. This is a condition in which there is a major discrepancy between intra-arterial and arm-cuff BPs, such that cuff pressures are high while simultaneous or nearly simultaneous intra-arterial readings are normal.

'Pseudohypertension' is a disorder to be distinguished from 'white coat' hypertension, a condition in which BP varies depending on the circumstances under which it is measured. There have been a number of bedside or laboratory tests for 'pseudohypertension', e.g. Osler manoeuvre, palpatory, oscillometric or intra-arterial assessment of forearm systolic BP, and Finapres or cuff-occlusion plethysmographic measurement of finger BP.[11–17]

BP readings are far more variable in the elderly, so more readings should be taken initially than for patients in the general population. BP should be measured in both the sitting and standing positions since there is a high frequency (as much as 30%) of a 20 mmHg fall in BP in patients with a systolic pressure over 160 mmHg. Standing BP should be used to guide treatment decisions. Prevalence of clinically significant secondary hypertension is low (probably in the 1–5% range).

AMBULATORY AND HOME BLOOD PRESSURE IN THE ELDERLY

Both home BP monitoring (HBPM) and ambulatory BP monitoring (ABPM) have become tools in the evaluation of hypertensive patients in clinical practice. The recent guidelines for the management of hypertension provide detailed suggestions regarding how and when to use ABPM,[18] and not only in the diagnostic work-up, but also for monitoring treatment. Although additional information beyond mere average 24-hour BP levels can be obtained, the clinical applicability for other variables is still under scrutiny.[19,20] The reproducibility of ABPM over a year has been found to be good in elderly normotensive subjects.[21]

In a population-based cohort of 70-year-old men, ABP was a significant predictor of cardiovascular morbidity, independent of office BP and other risk factors.[22] Similarly in older patients with isolated systolic hypertension (ISH), ABP was a significant predictor of cardiovascular risk over and above conventionally measured BP.[23]

It has been suggested that conventional BP measurements in the elderly can be inaccurate and misleading due to extreme BP variability,[18] leading to the potential risk of over-treatment. The white coat phenomenon, the difference between office BP and ABP, may be more pronounced in the elderly.[24] However, the reproducibility and, therefore, the clinical utility of the white coat effect has been questioned.[19] Another complication is the 'reversed white coat phenomenon', e.g. ABP greater than office BP, which was apparent in a substantial proportion of the patients in the second Australian National Blood Pressure Study.[25]

In most people, BP is reduced at night. The nocturnal dip in BP is less marked with increasing age,[19,26-28] and abolished in centenarians.[27,29] The importance of the dip in BP during sleep has been debated, and inconsistent findings are reported in older patients. In elderly subjects with Isolated Systolic Hypertension (ISH), an inverse association between reduction in BP during the night and cardiovascular risk has been observed.[22] For every 10% increment in night-to-day BP ratio the cardiovascular risk increased 41%. Kario et al. observed that a marked dip in BP was associated with more advanced cerebrovascular damage,[20] while a Swedish study questioned the usefulness of recognizing a non-dipping BP pattern in an elderly population as there was no association with either metabolic disturbances or target-organ damage.[30] A postprandial dip in BP has been observed in very old people.[28,29]

Despite shortcomings and inconsistency in interpretations, ABPM has advantages over conventionally measured BP as it characterizes the BP status more extensively through a number of measurements, both day and night, and is more closely linked to cardiovascular risk. Descriptive data from large cohorts of elderly subjects may provide the basis for reference values.[24,28,29,31] There is a paucity of data on HBPM in elderly subjects. Ongoing studies will contribute to proper reference values under standardized conditions and with validated devices, but are not specifically designed for older populations. In the Ohasama study, HBP had predictive power for mortality and stroke stronger than screening BP,[32,33] suggesting the potential usefulness of HBP measurements. However, physical and intellectual limitations, which are more evident in elderly subjects, may curtail more extensive use of HBPM.[18]

Both HBP and ABP reflect the age-dependent increase in systolic BP. ABP provides information about the altered BP rhythm with advancing age, with less pronounced nocturnal dip and more marked postprandial BP reduction. Both ABP and HBP have been shown to be closely associated with cardiovascular morbidity and mortality and appear superior to conventionally measured BP. While there are accumulating data on the use of ABPM in the elderly populations, data on HBPM are still lacking. Greater use of ABPM in the elderly might inform the selection of appropriate therapeutic options.

PHARMACOKINETICS AND PHARMACODYNAMICS OF ANTIHYPERTENSIVE DRUGS

It is well recognized that the elderly are more likely to suffer from conditions that benefit from the use of pharmacotherapy. However, in a small proportion of older patients prescribed drugs can cause morbidity. Notably, 11% of episodes of syncope in the elderly are drug-induced.[34] Nevertheless, it appears reasonable to treat elderly hypertensive patients, particularly those with evidence of target-organ damage.[35]

Pharmacokinetics

Glomerular filtration rate decreases with age but serum creatinine concentration may not be an appropriate measure in the elderly because of reduced muscle mass.[36] Therefore, calculated creatinine clearance, which takes account of age, gender and weight is recommended.[37] Renal function is relevant for medication that is predominantly excreted by the kidney, e.g. atenolol and ACE-inhibitors. Excretion of potassium sparing agents can also be affected by reduced clearance rate in elderly patients[38] and hyperkalaemia due to reduced renal function is a common problem.

Ageing is associated with a reduction in first-pass metabolism, probably due to a reduction in liver mass and blood flow.[39] As a result, the bioavailability of drugs undergoing extensive first-pass metabolism such as propanolol and labetolol can be significantly increased.[40] In contrast, several ACE-inhibitors such as enalapril and perindopril are prodrugs that need to be activated in the liver. Therefore, first-pass activation might be slowed or reduced with advancing age.[41]

A decrease in liver cytochrome P450 activity, secondary to reduced gene expression, has been observed in renal failure.[42] Therefore, the age-associated reduction in renal function might also potentially affect drug metabolism in the liver. Body mass reduction and relative increase in adipose tissue will affect the distribution of both lipophilic and hydrophilic drugs. The elimination half-lives of some drugs can be prolonged. This is especially relevant for those drugs metabolized by phase I reactions. The amount of free (active) drug is affected by the level of serum albumin, which decreases with age. There are no significant age-related differences in drug absorption rates.[43] However, sustained nifedipine is more slowly absorbed in the elderly than in the young.[34,44]

Pharmacodynamics

Between ages 20 and 80 years a 90% loss of vessel elasticity and distensibility[45] results in increased risk of hypovolaemia and hypotension. Baroreceptor sensitivity also decreases, leading to greater risk of orthostatic hypertension and drug-induced falls in BP, especially when altered baroreceptor function is associated with decreased body water, varicose veins, etc.[34,12]

Reduced β-adrenoceptor sensitivity has been documented in the elderly.[46] Monotherapy with β-blockers controlled BP in 75% of patients younger than 40 years, but in only 20% of patients 60 years of age and over.[47]

Many elderly patients are on long-term therapy with diuretics. Because of a decrease in total body water with advancing age, an equal volume of fluid loss in young and old patients represents more severe dehydration in the elderly. Combined with decrease in thirst, fluid intake, and cardiovascular reflexes in the elderly, hypovolaemia may contribute to deficits in hemoperfusion of vital organs. In addition, patients over 65 years of age, especially females, are at increased risk of developing hypokalaemia, hyponatraemia, and prerenal azotaemia, when treated with thiazides in combination with loop diuretics compared with younger patients.[48]

Diuretic therapy in the elderly is also complicated because the site of action of both loop and thiazide diuretics is the luminal cell membrane of the renal tubule. The intensity of the diuretic effect is not primarily related to diuretic concentration in plasma but to that in the tubular lumen. Reduction in the renal clearance of loop and thiazide diuretics in the elderly results in higher plasma levels and systematic toxicity, whereas the diuretic and natriuretic effect is decreased.[49] Hypokalaemia is common and may be exaggerated by dietary deficiency of potassium. Hyponatraemia can also arise in the elderly. Renal function deterioration can lead to unintended hypotension when using ACE-inhibitors and angiotensin receptor blockers. Hypotension can occur after the first dose due to venodilatation, especially when there is concomitant diuretic therapy. Medication with NSAIDs and COX-2 inhibitors attenuates BP lowering effects.

In the elderly there is a heightened BP lowering effect with some calcium channel blockers, such as verapamil.[50] Higher volume of distribution for lipid-soluble calcium antagonists like amlodipine and lacidipine enhances bioavailability.

TOTAL CARDIOVASCULAR RISK AND WHEN TO START DRUG TREATMENT FOR HYPERTENSION IN THE ELDERLY

The same general rules apply to the whole hypertensive population.[51-60] Calculation of total cardiovascular risk is recommended using methods such as those proposed by the 2007 European Society of Hypertension – European Society of Cardiology Guidelines.[37] There is limited information on treatment above the age of 80 years where controversy exists regarding mortality.[59] Treatment of hypertension in very old patients should be restricted to those with concomitant evidence of target-organ damage. Decisions regarding true primary prevention must await results from ongoing clinical trials.

TREATMENT OF HYPERTENSION IN THE ELDERLY BASED ON EVIDENCE FROM PLACEBO-CONTROLLED TRIALS

The 2007 European Society of Hypertension – European Society of Cardiology Guidelines[37] for the management of arterial hypertension conclude that randomized controlled trials leave little doubt that elderly patients benefit from anti-hypertensive treatment in terms of reduced cardiovascular morbidity and mortality, irrespective of whether they have systolic-diastolic hypertension or isolated systolic hypertension. Benefits in elderly patients[53,61-65] have been shown with representative agents from several classes, i.e. diuretics, β-blockers, calcium anatagonists, angiotensin converting enzyme inhibitors and angiotensin receptor blockers (Table 20.1).

Several studies[62,66-69] have shown major benefits from treating elderly patients with isolated systolic hypertension (Table 20.2).

TREATMENT OF HYPERTENSION IN THE ELDERLY BASED ON EVIDENCE FROM COMPARATIVE TRIALS

The first five large comparative trials comprising about 58 000 hypertensive patients did not show a difference in the primary cardiovascular endpoint when 'newer' drugs were compared with 'older' drugs (Fig. 20.1). The impression was thus that the most important aspect of management is to lower BP with a combination of well-tolerated drugs.[70-76] This conclusion can then

Table 20.1 Hypertension studies in the elderly (vs. placebo)

Study	Drugs	Stroke	Coronary heart disease	Total mortality
			Reduction %	
SHEP (n = 4736)	Chlorthalidone, atenolol	−36	−27	−13 (n.s.)
STOP (n = 1627)	HCTZ, atenolol, metoprolol or pindolol	−47	−13 (n.s.)	−43
MRC II (n = 4396)	HCTZ, atenolol	−25	−19 (n.s.)	−3 (n.s.)

n.s. = not significant

Table 20.2 Studies in isolated systolic hypertension (vs. placebo)

Study	Drugs	Stroke	Coronary heart disease	Total mortality
			Reduction %	
SHEP (n = 4736)	Chlorthalidone, atenolol	−36	−27	−13 (n.s.)
Syst-Eur (n = 4695)	Nitrendipine, enalapril, HCTZ	−42	−30 (n.s.)	−22 (n.s.)
Syst-China (n = 2394)	Nitrendipine, captopril, HCTZ	−38	+6 (n.s.)	−39

n.s. = not significant

be applied to all hypertensive patients, but is relevant to elderly hypertensives as the STOP-2 study[71] was designed to investigate, but did not show, differences in cardiovascular death between treatment based on diuretic/β-blocker in combination and treatment based on ACE-inhibitors and calcium antagonists. The NORDIL trial[72] was neutral for the primary endpoint, but diltiazem was associated with fewer strokes, a secondary endpoint, despite less BP lowering than with the diuretic/β-blocker combination, and this difference tended to be more pronounced in the elderly participants.[73]

The LIFE study[77] showed clear benefit of the ARB losartan over the β-blocker atenolol in patients with left ventricular hypertrophy; thiazide was

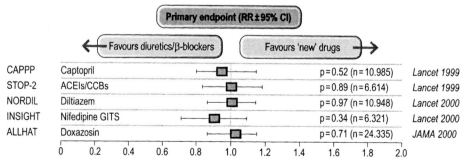

Fig. 20.1 Overview of primary outcome of the first five large comparative trials in hypertension. Except for the CAPPP study, the trials comprised large fractions or only (STOP-2) elderly patients.

used similarly as add-on treatment in both arms. The losartan benefits were particularly expressed in two pre-specified subgroups of patients: those with diabetes[78] and those with isolated systolic hypertension.[79] The Second National Australian Blood Pressure Study[80] conducted in the elderly showed benefits for ACE-inhibitors over thiazides and the SCOPE study[81] was neutral for the primary endpoint compared with control. The angiotensin receptor blocker candesartan was associated with fewer strokes, but also lower BP. The SHELL Study[82] showed no difference in outcome between calcium antagonists and diuretics in patients with isolated systolic hypertension, but was somewhat underpowered. In VALUE[83] the angiotensin receptor blocker valsartan and the calcium antagonist amlodipine prevented the primary cardiac endpoint to the same extent, although BP remained higher on valsartan. The VALUE findings[84] strongly suggest that BP should be controlled below 140/90 mmHg within 3–6 months to prevent new or worsening cardiovascular disease.

In ASCOT[85] it was shown that treatment with the combination of amlodipine plus the ACE-inhibitor perindopril was associated with reduced mortality and fewer cardiovascular endpoints than treatment with atenolol combined with bendroflumethiazide. However, the importance of somewhat lower BP throughout in the amlodipine-perindopril arm needs to be clarified.

TREATMENT OF ISOLATED SYSTOLIC HYPERTENSION IN THE ELDERLY

A large proportion of participants in the comparative outcome trials have been elderly patients with isolated systolic hypertension. There is general agreement that systolic BP should be treated to a target of less than 140 mmHg. To achieve this goal, a combination of various drugs is usually needed.[7,14,67–69,79,82,86] Most drugs are appropriate, although in light of findings from the LIFE study,[79] in which atenolol was less effective for the same BP control, a β-blocker may not be the most appropriate first drug of choice in these patients. ASCOT data[85] confirmed this finding from LIFE.

TREATMENT OF HYPERTENSION IN THE ELDERLY WITH CONCOMITANT DISEASE(S)

Initiation of antihypertensive treatment in elderly patients should follow the general guidelines.[37] Many patients will have other risk factors, target-organ damage and associated cardiovascular conditions, to which the choice of the first drug should be tailored.

TREATMENT OF RESISTANT HYPERTENSION IN THE ELDERLY

Treatment of resistant hypertension in elderly patients should follow the general guidelines with particular emphasis on not over-treating.[15,37] Occasionally patients receive multiple drugs in combination. Appropriate work-up for pseudohypertension, white coat hypertension and orthostatic hypotension (see above) is frequently needed. This is particularly appropriate in patients with no target-organ damage, no associated cardiovascular disease, low risk in general and in patients who report typical side effects of potential over-treatment like dizziness and light-headedness.

TARGET BLOOD PRESSURE IN THE ELDERLY AND THE BENEFITS OF ACETYLSALICYLIC ACID AND STATIN AS ADD-ON THERAPY

The Hypertension Optimal Treatment (HOT) study[87] aimed to study the relationship between three levels of target diastolic BP ($\leq$90, $\leq$85 or $\leq$80 mmHg) and cardiovascular morbidity and mortality in hypertensive patients, and to examine the effects of cardiovascular morbidity and mortality of a low dose (80 mg daily) of acetylsalicylic acid. The study was stopped in 1997 after an average of 3.8 years of follow-up (range 3.3–4.9 years), 71 051 patient-years and 683 patients with primary events (defined as cardiovascular death, myocardial infarction and stroke). The HOT study comprised a large group of elderly patients ($\geq$65 years) making it one of the largest randomized cardiovascular trials ever done in the elderly.[88] These subjects ($n = 5987$) averaged 70.6 + 3.9 years of age, 54% were women and their BPs were 175 ± 15/ 105 ± 4 mmHg at randomization, after previous treatment in 56% had been offset for 2 weeks. The achieved BPs (mmHg) and endpoint rates are summarized in Table 20.3.[88]

None of the differences in endpoints between target BP levels in Table 20.3 was statistically significant. Acetylsalicylic acid[88] lowered the event rate of myocardial infarction (2.5/1000 patient-years vs. 4.1/1000 patient-years on placebo, $n = 2974$ and $n = 3013$, respectively, RR = 0.62, 95% CI: 0.38–0.98, $p = 0.04$).

The HOT study (Fig. 20.2) has until now been the only large scale trial that has investigated how much BP should be lowered in older patients with essential hypertension. No significant difference was observed between treatment arms in the HOT study.[88] Thus, with the limitation that even this large study was underpowered, there is no trial evidence to support a very low BP target in elderly patients, i.e. a BP target much below 140/90 mmHg. However, with <140/90 mmHg as a reasonable treatment target in the older patient,

Table 20.3 Achieved blood pressures (mmHg) and endpoint rates (events/1000 patient-years) in subgroup of older patients in the HOT study ($\geq$65 years, $n = 5987$)

Target group	$\leq$90 mmHg	$\leq$85 mmHg	$\leq$80 mmHg
Diastolic blood pressure	83 ± 8	82 ± 7	80 ± 7
Systolic blood pressure	147 ± 16	145 ± 16	143 ± 15
Major cardiovascular events	16.9	13.0	15.2
Cardiovascular mortality	7.6	5.7	8.0
Stroke	7.8	6.6	6.7
Myocardial infarction	4.4	2.4	3.2
Total mortality	15.7	13.9	15.4

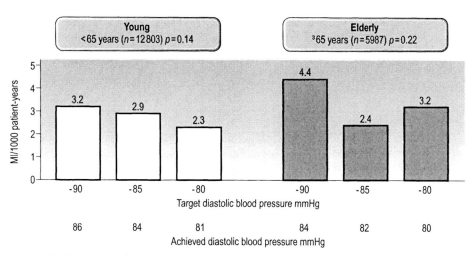

Fig. 20.2 Rates of myocardial infarction in blood pressure target groups of young and elderly participants in the HOT study.

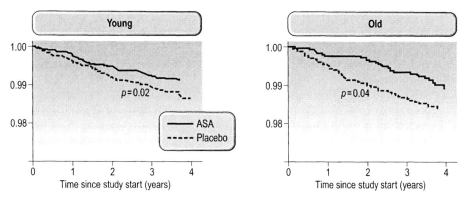

Fig. 20.3 Survival curves without myocardial infarction in young and elderly/old participants on placebo vs. acetylsalicylic acid in the HOT study.

over-treatment is also unlikely. The benefit of acetylsalicylic acid must be considered on an individual basis; the price to pay would be about one non-fatal major bleeding event per myocardial infarction prevented.[88] Only those with 10-year cardiovascular risk of 20% or greater are likely to benefit (Fig. 20.3).

Likewise, the effect of atorvastatin was at least as strong in the elderly patients as in the younger patients in the lipid lowering arm of the ASCOT study.[89]

TOLERABILITY AND COMPLIANCE WHEN TREATING HYPERTENSION IN THE ELDERLY: UPRIGHT BLOOD PRESSURE

General rules apply. As pointed out above, upright BP should probably always be taken at clinical visits.[15,37]

TREATMENT OF HYPERTENSION IN THE VERY OLD

Whereas trials in the elderly usually include patients who are at least 60 years old, a recent meta-analysis concluded that fatal and non-fatal cardiovascular events combined were significantly reduced in participants in randomized, controlled trials of antihypertensive drug treatment aged 80 years and over, but all-cause mortality was not reduced.[90] While we tend to extrapolate data from outcome trials in the 'young' elderly, patients of ages 60–80 years of age, to those above 80 years, this may be an over-simplification. In the very old patient the disease or condition may behave differently from that in the 'young' elderly or there may simply be a shortage of documentation because appropriate clinical trials have not been carried out. In very old hypertensive patients above 80 years there has been uncertainty about the relation between hypertension and cardiovascular morbidity.

O'Sullivan et al.[91] investigated whether hypertension in people above 80 years is associated with target-organ damage, more than that expected from the effects of ageing, and whether ambulatory BP could improve on conventional BP monitoring in predicting target-organ damage. Investigations included echocardiography, magnetic resonance imaging assessment of the brain, measurement of urinary albumin-creatinine ratio, aortic pulse wave velocity, and 24-hour ambulatory BP. The investigators compared 21 hypertensive with 22 normotensive subjects with a mean age of 84.3 years. In men, but not in women, left ventricular mass index was greater in hypertensives. Albuminuria and cerebral periventricular hyperintensity were greater in hypertensives while aortic stiffness did not differ. Ambulatory BP was positively associated with albuminuria and grade of cerebral effects, independent of its correlation with conventional BP. The conclusion was that in advanced old age, hypertension is associated with evidence of target-organ damage, and ambulatory BP can improve prediction of hypertensive target-organ damage in very old hypertensive subjects.

Uncertainty also surrounds treatment of hypertension in very old patients above 80 years of age. While in patients with severe organ damage or morbidity, antihypertensive treatment may be appropriate and reduce symptoms related to concomitant disease or complication, the benefit of treating very old hypertensives without obvious organ damage or disease is uncertain. Bulpitt et al.[92] reported outcome data of the HYVET-PILOT study. The investigators carefully selected and randomized 1283 patients in 10 European countries over the age of 80 years with a sustained BP of 160–219/90–109 mmHg to one of three treatments, a thiazide-based regimen, an angiotensin converting enzyme inhibitor regime or no treatment. The drug doses could be titrated and diltiazem slow-release added. Target BP was <150/80 mmHg and mean follow-up was 13 months. In the combined actively-treated groups the reduction instroke events was 53% and the reduction in stroke mortality was 43%. However, the estimate of total mortality suggested excess deaths with active treatment; in the HYVET-PILOT study treatment of 1000 patients for 1 year reduced stroke events by 19, but was associated with 20 extra non-stroke deaths. The preliminary results supported the need for a main HYVET trial, which is still ongoing.

In conclusion, there are yet unresolved issues in the diagnosis and treatment of hypertension in very old subjects above the age of 80 years. Recent studies[91,92] have advanced understanding of this important area. However, while awaiting more outcome data from ongoing research and eventually the full implications of utilizing ambulatory BP in this age group, treatment of uncomplicated hypertension in the very old requires careful clinical judgements including assessment of the many complicating factors discussed above.[93]

CONCLUSION

There is little doubt from randomized controlled trials that elderly patients benefit from antihypertensive treatment in terms of reduced cardiovascular morbidity and mortality, whether they have systolic-diastolic hypertension or isolated systolic hypertension. Whereas trials in the elderly usually include patients who are at least 60 years old, a recent meta-analysis concluded that fatal and non-fatal cardiovascular events combined were significantly reduced in participants in randomized, controlled trials of antihypertensive drug treatment aged 80 years and over, but all-cause mortality was not reduced. The larger randomized controlled trials of antihypertensive treatment versus placebo or no treatment in elderly patients with systolic-diastolic hypertension used a diuretic or a β-blocker as first-line therapy. In trials on isolated systolic hypertension, first-line drugs consisted of a diuretic or a dihydropyridine calcium channel blocker. In all these trials active therapy was superior to placebo or no treatment. Other drug classes have only been used in trials in which 'newer' drugs were compared with 'older' drugs. It appears that benefit has been shown in older patients for at least one representative agent of several drug classes, i.e. diuretics, β-blockers, calcium channel blockers, converting enzyme inhibitors and angiotensin receptor antagonists.

Initiation of antihypertensive treatment in elderly patients should follow the general guidelines. Many patients will have other risk factors, target-organ damage, and associated cardiovascular conditions, to which the choice of the first drug should be tailored. Furthermore, many patients will need two or more drugs to control BP, particularly since it is often difficult to lower systolic pressure to below 140 mmHg.

References

1. Dyer AR, Stamler J, Shekelle RB, et al. Hypertension in the elderly. *Med Clin North Am* 1997;61:513–529.
2. Harris T, Cook EF, Kannel WB, et al. Blood pressure experience and risk of cardiovascular disease in the elderly. *Hypertension* 1985;7:118–124.
3. Vokonas PS, Kannel WB, Cupples LA. Epidemiology and risk of hypertension in the elderly: the Framingham Study. *J Hypertens* 1988;6(Suppl1):S3–S9.
4. Mann SJ. Systolic hypertension in the elderly. *Arch Intern Med* 1992;152:1977–1984.
5. Bennet NE. Hypertension in the elderly. *Lancet* 1994;344:447–449.
6. Glynn RJ, Field TS, Rosner B, et al. Evidence for a positive linear relation between blood pressure and mortality in elderly people. *Lancet* 1995;345:825–829.
7. Chaudhry SI, Krumholz HM, Foody JM. Systolic hypertension in older persons. *JAMA* 2004;292:1074–1080.
8. Mich RA. Matrix properties of the aging arterial wall. *Monogr Surg Sci* 1965;2:261–341.
9. Learoyd BM, Taylor MG. Alterations with age in the viscoelastic properties of human arterial walls. *Circ Res* 1966;18:278–292.
10. Hall JE, Coleman TG, Guyton AC. The renin-angiotensin system. Normal physiology and changes in older hypertensives. *J Am Geriatr Soc* 1989;37:801–813.

11. Taguchi JT, Sumangool P. 'Pipe-stem' brachial arteries. A cause of pseudohypertension. *JAMA* 1974;228:733–734.

12. Sowers JR. Managing geriatric hypertension: a brief review. *Geriatrics* 1985;40:63–66.

13. National Health and Nutrition Examination Series (NHANES II), 1976–80.*Vital Health Statistics* 1986;11.

14. Pickering TG, James GD, Boddie C, et al. How common is white coat hypertension? *JAMA* 1988;259:225–228.

15. Rutan GH, Hermanson B, Bild DE, et al. Orthostatic hypertension in older adults. The Cardiovascular Health Study. *Hypertension* 1992;19:508–519.

16. Zweifler AJ, Tariq Shahab S. Pseudohypertension: a new assessment. *J Hypertens* 1993;11:1–6.

17. National High Blood Pressure Education Program Working Group. Report of hypertension in the elderly. *Hypertension* 1994;23:275–285.

18. O'Brien E, Asmar R, Beilin L, et al. European Society of Hypertension recommendations for conventional, ambulatory and home blood pressure measurement. *J Hypertens* 2003;21:821–848.

19. Stenehjem AE, Os I. Reproducibility of blood pressure variability, white-coat effect and dipping pattern in untreated, uncomplicated and newly diagnosed essential hypertension. *Blood Pressure* 2004;13:214–224.

20. Kario K, Matsuo T, Kobayashi H, et al. Nocturnal fall of blood pressure and silent cerebrovascular damage in elderly hypertensive patients. Advanced silent cerebrovascular damage in extreme dippers. *Hypertension* 1996;27:130–135.

21. Engfeldt P, Danielsson B, Nyman K, et al. 24-hour ambulatory blood pressure monitoring in elderly normotensive individuals and its reproducibility after one year. *J Hum Hypertens* 1994;8:545–550.

22. Bjørklund K, Lind L, Zethelius B, et al. Prognostic significance of 24-h ambulatory blood pressure characteristics for cardiovascular morbidity in a population of elderly men. *J Hypertens* 2004;22:1691–1697.

23. Staessen JA, Lutgarde T, Fagard R, et al. Predicting cardiovascular risk using conventional vs ambulatory blood pressure in older patients with systolic hypertension. *JAMA* 1999;282:539–546.

24. Wiinberg N, Høegholm A, Christensen HR, et al. 24-h ambulatory blood pressure in 352 normal Danish subjects, related to age and gender. *Am J Hypertens* 1995;8:978–986.

25. Wing LMH, Brown MA, Beilin LJ, et al. Reverse white-coat hypertension in older hypertensives. *J Hypertens* 2002;20:636–644.

26. Cuspidi C, Meani S, Salerno M, et al. Reproducibility of nocturnal blood pressure fall in early phases of untreated essential hypertension: a prospective observational study. *J Hum Hypertens* 2004;18:503–509.

27. Bertineri G, Grassi G, Rossi P, et al. 24-hour blood pressure profile in centenarians. *J Hypertens* 2002;20:1765–1769.

28. O'Sullivan C, Duggan J, Atkins N, O'Brien E. Twenty-four hour ambulatory blood pressure in community-dwelling elderly men and women, aged 60–102 years. *J Hypertens* 2003;21:1641–1647.

29. Jumabay M, Ozawa Y, Kawamura H, et al. Ambulatory blood pressure monitoring in Ulygur centenarians. *Circ J* 2002;66:75–79.

30. Bjørklund K, Lind L, Andrén B, Lithell H. The majority of nondipping men do not have increased cardiovascular risk: a population-based study. *J Hypertens* 2002;20:1501–1506.

31. Bjørklund K, Lind L, Lithell H. Twenty-four hour ambulatory blood pressure in a population of elderly men. *J Intern Med* 2000;248:501–510.

32. Okhubo T, Asayama K, Kikuya M, et al. How many times should blood pressure be measured at home for better prediction of stroke risk? Ten-year follow-up results from the Ohasama study. *J Hypertens* 2004;22:1099–1104.

33. Asayama K, Okhubo T, Kikuya M, et al. Prediction of stroke by self-measurement of blood pressure at home versus casual screening blood pressure measurement in relation to the Joint National Committee 7 Classification. *Stroke* 2004;35:2356–2361.

34. Robertson DRC, Walker DG, Renwick Ag, George CF. Age related changes in the pharmacokinetics and pharmacodynamics of nifedepine. *Br J Clin Pharmacol* 1988;25:297–305.

35. Duggan J. Benefits of treating hypertension in the elderly Should age affect treatment decisions? *Drugs Aging* 2001;18:631–638.

36. Fliser D, Bischoff I, Hanses A, et al. Renal handling of drugs in the healthy elderly. Creatinine clearance underestimates renal function and pharmacokinetics remain virtually unchanged. *Eur J Clin Pharmacol* 1999;55:205–211.

37. The Task Force for the Management of Arterial Hypertension of the European Society of Hypertension (ESH) and of the European Society of Cardiology (ESC). 2007 Guidelines for the Management of Arterial Hypertension. *J Hypertens* 2007;25:1105–1187.

38. Somogyi A, Hewson D, Muirhead M, Bochner F. Amiloride disposition in geriatric patients: importance of renal function. *Br J Clin Pharmacol* 1990;29:1–8.

39. Anantharuja A, Feller A, Chedid A. Aging liver. A Review. *Gerontology* 2002;48:343–353.
40. Castleden CM, George CF. The effect of ageing on the hepatic clearance of propranolol. *Br J Clin Pharmacol* 1988;25:297–305.
41. Todd PA. Perindopril. A review of its pharmacological properties and therapeutic use. *Drugs* 1991;42:90–114.
42. Pichette V, Leblond FA. Drug metabolism in chronic renal failure. *Curr Drug Metab* 2003;4:91–103.
43. Gainsborough N, Maskrey VL, Nelson ML, et al. The association of age with gastric emptying. *Age Ageing* 1993;22:37–40.
44. Scott M, Castelden CM, Adam HK, et al. The effect of ageing on the disposition of nifedepine and atenolol. *Br J Clin Pharmacol* 1998;25:289–296.
45. Lamy PP. Physiological changes due to age. *Drugs & Aging* 1991;1:385–404.
46. George CF. Medication in the elderly. *Ann Acad Med Singapore* 1987;16:277–280.
47. Buehler FR, Hulthen UL, Kiowske W, Bolli P. Beta blockers and calcium antagonists: cornerstones of antihypertensive therapy in the 1980s. *Drugs* 1983;25:50–57.
48. Howes LG. Hyponatraemia and hypokalaemia caused by indapamide. *Med J Aust* 2002;177:53–54.
49. Oberbauer R, Krivane K. Pharmacokinetics and pharmacodynamics of the diuretic bumetanide in the elderly. *Clin Pharmacol Ther* 1995;57:42–51.
50. Buehler FR. Age and cardiovascular response adaptation. *Hypertension* 1983;5(Suppl 111): 94–100.
51. Fotherby MD, Harper GD, Potter JF. General practitioner's management of hypertension in elderly patients. *Br Med J* 1992;305:750–752.
52. Beard K, Bulpitt C, Macie-Taylor H, et al. Management of elderly patients with sustained hypertension. *Br Med J* 1992;304:412–416.
53. Thijs L, Fagard R, Lijnen P, et al. A meta-analysis of outcome trials in elderly hypertensives. *J Hypertens* 1992;10:1103–1109.
54. O'Malley K, O'Brien E. Where are the guidelines for treating hypertension in elderly patients? *Br Med J* 1992;305:845–856.
55. Ekbom T, Lindholm LH, Odén A, et al. A five-year prospective, observational study of the withdrawal of antihypertensive treatment in elderly people. *J Int Med* 1994;235:581–588.
56. Lund-Johansen P. Stopping antihypertensive drug therapy in the elderly people – a dangerous experiment? *J Int Med* 1994;235:577–579.
57. Chalmers J. Hypertension in the elderly: benefits of treatment. *Blood Press* 1995;4(Suppl 3): 6–10.
58. Lever AF, Ramsay LE. Treatment of hypertension in the elderly. *J Hypertens* 1995;13:571–579.
59. Lindholm LH, Johannesson M. Cost-benefit aspects of treatment of hypertension in the elderly. *Blood Press* 1995;4(Suppl 3):11–14.
60. Gueyffier F, Bulpitt C, Boissel J-P, et al. Antihypertensive drugs in very old people: a subgroup meta-analysis of randomized controlled trials. *Lancet* 1999;353:793–796.
61. Amery A, Birkenhäger W, Brixko P, et al. Mortality and morbidity results from the European Working Party on High Blood Pressure in the Elderly trial. *Lancet* 1985;i: 1349–1354.
62. SHEP Collaborative Research Group. Prevention of stroke by antihypertensive drug tereatment in older persons with isolated systolic hypertension: final results of the Systolic Hypertension in the Elderly Program (SHEP). *JAMA* 1991;265:3255–3264.
63. Dahlöf B, Lindholm LH, Hansson L, et al. Morbidity and mortality in the Swedish Trial in Old Patients with Hypertension (STOP-Hypertension). *Lancet* 1991;338:1281–1285.
64. Medical Research Council Trial of Treatment of Hypertension in Older Adults: principal results. *BMJ* 1992;304:405–412.
65. Collins R, MacMahon S. Blood pressure, antihypertensive drug treatment and the risk of stroke and of coronary heart disease. *Br Med Bull* 1994;50:272–298.
66. Gong L, Zhang W, Zhu Y, et al. Shanghai trial of nifedipine in the elderly (STONE). *J Hypertens* 1996;16:1237–1245.
67. Staessen JA, Fagard R, Thijs L, et al; for the Systolic Hypertension in Europe (Syst-Eur) Trial Investigators. Randomised double-blind comparison of placebo and active treatment for older patients with isolated systolic hypertension. *Lancet* 1997;350:757–764.
68. Liu L, Wang JL, Gong L, et al; for the Syst-China Collaborative Group. Comparison of active treatment and placebo in older Chinese patients with isolated systolic hypertension. *J Hypertens* 1998;16:1823–1829.
69. Staesson JA, Gasowski J, Wang JG, et al. risks of untreated and treated isolated systolic hypertension in the elderly: meta-analysis of outcome trials. *Lancet* 2000;355:865–872.
70. Kjeldsen SE, Os I, Westheim A. INSIGHT and NORDIL. *Lancet* 2000;356:1229–1230.
71. Hansson L, Lindholm LH, Ekbom T, et al. Randomised trial of old and new antihypertensive drugs in elderly patients: cardiovascular mortality and morbidity in the Swedish Trial in Old Patients with Hypertension-2 study. *Lancet* 1999;354:1751–1756.

72. Hansson L, Hedner T, Lund-Johanson P, et al; for the NORDIL Study Group. Randomized trial of effects of calcium antagonists compared with diuretics and β-blockers on cardiovascular morbidity and mortality in hypertension: the Nordic Diltiazem (NORDIL) study. *Lancet* 2000;356:359–365.

73. Kjeldsen SE, Hedner T, Syvertsen JO, et al. Influence of age, gender and blood pressure levels on the principal endpoints of the Nordic Diltiazem (NORDIL) Study. *J Hypertens* 2002;20:1231–1237.

74. The INSIGHT Group. Morbidity and mortality in patients randomised to double-blind treatment with a long-acting calcium channel blocker or diuretic in the International Nifedipine GITS study: Intervention as a Goal in Hypertension Treatment (INSIGHT). *Lancet* 2000;356:366–377.

75. The ALLHAT Officers and Coordinators for the ALLHAT Collaborative Research Group. Major cardiovascular events on hypertensive patients randomized to doxazosin vs chlorthalidone. The Antihypertensive and Lipid-Lowering Treatment to Prevent Heart Attack Trial (ALLHAT). *JAMA* 2000;283:1967–1975.

76. The ALLHAT Officers and Coordinators for the ALLHAT Collaborative Research Group. Major outcomes in high-risk hypertensive patients randomized to angiotensin-converting enzyme inhibitor or calcium channel blocker vs. diuretic: The Antihypertensive and Lipid-Lowering Treatment to Prevent Heart Attack Trial (ALLHAT). *JAMA* 2002;288:2981–2997.

77. Dahlöf B, Devreux RB, Kjeldsen SE, et al. Cardiovascular morbidity and mortality in the Losartan Intervention for Endpoint reduction in hypertension study (LIFE): a randomised trial against atenolol. *Lancet* 2002;359:995–1003.

78. Lindholm LH, Ibsen H, Dahlöf B, et al; for the LIFE Study Group. Cardiovascular morbidity and mortality in patients with diabetes in the Losartan Intervention for Endpoint reduction in hypertension study (LIFE): a randomised trial against atenolol. *Lancet* 2002;358:1004–1010.

79. Kjeldsen SE, Dahlöf B, Devereux RB, et al; for the LIFE Study Group. Effects of losartan on cardiovascular morbidity and mortality in patients with isolated systolic hypertension and left ventricular hypertrophy. A losartan intervention for endpoint reduction (LIFE) substudy. *JAMA* 2002;288:1491–1498.

80. Wing LMH, Reid CM, Ryan P, et al. A comparison of outcomes with angiotensin-converting-enzyme inhibitors and diuretics for hypertension in the elderly. *N Engl J Med* 2003;348:583–592.

81. Lithell H, Hansson L, Skoog I, et al; for the SCOPE Study Group. The Study on Cognition and Prognosis in the Elderly (SCOPE). Principal results of a randomised double-blind intervention trial. *J Hypertens* 2003;21:875–886.

82. Malacco E, Mancia G, Rapelli A, et al. Treatment of isolated systolic hypertension. The SHELL Study results. *Blood Press* 2003;12:160–167.

83. Julius S, Kjeldsen SE, Weber M, et al. Cardiac events, stroke and mortality in high-risk hypertensives treated with valsartan or amlodipine: main outcomes of the VALUE Trial. *Lancet* 1993;363:2022–2031.

84. Weber M, Julius S, Kjeldsen SE, et al. Blood pressure dependent and independent effects of antihypertensive treatment on clinical events in the VALUE Trial. *Lancet* 2004;363:2049–2051.

85. Dahlöf B, Sever PS, Poulter NR, et al. Prevention of cardiovascular events with an amlodipne+perindopril strategy compared with an atenolol+thiazide strategy. Anglo-Scandinavian Cardiac Outcomes Trial – Blood Pressure – Lowering Arm (ASCOT-BPLA). *Lancet* 2005;366:895–906.

86. The SHEP Cooperative Research Group. Implications of the Systolic Hypertension in the Elderly Program. *Hypertension* 1993;21:335–343.

87. Hansson L, Zanchetti A, Carruthers SG, et al. Effects of intensive blood pressure lowering and low dose aspirin in patients with hypertension: principal results of the Hypertension Optimal Treatment (HOT) randomised trial. *Lancet* 1988;351:1755–1762.

88. Kjeldsen SE, Kolloch RE, Leonetti G, et al. Influence of gender and age on preventing cardiovascular disease by antihypertensive treatment and acetylsalicylic acid. The HOT study. *J Hypertens* 2000;18:629–642.

89. Sever PS, Dahlöf B, Poulter NR, et al; for the ASCOT Investigators. Prevention of coronary and stroke events with atorvastatin in hypertensive patients who have average or lower than average cholesterol concentrations, in the Anglo-Scandinavian Cardiac Outcomes Trial – Lipid Lowering Arm (ASCOT-LLA): a multicentre randomised controlled trial. *Lancet* 2003;361:1149–1158.

90. Gueyffier F, Bulptii C, Boissel JP, et al. Antihypertensive drugs in very old people: a subgroup analysis of randomised controlled trials. *Lancet* 1991;353:793–796.

91. O'Sullivan C, Duggan J, Lyons S, et al. Hypertensive target-organ damage in the very elderly. *Hypertension* 2003;42:130–135.

92. Bulpitt CJ, Beckett NS, Cooke J, et al. Results of the pilot study for the hypertension in the very elderly trial (HYVET-PILOT). *J Hypertens* 2003;21(12):2249–2250.

93. Kjeldsen SE, Os I. Hypertension in very old people. *J Hypertens* 2003;21:2249–2250.

21 | Hypertension and diabetes

Gordon T. McInnes

INTRODUCTION

Risk factors for cardiovascular disease are more likely to occur simultaneously than would be expected by chance.[1] In particular, the concordance of hypertension and diabetes is markedly increased in Westernized populations.[2] Male screenees for the Multiple Risk Factor Intervention Trial (MRFIT) with type 2 diabetes had a greater prevalence of systolic hypertension, as well as total cholesterol and cigarette smoking, compared with non-diabetic controls.[3]

The frequency of hypertension is increased in patients with diabetes.[4,5] In type 2 diabetes this is particularly so. The United Kingdom Prospective Diabetes Study (UKPDS) revealed a prevalence of hypertension (systolic blood pressure (BP) $\geq$160 mmHg and/or diastolic BP $\geq$90 mmHg, or antihypertensive drugs) of 39%.[6] Using more contemporary definitions of hypertension (BP $\geq$140/90 mmHg), the prevalence rates reach 70–80% in many European countries.[7,8] Some 75% of patients with type 2 diabetes have BP $\geq$130/80 mmHg or use antihypertensive treatment.

Hypertension in diabetes is characterized by an earlier onset of systolic hypertension and higher prevalence of isolated systolic hypertension at any age compared with people without diabetes. In type 2 diabetes, hypertension is more common in women than in men and the age-related increase in systolic BP is steeper in women.[9]

In type 1 diabetes, hypertension often reflects the onset of diabetic nephropathy[10] whereas most hypertensive individuals do not have albuminuria when type 2 diabetes develops.[11] The prevalence of hypertension (BP $\geq$140/90 mmHg) in type 2 diabetes and normoalbuminuria is very high (79%) and increases even further (to 90%) in the presence of microalbuminuria.[12] Hypertension approaches 100% of those with end-stage renal disease. In 55% of these subjects, BP is above 140/90 mmHg; only 12% have BP <130/85 mmHg, with very few with BP <130/80 mmHg.[13]

In Westernized populations, the prevalence of hypertension in adults is around 24%[14] and the age-adjusted prevalence is increasing. Hypertension is an independent risk predictor for the development of diabetes.[15–17] People with elevated BP are 2.5 times more likely than non-hypertensives to develop diabetes within 5 years.[18,19] Hypertension[11] and microalbuminuria independent of BP level[20] may precede the development of diabetes by several years.

There is a strong association between elevated BP and insulin resistance.[21–25] The prevalence of insulin resistance in hypertension has been estimated at 50%.[26] Several possible mechanisms have been proposed.[27] The consequent impaired fasting blood glucose is associated with increased cardiovascular risk,[28] particularly if accompanied by hypertension.[29]

In people with diabetes, cardiovascular disease risk is increased two- to fourfold compared with those with normal glucose tolerance.[30–32] One study[31] found that diabetic people without history of previous myocardial infarction had a risk of myocardial infarction as high as that in non-diabetic patients with such a history, although this finding has not been confirmed in other population-based studies.[33,34] The absolute risk of cardiovascular disease associated with any level of glycaemia is determined by the presence of other risk factors.[3] In both type 1 and type 2 diabetes, hypertension is a major predictor of macrovascular complications including coronary heart disease, stroke and peripheral vascular disease. Patients with hypertension and type 2 diabetes constitute a high-risk population.[8]

The coexistence of hypertension and diabetes is particularly pernicious because of the strong linkage of each with cardiovascular disease,[35,36] stroke,[6,35–41] progression of renal disease,[42–44] and diabetic retinopathy.[45] Concurrent hypertension and diabetes (type 1 and type 2) doubles the risk of developing microvascular and macrovascular complications including stroke and coronary heart disease, and the risk of mortality compared with hypertension alone.[7,10,40,46–51]

In Westernized countries diabetes and hypertension are the leading causes of end-stage renal disease, with a prevalence that has increased steadily over the last two decades while other causes have remained constant.[6] Renal function declines with time in both type 1 and type 2 diabetes. The rate of decline in renal function in diabetic nephropathy is a continuous function of arterial pressure down to systolic BP of approximately 125–130 mmHg and diastolic BP of 70–75 mmHg.[43,44,52–55] Deterioration in renal function is accelerated significantly when hypertension coexists. Systolic BP correlates better than diastolic BP with renal disease progression in diabetes.[5,43,44,52,53]

METABOLIC SYNDROME

Hypertension is frequently associated with insulin resistance (and concomitant hyperinsulinaemia), central obesity and a characteristic pattern of dislipidaemia (high triglycerides and low HDL-cholesterol).[56,57] The relationship between insulin resistance and hypertension is well established,[21–25] but, despite this association, insulin resistance contributes only modestly to the prevalence of hypertension.[58] This constellation of risk factors is known as the (cardiovascular) metabolic syndrome. There are various definitions,[59–61] but all agree on the essential components – glucose intolerance, obesity, hypertension and dyslipidaemia.

Insulin resistance, hyperinsulinaemia, diabetes, hypertension and dyslipidaemia are much more prevalent in people with central obesity than in non-obese subjects. Obesity causes cardiac and vascular disease through hypertension, type 2 diabetes and hyperlipidaemia; obesity is an independent predictor of cardiovascular risk factors, morbidity and mortality.[62–65] Obesity is also a cause of abnormal renal function.

Almost one-quarter of adults in the USA has the metabolic syndrome.[66] This frequency is likely to rise in the next several years primarily because of the rapid increase in obesity. People with the metabolic syndrome are at particularly high risk of cardiovascular disease because it envelops several inter-related risk factors.[67–72] Such individuals are also predisposed to the development of chronic kidney disease[73] and type 2 diabetes.[74]

Since people with the metabolic syndrome have increased risk of cardiovascular disease prior to the development of diabetes, the syndrome has become the focus for the primary prevention of cardiovascular disease. By broadening the clinical focus to include impaired glucose regulation outside the diabetic range, the scope and yield of cardiovascular disease prevention is increased. Management of underlying risk factors should be independent of risk status.

RISK STRATIFICATION

There is a clear relationship between higher levels of BP and increased cardiovascular morbidity and mortality in the general population.[75–79] Epidemiological studies demonstrate that increasing systolic and diastolic BP correlates with increasing risk with no evidence of 'threshold' below which lower levels are not associated with lower risks of stroke and coronary heart disease. The relationship between BP and cardiovascular events is graded and extends below the traditional hypertensive threshold.[79] Persons with systolic BP <120 mmHg have fewer cardiovascular events than their counterparts with systolic BP 120–129 mmHg or 130–139 mmHg.

Hypertension is both a cause and a consequence of renal disease. BP is a strong independent risk factor for end-stage renal disease.[80,81] Results from MRFIT showed that the increased risk of end-stage renal disease associated with higher BP was graded and continuous throughout the distribution of BP above the optimal level.[80]

In the diabetic population, hypertension increases the risk and accelerates the progression of coronary heart disease, left ventricular hypertrophy, congestive heart failure, cardiovascular disease, peripheral vascular disease and kidney disease. Population-based observational data suggest that, when compared with the non-diabetic population, cardiovascular disease risk is elevated in people with diabetes at every level of BP well into the conventional normotensive range.[3,37] Moreover, there appears to be no threshold below which risk declines substantially. From a pathophysiological perspective people with diabetes exhibit disturbances of BP regulation and vascular function that increase vulnerability to hypertensive injury.[8] In diabetes, antihypertensive therapy should be initiated if systolic BP is sustained ≥140 mmHg and/or diastolic BP is sustained at ≥90 mmHg.[9]

Metabolic syndrome

Presence of one component of the metabolic syndrome places individuals at higher risk of clustering with other components. The result is an additive or a more than additive effect on cardiovascular and renal outcomes. All those with the metabolic syndrome must be stratified in the highest risk category for cardiovascular and renal disease.

For asymptomatic individuals with no history of cardiovascular disease or diabetes, the blood glucose level should be viewed in the context of total cardiovascular disease risk based on the Framingham risk algorithm.[9] Apparently healthy individuals with cardiovascular disease risk ≥20% over 10 years should receive appropriate risk-factor intervention. Risk assessment is not appropriate in those with type 2 diabetes because the vast majority (i.e. those aged over 50 years or diagnosed for at least 10 years) probably have a risk of cardiovascular disease equivalent to people who have had a myocardial infarction and, therefore, should be considered as for secondary prevention.[61]

The incidence of cardiovascular disease in Asians is much lower than in whites.[82] The Framingham risk equation overestimates risk of coronary heart disease in Asians[83] and may be inappropriate in that population.

STRATEGIES TO REDUCE CARDIOVASCULAR RISK

Since all patients with hypertension and diabetes are at the highest risk of cardiovascular and renal events, it is imperative to devise preventive and therapeutic strategies to reduce such events and disease progression.

Non-pharmacological interventions

Lifestyle intervention inspires a sense of wellbeing, may be less expensive than pharmacological interventions and has no known harmful effects. A variety of lifestyle modifications reduces BP and the incidence of hypertension.[84–87] Non-pharmacological interventions include weight loss in overweight,[85,87] exercise programmes,[87] moderation of alcohol intake,[88] a diet with increased fruit and vegetables and reduced saturated fat content,[86] reduction in dietary sodium intake[86,89] and increased dietary potassium intake[90] (Table 21.1). When adherence is optimal, systolic BP is reduced by >10 mmHg.[86] Reductions are more modest in clinical practice[84] and studies were not designed or powered to evaluate changes in overall or cardiac mortality. However, in long-term, large-scale population studies, even small reductions in BP are associated with reduced cardiovascular disease risk.[91]

Lifestyle modification should be advocated for all people with high BP and those with borderline or high-normal BP. Such interventions are recommended

Table 21.1 Lifestyle measures recommended in management of hypertension

Maintain normal weight for adults (body mass index 20–25 Kg/m²)
Reduce salt intake to <100 mmol/day (<6 g NaCl or <2.5 g sodium/day)
Limit alcohol consumption to ≤3 units/day for men or ≤2 units/day for women
Engage in regular aerobic physical exercise (brisk walking rather than weightlifting) for ≥30 minutes/day, ideally on most days of the week but at least on 3 days/week
Consume at least five portions/day of fresh fruit and vegetables
Reduce intake of total and saturated fat

(Modified from ref. (9).)

even when antihypertensive drugs are prescribed as the BP effects of drugs are complemented and, thus, the dose or number of drugs required to control BP is reduced.

Dietary modification
A key component of management is to avoid overweight, particularly by calorie restriction and decrease of sodium intake because of the strong relationship between obesity, hypertension, sodium sensitivity and insulin resistance.[92]

Physical activity and weight loss
The increasingly sedentary lifestyle of the general population has contributed to an epidemic of obesity and the metabolic syndrome. A graded exercise programme is strongly recommended.[87,93]

Tobacco cessation
The combination of smoking and diabetes enhances the risk of microvascular and macrovascular disease as well as premature mortality. Patients with diabetes should be counselled about smoking cessation, the enhanced risks of smoking and diabetes for morbidity and mortality, and the proven efficacy and cost-effectiveness of cessation strategies.[94,95]

Pharmacological interventions

Several drug therapies are of proven value in reducing cardiovascular risk in people with diabetes and hypertension.

Blood pressure control
Effective BP control has considerable and immediate benefit in patients with diabetes.[41,96–98] In trials which included patients with diabetes, BP lowering reduced or prevented an aggregate of major cardiovascular events including heart failure, cardiovascular death and total mortality. Antihypertensive therapy diminishes the risk of macrovascular complications by around 20%. Reducing BP also reduces progression of retinopathy, albuminuria and progression to nephropathy. Clinical trials with diuretics, β-blockers, ACE inhibitors, angiotensin receptor blockers and calcium channel blockers have demonstrated benefit of treatment of hypertension in type 2 diabetes.[6,38,40,46,99–101] Although no major trial has assessed the effect of BP lowering on cardiovascular morbidity and mortality exclusively in hypertensive patients with type 1 diabetes, these patients are generally managed in a similar manner.

In 492 type 2 diabetes patients with isolated systolic hypertension in the Systolic Hypertension European (SYST EUR) trials[46] all-cause mortality, all cardiovascular endpoints, fatal and non-fatal stroke, and fatal and non-fatal cardiac endpoints were all reduced by antihypertensive therapy. The reduction in relative hazard ratios was greater for all outcomes in diabetics compared with non-diabetics ($n = 4203$) and, for most, these were significant treatment–diabetes interactions. A BP reduction of 8.6/3.9 mmHg was associated with a 69% reduction in cardiovascular disease in the type 2 diabetes subgroup compared with a 26% reduction in non-diabetic individuals (Fig. 21.1). Similar benefits were seen in the diabetes subgroup in the Systolic Hypertension in the Elderly

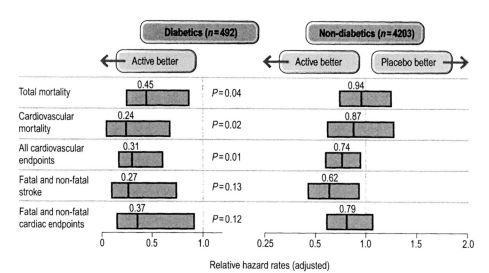

Fig. 21.1 Syst-Eur relative hazard ratios. Active treatment vs. placebo. *(From Syst-Eur - Systolic Hypertension European trial, ref. (46).)*

Program (SHEP);[102] the 5-year cardiovascular disease event rate was reduced by 34% compared with the overall reduction.

Randomized controlled trials that have included large diabetes populations have demonstrated impressive improvements in cardiovascular disease outcomes, especially stroke and microvascular complications, when rigorous BP targets are achieved.[6,38,40,41,46,103,104] The importance of tight BP control in diabetes was illustrated in UKPDS.[6] Tight BP control (<150/85 mmHg) was associated with an outcome benefit greater than that with less tight control (<180/105 mmHg). Lowering BP to a mean of 144/82 mmHg significantly reduced stroke, diabetic-related deaths and heart failure. A 10/15 mmHg difference over 8.4 years resulted in a 21% reduction in myocardial infarction (non-significant) and significant reduction in stroke (44%), all macrovascular endpoints (35%) and microvascular disease (25%). There was a continuous relationship between the risk of these outcomes and systolic BP, with no evidence of a threshold for these complications down to systolic BP 130 mmHg. The lowest risk was in those with systolic BP <120 mmHg. The relative risk reductions with tight BP control were greater in magnitude than those for intensive glucose control in prevention of stroke, any type 2 diabetes endpoint, any type 2 diabetes-related death and microvascular complications.[6,11]

The exquisite sensitivity of patients with type 2 diabetes and hypertension to tight BP control was confirmed in the Hypertension Optimal Treatment (HOT) trial.[40] In 1501 patients with hypertension and type 2 diabetes, there was a stepwise reduction in cardiovascular events in those randomized to diastolic BP targets ≤90 mmHg, ≤85 mmHg and ≤80 mmHg (Fig. 21.2). The relative risk reduction for major cardiovascular events (non-fatal myocardial infarction, non-fatal stroke and cardiovascular deaths) from ≤90 mmHg to ≤80 mmHg was 51%. Since achieved BP was 85 mmHg and 81 mmHg in those randomized to ≤90 mmHg and ≤80 mmHg respectively, the reduction resulted from a difference in diastolic BP of only 4 mmHg.

In hypertensive patients with diabetes, the greater the BP lowering, the greater the benefit for cardiovascular events with no BP threshold level below

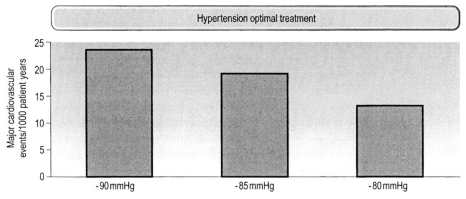

Fig. 21.2 Hypertension Optimal Treatment (HOT) Trial: Diabetes Population. *(From ref. (40).)*

which risk no longer declines.[104] Several trials have shown that in diabetes mellitus, reduction of diastolic BP to about 80 mmHg and systolic BP to about 130 mmHg is associated with further reduction in cardiovascular events and diabetes mellitus-related microvascular complications compared with less stringent BP control.[6,37,105]

The BP target for those with diabetes is lower than that for individuals without diabetes. Evidence from intervention trials in people with diabetes and extrapolation from epidemiological studies supports a 'lower the better' policy for optimal BP[40,41] with a target of <130/80 mmHg.[9,106,107] The optimal BP is the lowest tolerated. There is no need to modify the target for gender or age. US guidelines recommend a less rigorous target,[2,108] but acknowledge that the available data in support of the optimal target are sparse.

Despite best practice, the BP target of <130/80 mmHg is difficult to achieve, particularly in an older population.[9,105,109,110] Control of diastolic BP is less problematic and the focus should be on systolic BP control since many (especially those with type 2 diabetes) have isolated systolic hypertension. An audit standard of <140/80 mmHg is suggested.[9] Thereafter, further cardiovascular benefits can be expected if BP is lowered to the optimal target of <130/80 mmHg, especially in diabetic nephropathy or retinopathy.

All patients with grade 1 hypertension (sustained systolic BP of 140–159 mmHg or diastolic BP of 90–99 mmHg or both) or higher and diabetes should be offered treatment with antihypertensive drugs.[9] The composition of the treatment regimen has been an area of great controversy, myths and misconceptions.[105] The evidence for superiority or inferiority of different drug classes is vague and contradictory. Most comparisons come from relatively small studies or substudies of larger trials with inadequate power to test for the small difference to be expected. There is controversy about the safety and efficacy of calcium channel blockers[111] and reluctance to use thiazides and thiazide-like diuretics because of perceived effects on insulin sensitivity and metabolic indices. Many of these concerns have been allayed by the results of recent clinical trials.[38,40,46,99,100,102,104,112]

Choice of agents

Calcium channel blockers   Calcium channel blocker-based therapy appears equivalent to conventional therapy (based on diuretics or β-blockers) in cardiovascular risk reduction.[38,99,112] In the International Verapamil SR – Trandolapril

(INVEST) study,[112] there was no difference between verapamil and atenolol for the primary outcome (all-cause mortality plus non-fatal myocardial infarction plus non-fatal stroke) in the diabetes subgroup (6400 of 22 576 participants). Similar results were achieved in the diabetic subgroup of the Controlled Onset Verapamil Investigation of Cardiovascular End Points (CONVINCE).[99]

In the diabetes subgroup of the Antihypertensive and Lipid Lowering Treatment to Prevent Heart Attack Trials (ALLHAT), the dihydropyridine, amlodipine, was equivalent to chlorthalidone in reducing the primary endpoint of fatal coronary heart disease and myocardial infarction, although the calcium channel blocker was significantly inferior in protection against heart failure.[38] The Appropriate Blood Pressure Control in Diabetes (ABCD) study was stopped prematurely because nisoldipine was inferior to lisinopril in reducing the incidence of ischaemic cardiac events.[111] However, in normotensive diabetes in the second ABCD study (ABCD2), nitrendipine was equivalent to lisinopril in stroke prevention and in retardation of the development of albuminuria.[104]

ACE inhibitors In UKPDS,[113] ACE inhibitor (captopril) and β-blocker (atenolol)-based therapy were equally effective for all outcome measures, including diabetes-related death, myocardial infarction and all microvascular endpoints. However, patients randomized to atenolol had slightly better BP control (−1 mmHg systolic and −2 mmHg diastolic).

In a subgroup analysis of the Captopril Prevention Project (CAPPP), captopril was superior to a diuretic/β-blocker regimen in preventing cardiovascular events in hypertensive diabetic patients.[114] In the Fosinopril versus Amlodipine Cardiovascular Events randomised Trial (FACET), fosinopril and amlodipine reduced fasting blood sugar, serum insulin and microalbuminuria by similar magnitudes,[115] but, despite greater BP reduction on amlodipine, fosinopril was associated with a 51% lower incidence of the combination of death, myocardial infarction, hospitalized angina and stroke. The combined results of ABCD, CAPPP and FACET showed a significant benefit of ACE inhibition compared with alternative treatments on the outcomes of acute myocardial infarction (63%), cardiovascular events (51%) and all-cause mortality (62%). None of these differences was explained by differences in BP.[116]

The Heart Outcomes Prevention Evaluation (HOPE) provided further support for the use of ACE inhibitors. In the hypertensive and normotensive diabetes subpopulation,[117] treatment with ramipril added to standard therapy reduced combined myocardial infarction, stroke and cardiovascular death by about 25% and stroke by 33% compared with placebo plus conventional therapy. Combined microvascular events were reduced by 16%. To what extent this was independent of the 2.2/1.4 mmHg difference in BP remains controversial.

Despite these findings, the evidence for ACE inhibitors as first-line therapy is limited. In ALLHAT,[38] an ACE inhibitor did not show superiority over a thiazide-like diuretic in over 12 000 individuals with type 2 diabetes. Indeed, the ACE inhibitor showed a trend for elevated risk of cardiovascular disease. However, ALLHAT has been much criticized because of flaws in design and the comparability of the groups.[118]

The superiority of ACE inhibitors rests largely on two comparisons, with diuretics/β-blockers[114] or calcium channel blockers,[111] or on analysis of cause-specific events for which the trial power is low. In type 1 diabetes mellitus, there is evidence for renoprotection with ACE inhibitors, but no substantive data confirming cardioprotection with ACE inhibitor, beyond the impact of BP control.[119]

Angiotensin receptor blockers In the diabetic subpopulation ($n = 1195$) of the Losartan Intervention For Endpoint (LIFE) reduction study of hypertensive patients with ECG evidence of left ventricular hypertrophy,[120] therapy based on losartan was superior to atenolol-based therapy for the primary composite endpoint (25% reduction) and all-cause mortality (39% reduction). There was also significant reduction in cardiovascular mortality (37%), heart failure (41%) and stroke. Regression of left ventricular hypertrophy was twice as great with losartan compared with atenolol.[121,122]

Similar results were seen in the Reduction of Endpoints in NIDDM with the Angiotensin Antagonist Losartan (RENAAL) study,[96] which included 1513 type 2 diabetes mellitus patients with early renal insufficiency and microalbuminuria. Compared with conventional therapy, losartan reduced new onset congestive heart failure with a trend to reduced myocardial infarction.

The use of renin–angiotensin system blockade in type 2 diabetes is well supported.[120] The evidence for cardiovascular protection with angiotensin receptor blockers is more substantial than that for ACE inhibitors.

Treatment strategies Almost all patients with hypertension and diabetes require combinations of BP-lowering drugs to achieve the recommended BP targets.[5,108] Three or more drugs may be needed.[105,109] Clinical trial data support the combined use of a renin–angiotensin system blocking drug and a thiazide diuretic to reduce cardiovascular events.[19,44,45,52,96–98,120] Many patients will gain additional benefits from both β-blockers and calcium channel blocker therapy to achieve lower BP goals. For example, when combined with an ACE inhibitor, the calcium channel blocker, amlodipine, reduced BP and also morbidity and mortality in type 2 diabetes with hypertension.[115] However, α-blockers are probably less effective than other antihypertensive agents in reducing BP in type 2 diabetes.[123]

Combination therapy is likely to include a thiazide or thiazide-like diuretic.[38] In patients with renal impairment, a loop diuretic may be required as an alternative to, or in addition to a thiazide or a thiazide-like diuretic.[9] When there are no cost disadvantages, the combined drugs should be used as a fixed-dose combination to reduce the number of medications.

Role of renin–angiotensin system in diabetes mellitus and vascular complications
Local formation of angiotensin II by tissue-based renin–angiotensin systems in cardiac, renal and vascular tissues represents an important pathophysiological mechanism that is upregulated in diabetes. Short-term moderate hyperglycaemia without glycosuria during the early stages of diabetes is linked with increased plasma renin activity, mean arterial pressure and renal vascular resistance[124] with activation of circulating and local renin–angiotensin systems. In animal models of diabetes, inhibition of the renin–angiotensin system with ACE inhibitor[125] or angiotensin receptor blocker[126] has been shown to prevent atherosclerosis independent of BP reduction.

Improvement in insulin sensitivity follows ACE inhibition,[127–130] particularly in hypertensives with type 2 diabetes.[131,132] Many of the initial reports were based on uncontrolled studies or flawed study design, indirect measures of insulin sensitivity or studies in patients receiving potentially confounding medications.[133] Nevertheless, data suggest that treatment of type 2 diabetes with ACE inhibition may improve glycaemic control[117] or even induce hypoglycaemia when used with insulin[134] or oral hypoglycaemic agents.[135,136]

Blockers of the renin–angiotensin system may be more effective than other antihypertensives for the same BP reduction in regression of left ventricular mass.[121,122] Renin–angiotensin system blockade may also reverse endothelial dysfunction in patients with coronary heart disease, hypertension and diabetes, and may favourably affect fibrinolytic balance, possibly by attenuation of angiotensin II and enhancement of bradykinin.[137,138]

More specific outcome trials in diabetes are needed to dispel the myths that seem to limit widespread use of drugs that block the renin–angiotensin system in diabetes.[139] These include fear of precipitating azotaemia with or without pre-existing renal disease; fear of haemodynamic instability, particularly in patients with suspected autonomic neuropathy; fear of hyperkalaemia; fear of precipitating renal failure due to exacerbation of bilateral renal artery stenosis, which is more common in diabetes.

Microalbuminuria and macroalbuminuria

Microalbuminuria is one of the most important factors in predicting progression to macroalbuminuria or overt nephropathy in type 1 and type 2 diabetes.[52,140] Microalbuminuria is also predictive of cardiovascular mortality in both diabetic and non-diabetic populations.[103,140,141] The presence of microalbuminuria indicates widespread disturbance of endothelial function, resulting in enhanced risk of atherosclerosis.[142] Thus, it may serve as a useful biomarker for systemic vascular disease.

In microalbuminuria, a lower BP target should be considered. Subgroup analyses of type 2 diabetes in major outcome trials indicate that more intensive BP control (systolic BP < 130 mmHg) with blockade of the renin–angiotensin aldosterone system as part of the regimen, provides the optimal strategy for both cardiovascular risk reduction[114,115] and prevention of progression from microalbuminuria to macroalbuminuria, and from macroalbuminuria to overt nephropathy.[117] Normalization of urine albumin excretion may serve as a clinical clue to optimal BP control.

Correction of dyslipidaemia

The evidence for cholesterol reduction in diabetes comes predominantly from subgroup analyses of clinical trials that included people with diabetes. In those with established cardiovascular disease, gemfibrozil and statins have shown significant reduction in coronary heart disease and cardiovascular events.[143–148] In primary prevention, benefits have been shown with gemfibrozil[143,149] and a statin in a hypertensive population.[150] In the only trial of primary prevention exclusively in diabetes, there was reduction in acute coronary events and strokes with atorvastatin.[151]

The primary target is lowering LDL-cholesterol and recent evidence supports rigorous goals.[150,151] Statins are the preferred pharmacological agents.[9] Reduction in LDL-cholesterol should take primacy. Once LDL-cholesterol levels have been lowered, attention should be given to treatment of residual hypertriglyceridaemia and low HDL-cholesterol.[152]

British and European guidelines are consistent.[9,106] All hypertensive patients up to 80 years of age with type 2 diabetes should be considered for lipid lowering with a threshold total cholesterol ≥ 3.5 mmol/L. Target lipid concentrations are total cholesterol <4.0 mmol/L (or 25% reduction) and LDL-cholesterol <2.0 mmol/L (or 30% reduction), whichever is greater. Type 2 diabetes patients benefit from statin therapy irrespective of baseline total cholesterol.[145,151] Use of statins in type 2 diabetes with hypertension should be routine.[9] There is less evidence in type 1 diabetes, but treatment should be as for type 2 diabetes.

Aspirin therapy

Concerns about the safety of aspirin in diabetes appear to be unfounded.[153] Low-dose aspirin is recommended in diabetes whether or not there is evidence of large vessel disease. The British Hypertension Society recommends aspirin 75 mg for all with hypertension and diabetes, unless contraindicated;[9] BP should be controlled to audit standards ($<150/90$ mmHg) for the general hypertensive population.

Glycaemic control

Improved glycaemic control is associated with reduced cardiovascular events,[110,154] as well as microvascular complications in type 1 and type 2 diabetes. Neither the Diabetes Control and Complications Trial (DCCT)[154] nor UKPDS[110] proved definitively that intensive therapy to lower blood glucose levels reduced the risk of cardiovascular complications compared with less-intensive therapy, although DCCT was underpowered for cardiovascular disease. A practical HbA_{IC} target is $\leq 6.5\%$ (audit standard $\leq 7.5\%$).

Choice of treatment in type 2 diabetes with hypertension may be critical. Rosiglitazone improves plasma glucose and BP in type 2 diabetes probably by attenuation of hyperinsulinaemia and sympathetic activity, while glibenclamide, for the same plasma glucose control, worsens BP control, possibly by elevation of insulin levels and activation of the sympathetic system.[155]

Two large outcome studies, the Prospective Pioglitazone Clinical Trial in Macrovascular Events (PROACTIVE)[156] and the Diabetes Reduction Assessment with Ramipril and Rosiglitazone Medication (DREAM),[157] have examined the long-term effects of thiazolidinediones compared with placebo. In both studies, blood glucose and BP were reduced significantly but, while in PROACTIVE there was a trend to reduced cardiovascular events, no such benefit was observed in DREAM. Further studies are required.

Multifactorial intervention

There is limited evidence from a small study in patients with type 2 diabetes[158] that more intensive intervention incorporating modifications in lifestyle, glycaemia, BP, dyslipidaemia and microalbuminuria (ACE inhibitor or angiotensin receptor blocker) is superior to conventional therapy. Cardiovascular events were reduced 53%, stroke 85%, amputations 50%, nephropathy 61%, retinopathy 56% and autonomic neuropathy 67% (all significant). This approach is similar to current guidelines for management of people with diabetes and hypertension.

STRATEGIES TO REDUCE KIDNEY DISEASE RISK

Non-pharmacological interventions

Lifestyle intervention should focus on dietary modification, including low-saturated-fat and low-salt diets, weight reduction and increased physical activity, cessation of tobacco use and moderation of alcohol consumption (see Non-pharmacological interventions, p. 524). Because the majority of patients with type 2 diabetes have hypertension, non-pharmacological interventions to assist reduction in BP will help preserve kidney function.

Increasing salt intake attenuates the antihypertensive and anti-proteinuria effects of ACE inhibitors and angiotensin receptor blockers.[159] Thus, salt restriction should be encouraged in hypertensive diabetic patients, although clinical trials are needed to inform guidelines.

Moderate protein restriction reduces albuminuria, progression of renal disease and improves outcome in type 1 and type 2 diabetes. This benefit is additive to those of antihypertensive treatments.[160]

Pharmacological interventions

Blood pressure control

Strict control of BP is the most important factor in preventing the development of diabetic nephropathy and end-stage renal disease, and the progression of diabetic nephropathy to end-stage renal disease.[43,44,52,108] Multiple placebo-controlled trials have shown significant reductions in proteinuria and slowing of progression of renal damage in type 1 and type 2 diabetes.[96–98]

Compared with lesser control, more intensive BP lowering significantly reduces the progression of retinopathy, albuminuria and progression of nephropathy.[6,41,46,102,104,123,161] A modest 4/2 mmHg reduction in BP in type 1 and type 2 diabetes mellitus with baseline BP 124/77 mmHg resulted in 50% reduction in progression from microalbuminuria to clinical proteinuria.[161] In UKPDS,[6] lowering BP by 10/5 mmHg to a mean of 144/82 mmHg significantly reduced microvascular complications compared with less aggressive treatment. There was a continuous relation between microvascular outcomes and systolic BP with no evidence of a threshold above a systolic BP of 130 mmHg.

These clinical data support the advantage of lower BP goals in prevention of renal disease progression in diabetes mellitus. BP control to levels lower than those necessary for the general population is a major therapeutic initiative in diabetic nephropathy.[96–98,119,161] Current guidelines recommend a BP goal for diabetes with any evidence of kidney damage of <130/80 mmHg[2,9,106,107] and lower if there is proteinuria > 1 g per 24 hours.

The average number of drugs required to achieve optimal BP control in patients with chronic kidney disease is estimated to be 2.6–3.4.[162] If initial BP is more than 20/10 mmHg above goal, it may be best to consider initiating therapy with two agents.

A meta-analysis of 100 studies comprising 2494 patients with both type 1 and type 2 diabetes with proteinuria indicated that antihypertensive agents reduced urine albumin excretion compared with placebo with a rank order of benefit: ACE inhibitor > calcium channel blocker > diuretic.[163] Angiotensin receptor blockers also reduce the incidence of new proteinuria compared with other agents.[120] The finding of even microalbuminuria in type 1 and type 2 diabetes is an indication for antihypertensive therapy that should include a blocker of the renin–angiotensin system irrespective of BP level.[106] In patients with high-normal BP, who may sometimes achieve BP goal by monotherapy, an angiotensin receptor blocker (or ACE inhibitor) should be the first drug used. Aldosterone receptor antagonists might also have a role, but need to be studied in more detail.[164]

Thiazides, or loop diuretics if there is renal insufficiency, facilitate the antihypertensive effects of ACE inhibitors and angiotensin receptor blockers. Likewise, calcium channel blockers have robust antihypertensive effects. Dihydropyridine calcium channel blockers increase or do not change proteinuria, and do not reduce progression of renal disease compared with angiotensin receptor blockade,[97] while non-dihydropyridines may be as effective as ACE inhibitors in reducing albuminuria.[165] However, in the Bergamo Nephrologic Diabetic Complications Trial (BENEDICT), despite equivalent BP and glycaemic control, verapamil was less effective than trandolapril in attenuation of urinary albumin extraction,[166] although the combination was highly effective in BP control and reducing albuminuria.

In UKPDS,[113] there was no difference between atenolol and captopril in microalbuminura, or for conversion of microalbuminuria to macroalbuminura. However, the low prevalence of nephropathy in the population makes it unclear whether either drug was protective in progression of nephropathy.

Microalbuminuria Microalbuminuria (incipient nephropathy) is highly predictive of diabetic nephropathy and worsening renal function. Approximately 30% of people with type 2 diabetes have microalbuminuria, especially those with hypertension and other features of the metabolic syndrome.

A series of studies in microalbuminuric patients provides clear evidence of an advantage of lower BP goals combined with renin–angiotensin system blockade. In normotensive individuals with type 1 and type 2 diabetes, captopril-based therapy significantly reduced progression to clinical proteinuria compared with placebo.[161] In 94 patients with mean post-treatment BP 130/ 80 mmHg, enalapril for 7 years was associated with 42% reduction in nephropathy compared with placebo.[167] Similarly, angiotensin receptor blocker therapy provoked a 70% reduction in progression of microalbuminuria to clinical proteinuria compared with placebo in hypertensive patients with type 2 diabetes.[98] In type 2 diabetes, a comparison of valsartan and amlodipine demonstrated a BP-independent anti-microalbuminuric effect of the angiotensin receptor blocker.[168]

Type 1 diabetes In type 1 diabetes, BP reduction with ACE inhibition slows the rate of decline of renal function in overt diabetic nephropathy[119] and delays progression from microalbuminuria to overt nephropathy.[52,169,170] Smaller studies have confirmed that even among patients with initial BP < 130/ 80 mmHg, addition of an ACE inhibitor reduces proteinuria.[161,171] ACE inhibition also slows progression of diabetic retinopathy in normotensive patients.[172]

ACE inhibitors are recommended as initial therapy in incipient and overt diabetic nephropathy. If there is ACE inhibitor cough, an angiotensin receptor blocker is the recommended alternative. ACE inhibitor dose should be titrated to the maximum recommended and tolerated. Add-on drugs include low dose thiazide/thiazide-like diuretics, calcium channel blockers and β-blockers.[9] A similar approach is recommended in persistent microalbuminuria.[119,169,173] It remains unclear whether the benefit accrues from blockade of the renin–angiotensin system per se or the associated BP reduction.

Type 2 diabetes In type 2 diabetes, hypertension accelerates and antihypertensive therapy slows the decline of renal function.[169,174] ACE inhibitors have an anti-proteinuric action and delay progression from microalbuminuria to overt nephropathy.[169,170,175] It is less clear whether there is a specific renoprotective action beyond BP reduction.

There is good evidence that angiotensin receptor blocker-based therapy can delay progression of microalbuminuria to overt nephropathy (proteinuria)[98] and progression of overt nephropathy to end-stage renal disease.[96,97] Several studies have confirmed the renoprotective effect of angiotensin receptor blockers in nephropathy associated with type 2 diabetes. The RENAAL study[96] included type 2 diabetes patients with early renal insufficiency and microalbuminuria; compared with conventional therapy, losartan-based therapy reduced proteinuria and end-stage renal disease (Fig. 21.3). The Irbesartan Diabetic Nephropathy Trial (IDNT)[97] also demonstrated a significant benefit of a multi-drug regimen including irbesartan compared with conventional multi-drug therapy or an amlodipine-based regimen in reducing the composite endpoint of a doubling in serum creatinine, end-stage renal disease or death in patients with type 2 diabetes, clinical proteinuria and early renal insufficiency (Fig. 21.4). The benefit of angiotensin receptor blocker-based therapy in delaying progression of diabetic nephropathy is complementary to the more substantial benefits achieved by improved BP control.

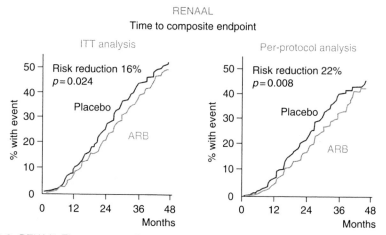

Fig. 21.3 RENAAL Time to composite endpoint. Composite endpoint = doubling of serum creatinine, end-stage renal disease or death. *(From ref. (96).)*

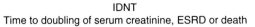

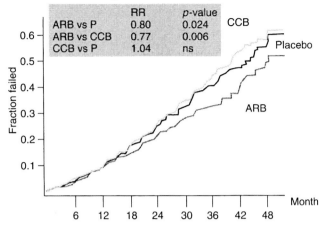

Fig. 21.4 IDNT Time to doubling of serum creatinine, end-stage renal disease or death. *(From ref. (97).)*

Blockade of the renin–angiotensin system in diabetic nephropathy

At least in type 2 diabetes, there is evidence for activation of the intrarenal renin–angiotensin system despite low levels of circulating renin.[176] Blockade of the renin–angiotensin system results in selective dilation of the efferent arterioles in the kidney and hence reduced glomerular pressure and reduced albumin excretion rate.[177] In addition, blockade of growth promoting, profibrotic, non-haemodynamic actions of angiotensin may contribute to renal protection.

In a relatively small study of 409 patients with type 1 diabetes and nephropathy, most with hypertension, captopril-based therapy was superior to placebo-based therapy (with other antihypertensive agents added as needed) in reducing measures of renal dysfunction over a 5-year period of follow-up.[119] To what extent this benefit reflects ACE inhibition or better BP control in the captopril arm remains uncertain.

ACE inhibitors are effective in reducing albumin excretion rate and BP in type 2 diabetes and nephropathy[163] and in reducing microalbuminuria in normotensive non-obese type 2 diabetes.[178] ACE inhibition even confers long-term renal protection in hypertensive and non-hypertensive patients with type 2 diabetes who have not yet developed microalbuminuria.[160,178] The extent of ACE inhibition appears important since very low dose ramipril had no outcome benefit in type 2 diabetes mellitus with persistent microalbuminuria or proteinuria despite BP reduction.[179]

A series of trials has demonstrated the renoprotective effect of angiotensin receptor blockers in patients with type 2 diabetes, hypertension and nephropathy.

RENAAL was a comparison of losartan plus other antihypertensives and placebo plus other antihypertensives.[96] The endpoint was doubling of serum creatinine, end-stage renal disease or death. In 1512 patients followed-up for 4 years, the time to the composite endpoint was improved significantly in the losartan arm. Risk reduction was 16% in the intention to treat analysis and 22% in the per protocol analysis. End-stage renal disease was reduced

28% on losartan, but there was no advantage for two pre-defined secondary cardiovascular endpoints. The design of RENAAL ensured better BP control in the losartan arm.

IDNT was a comparison of irbesartan plus other antihypertensives, placebo plus other antihypertensives and amlodipine plus other antihypertensives. The endpoint was doubling of serum creatinine, end-stage renal disease or death.[97] In 1554 patients followed-up for 4 years, time to doubling serum creatinine, end-stage renal disease or death was improved significantly in the irbesartan arm compared with the 'placebo' or the amlodipine arm. Relative risks were 0.80 for angiotensin receptor blocker compared with 'placebo'; 0.77 compared with amlodipine and 1.04 for the calcium channel blocker versus 'placebo'. BP over time was lower in the angiotensin receptor blocker group than in the 'placebo' group, but there was no difference between the irbesartan and amlodipine arms. The angiotensin receptor blocker exhibited no advantages for secondary cardiovascular endpoints.

IRMA2 (Irbesartan Microalbuminuria Type II Diabetes in Hypertensive Patients) compared irbesartan and placebo in 590 type 2 diabetes patients with microalbuminuria.[98] The endpoint was overt proteinuria. Over 2 years' follow-up, the population with progression to overt nephropathy (overt proteinuria) was reduced in a dose-dependent manner by irbesartan 150–300 mg daily compared with placebo. Irbesartan treatment led to 68% reduction in progression to nephropathy, 54% reduction in urine albumin excretion and 1.7 times greater regression to normoalbuminurua. Glomerular filtration rate was preserved on irbesartan. The importance of BP control on these outcomes is unclear.

The smaller Microalbuminuria Reduction with Valsartan (**MARVAL**) study compared treatment based on valsartan and treatment based on amlodipine in type 2 diabetes with microalbuminuria.[168] Valsartan was associated with 44% reduction in albumin excretion rate compared with 8.5% reduction on amlodipine despite equivalent BP reduction.

Thus, angiotensin receptor blocker therapy prevents progression of microalbuminuria to overt nephropathy (IRMA2/MARVAL) and of overt nephropathy to end-stage renal disease (IDNT/RENAAL).

Angiotensin receptor blockers and ACE inhibitors reduce urinary albumin excretion.[180] Until recently, there was no direct comparison of ACE inhibitors and angiotensin receptor blockers in diabetes. The Diabetics Exposed to Telmisartan and Enalapril (DETAIL) study[181] was a prospective, double-blind study in 250 patients with type 2 diabetes and early nephropathy, mostly with hypertension, randomized to telmisartan 80 mg or enalapril 20 mg daily. After 5 years, the decrement in glomerular filtration rate did not differ significantly between the groups. The findings satisfied the non-inferiority criteria, although there was a trend in favour of enalapril. Although BP changes were similar, these favoured telmisartan. There were no differences for secondary endpoints including serum creatinine, urinary albumin excretion, end-stage renal disease, cardiovascular deaths or deaths from all causes. This study supports equivalence of angiotensin receptor blockers and ACE inhibitors in renoprotection in type 2 diabetes, but was underpowered to detect small differences.

In patients with type 2 diabetes and nephropathy, dual blockade of the renin–angiotensin system with ACE inhibition plus angiotensin receptor blockade significantly reduces albuminuria and may be renoprotective even when the doses of the agents are reduced by one half.[182] In the Candesartan and Lisinopril Microalbuminuria (CALM) study, combination treatment with lisinopril 20 mg plus candesartan 16 mg daily reduced BP and urinary albumin excretion rate to a greater extent than either drug alone.[183] The combination was well tolerated with only a small increase in serum potassium (0.3 mmol/L).

The mechanism of action of the two classes appears complementary,[182] and several studies suggest a beneficial effect of the combination in diabetic kidney disease, including reduction in albuminuria of 16–43%.[182–184] However, it is uncertain whether the combination per se is superior to full-dose monotherapy. The combination resulted in greater BP reduction in most studies[183,184] and this may explain the benefit. The answer may be provided by the results of the Ongoing Telmisartan Alone and in Combination with Ramipril Global End point Trial (ONTARGET), which compares ACE inhibitor, angiotensin receptor blocker and the combination in a population that includes type 2 diabetes.[185]

Preventing (or delaying) the development of microalbuminuria is a key treatment goal for renoprotection.[6,110,154] ACE inhibitors and angiotensin receptor blockers appear to be the most effective agents.[96,97,119,171] There is continued doubt and uncertainty about whether the small differences in BP in several major outcome trials fully or only partly explain the observed reductions in renal outcomes.

Much of the evidence relating to ACE inhibition in diabetic nephropathy was obtained in type 1 diabetes. Type 2 diabetic nephropathy is a very different problem. Blockade of the renin–angiotensin system by whatever means is highly effective. ACE inhibitors are less expensive but the evidence base is less strong.

It has been suggested that, while ACE inhibitors and angiotensin receptor blockers have similar effects on renal outcomes, the latter class may be associated with increased risk of myocardial infarction[186] and all-cause mortality.[187] The value of angiotensin receptor blockers for renoprotection in overt type 2 diabetic nephropathy is well documented. These agents should be the standard of care. The citation of incomplete or misleading data[186,187] in support of an alarmist position should not alter this therapeutic approach.

Correction of dyslipidaemia

Lipid-lowering has a moderately favourable effect.[188,189] Treatment with atorvastatin in addition to a regimen including ACE inhibitor or angiotensin receptor blocker reduces proteinuria and the rate of progression of kidney disease in patients with chronic kidney disease, proteinuria and hypercholesterolaemia.[190] Although not all patients had diabetes, the benefit might be extrapolated to that population. Intensive strategies to control BP, lipids and glucose demonstrated benefit for the development of nephropathy, autonomic neuropathy and cardiovascular deaths[158] (Fig. 21.5).

Glycaemic control

Meticulous control of glycaemia preserves kidney function and delays development of renal damage in diabetes mellitus.[158] Thus, strict glycaemic control should accompany optimal BP control. The treatment goals are a random blood sugar ≤ 6.0 mmol/L and $HbA_{IC} \leq 6.5\%$.[191]

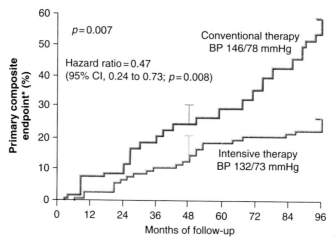

* Primary composite endpoint = composite of death from cardiovascular causes, non-fatal myocardial infarction, non-fatal stroke, revascularization and amputation

Fig. 21.5 Intensive strategies to control blood pressure, lipids and glucose. Kaplin-Maier estimates for the composite endpoint of nephropathy, retinopathy, neuropathy and death from cardiovascular causes. *(From ref. (158).)*

RISK OF DIABETES MELLITUS WITH ANTIHYPERTENSIVE DRUGS

Individuals with hypertension, whether treated or untreated, are at increased risk of developing type 2 diabetes. In treated hypertensive subjects, compared with those who received no antihypertensive therapy, the risk of development of diabetes was not significantly altered with ACE inhibitors, calcium channel blockers or thiazide diuretics. Only those treated with β-blockers were at increased risk of developing diabetes.[18]

Epidemiological studies and clinical trials support a causal link between use of β-blockers and type 2 diabetes.[192] β-blockers can adversely affect glucose homeostasis including worsening of insulin sensitivity. The diabetic potential of β-blockers may be partly related to weight gain.[27]

Thiazide and thiazide-like diuretics are also cited frequently as predisposing to diabetes.[193,194] Short-term metabolic studies raised concerns about the metabolic potential of these agents.[195] Subsequently, epidemiological studies and clinical trials suggested a causal link between use of thiazides and type 2 diabetes.[192] However, the studies that have suggested an increased risk of new-onset diabetes with thiazides have limitations: small numbers of patients, short follow-up, suboptimal definition of new-onset diabetes, lack of adequate comparison group, highly selected patients and failure to allow for confounders.[18] In ALLHAT,[38] there was a tendency for chlorthalidone to increase hyperglycaemia, but the effect was small and not associated with increased cardiovascular events.

Calcium channel blockers are generally considered to be metabolically neutral.[38,100,196] In INVEST,[197] verapamil-based therapy reduced new-onset diabetes compared with atenolol-based therapy, but the effect was modest compared with that of inhibitors of the renin–angiotensin system.

Early experience with ACE inhibitors suggested no detrimental effect on fasting blood glucose after long-term administration.[198] The Swedish Trial in Old Patients with Hypertension-2 (STOP-2) study failed to show a protective effect of ACE inhibition against type 2 diabetes mellitus.[199] The study population was elderly (average age 76 years) and the criteria for definition of diabetes were not specified. In CAPPP,[200] there was significant reduction in new-onset diabetes in the captopril group compared with conventional therapy. It is not clear whether this represented a protective effect of the ACE inhibitor or an adverse effect of β-blockade or thiazide. The scientific value of CAPPP is reduced by a flaw in the randomization procedure, which resulted in an imbalance of baseline BP and the prevalence of diabetes:[201] this may have influenced the incidence of new onset diabetes. In HOPE,[41] there was significant reduction in new-onset diabetes with ramipril compared with standard therapy. However, while the data on new-onset diabetes were prospective, new-onset diabetes was not a primary or even a secondary endpoint, and the analysis was post hoc; the findings should be interpreted with caution. In ALLHAT,[38] lisinopril-based therapy was associated with 30% reduced new-onset diabetes compared with therapy based on chlorthalidone and 17% compared with amlodipine-based therapy. This study provides the best evidence for an anti-diabetagenic effect of ACE inhibitors in hypertension.

In LIFE,[202,203] losartan-based therapy was associated with a significant 25% reduction in new-onset diabetes compared with therapy based on atenolol; 70% of the time each group received concomitant thiazide therapy. Whether this finding is due to improved insulin resistance with the angiotensin receptor blocker or a decrease in insulin sensitivity with atenolol, or both, remains uncertain. A similar reduction in new-onset diabetes has been seen with candesartan.[204,205] In the Study on Cognition and Prognosis in the Elderly (SCOPE),[204] the reduction in new-onset diabetes with candesartan was not significant, but of a similar magnitude to that with losartan in LIFE.[202,203] In the Valsartan Long-term Use Evaluation (VALUE), valsartan-based therapy was associated with a 23% reduction in new-onset diabetes compared with amlodipine.[206] Although the results of VALUE do not establish that angiotensin receptor blockade per se reduces or delays the onset of type 2 diabetes, the lower incidence of new-onset diabetes in valsartan-treated subjects might well reflect an anti-diabetic effect of angiotensin receptor blockers. The Antihypertensive Treatment and Lipid Profile in a North of Sweden Efficacy Evaluation (ALPINE)[207] confirmed the results of larger trials demonstrating a more favourable metabolic profile and lower risk of new-onset diabetes in hypertensive patients treated with an angiotensin receptor blocker compared with thiazides. Costs are greater in the short term, but favourable health benefits in the long term are possible.

Recent outcome studies have reported an increased incidence of diabetes in patients treated with β-blocker or diuretics compared with angiotensin receptor blockers, ACE inhibitors or calcium channel blockers, especially when β-blockers and diuretics are combined. β-blocker/diuretic combination therapy has been associated with around 20% increase in diabetes over trial periods of approximately 5 years in comparison with therapy based on ACE inhibitors or angiotensin receptor blockers.[208]

The shortcomings of the evidence must be considered. Although the major antihypertensive classes appear to exert differential effects on diabetes mellitus incidence, the data are far from conclusive.[192] None had diabetes mellitus as a primary endpoint, and the evidence from randomized trials is limited by sources of bias, including treatment contamination and the bias of post-hoc analysis. The data from the highest quality studies suggest that diabetes is unchanged or increased by thiazides and β-blockers, and unchanged or decreased by ACE inhibitors, calcium channel blockers or angiotensin receptor blockers.

Both diuretics and β-blockers may exert detrimental metabolic effects leading to increased incidence of type 2 diabetes.[192] Glucose intolerance with thiazides has been attributed to potassium depletion.[209] Hypokalaemia can impair glucose tolerance by interfering with insulin release by the pancreas. In-vitro studies, and studies in animals and humans, have suggested a possible relationship between the renin–angiotensin system and the pathogenesis of insulin resistance.[210] Both animal and human studies have shown improvement in insulin resistance by inhibition of angiotensin II.[211] Almost half of the studies of ACE inhibitors in hypertensive non-diabetic individuals demonstrated a slight, but significant, increase in insulin sensitivity as assessed by insulin-stimulated glucose disposal during englycaemic hyperinsulinaemic clamp studies, while the other half failed to reveal any significant changes.[212] Several clinical trials suggest that angiotensin receptor blockers have a protective effect on glucose metabolism.[27,202–206,209] However, most placebo- controlled trials failed to show an anti-diabetic effect.[210] The effects of angiotensin receptor blockers on insulin sensitivity are neutral in most studies.[27]

The potential mechanisms of improvement of glucose tolerance and insulin sensitivity through inhibition of the renin–angiotensin system are complex[27] (Table 21.2). These may include improved blood flow and microcirculation in skeletal muscle and thereby enhancement of insulin and glucose delivery to insulin sensitive tissue,[212] facilitation of insulin signally at the cellular level,[210] and improvement of insulin secretion by the β-cells via a direct effect in blood flow to the endocrine pancreas.[213] Blockade of the renin–angiotensin system may promote recruitment and differentiation of adipocytes, which would counteract the ectopic deposition of lipid in other tissues (liver, muscle, pancreas), thereby improving insulin sensitivity.[214]

Table 21.2 Potential anti-diabetic mechanisms mediated by inhibitors of the renin–angiotensin system

---

Adverse effects of angiotensin II blocked by ACE inhibitors and angiotensin receptor blockers
- insulin signalling
- tissue blood flow
- oxidative stress
- sympathetic activity
- adipogenesis

Beyond effects on the renin–angiotensin system
- enhanced glucose metabolism by activation of bradykinin/nitric oxide pathways (ACE inhibitors)
- improved glucose and lipid metabolism by activation of $PPAR_\delta$

$PPAR_\delta$ = peroxisome proliferator activated receptor gamma
(Modified from ref. (211).)

The availability of drugs that have anti-diabetic as well as antihypertensive properties should be of considerable clinical value. In ALLHAT,[38] less new-onset diabetes did not translate into fewer cardiovascular events in the lisino-pril group. However, the complications of diabetes were reduced significantly in the ramipril group compared with conventional therapy in HOPE.[41] In long-term observational studies, new-onset diabetes has the same high cardiovascular risk as that in patients with diabetes at the outset, but some years of follow-up are needed before the prognostic curves separate.[215–219] In treated hypertensives, the risk of subsequent cardiovascular events was not dissimilar from that in previously known diabetes;[219] risk was almost three-times that in those who did not develop diabetes, although only 63 events were recorded in this study. The average time to an event was 6 years. Since typical outcome trials in hypertension have an average follow-up of 5 years, the average duration of new-onset diabetes is only 2.5 years, leading to underestimation of the implications for cardiovascular risk.

Patients with increased fasting glucose are more likely to develop diabetes when exposed to drugs that worsen glucose tolerance.[220] The British Hypertension Society[9] recommends caution when using the combination of β-blockers and thiazide diuretics in patients at high risk of developing diabetes: impaired glucose tolerance, strong family history of diabetes mellitus, obesity, metabolic syndrome and those of South Asian or Afro-Caribbean descent.

CONCLUSIONS

Adults with diabetes have experienced a 50% reduction in the rate of incident cardiovascular disease, although persons with diabetes have remained at a consistent twofold increased risk for cardiovascular events compared with those without diabetes.[221] Patients with diabetes have benefited in a similar manner to those without diabetes during the decline in cardiovascular disease rates over the last several decades. When comparing cardiovascular risk factors from earlier and later periods, there are significant declines for important cardiovascular disease risk factors including systolic BP. Ongoing efforts remain necessary to promote rigorous cardiovascular disease risk reduction among adults with diabetes. In the US,[222] 18% have poor glycaemic control, 34% have BP of >140/90 mmHg and 58% have elevated LDL-cholesterol. Given the increasing prevalence of diabetes,[221] it is critical to make efforts to implement the findings from clinical trials to promote cardiovascular disease risk factor reduction.

The strategy for patients with diabetes or the metabolic syndrome should combine early detection of combined risk factors and target organ damage, and preventive approaches including lifestyle modification and multi-targeted pharmacological intervention. All such patients should have assessment of obesity, tobacco use, BP, lipid status and urine albumin excretion.

The risk of premature cardiovascular disease is even higher in type 1 diabetes than in type 2 diabetes. Therefore, cardiovascular risk reduction should be integral to the management of type 1 diabetes. This should include attention to lifestyle in childhood, with antihypertensive drugs and lipid-lowering therapy in adulthood.

Pharmacological interventions in all people with diabetes should include BP control to a goal of <130/80 mmHg and normalization of urine albumin excretion with a multi-drug regimen including an ACE inhibitor in type 1 diabetes mellitus or an angiotensin receptor blocker in type 2 diabetes mellitus, correction of dyslipidaemia with a statin to achieve target LDL-cholesterol, and thereafter reduction in triglycerides and increase in HDL-cholesterol, low-dose aspirin and glycaemic control. Diabetic patients will derive greater cardiovascular and renal risk reduction benefits from these approaches if these are instituted early. This requires multiple medications, good compliance and a multidisciplinary effort.

The challenging task for patient and doctor is to achieve the defined goals of therapy. Poor adherence to guidelines and inability to reach defined targets are common.[222] Nevertheless, the use of a comprehensive multi-factorial cardiovascular and renal risk approach tailored to expected risk benefits in the individual patient is bound to reduce the risk of cardiovascular and renal disease in diabetes. The criteria are attention to all risk factors, including BP, with a low threshold for intervention, rigorous targets and multiple antihypertensive agents, including the use of agents to block the renin–angiotensin system. Effective cardiovascular and renal disease care requires a multi-professional approach, involvement of the individual, integration with the management of other diabetes complications, and other therapies including aspirin and lipid-lowering drugs, particularly statins.

References

1. Betteridge DJ. The interplay of cardiovascular risk factor in the metabolic syndrome and type 2 diabetes. *Eur Heart J* 2004;6(Suppl G):G3–G7.
2. Chobanian AV, Bakris GL, Black HL, et al. Seventh report of the Joint National Committee on prevention, detection, evaluation, and treatment of high blood pressure. *Hypertension* 2003;42:1206–1252.
3. Stamler J, Vaccaro O, Neaton J, et al. Diabetes, other risk factors, and 12-year cardiovascular mortality for men screened for the Multiple Risk Factor Intervention Trial. *Diabetes Care* 1993;16:434–439.
4. Simonson DC. Etiology and prevalence of hypertension in diabetic patients. *Diabetes Care* 1988;11:821–827.
5. Sowers JR, Haffner S. Treatment of cardiovascular and renal risk factors in the diabetic hypertensive. *Hypertension* 2002;40:781–788.
6. UK Prospective Diabetes Study Group. Tight blood pressure control and risk of macrovascular and microvascular complications in type 2 diabetes: UKPDS 38. *BMJ* 1998;317:703–713.
7. Sowers JR, Epstein M, Frohlich ED. Diabetes, hypertension and cardiovascular disease. *Hypertension* 2001;37:1053–1059.
8. Williams B. The unique vulnerability of diabetic patients to hypertensive injury. *J Hum Hypertens* 1999;13:S3–S8.
9. Williams B, Poulter NR, Brown MJ, et al. Guidelines for management of hypertension: report of the fourth working party of the British Hypertension Society, 2004 – BHS IV. *J Human Hypertens* 2004;18:139–185.
10. Epstein M, Sowers JR. Diabetes mellitus and hypertension. *Hypertension* 1992;19:403–418.
11. Hypertension in Diabetes Study (HDS). I: prevalence of hypertension in newly presenting type 2 diabetic patients and the association with risk factors for cardiovascular and diabetic complications. *J Hypertens* 1993;11:309–317.
12. Tarnow L, Rossing P, Gall MA, et al. Prevalence of arterial hypertension in diabetic patients before and after JNC-V. *Diabetes Care* 1994;17:1247–1251.
13. Harris M. Health care and health status and outcomes for patients with type 2 diabetes. *Diabetes Care* 2000;23:754–758.
14. Burt VL, Whelton P, Roccella EJ, et al. Prevalence of hypertension in the US adult population. Results from the Third National Health and Nutrition Examination Survey, 1988–1991. *Hypertension* 1995;25:305–313.
15. Medalie JH, Papier CM, Goldbourt U, et al. Major factors in the development of diabetes mellitus in 10,000 men. *Arch Intern Med* 1975;135:811–817.

16. Morales PA, Mitchell BD, Valdez RA, et al. Incidence of NIDDM and impaired glucose tolerance in hypertensive subjects: the San Antonio Heart Study. *Diabetes* 1993;42:154–161.

17. Skarfors ET, Selinus KI, Lithell HO. Risk factors for developing non-insulin dependent diabetes: a 10 year follow up of men in Uppsala. *BMJ* 1991;303:755–760.

18. Gress TW, Nieto FJ, Shahar E, et al. Hypertension and antihypertensive therapy as risk factors for type 2 diabetes mellitus. Atherosclerosis Risk in Communities Study. *N Engl J Med* 2000;342:905–912.

19. Sowers JR, Bakris GL. Antihypertensive therapy and the risk of type 2 diabetes mellitus. *N Engl J Med* 2000;342:969–970.

20. Mykkanen L, Haffner SM, Kuusisto J, et al. Microalbuminuria precedes the development of NIDDM. *Diabetes* 1994;43:552–557.

21. Bühler FR, Julius S, Reaven GM, et al. A dimension in hypertension: role of insulin resistance. *J Cardiovasc Pharmacol* 1990;15(Suppl 5):S1–S3.

22. Ferrannini E, Buzzigoli C, Bonadonna R, et al. Insulin resistance in essential hypertension. *N Engl J Med* 1987;317:350–357.

23. Ferrari P, Weidmann P. Insulin, insulin sensitivity and hypertension. *J Hypertens* 1990;8:491–500.

24. Modan M, Halkin H, Almog S, et al. Hyperinsulinemia: a link between hypertension, obesity and glucose intolerance. *J Clin Invest* 1985;75:809–817.

25. Swislocki ALM, Hoffman BB, Reaven GM. Insulin resistance, glucose intolerance and hyperinsulinemia in patients with hypertension. *Am J Hypertens* 1989;2:419–423.

26. Reaven GM. Intensive blood pressure/glucose control in type 2 diabetes: why is it so difficult to decrease coronary heart disease? *J Hum Hypertens* 1999;13:S19–S23.

27. Scheen AJ. Prevention of type 2 diabetes mellitus through inhibition of the renin-angiotensin system. *Drugs* 2004;64:2537–2565.

28. Coutinho M, Gerstein HC, Wang Y, Yusuf S. The relationship between glucose and incident cardiovascular events. A metaregression analysis of published data from 20 studies of 95,783 individual followed for 12.4 years. *Diabetes Care* 1999;22:233–240.

29. Henry P, Thomas F, Benetos A, Guize L. Impaired fasting glucose, blood pressure and cardiovascular disease mortality. *Hypertension* 2002;40:458–463.

30. Alderberth AM, Rosengren A, Wilhelmsen L. Diabetes and long-term risk of mortality from coronary and other causes in middle-aged Swedish men. A general population study. *Diabetes Care* 1998;21:539–545.

31. Haffner SM, Lehto S, Ronnemaa T, et al. Mortality from coronary heart disease in subjects with type 2 diabetes and in non diabetic subjects with and without prior myocardial infarction. *N Engl J Med* 1998;339:229–234.

32. Laakso M, Lehto S. Epidemiology of macrovascular diseases in diabetes. *Diabetes Rev* 1997;5:294–315.

33. Cho E, Rimm EB, Stampfer MJ, et al. The impact of diabetes mellitus and prior myocardial infarction on mortality from all causes and from coronary heart disease in men. *J Am Coll Cardiol* 2002;40:954–960.

34. Lee CD, Folsom AR, Pankow JS, et al. Cardiovascular events in diabetic and nondiabetic adults with or without history of myocardial infarction. *Circulation* 2004;109:855–860.

35. Davis TM, Millns H, Stratton IM, et al. Risk factors for stroke in type 2 diabetes mellitus. United Kingdom Prospective Diabetes Study (UKPDS) 29. *Arch Intern Med* 1999;159:1097–1103.

36. Fagan TC, Sowers J. Type 2 diabetes mellitus: greater cardiovascular risks and greater benefits of therapy. *Arch Intern Med* 1999;159:1033–1034.

37. Adler AI, Stratton IM, Neil HA, et al. Association of systolic blood pressure with macrovascular and microvascular complications of type 2 diabetes: UKPDS 36: prospective observational study. *BMJ* 2000;321:412–419.

38. The ALLHAT Officers and Coordinators for the ALLHAT Collaborative Research Group. Major outcomes in high-risk hypertensive patients randomized to angiotensin-converting enzyme inhibitor or calcium channel blocker vs diuretic. The Antihypertensive and Lipid-Lowering Treatment to Prevent Heart Attack Trial (ALLHAT). *JAMA* 2002;288:2981–2997.

39. Goldstein LB, Adams R, Becker K, et al. Primary prevention of ischemic stroke: a statement for health professionals from the Stroke Council of the American Heart Association. *Circulation* 2001;103:163–182.

40. Hansson L, Zanchetti A, Carruthers SG, et al. Effects of intensive blood-pressure lowering and low-dose aspirin in patients with hypertension: principal results of the Hypertension Optimal Treatment (HOT) randomised trial. HOT Study Group. *Lancet* 1998;351:1755–1762.

41. Heart Outcomes Prevention Evaluation Study Investigators. Effects of an angiotensin-converting-enzyme inhibitor, ramipril, on cardiovascular events in high-risk patients. *N Engl J Med* 2000;342:145–153.

42. Bakris GL, Williams M, Dworkin L, et al. Preserving renal function in adults with hypertension and diabetes: a consensus approach. National Kidney Foundation Hypertension and Diabetes Executive Committees Working Group. *Am J Kidney Dis* 2000;36:646–661.

43. Maki DD, Ma JZ, Louis TA, Kasiske BL. Long-term effects of antihypertensive agents on proteinuria and renal function. *Arch Intern Med* 1995;155:1073–1080.

44. Nelson RG, Bennett PH, Beck GJ, et al. Development and progression of renal disease in Pima Indians with non-insulin-dependent diabetes mellitus. Diabetic Renal Disease Study Group. *N Engl J Med* 1996;335:1636–1642.

45. Kohner EM, Eldington SJ, Stratton IM, et al. United Kingdom Prospective Diabetes Study, 30: diabetic retinopathy at diagnosis of non-insulin-dependent diabetes mellitus and associated risk factors. *Arch Opthalmol* 1998;116:297–303.

46. Tuomilehto J, Rastenyte D, Birkenhager WH, et al; for the Systolic Hypertension in Europe Trial Investigators. Effects of calcium channel blockers in older patients with diabetes and systolic hypertension. *N Engl J Med* 1999;340:677–684.

47. Alderman MH, Cohen H, Madhaven S. Diabetes and cardiovascular events in hypertensive patients. *Hypertension* 1999;33:1130–1134.

48. Gerber LM, Madhaven S, Alderman MH. Coincident hypertension: deleterious effects on patients with hyperglycaemia. *NY State J Med* 1983;83:693–696.

49. Grossman E, Messerli FH. Diabetes and hypertensive heart disease. *Ann Intern Med* 1996;125:304–310.

50. Jarrett RJ, McCartney P, Keen H. The Bedford survey: 10-year mortality rates in newly diagnosed diabetics and hyperglycaemic controls and risk indices for coronary heart disease in borderline diabetics. *Diabetologia* 1982;22:79–84.

51. Pell S, D'Alonzo CA. Some aspects of hypertension in diabetes mellitus. *JAMA* 1967;202:104–110.

52. Mogensen CE, Keane WF, Bennett PH, et al. Prevention of diabetic renal disease with special reference to microalbuminuria. *Lancet* 1995;346:1080–1084.

53. Parving HH, Andersen AR, Smidt UM, et al. Effect of antihypertensive treatment on kidney function in diabetic nephropathy. *BMJ* 1987;294:1443–1447.

54. Dillon JJ. The quantitative relationship between treated blood pressure and progression of diabetic renal disease. *Am J Kidney Dis* 1993;22:798–802.

55. Walker WG. Hypertension-related renal injury: a major contributor to end-stage renal disease. *Am J Kidney Dis* 1993;22:164–173.

56. Reaven G. Metabolic syndrome: pathophysiology and implications for management of cardiovascular disease. *Circulation* 2002;106:286–288.

57. Reaven GM, Lithell H, Landsberg L. Hypertension and associated metabolic abnormalities–the role of insulin resistance and the sympathoadrenal system. *N Engl J Med* 1996;334:378–381.

58. Hanley AJ, Karter AJ, Festa A, et al. Factor analysis of metabolic syndrome using directly measured insulin sensitivity. The Insulin Resistance Atherosclerosis Study. *Diabetes* 2002;51:2642–2647.

59. Alberti KG, Zimmet PZ. Definition, diagnosis and classification of diabetes mellitus and its complications. Part 1: diagnosis and classification of diabetes mellitus. Provisional report of a WHO consultation. *Diabet Med* 1998;15:539–553.

60. Balkau B, Charles MA. Comment of the provisional report from the WHO consultation. European Group for the Study of Insulin Resistance (EGIR). *Diabet Med* 1999;16:442–443.

61. Executive Summary of the Third Report of The National Cholesterol Education Program (NCEP). Expert Panel on Detection, Evaluation, And Treatment of High Blood Cholesterol in Adults (Adult Treatment Panel III). *JAMA* 2001;285:2486–2497.

62. Calle EE, Thun MJ, Petrelli JM, et al. Body-mass index and mortality in a prospective cohort of US adults. *N Engl J Med* 1999;341:1097–1105.

63. Katzmarzyk PT, Craig CL, Bruchard C. Underweight, overweight and obesity: relationships with mortality in the 13-year follow-up of the Canada Fitness Survey. *J Clin Epidemiol* 2001;54:916–920.

64. Seidell JC, Visscher TL, Hoogeveen RT. Overweight and obesity in the mortality rate data: Current evidence and research issues. *Med Sci Sports Exerc* 1999;31:S597–S601.

65. Stevens J, Cai J, Pamuk ER, et al. The effect of age on the association between body-mass index and mortality. *N Engl J Med* 1998;338:1–7.

66. Ford ES, Giles WH, Dietz WH. Prevalence of the metabolic syndrome among US adults: findings from the third National Health and Nutrition Examination Survey. *JAMA* 2002;287:356–359.

67. Hsia J, Bittner V, Tripputi M, Howard BV. Metabolic syndrome and coronary angiographic disease progression: the Women's Angiographic Vitamin and Estrogen trial. *Am Heart J* 2003;146:439–445.

68. Isomaa B, Almgren P, Tuomi T, et al. Cardiovascular morbidity and mortality associated with the metabolic syndrome. *Diabetes Care* 2001;24:683–689.
69. Laaksonen DE, Lakka HM, Niskanen LK, et al. Metabolic syndrome and development of diabetes mellitus: application and validation of recently suggested definitions of the metabolic syndrome in a prospective cohort study. *Am J Epidemiol* 2002;15:1070–1077.
70. Lakka HM, Laaksonen DE, Lakka TA, et al. The metabolic syndrome and cardiovascular disease mortality in middle-aged men. *JAMA* 2002;2709–2716.
71. Liese AD, Mayer-Davis EJ, Haffner SM. Development of the multiple metabolic syndrome: an epidemiologic perspective. *Epidemiol Rev* 1998;20:157–172.
72. Reaven GM. Banting lecture 1988. Role of insulin resistance in human disease. *Diabetes* 1988;37:1595–1607.
73. Chen J, Muntner P, Hamon LL, et al. The metabolic syndrome and chronic kidney disease in US adults. *Ann Intern Med* 2004;140:167–174.
74. Haffner SM. The prediabetic problem: development of non-insulin-dependent diabetes mellitus and related abnormalities. *J Diabet Complic* 1997;11:69–76.
75. Franklin S, Gustin W, Wong N, et al. Hemodynamic patterns of age-related changes in blood pressure: The Framingham Heart Study. *Circulation* 1997;96:308–315.
76. Franklin S, Shehzad A, Khan B, et al. Is pulse pressure useful in predicting risk for coronary heart disease? The Framingham Heart Study. *Circulation* 1999;100:354–360.
77. National High Blood Pressure Education Program Working Group. National High Blood Pressure Education Program Working Group Report on Hypertension in the Elderly. *Hypertension* 1994;23:275–285.
78. Prospective Studies Collaboration. Age-specific relevance of usual blood pressure to vascular mortality: a meta-analysis of individual data for one million adults in 61 prospective studies. *Lancet* 2002;360:1903–1913.
79. Vasan RS, Larson MG, Leip EP, et al. Impact of high-normal pressure on the risk of cardiovascular disease. *N Engl J Med* 2001;345:1291–1297.
80. Klag MK, Whelton PK, Randall BL, et al. A prospective study of blood pressure and incidence of end-stage renal disease in 332,544 men. *N Engl J Med* 1996;334:13–18.
81. Hunsicker LG, Adler S, Esler A, et al. Predictors of the progression of renal disease in the Modification of Diet in Renal Disease Study. *Kidney Int* 1997;51:1908–1919.
82. Van den Hoogen PCW, Feskens EJM, Nagekerke NJD, et al; for the Seven Countries Study Research Group. The relation between blood pressure and mortality due to coronary heart disease among men in different parts of the world. *N Engl J Med* 2000;342:1–8.
83. Liu J, Hong Y, D'Agostini Jr. RB, et al. Predictive value for the Chinese population of the Framingham CHD risk assessment tool compared with the Chinese Multi-Provincial Cohort Study. *JAMA* 2004;291:2591–2599.
84. Ebrahim S, Smith GD. Lowering blood pressure : A systematic review of sustained effects of non-pharmacological interventions. *J Public Health Med* 1998;20:4441–4448.
85. He J, Whelton PK, Appel LJ, et al. Long-term effects of weight loss and dietary sodium restriction on incidence of hypertension. *Hypertension* 2000;35:544–549.
86. Sacks FM, Svetkey LP, Vollmer WM, et al; for the DASH-Sodium Collaborative Research Group. Effects on blood pressure of reduced dietary sodium and the Dietary Approaches to Stop Hypertension (DASH) diet. *N Engl J Med* 2001;344:3–10.
87. Whelton PK, He J, Appel LJ, et al. Primary prevention of hypertension. Clinical and public health advisory from the National High Blood Pressure Education Program. *JAMA* 2002;288:1882–1888.
88. Xin X, He J, Frontini MG, et al. Effects of alcohol reduction on blood pressure: a meta-analysis of randomised controlled trials. *Hypertension* 2001;38:1112–1117.
89. Whelton PK, Appel LJ, Espeland MA, et al. Sodium reduction and weight loss in the treatment of hypertension in older persons: a randomized controlled trial of non-pharmacological intervention in the elderly (TONE). TONE Collaborative Research Group. *JAMA* 1998;279:839–846.
90. He J, Whelton PK. What is the role of dietary sodium and potassium in hypertension and target organ injury? *Am J Med Sci* 1999;317:152–159.
91. Cook NR, Cohen J, Hebert PR, et al. Implications of small reductions in diastolic blood pressure for primary prevention. *Arch Intern Med* 1995;155:701–709.
92. Rocchini AP. Obesity hypertension, salt sensitivity and insulin resistance. *Nutr Metab Cardiovasc Dis* 2000;10:287–294.
93. Wasserman DH, Zinman B. Exercise in individuals with IDDM. *Diabetes Care* 1994;17:924–937.
94. Haire-Joshu D, Glasgow RE, Tibbs TL. Smoking and diabetes. *Diabetes Care* 1999;22:1887–1898.
95. Kawachi I, Colditz GA, Stampfer MJ, et al. Smoking cessation and time course of increased risks of coronary heart disease in middle aged women. *Arch Intern Med* 1994;154:169–175.

96. Brenner BM, Cooper ME, De Zeeuw D, et al; for the RENAAL Study Investigators. Effects of losartan on renal and cardiovascular outcomes in patients with type 2 diabetes and nephropathy. *N Engl J Med* 2001;345:861–869.

97. Lewis EJ, Hunsicker LG, Clarke WR, et al; for the Collaborative Study Group. Renoprotective effect of the angiotensin-receptor antagonist irbesartan in patients with nephropathy due to type 2 diabetes. *N Engl J Med* 2001;345:851–860.

98. Parving H-H, Lehnert H, Bröchner-Mortensen J, et al; for the Irbesartan in Patients with Type 2 Diabetes and Microalbuminuria Study Group. The effect of irbesartan on the development of diabetic nephropathy in patients with type 2 diabetes. *N Engl J Med* 2001;345:870–878.

99. Black HR, Elliott WJ, Grandits G, et al. Principal results of the Controlled Onset Verapamil Investigation of Cardiovascular End Points (CONVINCE) trial. *JAMA* 2003;289:2073–2082.

100. Brown MJ, Palmer CR, Castaigne A, et al. Morbidity and mortality in patients randomised to double-blind treatment with a long-acting calcium channel blocker or diuretic in the International Nifedipine GITS Study: Intervention as a Goal in Hypertension Treatment (INSIGHT). *Lancet* 2000;356:366–377.

101. Staessen JA, Fagard R, Thijs L, et al. Randomised double-blind comparison of placebo and active treatment for older patients with isolated systolic hypertension. The Systolic Hypertension in Europe (Syst-Eur) Trial Investigators. *Lancet* 1997;350:757–764.

102. Curb JD, Pressel SL, Cutler JA, et al. Effect of diuretic-based antihypertensive treatment on cardiovascular disease risk in older diabetic patients with isolated systolic hypertension. *JAMA* 1996;276:1886–1892.

103. Mann JF, Gerstein HC, Pogue J, et al. Renal insufficiency as a predictor of cardiovascular outcomes and the impact of ramipril: the HOPE randomized trial. *Ann Intern Med* 2001;134:629–636.

104. Schrier RW, Estacio RO, Esler A, Mehler P. Effects of aggressive blood pressure control in a normotensive type 2 diabetic patients on albuminuria, retinopathy and strokes. *Kidney Int* 2002;61:1088–1097.

105. Zanchetti A, Ruilope LM. Antihypertensive treatment in patients with type 2 diabetes mellitus: what guidance from recent randomized controlled trials? *J Hypertens* 2002;20:2099–2110.

106. Guidelines Committee. European Society of Hypertension–European Society of Cardiology guidelines for the management of arterial hypertension. *J Hypertens* 2003;21:1011–1053.

107. World Health Organization, International Society of Hypertension Working Group. World Health Organization (WHO)/International Society of Hypertension (ISH) statement on management of hypertension. *J Hypertens* 2003;21:1983–1992.

108. American Diabetes Association. Diabetic nephropathy. *Diabetes Care* 2002;25:S85–S89.

109. Mancia G, Grassi G. Systolic and diastolic blood pressure control in antihypertensive drug trials. *J Hypertens* 2002;29:1461–1464.

110. UK Prospective Diabetes Study Group. Intensive blood-glucose control with sulphonylureas or insulin compared with conventional treatment and risk of complications in patients with type II diabetes: UKPDS33. *Lancet* 1998;352:837–853.

111. Estacio RO, Jeffers BW, Hiatt WR, et al. The effect of nisoldipine as compared with enalapril on cardiovascular outcomes in patients with non-insulin-dependent diabetes and hypertension. *N Engl J Med* 1998;338:645–652.

112. Bakris GL, Gaxiola E, Messerli FH, et al. Clinical outcomes in the diabetes cohort of the International Verapamil SR-Trandolapril Study. *Hypertension* 2004;44:637–642.

113. UK Prospective Diabetes Study Group. Efficacy of atenolol and captopril in reducing risk of macrovascular and microvascular complications in type 2 diabetes: UKPDS 39. *BMJ* 1998;317:713–720.

114. Niskanen L, Hedner T, Hansson L, et al. Reduced cardiovascular morbidity and mortality in hypertensive diabetic patients on first-line therapy with an ACE inhibitor compared with a diuretic/beta-blocker-based treatment regimen: a subanalysis of the Captopril Prevention Project. *Diabetes Care* 2001;24:2091–2096.

115. Tatti P, Pahor M, Byington RP, et al. Outcome results of the Fosinopril versus Amlodipine Cardiovascular Events randomized Trial in patients with hypertension and NIDDM. *Diabetes Care* 1998;21:597–605.

116. Pahor M, Psaty BM, Alderman MH, et al. Therapeutic benefits of ACE inhibitors and other antihypertensive drugs in patients with type 2 diabetes. *Diabetes Care* 2000;23:888–892.

117. Heart Outcomes Prevention Evaluation (HOPE) Study Investigators. Effect of ramipril on cardiovascular and microvascular outcomes in people with diabetes mellitus: results of the HOPE study and MICRO-HOPE substudy. *Lancet* 2000;355:253–259.

118. McInnes GT. Size isn't everything – ALLHAT in perspective. *J Hypertens* 2003;21:459–461.

119. Lewis EJ, Hunsicker LG, Blain RP, Rohde ED and the Collaborative Study Group. The effect of angiotensin-converting enzyme inhibition on diabetic nephropathy. *N Engl J Med* 1993;329:1456–1462.

120. Lindholm LH, Ibsen H, Dahlöf B, et al; for the LIFE study group. Cardiovascular morbidity and mortality in patients with diabetes in the Losartan Intervention For Endpoint reduction in hypertension study (LIFE): a randomised trial against atenolol. *Lancet* 2002;359:1004–1010.

121. Kjeldsen SE, Dahlöf B, Devereux RB, et al; for the LIFE Study Group. Effects of losartan on cardiovascular morbidity and mortality in patients with isolated systolic hypertension and left ventricular hypertrophy: a Losartan Intervention for Endpoint Reduction (LIFE) substudy. *JAMA* 2002;288:1491–1498.

122. Okin PM, Devereux RB, Jern S, et al. Losartan Intervention for Endpoint Reduction in Hypertension Study Investigators. Regression of electrocardiographic left ventricular hypertrophy by losartan versus atenolol: the Losartan Intervention for Endpoint Reduction in Hypertension (LIFE) Study. *Circulation* 2003;108:684–690.

123. Beckman JA, Creager MA, Libby P. Diabetes and atherosclerosis: epidemiology, pathophysiology and management. *JAMA* 2002;287:2570–2581.

124. Miller JA, Floras JS, Zinman B, et al. Effect of hyperglycaemia on arterial pressure, plasma renin activity and renal function in early diabetes. *Clin Sci* 1996;90:189–195.

125. Candido R, Jandeleit-Dahm KA, Cao Z, et al. Prevention of accelerated atherosclerosis by angiotensin-converting enzyme inhibition in diabetic apolipoportein C-deficient mice. *Circulation* 2002;106:246–253.

126. Candido R, Allen TJ, Lassila M, et al. Irbesartan but not amlodipine suppresses diabetes-associated atherosclerosis. *Circulation* 2004;109:1536–1542.

127. Berne C, Pollare T, Lithell H. Effects of antihypertensive treatment on insulin sensitivity with special reference to ACE inhibitors. *Diabetes Care* 1991;14:39–47.

128. Donnelly R. Angiotensin-converting enzyme inhibitors and insulin sensitivity: metabolic effects in hypertension, diabetes and heart failure. *J Cardiovasc Pharmacol* 1992;20(Suppl 11): S38–S44.

129. Ferrannini E, Seghieri G, Muscelli E. Insulin and the renin-angiotensin-aldosterone system: influence of ACE inhibitors. *J Cardiovasc Pharmacol* 1994;24(Suppl 3):S61–S69.

130. Pollare T, Lithell H, Berne C. A comparison of the effects of hydrochlorothiazide and captopril on glucose and lipid metabolism in patients with hypertension. *N Engl J Med* 1989;321:868–873.

131. Torlone E, Rambotti AM, Perriello G, et al. ACE-inhibition increases hepatic and extrahepatic sensitivity to insulin in patients with type 2 (non-insulin-dependent) diabetes mellitus and arterial hypertension. *Diabetologia* 1991;34:119–125.

132. Torlone E, Britta M, Rambotti AM, et al. Improved insulin action and glycaemic control after long-term angiotensin-converting enzyme inhibition in subjects with arterial hypertension and type 2 diabetes. *Diabetes Care* 1993;16:1347–1355.

133. Petrie JR, Morris AD, Ueda S, et al. Trandolapril does not improve insulin sensitivity in patients with hypertension and type 2 diabetes : a double-blind, placebo-controlled cross-over trial. *J Clin Endocrinol Metab* 2000;85:1882–1889.

134. Herings RMC, de Boer A, Stricker BHC, et al. Hypoglycemia associated with use of inhibitors of angiotensin converting enzyme. *Lancet* 1995;345:1195–1198.

135. Morris AD, Boyle DI, McMahon AD, et al. ACE inhibitor use is associated with hospitalisation for severe hypoglycemia in patients with diabetes. DARTS-MEMO Collaboration. Diabetes Audit and Research in Tayside, Scotland. Medicines monitoring unit. *Diabetes Care* 1997;20:1363–1367.

136. Thamer M, Ray NF, Taylor T, et al. Association between antihypertensive drug use and hypoglycemia: a case-control study of diabetic users of insulin or sulfonylureas. *Clin Ther* 1999;21:1387–1400.

137. Hornig B, Kohler C, Drexter H. Role of bradykinin in mediating vascular effects of angiotensin-converting enzyme inhibitors in humans. *Circulation* 1997;25:1115–1118.

138. Mancini CBJ, Henry GC, Macaya C, et al. Angiotensin-converting enzyme inhibition with quinapril improves endothelial vasomotor dysfunction in patients with coronary artery disease. *Circulation* 1996;94:258–265.

139. Lim HS, MacFadyen RJ, Lip GYH. Diabetes mellitus, the renin-angiotensin-aldosterone system, and the heart. *Arch Intern Med* 2004;164:1734–1748.

140. Mogensen C. Microalbuminuria predicts clinical proteinuria and early mortality in maturity-onset diabetes. *N Engl J Med* 1984;310:356–360.

141. Agrawal B, Berger A, Wolf K, et al. Microalbuminuria screening by reagent predicts cardiovascular risk in hypertension. *J Hypertens* 1996;14:223–228.

142. Ruilope L, Rodicio J. Microalbuminuria in clinical practice: a current survey of world literature. *Kidney Int* 1995;4:211–216.

143. Frick MH, Elo O, Haapa K, et al. Helsinki Heart Study: a primary-prevention trial with gemfibrozil in middle-aged men with dyslipidemia. Safety of treatment, changes in risk factors and incidence of coronary heart disease. *N Engl J Med* 1987;317:1237–1245.

144. Goldberg RB, Mellies MJ, Sacks FM, et al. Cardiovascular events and their reduction with pravastatin in diabetic and glucose-intolerant myocardial infarction survivors with average cholesterol levels: subgroup analyses in the Cholesterol And Recurrent Events (CARE) trial. The Care Investigators. *Circulation* 1998;98:2513–2519.

145. Heart Protection Study Group. MRC/BHF Heart Protection study of cholesterol lowering with simvastatin in 20,536 high-risk individuals: a randomised placebo-controlled trial. *Lancet* 2002;360:7–22.

146. Pyorala K, Pedersen TR, Kjekshus J, et al. Cholesterol lowering with simvastatin improves prognosis of diabetic people with coronary heart disease. A subgroup analysis of the Scandinavian Simvastatin Survival Study (4S). *Diabetes Care* 1997;20:614–620.

147. Rubins HB, Robins SJ, Collins D, et al. Gemfibrozil for the secondary prevention of coronary heart disease in men with low levels of high-density lipoprotein cholesterol. Veterans Affairs High-Density Lipoprotein Cholesterol Intervention Trial Study Group. *N Engl J Med* 1999;341:410–418.

148. The Long-Term Intervention with Pravastatin in Ischaemic Disease (LIPID) Study Group. Prevention of cardiovascular events and death with pravastatin in people with coronary heart disease and a broad range of initial cholesterol levels. *N Engl J Med* 1998;339:1349–1357.

149. Koskinen P, Manttari M, Manninen V, et al. Coronary heart disease incidence in NIDDM patients in the Helsinki Heart Study. *Diabetes Care* 1992;15:820–825.

150. Sever PS, Dahlöf B, Poulter NR, et al. Prevention of coronary and stroke events with atorvastatin in hypertensive patients who have average or lower-than-average cholesterol concentration in the Anglo-Scandinavian Cardiac Outcomes Trial in Lipid Lowering Arm (ASCOT-LLA): a multicentre randomised controlled trial. *Lancet* 2003;361:1149–1158.

151. Colhoun H, Betteridge D, Durrington P, et al. On behalf of the CARDS investigators. Primary prevention of cardiovascular disease with atorvastatin in type 2 diabetes in the Collaborative Atorvastatin Diabetes Study (CARDS): multicentre randomised placebo-controlled trial. *Lancet* 2004;364:685–696.

152. Haffner SM. Management of dyslipidemia in adults with diabetes. *Diabetes Care* 1998;21:160–178.

153. Antithrombotic Trialists' Collaboration. Collaborative meta-analysis of randomised trials of antiplatelet therapy for prevention of death, myocardial infarction and stroke in high risk patients. *BMJ* 2002;324:71–86.

154. The Diabetes Control and Complications Trial Research Group. The effect of intensive treatment of diabetes on the development and progression of long-term complications in insulin-dependent diabetes mellitus. *N Engl J Med* 1993;329:977–986.

155. Yosefy C, Magen E, Kiselevich A, et al. Rosiglitazone improves, while glibenclamide worsens blood pressure control in treated hypertensive diabetic and dyslipidemic subjects via modulation of insulin resistance and sympathetic activity. *J Cardiovasc. Pharmacol* 2004;44:215–222.

156. Dormandy J, Charbonnel B, Eckland DJ, et al. Secondary prevention of macrovascular events in patients with type 2 diabetes in the PROactive study (PROspective pioglitAzone Clinical Trial In macroVascular Events): a randomised controlled trial. *Lancet* 2005;366:1279–1289.

157. The DREAM (Diabetes REduction Assessment with ramipril and rosiglitazone Medication) Trial Investigators. Effect of rosiglitazone on the frequency of diabetes in patients with impaired glucose tolerance or impaired fasting glucose: a randomised controlled trial. *Lancet* 2006;368:1096–1105.

158. Gaede P, Vedel P, Larsen N, et al. Multifactorial intervention and cardiovascular disease in patients with type 2 diabetes. *N Engl J Med* 2003;348:383–393.

159. Heeg J, de Jong P, Van der Hem G, et al. Efficacy and variability of the antiproteinuric effect of ACE inhibition by lisinopril. *Kidney Int* 1989;36:272–279.

160. Pedrini M, Levey A, Lau J, et al. The effect of dietary protein restriction on the progression of diabetic and nondiabetic renal disease: a meta-analysis. *Ann Intern Med* 1996;124:627–632.

161. Viberti G, Mogensen C, Groop L, et al; for the European Microalbuminuria Captropril Study Group. Effect of captopril on progression to clinical proteinuria in patients with insulin-dependent diabetes mellitus and microalbuminuria. *JAMA* 1994;271:275–279.

162. Bakris GL. Maximising cardiorenal benefits in the management of hypertension: achieve blood pressure goals. *J Clin Hypertens* 1999;1:141–147.

163. Kasiske BL, Kalil RS, Ma JZ, et al. Effect of antihypertensive therapy on the kidney in patients with diabetes: a meta-regression analysis. *Ann Intern Med* 1993;118:129–138.

164. Sato A, Hayashi K, Naruse M, et al. Effectiveness of aldosterone blockade in patients with diabetic nephropathy. *Hypertension* 2003;41:64–68.

165. Bakris GL, Copley JB, Vicknair N, et al. Calcium channel blockers versus other antihypertensive, therapies on progression of NIDDM associated nephropathy. *Kidney Int* 1996;50:1641–1650.

166. Ruggenenenti P, Fassi A, Ilieva AP, et al; for the Bergamo Nephrologic Diabetes Complications Trial (BENEDICT) Investigators. Preventing microalbuminuria in type 2 diabetes. *N Engl J Med* 2004;351:1941–1951.

167. Ravid M, Savin H, Jutrin I, et al. Long-term stabilising effect of angiotensin-converting enzyme inhibition on plasma creatinine and on proteinuria in normotensive type II diabetic patients. *Ann Intern Med* 1993;118:577–581.

168. Viberti G, Wheeldon NM for the MicroAlbuminuria Reduction with VALsartan (MARVAL) Study Investigators. Microalbuminuria reduction with valsartan in patients with type 2 diabetes mellitus. A blood pressure-independent effect. *Circulation* 2002;106:672–678.

169. Cooper ME. Pathogenesis, prevention and treatment of diabetic nephopathy. *Lancet* 1998;352:213–219.

170. Parving HH. Initiation and progression of diabetic nephropathy. *N Engl J Med* 1996;335:1682–1683.

171. Parving H, Hommel E, Jensen B, et al. Long-term beneficial effects of ACE inhibition on diabetic nephropathy in normotensive type 1 diabetic patients. *Kidney Int* 2001;60: 228–234.

172. Chaturvedi N, Sjolie A-K, Stephenson JM, et al; for the EUCLID Study Group. Effect of lisinopril on progression of retinopathy in normotensive people with type I diabetes. *Lancet* 1998;351:28–31.

173. The EUCLID Study Group. Randomised placebo-controlled trial of lisinopril in normotensive patients with insulin-dependent diabetes and normoalbuminuria or microalbuminuria. *Lancet* 1997;349:1787–1792.

174. Gall MA, Houguard P, Borch-Johnsen K, Parving HH. Risk factors for development of incipient and overt diabetic nephropathy in patients with non-insulin dependent diabetes mellitus: prospective observational study. *BMJ* 1997;314:783–788.

175. Ravid M, Leug R, Rachmanni R, Lisner M. Long-term renoprotective effect of angiotensin converting enzyme inhibitors in non-insulin dependent diabetes: a seven year follow-up. *Arch Intern Med* 1996;156:286–289.

176. Price DA, Porter LE, Gordon M, et al. The paradox of the low-renin state in diabetic nephropathy. *J Am Soc Nephrol* 1999;10:2382–2389.

177. Sharma AM. Is there a rationale for angiotensin blockade in the management of obesity hypertension? *Hypertension* 2004;44:12–19.

178. Ravid M, Brosh D, Levi Z, et al. Use of enalapril to attenuate decline in renal function in normotensive, normoalbuminuric patients with type 2 diabetes mellitus: a randomized, controlled trial. *Ann Intern Med* 1998;128:982–988.

179. Marre M, Lievre M, Chatellier G, et al. On behalf of the DIABHYCAR Study Investigators. Effects of low dose ramipril on cardiovascular and renal outcomes in patients with type 2 diabetes and raised excretion of urinary albumin: randomised, double blind, placebo controlled trial (the DIABHYCAR Study). *BMJ* 2004;328:495–499.

180. Lacourciere Y, Belanger A, Godin C, et al. Long-term comparison of losartan and enalapril on kidney function in hypertensive type 2 diabetes with early nephropathy. *Kidney Int* 2000;58:762–769.

181. Barnett AH, Bain SC, Bouter P, et al; for the Diabetics Exposed to Telmisartan and Enalapril Study Group. Angiotensin-receptor blockade versus converting-enzyme inhibition in type 2 diabetes and nephropathy. *N Engl J Med* 2004;351:1952–1961.

182. Fujisawa T, Ikegami H, Ono M, et al. Combination of half doses of angiotensin type 1 receptor antagonist and angiotensin-converting enzyme inhibitor in diabetic nephropathy. *Am J Hypertens* 2005;18:13–17.

183. Mogensen CE, Neldam S, Tikkanen I, et al. Randomised controlled trial of dual blockade of renin-angiotensin system in patients with hypertension, microalbuminuria, and non-insulin dependent diabetes: the candesartan and lisinopril microalbuminuria (CALM) study. *BMJ* 2000;321:1440–1444.

184. Jacobsen P, Andersen S, Rossing K, et al. Dual blockade of the renin-angiotensin system versus maximal recommended dose of ACE inhibition in diabetic nephropathy. *Kidney Int* 2003;63:1874–1880.

185. Zimmermann M, Unger T. Challenges in improving prognosis and therapy: The Ongoing Telmisartan Alone and in Combination with Ramipril Global End point Trial Program. *Expert Opin Pharmacother* 2004;5:1201–1208.

186. Verma S, Strauss M. Angiotensin receptor blockers and myocardial infarction. *BMJ* 2004;329:1248–1249.

187. Strippoli GFM, Craig M, Deeks JJ, et al. Effects of angiotensin converting enzyme inhibitors and angiotensin II receptor antagonists on mortality and renal outcomes in diabetic nephropathy: systematic review. *BMJ* 2004;329:823–838.

188. Fried LF, Orchard TJ, Kasiske BL. Effect of lipid reduction on the progression of renal disease: a meta-analysis. *Kidney Int* 2001;59:260–269.

189. Sica DA, Gehr TW. 3-Hydroxy-3-methylglutaryl coenzyme A reductase inhibitors and rhabdomyolysis: consideration in the renal failure patient. *Curr Opin Nephrol Hypertens* 2002;11:123–133.

190. Bianchi S, Bigazzi R, Caiazza A, et al. A controlled, prospective study of the effects of atorvastatin in proteinuria and prognosis of kidney disease. *Am J Kidney Dis* 2003;41:565–570.

191. European Diabetes Policy Group 1999. A desktop guide to type 2 diabetes mellitus. *Diabetes Med* 1999;16:716–730.

192. Padwal R, Laupacis A. Antihypertensive therapy and evidence of type 2 diabetes. *Diabetes Care* 2004;27:247–255.

193. Lithell HO. Effect of antihypertensive drugs on insulin, glucose, and lipid metabolism. *Diabetes Care* 1991;14:203–209.

194. Opie LH, Schall R. Old antihypertensives and new diabetes. *J Hypertens* 2004;22:1453–1458.

195. Shapiro APJ, Benedeck TG, Small JL. Effect of thiazides on carbohydrate metabolism in patients with hypertension. *N Engl J Med* 1961;265:1028–1033.

196. Hansson L, Hedner T, Lund-Johannsen P, et al; for the NORDIL Study Group. Randomised trial of efforts of calcium antagonists compared with diuretics and β-blockers on cardiovascular morbidity and mortality in hypertension: the Nordic Diltiazem (NORDIL) Study. *Lancet* 2000;356:359–365.

197. Pepine CJ, Handberg EM, Cooper-De Hoff RM, et al. A calcium antagonist vs a non-calcium antagonist hypertension treatment strategy for patients with coronary artery disease: the International Verapamil-Trandolapril Study (INVEST): a randomised controlled trial. *JAMA* 2003;290:2805–2816.

198. Neaton JD, Grimm RH, Prineas RJ, et al. Treatment of Mild Hypertension Study. Final results. Treatment of Mild Hypertension Study Research Group. *JAMA* 1993;270:713–724.

199. Hansson L, Lindholm LH, Ekbom T, et al. Randomised trial of old and new antihypertensive drugs in elderly patients: cardiovascular mortality and morbidity. The Swedish Trial in Old Patients with Hypertension-2 study. *Lancet* 1999;354:1751–1756.

200. Hansson L, Lindholm LH, Niskanen L, et al. Effect of angiotensin-converting enzyme inhibition compared with conventional therapy on cardiovascular morbidity and mortality in hypertension: the Captopril Prevention Project (CAPPP) randomised trial. *Lancet* 1999;353:611–616.

201. Peto R. Failure of randomisation by "sealed" envelope. *Lancet* 1999;354:73.

202. Dahlöf B, Devereux RB, Kjeldson SE, et al; for the LIFE study group. Cardiovascular morbidity and mortality in the Losartan Intervention For Endpoint reduction in hypertension study (LIFE): a randomised trial against atenolol. *Lancet* 2002;359:995–1003.

203. Lindholm LH, Ibsen H, Borch-Johnsen K, et al; for the LIFE Study Group. Risk of new-onset diabetes in the Losartan Intervention For Endpoint reduction in hypertension study. *J Hypertens* 2002;20:1879–1886.

204. Lithell H, Hansson L, Skoog I, et al; for the SCOPE Study Group. The Study of Cognition and Prognosis in the Elderly (SCOPE): principal results of randomised double-blind intervention trial. *J Hypertens* 2003;21:875–886.

205. Pfeffer MA, Swedberg K, Granger CB, et al. CHARM Investigators and Committees: Effects of candesartan on mortality and morbidity in patients with chronic heart failure: the CHARM-Overall programme. *Lancet* 2003;362:759–766.

206. Julius S, Kjeldsen SE, Weber M, et al; for the VALUE trial group. Outcomes in hypertensive patients at high cardiovascular risk treated with regimens based on valsartan or amlodipine: the VALUE randomised trial. *Lancet* 2004;363:2022–2031.

207. Lindholm LH, Persson M, Alaupovic P, et al. Metabolic outcomes during 1 year in newly detected hypertensives: results of the Antihypertensive Treatment and Lipid Profile in a North of Sweden Efficacy Evaluation (ALPINE study). *J Hypertens* 2003;21:1563–1574.

208. Mason JM, Dickinson HO, Nicolson DJ, et al. The diabetogenic potential of thiazide-type diuretics and beta-blocker combinations in patients with hypertension. *J Hypertens* 2005;23:1777–1781.

209. Helderman JH, Elahi D, Anderson DK, et al. Prevention of the glucose intolerance of thiazide diuretics by maintenance of body potassium. *Diabetes* 1983;32:106–111.

210. Kurtz TW, Pravenec M. Antidiabetic mechanisms of angiotensin-converting enzyme inhibitors and angiotensin II receptor antagonists: beyond the renin-angiotensin system. *J Hypertens* 2004;22:2253–2261.

211. Hovens MMC, Tamsma JK, Beishuizen ED, Huisman MV. Pharmacological strategies to reduce cardiovascular risk in type 2 diabetes mellitus. An update. *Drugs* 2005;65:433–445.

212. Julius S, Gudbrandsson T, Jamerson KA, et al. The haemodynamic link between insulin resistance and hypertension. *J Hypertens* 1991;9:983–986.

213. Carlsson P-O, Berne C, Jansson L. Angiotensin II and the endocrine pancreas: effects on islet blood flow and insulin secretion in rats. *Diabetologia* 1998;41:127–133.

214. Sharma AM, Janke J, Gorzelniak K, et al. Angiotensin blockade prevents type 2 diabetes by promotion of fat cells. *Hypertension* 2002;40:609–611.

215. Bartnik M, Malmberg K, Norhammar A, et al. Newly detected abnormal glucose tolerance: an important predictor of long-term outcome after myocardial infarction. *Eur Heart J* 2004;25:1990–1997.

216. Dunder K, Lind L, Zethelius B, et al. Increase in blood glucose concentration during antihypertensive treatment as a predictor of myocardial infarction: population based cohort study. *BMJ* 2003;326:681–684.

217. Eberly LE, Cohen JD, Prineas RP, Yang L; for the MRFIT Research Group. Impact of incident diabetes and incident non fatal cardiovascular disease on 18-year mortality. *Diabetes Care* 2003;26:848–854.

218. Kostis JB, Wilson AC, Freudenberger RS, et al; for the SHEP Collaborative Research Group. Long-term effect of diuretic-based therapy on fatal outcomes in subjects with isolated systolic hypertension with and without diabetes. *Am J Cardiol* 2005;45:29–35.

219. Verdecchia P, Reboldi G, Angeli F, et al. Adverse prognostic significance of new diabetes in treated hypertensive subjects. *Hypertension* 2004;43:963–969.

220. Von Eckardstein A, Schulte H, Assmann G. Risk for diabetes mellitus in middle-aged Caucasian male participants of the PROCAM study: implications for the definition of impaired fasting glucose by the Am Diabetes Association. *J Clin Endocrinol Metab* 2000;85:3101–3108.

221. Fox CS, Coady S, Sorlie PD, et al. Trends in cardiovascular complications of diabetes. *JAMA* 2004;292:2495–2499.

222. Saadine JB, Engelgau MM, Beckles GL, et al. A diabetes report card for the United States: quality of care in the 1990s. *Ann Intern Med* 2002;136:565–574.

22 | Ethnic considerations in hypertension

Donna S. Hanes, Charlotte Jones-Burton and Matthew R. Weir

CLINICAL PHARMACOLOGY AND THERAPEUTICS OF HYPERTENSION **VOL 25**

INTRODUCTION

Ethnic variations in blood pressure (BP) have been documented in the medical literature for three-quarters of a century. In 1932, Adams first reported a 7 mmHg higher systolic BP among African-American workmen compared to white workmen in New Orleans.[1] Since then, numerous population-based studies have confirmed that African-Americans, indeed, have higher rates of hypertension, even during childhood years.[2] Moreover, the subsequent cardiovascular and renal injury due to hypertension is more severe in African-Americans. Increasing interest is now focusing on other ethnic/racial minorities, particularly non-black Hispanics, Asians and American Indians, who are making up a more substantial part of the general population of the USA. Currently, the rates of hypertension appear to be similar to those in African-Americans.

Hypertension is the most common primary diagnosis worldwide. In the USA it affects 65 million adults. Racial and ethnic minorities are disproportionately represented in this number. Recently, Vasan reported follow-up data on the Framingham population indicating that even patients with 'normal' (<140/90 mmHg) BP were at higher risk for cardiovascular events compared to those with optimal control (<120/80 mmHg).[3] The normotensive patients were also twice as likely to develop high BP over 4 years, warranting more aggressive efforts of detection and management at early stages.[3] In view of the increased prevalence of hypertension among some ethnic groups and the enormous impact that modification of BP can have on morbidity and mortality, it is prudent for healthcare providers to individualize management strategies with race/ethnicity in mind. Furthermore, from a societal perspective, these groups should be targeted for screening in an effort to increase the awareness of their increased risk of mortality.[4]

This chapter will: (1) summarize what we currently know about the epidemiology of hypertension among ethnic groups, (2) examine the association of increased disease rates with lower socioeconomic status, (3) highlight genetic and pathophysiological derangements that contribute to a slightly different disease in African-Americans than that seen in whites, (4) report the results of recent clinical hypertension trials in ethnic subgroups, and (5) offer a comprehensive management approach to ethnic patients with hypertension that will facilitate achieving appropriate BP goals and minimize target organ injury.

CLINICAL EPIDEMIOLOGY

The overall prevalence of hypertension among people over the age of 18 is estimated to be 31.1% of the US population, a 30% increase over the last 10 years.[5,6] Currently, 48 million non-Hispanic whites, nine million non-Hispanic blacks, three million Mexican Americans and five million other adults have hypertension.[6] However, the incidence, severity and response to treatment of hypertension vary considerably by age and race as well as geographic location. The Third National Health and Nutrition Examination Survey (NHANES III) demonstrated that among all men aged 49–59 years, the rates of hypertension in Southern states far exceed the prevalence in the north, regardless of race.[5]

African-Americans

Although African-Americans make up only 12% of the population, 32.4% have hypertension, compared with 23.3 % of non-Hispanic whites. Among individuals aged 60–79 years, the prevalence in African-Americans is exceedingly high, such that by the age of 65 years, 65% of African-American men and 75% of African-American women are hypertensive (Fig. 22.1). Furthermore, severe hypertension is five times more common in African-Americans.

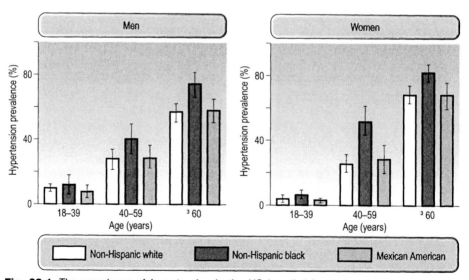

Fig. 22.1 The prevalence of hypertension in the US by ethnicity. *(Adapted from reference #5, permission requested.)*

These trends have been reported in children as young as 6 years and persist through adolescence, although environmental factors and differences in body mass contribute to this effect. The National Heart, Lung, and Blood Institute (NHLBI) recently released data demonstrating an average increase in systolic and diastolic BP in children of 2 mmHg over the last 15 years. This trend was found across all ethnic groups studied. Although this may not appear significant, it could have serious consequences, as it corresponds to a 10% greater risk of developing hypertension as an adult.[7]

The morbidity and mortality of hypertension in African-Americans far exceeds that of other groups. Although heart disease and stroke rates have declined in the last decade, the age-adjusted rates for African-Americans remain higher (Fig. 22.2). Recent literature suggests that the age-adjusted heart disease rate is 29% higher among African-Americans, with over 50% greater mortality. In 2001, the death rates per 100 000 population due to high BP were 13.7 for white males, 47.8 for black males, 13.4 for white females, and 38.9 for black females (Fig. 22.2). The stroke rate is 40% higher, with 80% greater mortality, and the risk for the development of hypertensive-related end-stage renal disease (ESRD) is no less than 320% higher among African-Americans than in the general population. These differences may be, in part, related to underlying genetic factors, but also underscores the importance of the socioeconomic barriers to care and inadequate treatment among minorities. For example, 65% of hypertensive African-American men under the age of 50 are aware that they have hypertension, but only 32% are treated and only 18% achieve adequate control. Similarly, 75% of African-American women are aware of their hypertension, but the control rate only reaches 23%. In comparison, in the general hypertensive population, 53% of patients are treated and 24% achieve adequate control.

Hispanic Americans

Historically, use of the term 'minority' in the hypertension literature has focused on African-Americans. There is little published information about this disease in other minorities. Persons of Hispanic or Latino descent currently make up approximately 6.5% of the US population, and represent the fastest growing segment. At this rate, Hispanics may surpass African-Americans as

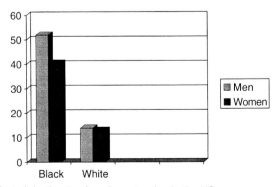

Fig. 22.2 Age adjusted death rates from hypertension in the US.

the largest US minority group. Most of the studies on hypertension in Hispanics are on Mexican Americans, which may not be generalizable to all Hispanics. One of the greatest problems studying this segment of the population is that, traditionally, Hispanics included anyone whose primary language was Spanish. As pointed out by Pickering, a white Cuban exile living in Miami will have very little in common with a Mexican immigrant living in Texas. Yet they are included in the same category for study purposes.[8,9]

Early studies suggested that Hispanics do not experience increased death rates compared with whites, despite their relatively lower socioeconomic status.[9,10] According to the National Center for Health Statistics, the age-adjusted death rate for whites is 121.9 per 100 000, versus 183.3 for African-Americans and 82.4 for Hispanics. The corresponding numbers for stroke are 23.3, 41.4 and 19. Interestingly, Hispanics experience lower death rates despite being 25% less likely than non-Hispanics to be treated with antihypertensive medications.[11]

The available data regarding hypertension in the Hispanic population are surprisingly sparse. In comparison with African-Americans, who have the highest prevalence of hypertension (33%), Mexican Americans have the lowest prevalence (20.7%); whites occupy an indeterminate position (28.9%). These lower rates do not correlate with better hypertension control since only 40% of Mexican Americans were receiving antihypertensive treatment, compared with 63% for whites and 60% for African-Americans. Data from NHANES III also indicate significant racial, ethnic and socioeconomic disparities in the clustering of cardiovascular risk factors, including diabetes, dyslipidaemia, hypertension and smoking.[12] Twenty per cent of non-Hispanic whites had no cardiac risk factors, versus 18% of Mexican Americans and 13% of non-Hispanic blacks. Non-Hispanic blacks were twice as likely to have four to five risk factors. Thus, the relationship between hypertension, ethnicity and socioeconomic status is complex and warrants further study.

Mexican Americans also have a greater prevalence of diabetes and obesity compared with blacks and non-Hispanic whites. The issues surrounding mortality rates from these causes have not been fully established, but are clearly linked to income. Hispanic males, aged 25–64 years, experience a twofold increase in mortality when family income drops from >$17 000 per year to <$10 000 per year.[13]

Non-Mexican Hispanics

Non-Mexican Hispanics fare as poorly as their Mexican counterparts. In small studies, <50% of Puerto Ricans with hypertension knew they were hypertensive and only 22% of those individuals achieved adequate BP control.[14] Similarly, only 28% of Cuban hypertensives reach target BP. Among all the subgroups of Hispanics, prevalence of hypertension in the USA significantly exceeds that of Hispanics in their native countries, possibly because of increased salt ingestion and psychological stress.

Because Hispanics tend to have obesity, dyslipidaemia and insulin resistance rates greater than in other groups, efforts to characterize the underlying pathophysiology are underway. Compared with normotensives, hypertensive Mexican Americans have higher plasma norepinephrine levels, greater ventricular wall mass, and more increased carotid wall thickness. These findings contrast with observations in African-Americans, who have lower sympathetic tone.[15] The clinical implications may be that hypertensive Latinos benefit significantly from preferential blockage of sympathetic tone. Clinical trials that optimize antihypertensive treatment in this group are eagerly awaited.

The San Antonio Heart Study is one of the few studies examining the prevalence of hypertension in a more homogenous population.[16] This large, prospective study was important for several reasons. It demonstrated that Mexican Americans had rates of obesity and type 2 diabetes significantly higher than in whites. It also helped resolve the 'Hispanic paradox' in which earlier studies found lower death rates in Hispanics compared with whites, despite the higher incidence of other cardiac risk factors. This study demonstrated a 60% higher mortality rate from cardiovascular disease in Hispanics compared with whites.

From a clinical perspective, very little has been published about the nature of hypertension in Hispanics, or the response to therapy. The Hispanic Health and Nutrition Examination Survey (1982–1984) demonstrated that dietary intake and specific nutrients did not significantly correlate with hypertension in Mexican, Cuban and Puerto Rican women. As expected, age and body mass composition were strongly correlated with hypertension.[17,18] Many studies have demonstrated that African-Americans are more likely than whites to have a non-dipping diurnal BP, which correlates with increased target organ injury. The only study performed in Mexican Americans showed that men, but not women, were more likely to be non-dippers than whites.[19]

Asian Americans

While little is known about hypertension in Hispanics, even less is known about the disease in Asian Americans. One large study from California found that Filipino men and women had the highest prevalence of hypertension, whereas Japanese and other Asian men had rates similar to those in Caucasians.[20] Furthermore, the prevalence of overweight and obesity among Filipino women has increased nearly sixfold from 6% in 1983, to 35% in 1999.[21] This dramatic trend of increasing weight represents a serious health concern in light of the strong association between excess weight and hypertension. In Japanese Americans, visceral adiposity has recently been shown to be predictive of incident hypertension.[22] Moreover, the incidence of insulin resistance and the metabolic syndrome rises linearly with BP in Japanese.[23]

Japanese men living in Japan experience coronary heart disease death rates significantly lower than do those residing in the USA, despite higher incidence rates of smoking and hypertension. This has been attributed to lower risk from other risk factors. In Japan, serum haemoglobin A1c, body mass index, and serum total and low-density lipoprotein levels are lower, and high-density lipoprotein levels are higher than those in the US Japanese population.[24]

Among younger adults, one study demonstrated that Asian girls had the highest prevalence of hypertension (13% versus 7% in non-Asians) and 23% of Asian boys were hypertensive versus 18% of others.[25] Other studies have not confirmed this finding, but have demonstrated that the frequency of obesity and smoking in younger Asians is increasing at an alarming rate.[2]

THE INFLUENCE OF SOCIOECONOMIC STATUS ON HEALTH

Ethnic minorities include a disproportionate number of persons with lower economic status, education and health status. Compared with Caucasians, African-Americans and Hispanics are 200 and 300%, respectively, less likely to complete 12 years of school. This lack of education correlates with a lower income level. Deprivation undoubtedly contributes to health disparities in the USA as it forces people to live in unsafe and crowded environments, and denies access to healthy eating habits and regular medical care. Lower socio-economic status is correlated with increased cardiac risk factors and coronary disease mortality as well as end-stage renal disease.[26,27]

There is compelling evidence supporting the association between lifestyle and health status. Epidemiological studies frequently use education and income as surrogate markers and predictors of dietary patterns, environment and level of physical activity, in addition to health-related seeking behaviours and access to medical care. The Hypertension Detection and Follow-up Program (HDFP) recruited over 40 000 participants to assess the impact of economic status on the incidence, prevalence and outcome of hypertension in African-Americans.[28] In this community-based study, the incidence of hypertension was twofold greater in African-Americans. Moreover, in both African-Americans and whites there was an inverse relationship between level of education and the prevalence of hypertension. However, even whites with the lowest level of education had less hypertension than the most, well-educated blacks. Further, when free medical information and medications were dispensed in a stepped-care subgroup, the inverse correlation between educational level and mortality was eliminated, implying that the poor prognosis associated with being African-American may partially be eliminated by improving access to care.[13]

Ooi et al. confirmed this finding in a New York population.[29] When African-Americans and whites were given equal access to care through their worksite, the African-Americans achieved similar BP reductions and actually experienced a lower rate of cardiovascular disease. This finding was not reproduced when examining the impact of improved diabetes management in ethnic minorities.[30]

The Treatment of Mild Hypertension Study (TOMHS) was a multi-centred, randomized, placebo-controlled trial examining the efficacy of different classes of antihypertensive medications in adults with stage I (mild) diastolic hypertension.[31] Subsequent analysis of the data revealed that there were discrepant levels of urinary sodium and potassium between African-Americans and whites, and these differences correlated with socioeconomic levels. Specifically, African-Americans, but not whites, had higher urinary sodium levels and sodium to potassium ratios; this was particularly apparent among those with lower incomes and educational levels. It has been suggested that, if the finding reflects widespread ethnic differences in dietary electrolyte intakes, it may partially explain the higher prevalence of hypertension and target organ damage among African-Americans.

Whether racial discrimination influences access-related outcomes is controversial and difficult to examine in clinical trials. More insight about such racial disparities should be gained from the ongoing Jackson Heart Study. This is an NHLBI-sponsored, prospective cohort of over 6500 African-American men and women from Jackson, MI, including over 400 families.[32] This study is designed to track the cardiovascular-health-related progress of African-Americans over their lifetime; the study design parallels that of the Framingham Study. It is the largest study of African-Americans in the world, and will likely yield vast amounts of information.

PATHOPHYSIOLOGY OF HYPERTENSION

Since the highest rates of hypertension occur in African-Americans there may be a distinct, definable, difference between African-Americans and whites in the basic pathophysiological mechanisms of primary hypertension. Currently, there is little evidence to support this theory, but there are several intriguing findings. Compared with whites, African-Americans have earlier and more severe arterial stiffness, which may predispose to earlier vascular injury.[33] There is also a greater frequency of salt-sensitivity among African-Americans. In many sub-Saharan black populations where the salt intake does not exceed 50 mmol/day, there is no hypertension and BP does not rise with age. This may suggest that extreme salt restriction would significantly lessen the burden of hypertension. Even lowering dietary salt in African-American high school students can significantly lower BP.

The salt-induced rise in BP in African-Americans exceeds that found in whites and Hispanics. Consequently, African-Americans experience an earlier rise in BP compared with whites as dietary salt increases. In both the acute and chronic setting, normotensive and hypertensive African-Americans have BP responsiveness to salt greater than that of whites. Moreover, those persons who do have a salt-related pressure increment tend to have delayed renal sodium excretion and lower plasma renin (Table 22.1).[34]

ROLE OF GENETICS

Historically, investigators have focused on the 'Slavery Hypothesis' as an explanation for the ethnic variation in the incidence of hypertension, particularly among African-Americans.[35] This theory suggests that the enhanced

Table 22.1 Proposed pathogenetic markers in hypertensive blacks

Genotypic variations: renin, angiotensin, angiotensinogen, kallikrein, renal sodium channel
Hormonal and physiological differences
Deficiency in natriuretic vasodilatory renal system
Sympathetic nervous dysfunction or greater sensitivity
Higher plasma volume and lower renin
Increased salt sensitivity
Reduced NO production
Increased sodium:potassium ratio in the urine
Increased arterial stiffness
Differences in erythrocyte cation transport
Delayed renal sodium excretion
Earlier rise in blood pressure
Decreased potassium intake

ability to conserve sodium in the kidney offered a survival advantage to African blacks living in a dry, hot environment devoid of access to salt. This salt avidity also facilitated survival during the transatlantic crossing, which was plagued by dehydration from gastrointestinal losses and a lack of food and water. Subsequently, when the slaves reached America, the cooler environment and easy access to salt perpetuated increased salt reabsorption and hypertension. While attractive, there are no data to support this hypothesis.

Although members of specific ethnic groups would be expected to share similar genes, a role in the causality of hypertension has not been established. Certainly in African-Americans and Hispanics such associations have been described, but understanding of the complex interplay between specific genes and the environment is still in its infancy.[36] There are data to support specific genetic associations of hypertension in African-Americans and Hispanics, but these do not appear to differ from those in other groups.[37] Researchers are actively seeking specific mutations in the genes for renin, angiotensinogen, angiotensin, kallikrein and others to explain ethnic differences in hypertension.

A particularly attractive candidate gene to explain ethnic variation, at least in part, may be that related to the epithelial sodium channel (EnaC), located in the cortical collecting duct of the nephron. This channel is responsible for reabsorption of sodium from the urine. Potentiation of this channel's activity will lead to increased sodium reabsorption, increased effective circulating blood volume, and low renin, salt-sensitive hypertension. Certain polymorphisms of this gene have been identified. One allele in particular is present in up to 6% of persons of African descent, but absent in whites.[38] Intuitively, this may help explain the remarkable antihypertensive effectiveness of drugs that block sodium reabsorption, such as diuretics and calcium antagonists, in African-Americans.

Other abnormalities in sodium transport have also been described in African-Americans. They tend to have higher intracellular sodium content, increased fibroblast sodium-hydrogen antiport activity and reduced RBC sodium-potassium co-transport.[39] What contribution these abnormalities have to the development of hypertension remains unknown, as such changes may not represent primary abnormalities, but may be secondary to volume expansion.

African-Americans also exhibit a nocturnal natriuresis greater than do whites.[40] Normally, there is a significant day–night variation in sodium excretion, which parallels BP changes. In normotensive persons, the lowest BPs at night occur during the period of greatest sodium reabsorption. It seems likely that decreased BP drives reduced sodium excretion. An associated finding involves the loss of nocturnal 'dip' of BP frequently seen in African-Americans. Indeed, even in normotensive African-Americans, there is a significant loss of the nocturnal BP decline that is associated with increased urinary sodium excretion, both of which are associated with low renin.[41]

It has been suggested that increased sodium consumption and decreased potassium intake among African-Americans may contribute to differences in BP. In keeping with this alternative theory, it has been demonstrated that dietary salt restriction helps reduce BP in all ethnic groups, and controlling for salt sensitivity diminishes race-related differences in the antihypertensive response to therapy.[42]

Another hypothesis for the clinical differences in BP is that while ethnic minorities do not have enhanced sympathetic system neuroendocrine activation, despite increased life stresses, they may have greater tissue sensitivity to adrenergic stimulation compared with whites. African-Americans have exaggerated vascular responses to physical stressors. This response does not appear to be mediated by the α_2-adrenergic receptor.[43]

Recent efforts to explain ethnic disparities in BP have started to focus on the early target organ injury from hypertension. Impairment of arterial dilatation occurs earlier than arterial wall thickening in the atherosclerotic process. African-Americans have accelerated large arterial wall stiffness and this occurs earlier in the process of hypertension compared with whites.[33] It is possible that this is a result of impaired nitric oxide (NO) balance. African-Americans have enhanced inactivation of vasodilatory NO within the endothelium in the presence of oxidative stress.[44] Clinically, this theory explains why African-Americans tend to have a blunted coronary vasodilatory response when compared to whites.[45]

TARGET ORGAN DAMAGE

Whatever the mechanism for the development of more severe hypertension, there is unequivocal evidence that there is a strong and independent relationship between hypertension and stroke, coronary artery disease, congestive heart failure and end-stage kidney disease.[46]

Left ventricular hypertrophy

The early cardiac response to increased systemic pressure includes the development of left ventricular hypertrophy (LVH), which subsequently leads to congestive heart failure (CHF). A 20 mmHg increase in BP increases the relative risk of LVH by 43% in men, and 25% in women.[47] Although the prevalence of CHF appears to be similar in all ethnic groups, African-Americans with LVH have up to 50% higher risk of hospitalization compared with non-blacks, and over two-fold higher mortality, even in the absence of coronary disease.[48] For women, the risk is even greater. Furthermore, hypertensive African-American men are more than twice as likely as hypertensive whites to develop LVH.[49]

LVH is not only a risk factor for coronary heart disease and death, but also for ischaemic stroke. Concentric hypertrophy as a result of hypertension is associated with a 2.5-fold higher risk for ischaemic stroke, after adjustment for other risk factors. Since stroke is a leading cause of death, the potential to reverse LVH may have enormous health implications.

African-Americans are burdened by a disproportionate accumulation of risk factors for stroke, including diabetes, and may develop more severe complications. They tend to have more subarachnoid haemorrhages, lacunar infarcts and large intracranial occlusive disease, as well as a higher incidence of cerebral infarction. Younger patients have a risk for ischaemic stroke two-to threefold higher than whites, and are more likely to die as a result.[50]

Renal disease

The burden of kidney disease among African-Americans and other minorities illustrates the huge ethnic disparity that results from hypertension.[51] Not only do African-Americans have the highest rate of end-stage renal disease, they also have much higher rates of chronic kidney disease. From the NHANES III population, it is estimated that 19.5 million (or 11%) have chronic kidney disease (CKD), defined as an estimated glomerular filtration rate (EGFR) of less than 60 mL/minute/1.73 m^2 or the presence of albuminuria.[52] Extrapolating these data to the population as a whole, and applying the definitions of the National Kidney Foundation Kidney Disease Outcome Quality Initiative CKD staging criteria, the absolute number of patients with prevalent CKD can be estimated (Table 22.2).[53] There are approximately 5.9 million individuals (30.3%) with stage 1 disease (EGFR >90 mL/minute/1.73 m^2 or with microalbuminuria), 5.3 million (27.2%) with stage 2 disease (EGFR 60–89 mL/minute/1.73 m^2), 7.6 million (39%) with stage 3 disease (EGFR 30–59 mL/minute/1.73 m^2), 400 000 persons (2.1%) with stage 4 disease (EGFR 15–29 mL/minute/1.73 m^2), and 300 000 (1.5%) with stage 5 (kidney failure) (EGFR less than 15 mL/minute/1.73 m^2).

Although the incidence of kidney disease is increasing among all ethnic subgroups, the burden of disease is much more striking among minorities. Data from the United States Renal Disease Study (USRDS) show that African-Americans compared with whites have four times the incidence of kidney disease, followed in descending order by Native Americans, Asian Americans and non-Hispanic whites. While African-Americans comprise only 13% of the population, they represent 32% of the prevalent ESRD patients. Non-Hispanic blacks also have a high prevalence of CKD. In addition, African-Americans have a greater prevalence of risk factors for renal disease progression, such as anaemia, lower income, smoking, lead exposure and obesity.

A possible mechanism whereby African-Americans develop more severe renal injury secondary to hypertension involves renal sodium handling. Habitual consumption of salt causes chronic intermittent renal tubular hyperperfusion at the macula densa, resulting in resetting of the operating point for tubuloglomerular feedback. This resetting causes an imbalance between the afferent and efferent arteriole tone, a rise in glomerular capillary pressure, and subsequent glomerular hyperfiltration and injury.[54]

African-Americans, Hispanics, Native Americans and Asians not only have a greater prevalence of kidney disease, they have to face more barriers to high-quality care. These ethnic minorities are less likely to receive renal transplantation at initiation of renal replacement therapy.[55]

The Modification of Diet and Renal Disease Study provided suggested evidence that not only are African-Americans at higher risk for progression of kidney disease, but also that they benefit from rigorous control of BP.[56] In this study, the rate of loss of renal function as measured by iodothalamate

Table 22.2 Estimated prevalence of chronic kidney disease in the USA

Estimated glomerular filtration rate (mL/minute/1.73 m^2)	Estimated no. of affected individuals (millions)	% population
>90	5.9	33
60–89	5.3	27
30–59	7.6	39
15–29	0.4	2.1
<15	0.3	1.5

clearance over 3 years was 11 mL/minute in whites, but 18 mL/minute in African-Americans. This rate was reduced by 50% in those patients who achieved tight BP control (a mean arterial pressure <92 mmHg). This is particularly important as cardiovascular mortality is 10–30 times higher in patients with ESRD than the general population.

Even early kidney disease is an independent risk factor for cardiovascular mortality. In the Heart Outcomes Prevention Evaluation (HOPE) Study, cardiovascular disease was proportional to the level of urinary protein excretion.[57] Moreover, proteinuria was a predictor of cardiovascular disease mortality more powerful than known CAD or diabetes. In African-Americans, reduction in renal function predicts LV wall mass, and the associated lower haemoglobin level independently predicts increased LV diameter.[58] These findings explain, in part, the excessive cardiovascular disease risk observed among individuals with kidney disease.

Two landmark trials have provided insight into the management of hypertension in African-Americans: The African-American Study of Kidney (AASK) Disease and the Antihypertensive and Lipid Lowering Treatment to Prevent Heart Attack Trial (ALLHAT).[59,60] These are among the first clinical trials to include large enough numbers of minority patients to provide meaningful data.

AASK was a randomized, double-blind trial designed to answer two questions: does tight control of BP halt the progression of renal disease, and are certain antihypertensive agents more renoprotective in African-Americans with hypertensive kidney disease? One thousand and ninety four patients were enrolled, and randomized to a calcium blocker, an ACE inhibitor, or a β-blocker. At the completion of the trial, patients with proteinuria treated with the ACE inhibitor had a 36% reduction in the rate of loss of renal function compared with those assigned to the calcium channel blocker group. Similar renal function benefits were achieved with the β-blocker. However, a statistically significant reduction in the risk for reaching secondary endpoints (a decline in GFR, ESRD or death) was only achieved in patients randomized to the ACE inhibitor. This was the first trial to demonstrate the efficacy of inhibition of the renin–angiotensin–aldosterone system (RAAS) as first-line therapy for hypertension in the setting of renal disease in African-Americans (Fig. 22.3).

The AASK trial refuted the common clinical practice of avoiding ACE inhibitors in African-Americans due to a perceived reduced potency. It was clearly demonstrated that these drugs are effective, but frequently it is necessary to use higher doses. Furthermore, the AASK trial demonstrated that African-Americans can achieve target BP levels in the setting of persistent and rigorous treatment. Other studies have demonstrated that renoprotection in diabetics from minority groups can be achieved with amlodipine in the setting of concurrent angiotensin receptor blocker use (Fig. 22.4).[61] All of these trials highlighted that the majority of patients required multiple agents (three to four) to control BP.

ALLHAT is the largest antihypertensive trial to date. Although the target was to enroll 55% African-Americans, the final number was approximately 15 000 (35%). This provided adequate power for meaningful interpretation. Patients were randomized to one of three initial therapies: (1) a thiazide-like diuretic (chlorthalidone), (2) an ACE inhibitor (lisinopril) or (3) a calcium channel blocker (amlodipine). Additional drugs from other classes were added as needed.

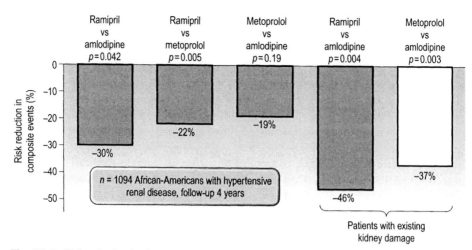

Fig. 22.3 Risk reduction in glomerular filtration rate, end stage renal disease, or death demonstrating the superiority of the ACE inhibitor over a beta-blocker or calcium antagonist in African-American patients with hypertensive renal disease. *(Adapted from reference #59.)*

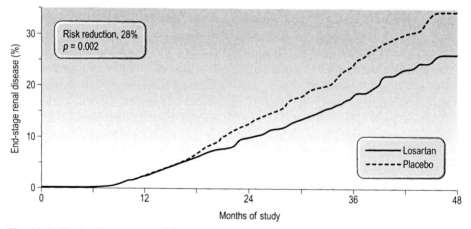

Fig. 22.4 Kaplan-Meier curves of the percentage of patients developing end stage renal disease over 3.4 years in the RENAAL trial. *(Adapted from reference #61.)*

Initial data from all patients showed a greater reduction in systolic BP with chlorthalidone compared with lisinopril (2 mmHg difference) or amlodipine (1 mmHg difference). The difference was even more marked in the African-Americans, where chlorthalidone resulted in a BP reduction 4 mmHg greater than with lisinopril.[62] The rate of the primary outcome of fatal coronary heart disease or non-fatal myocardial infarction was equivalent in the three arms; but the rate of stroke was 15% higher among patients in the lisinopril group. Events in African-Americans accounted for most of the increased risk. It has been suggested that the 4 mmHg difference in BP between the two groups was responsible for this outcome.[62]

These results suggest that a thiazide-like diuretic may be more effective than ACE inhibitors in African-Americans, and should be included in every antihypertensive drug regimen. Since diuretics potentiate the effects of ACE inhibitors in African-Americans and most patients require more than one medication, the combination is probably much more effective than either agent alone.

ALLHAT also showed that BP control was worse in African-Americans than in non-blacks.[63] The overall control rate in the whole population was 65.6%, but in African-American men, it was 63.3% versus 70% in non-African-American men and 58.8% in African-American women versus 65.2% in white women. Whether this difference is explained by varying pathophysiology or lifestyles is unknown. The greater degree of salt sensitivity in the African-American population may have contributed to less effective BP control, but the inadequate use of multi-drug regimens is likely to have been an important contributory factor.

CLINICAL MANAGEMENT OF HYPERTENSION IN ETHNIC POPULATIONS

The purpose of treating hypertension is to avoid target organ injury, and reduce morbidity and mortality. In order to achieve adequate BP control in any patient, hypertension must be identified and appropriate drugs selected, and taken. Importantly, most patients will require combination therapy (two to four drugs) to reach targeted levels. It is prudent to inform the patients of this when initiating therapy, so dose adjustments or the need to add other drugs is no surprise. Patients at high risk for cardiovascular injury, including ethnic minority groups, should have lower BP targets.[64] Otherwise there is no evidence that BP targets should be lowered. As stated previously, the JNC7 recommends BP be lowered to <140/70 mmHg in uncomplicated hypertension, and <130/80 mmHg in those patients with kidney disease or diabetes. The Working Group of the Institute for Study of Hypertension in Blacks (ISHIB) recommends starting with combination therapy in African-Americans when SBP or DBP is greater than 15 mmHg and 10 mmHg, respectively, above target. There is no evidence at present that treatment in other minority groups should differ from that in whites.

Selection of drugs

In general, the selection of antihypertensive drug should be dictated by concurrent co-morbidities, as described in the JNC7 report.[64,65] However, it is important to consider the high incidence of obesity in ethnic minorities, and the potential for adverse drug reactions. Hispanic and American Indian patients may have a greater likelihood of developing insulin resistance or diabetes with hyperlipidaemia when treated with thiazides or β-blockers.[13] If such therapy is selected, the dose should be the lowest possible. Trials in Hispanics have confirmed declines in hyperlipidaemia and new-onset diabetes in patients treated with calcium antagonists and ACE inhibitors compared with thiazide diuretics. Moreover, the HOPE, ALLHAT, and VALUE trials demonstrated a lower incidence of new diabetes occurring in patients receiving ACE inhibitors or angiotensin receptor blockers (ARBs) as part of their medication regimen.[57,60,67]

Multiple studies confirm that there is no significant difference between whites, Hispanics or Asians in the antihypertensive response to various medications. However, there is widespread belief that there are different responses in African-Americans. Many studies show that African-Americans respond to diuretics better than do whites, and respond less well, if not poorly, to β-blockers and ACE inhibitors (Fig. 22.5). Clinical trials have shown that there is a different BP response pattern to ACE inhibitors in different ethnic groups, even after controlling for salt sensitivity (Fig. 22.6).[42] African-Americans do not respond as well as Caucasians and Hispanics whether on high- or low-salt diets (Fig. 22.7).

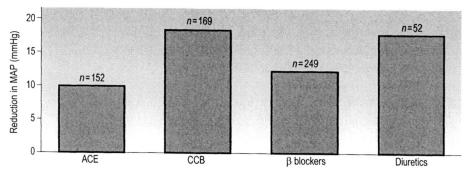

Fig. 22.5 Average mean reduction in blood pressure from prospective trials involving African-Americans.

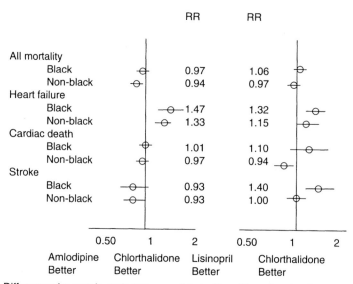

Fig. 22.6 Differences by race in endpoints associated with antihypertensive therapy with lisinopril, amlodipine and chlorthalidone. RR=relative risk. (*Adapted from reference #60.*)

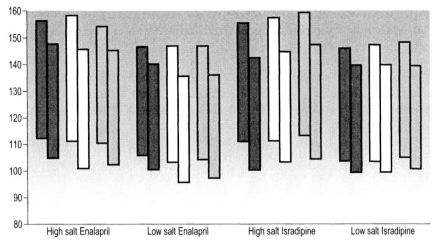

Fig. 22.7 Blood pressure reductions (placebo in the First column, drug therapy in the second column, in mmHg) with enalapril and isradipine (low and high Dose combined) in salt-sensitive black (diagonal bars), White (hollow bars), and Hispanic (horizontal bars) on high and low salt diets. (*Adapted from reference #42, with permission.*)

Such discrepancies in response have led many practitioners to avoid using ACE inhibitors/angiotensin receptor antagonists (ARB) even when they would be appropriate. These notions are not well founded since there is substantial evidence that ACE inhibitors/ARBs are effective in African-Americans if higher doses are used or they are combined with a thiazide diuretic or calcium antagonist.[66,67] Yet, even in large clinical trials, African-Americans are frequently under-dosed with ACE inhibitors or ARBs, thus perpetuating less favourable clinical outcomes. Currently, potential differences in antihypertensive efficacy are not valid reasons to withhold treatment with these drugs from patients with other compelling indications for their use, such as diabetes, proteinuria, CHF or renal disease.[64,65]

Does treatment of hypertension confer the same protection across ethnic groups?

Treatment of hypertension has resulted in a marked decline in cardiovascular death rates over the last 40 years. This trend is true regardless of gender, socioeconomic status or race. However, there is significant racial disparity in the magnitude of the decline. According to NHANES III, both African-Americans and whites achieved a 58% reduction in cerebrovascular accidents, but blacks had only a 25% reduction in cardiac events. Data are not available for Hispanic or Asian groups.

CONCLUSIONS

Ethnic variations in the incidence of hypertension and response to therapy are important clinical concerns. More needs to be learned about possible genetic and biological differences in the disease process and how this may help in specific treatment strategies. In the meantime, early identification and education of people at high risk, proper lifestyle modification and careful use of medications to achieve appropriate BP goals are the key mandates.

References

1. Adams JM. Some racial differences in blood pressure and morbidity in groups of white and colored workmen. *Am J Med Sci* 1932;184:342.
2. Sorof JM, Lai D, Poffenbarger T, et al. Overweight, ethnicity, and the prevalence of hypertension in school-aged children. *Pediatrics* 2004;113:475–482.
3. Vasan RS, Larson MG, Leip EP, et al. Impact of high-normal blood pressure on the risk of cardiovascular disease. *N Engl J Med* 2001;345:1291–1297.
4. McGill JB, Brown WW, Chen SC, et al. Kidney Early Evaluation Program (KEEP). Findings from a community-screening program. *Diabetes Educ* 2004;30:196–198.
5. Burt VL, Whelton P, Rocca EJ, et al. Prevalence of hypertension in the US adult population. Results from the Third National Health and Nutrition Examination Survey, 1988–1991. *Hypertension* 1995;25:305–313.
6. Fields LE, Burt VL, Cutler JA, et al. The burden of adult hypertension in the United States: 1999 to 2000. *Hypertension* 2004;44:398–404.
7. Muntner P, He J, Cutler JA, et al. Trends in blood pressure among children and adolescents. *JAMA* 2004;291:2107–2113.
8. Vergara C, Martin AM, Wang F, et al. Awareness about factors that affect the management of hypertension in Puerto Rican patients. *Conn Med* 2004;68(5):269–276.
9. Pickering TG. Hypertension in Hispanics. *J Clin Hypertension* 2004;6(5):279–282.
10. McGruder HF, Malarcher AM, Antione TL, et al. Racial and ethnic disparities in cardiovascular risk factors among stroke survivors. Unites States 1999 to 2001. *Stroke* 2004;10 [Epub ahead of print].
11. Raji MA, Kuo YF, Salazar JA, et al. Ethnic differences in antihypertensive medication use in the elderly. *Ann Pharmacother* 2004;38:209–214.
12. Sharma S, Malarcher AM, Giles WH, et al. Racial, ethnic and socioeconomic disparities in the clustering of cardiovascular disease risk factors. *Ethn Dis* 2004;14(1):43–48.
13. Jamerson K, DeQuattro V. The impact of ethnicity on response to antihypertensive therapy. *Am J Med* 1996;101:22S–32S.
14. Barrios E, Iler E, Mulloy K, et al. Hypertension in the Hispanic and black population in New York City. *J Natl Med Assoc* 1987;79:749–752.
15. Li D, DeQuattro V, Hseuh W, et al. Neurogenic factors, insulin and salt, on cardiovascular hypertrophy of hypertensives and their offspring. *Am J Hypertens* 1996;9:124A.
16. Haffner SM. Obesity and the metabolic syndrome: the San Antonio Heart Study. *Br J Nutr* 2000;83:S67–S70.
17. Goslar PW, Macera CA, Castellanos LG, et al. Blood pressure in Hispanic women: the role of diet, acculturation, and physical activity. *Ethn Dis* 1997;7:106–113.
18. Afghani A, Abbott AV, Wiswell RA, et al. Central adiposity, aerobic fitness, and blood pressure in premenopausal Hispanic women. *Int J Sports Med* 2004;25:599–606.
19. Hyman DJ, Ogbonnaya K, Taylor AA, et al. Ethnic differences in nocturnal blood pressure decline in treated hypertensives. *Am J Hypertens* 2000;13(8):884–891.
20. Klatsky AL, Armstrong MA. Cardiovascular risk factors among Asian Americans living in Northern California. *Am J Public Health* 1991;81:1423–1428.
21. Adair LS. Dramatic rise in overweight and obesity in adult Filipino women and risk of hypertension. *Obesity Research* 2004;12:1335–1341.
22. Hyashi T, Boyko EJ, Leonetti DL, et al. Visceral adiposity is an independent predictor of incident hypertension in Japanese Americans. *Ann Intern Med* 2004;140:992–1000.
23. Kanauchi M, Kanauchi K, Hashimoto T, et al. Metabolic syndrome and new category 'pre-hypertension' in a Japanese population. *Curr Med Res Opin* 2004;20:1365–1370.
24. Ueshima H, Okayama A, Saitoh S, et al. INTERLIPID Research Group. Differences in cardiovascular disease risk factors between Japanese in Japan and Japanese-Americans in Hawaii: the INTERLIPID study. *J Hum Hypertens* 2003;17:631–639.
25. Hohn AR, Dwyer KM, Dwyer JH. Blood pressure in youth from four ethnic groups: the Pasedena Prevention Project. *J Pediatr* 1994;125:368–373.
26. Keil JE, Sutherland SE, Knapp RG, et al. Does equal socioeconomic status in black and white men equal risk of mortality? *Am J Public Health* 1992;82:1133–1136.
27. Klag MJ, Whelton PK, Randall BL, et al. End stage renal disease in African-American and white men:16-year MRFIT findings. *JAMA* 1997;277:1293–1298.

28. Hypertension Detection and Follow-up Program Cooperative Group. Race, education and the prevalence of hypertension. *Am J Epidemiol* 1977;106:351–361.

29. Ooi WL, Budner NS, Cohen H, et al. Impact of race on treatment response and cardiovascular disease among hypertensives. *Hypertension* 1989;14:227–234.

30. Harris MI. Racial and ethnic differences in health care access and health outcomes for adults with type II diabetes. *Diabetes Care* 2001;24:454–459.

31. Ganguli MC, Grimm RH, Svendsen KH, et al. Higher education and income are related to a better Na:K ratio in blacks. Baseline results from the Treatment of Mild Hypertension Study (TOMHS) data. *Am J Hypertens* 1997;10:979–984.

32. Sempos CT, Bild DE, Manolio TA. Overview of the Jackson Heart Study: A study of cardiovascular disease in African-American men and women. *Am J Med Sci* 1999;317:142–146.

33. Din-Dzietham R, Couper D, Evans G, et al. Arterial stiffness is greater in African Americans than in whites. *Am J Hypertens* 2004;17:304–313.

34. Falkner B. Differences in blacks and whites with essential hypertension: biochemistry and endocrine. State of the Art Lecture. *Hypertension* 1990;15:681–686.

35. Kaplan NM. Primary hypertension: natural history, special populations, and evaluation. In: *Clinical hypertension, 6th edn.* Philadelphia: Williams and Wilkins; 1985:129.

36. Kammerer CM, Gouin N, Samollow PB, et al. Two quantitative trait loci affect ACE activities in Mexican Americans. *Hypertension* 2004;43:466–470.

37. Bouzekri N, Zhu X, Jiang Y, et al. Angiotensin I-converting enzyme polymorphisms, ACE level and blood pressure among Nigerians, Jamaicans, and African Americans. *Eur J Hum Genet* 2004;12:460–468.

38. Nesbitt S, Victor RG. Pathogenesis of Hypertension in African Americans. *CHF* 2004;10:24–29.

39. Kaplan N. Primary hypertension: natural history, special populations, and evaluation. In: *Clinical hypertension, 6th edn.* Baltimore: Willliams and Wilkens; 1994:109–143.

40. Luft FC, Weinberger MH, Grim CE. Nocturnal urinary electrolyte excretion and its relationship to the renin system and sympathetic activity in normal and hypertensive man. *J Lab Clin Med* 1980;95:395.

41. Harshfield GA, Hwang C, Grim CE. Circadian variation of blood pressure in blacks: influence of age, gender and activity. *J Human Hypertension* 1990;4:43.

42. Weir MR, Chrysant SG, McCarron DA, et al. Influence of race and dietary salt on the antihypertensive efficacy of an angiotensin-converting enzyme inhibitor or a calcium channel antagonist in salt sensitive hypertensives. *Hypertension* 1998;31:1088–1096.

43. Muszkat M, Sofowora GG, Wood AJ, et al. Alpha-adrenergic receptor induced vascular constriction in blacks and whites. *Hypertension* 2004;43:31–35.

44. Kalinowski L, Dobrucki IT, Malinski T. Race-specific differences in endothelial function: predisposition of African-Americans to vascular diseases. *Circulation* 2004;109:2511–2517.

45. Houghton JL, Strogatz DS, Torosoff MT. African-Americans with LVH demonstrate depressed sensitivity of the coronary microcirculation to stimulated relaxation. *Hypertension* 2003;42:267–276.

46. Flack JM, Neaton JD, Daniels B, et al. Ethnicity and renal disease: lessons from the Multiple Risk Factor Intervention Trial and the Treatment of Mild Hypertension Study. *Am J Kidney Dis* 1993;21:31–40.

47. Levy D, Larson MG, Vason RS. The progression from hypertension to congestive heart failure. *JAMA* 1996;275:1557–1562.

48. Alexander M, Grumbach K, Selby J. Hospitalization for congestive heart failure: explaining racial differences. *JAMA* 1995;274:1037–1042.

49. Kizer JR, Arnett DK, Bella JN, et al. Differences in left ventricular structure between black and white hypertensive adults: the Hypertension Genetic Epidemiology Network Study. *Hypertension* 2004;43:1182–1188.

50. www.strokecenter.org/pat/stats.htm.

51. US Renal Data System. *USRDS Annual Data Report.* Bethesda, MD: The National Institutes of Health, National Institute of Diabetes and Digestive and Kidney Diseases.

52. Weiner DE, Tighiouart H, Amin MG, et al. Chronic kidney disease as a risk factor for cardiovascular disease and all-cause mortality: a pooled analysis of community-based studies. *J Am Soc Nephrol* 2004;15:1307–1315.

53. http://www.kidney.org/professionals/kdoqui/index.cfm

54. Aviv A, Hollenberg NK, Weder AB. Sodium glomerulopathy: tubuloglomerular feedback and renal injury in African-Americans. *Kidney Intern* 2004;65:361–368.

55. Lopes AA. Relationships of race and ethnicity to progression of kidney dysfunction and clinical outcomes in patients with chronic kidney failure. *Adv Ren Replace Ther* 2004;11:14–23.

56. Hunsicker LG, Adler S, Caggiula A. Predictors of the progression of renal disease in the Modification of Diet in Renal Disease Study. *Kidney Int* 1997;51:1908–1919.

57. The Heart Outcomes Prevention Evaluation Study Investigators. Effects of an angiotensin-converting-enzyme inhibitor, ramipril, on cardiovascular events in high-risk patients. *N Engl J Med* 2000;342:145–153.

58. Astor BC, Arnett DK, Brown A, et al. Association of kidney function and hemoglobin with left ventricular morphology among African-Americans: the atherosclerosis risk in communities (ARIC) study. *Am J Kidney Dis* 2004;43:836–845.

59. Agodoa L. African-American Study of Kidney Disease and Hypertension (AASK)-Clinical trial update. *Ethn Dis* 1998;8:249–253.

60. ALLHAT Officers and Coordinators for the ALLHAT Collaborative Research Group: major outcomes in high-risk hypertensive patients randomized to angiotensin-converting enzyme inhibitor or calcium channel blocker vs diuretic: The antihypertensive and lipid-lowering treatment to prevent heart attack trial (ALLHAT). *JAMA* 2002;288:2981–2997.

61. Brenner BM, Cooper ME, deZeeu D, et al. Effects of losartan on renal and cardiovascular outcomes in patients with type 2 diabetes and nephropathy. *N Engl J Med* 2001;345:861–869.

62. Ferdinand KC. Recommendations for the management of special populations: racial and ethnic populations. *Am J Hypertens* 2003;16:50S–54S.

63. Cushman WC, Ford CE, Cutler JA, et al; for the ALLHAT Collaborative Research Group: Success and predictors of blood pressure control in diverse North American settings: the antihypertensive and lipid-lowering treatment to prevent heart attack trial (ALLHAT). *J Clin Hypertens* 2002;4:343–405.

64. Chobanian AV, Bakris GL, Black HR, et al. The seventh report of the Joint National Committee on Prevention, Detection, Evaluation and Treatment of High Blood Pressure: the JNC 7 report. *JAMA* 2003;289:2560–2572.

65. Materson BJ. High blood pressure in African-Americans. *Arch Intern Med* 2003;163:521–522.

66. Cohn JN, Julius S, Neutel J, et al. Clinical experience with perindopril in African-American hypertensive patients: a large United States community trial. *Am J Hypertens* 2004;17:134–138.

67. Julius S, Kjeldsen SE, Weber M, et al. Outcomes in hypertensive patients at high cardiovascular risk treated with regimens based on valsartan or amlodipine: the VALUE randomized trial. *Lancet* 2004;363:2022–2023.

Index

Please note that page references relating to non-textual content such as Boxes, Figures or Tables, where situated away from text, are in *italic* print.

571

Q

R

S